CRITICAL CARE SECRETS

Third Edition

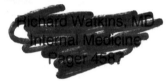

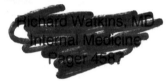

POLLY E. PARSONS, M.D.

Professor, Department of Medicine
University of Vermont College of Medicine
Director, Pulmonary and Critical Care Medicine
Chief of Critical Care Services
Fletcher Allen Health Care
Burlington, Vermont

JEANINE P. WIENER-KRONISH, M.D.

Professor of Anesthesia and Medicine
Vice-Chairman, Department of Anesthesia and Perioperative Care
Investigator, Cardiovascular Research Institute
University of California, San Francisco
San Francisco, California

HANLEY & BELFUS, INC./Philadelphia

Publisher: HANLEY & BELFUS, INC.
                    Medical Publishers
                    210 South 13th Street
                    Philadelphia, PA 19107
                    (215) 546-7293; 800-962-1892
                    FAX (215) 790-9330
                    Web site: http://www.hanleyandbelfus.com

Note to the reader: Although the information in this book has been carefully reviewed for correctness of dosages and indications, neither the authors nor the editors nor the publisher can accept any legal responsibility for any errors or omissions that may be made. Neither the publisher nor the editors make any warranty, expressed or implied, with respect to the material contained herein. Before prescribing any drug, the reader must review the manufacturer's current product information (package insert) for accepted indications, absolute dosage recommendations, and other information pertinent to the safe and effective use of the product described.

Library of Congress Control Number: 2002110366

CRITICAL CARE SECRETS, 3rd edition   ISBN 1-56053-507-5

Last digit is the print number: 9   8   7   6   5   4   3   2   1

CONTENTS

XII. PHARMACOLOGY

XIII. SURGERY AND TRAUMA

XIV. PERIOPERATIVE CARE

XV. SEDATION AND PAIN MANAGEMENT

XXI. ETHICS

XXII. ADMINISTRATION

CONTRIBUTORS

Olivia Vynn Adair, M.D.
Clinical Assistant Professor, Department of Cardiology, University of Colorado Health Sciences Center, Denver, Colorado

Hasan B. Alam, M.D.
Assistant Professor of Surgery, Uniformed Services University of the Health Sciences, Bethesda, Maryland; Attending Surgeon, Trauma/Surgical Critical Care and Director of Surgical Research, Washington Hospital Center, Washington, DC

Gil Allen, M.D.
Fellow and Clinical Instructor, Pulmonary and Critical Care, University of Vermont; Fletcher Allen Hospital, Burlington, Vermont

Suzanne Z. Barkin, M.D.
Associate Professor of Radiology, Department of Radiology, University of Colorado Health Sciences Center; Section Chief, Pediatric Radiology, Denver Health Medical Center, Denver, Colorado

Carolyn Bekes, M.D.
Professor of Medicine, Department of Medicine, Robert Wood Johnson Medical School; Senior Vice President for Academic Affairs, Chief Medical Officer, The Cooper Health System, Camden, New Jersey

Tomas Berl, M.D.
Professor of Medicine, and Head, Division of Renal Disease, Department of Medicine, University of Colorado School of Medicine, University Hospital, Denver, Colorado

Mary Bessesen, M.D.
Associate Professor of Medicine, Division of Infectious Diseases, University of Colorado Health Sciences Center; University of Colorado Hospital, Denver Veterans Affairs Medical Center, Denver, Colorado

Philip E. Bickler, M.D.
Professor, Anesthesia and Perioperative Care, University of California, San Francisco; UCSF Medical Center, San Francisco, California

Walter L. Biffl, M.D.
Assistant Professor of Surgery, Denver Health Medical Center and University of Colorado Health Sciences Center, Denver, Colorado

Raymond N. Blum, M.D.
Assistant Clinical Professor, Department of Infectious Diseases, University of Colorado Health Sciences Center, Denver, Colorado

James P. Bonar, M.D.
Assistant Professor of Surgery, Department of Surgery, University of Maryland School of Medicine; Surgeon, R.A. Cowley Shock Trauma Center, Baltimore, Maryland

David Bonovich, M.D.
Assistant Clinical Professor of Neurology, Department of Neurology, University of California, San Francisco; Moffitt-Long Hospital and San Francisco General Hospital, San Francisco, California

Mark W. Bowyer, M.D., F.A.C.S., D.M.C.C., Colonel, U.S. Air Force M.C.
Associate Professor of Surgery, Chief, Division of Trauma and Combat Surgery, Uniformed Services University of the Health Sciences, Bethesda, Maryland; Attending Surgeon, Trauma/Surgical Critical Care, Washington Hospital Center, Washington, DC

Daniel H. Burkhardt, M.D.
Assistant Professor, Department of Anesthesia and Perioperative Care, University of California, San Francisco; Moffitt-Long Hospital, San Francisco, California

David Burris, M.D., D.M.C.C.
Vice-Chairman, Department of Surgery, Uniformed Services University of the Health Sciences, Bethesda, Maryland; Walter Reed Army Medical Center, Washington, DC

William B. Cammarano, M.D.
Partner, Tacoma Anesthesia Associates; Tacoma General Hospital and Mary Bridge Children's Hospital, Tacoma, Washington

Lundy J. Campbell, M.D.
Resident in Anesthesia, Department of Anesthesia, University of California, San Francisco, San Francisco, California

E. Michael Canham, M.D.
Assistant Clinical Professor of Medicine, Pulmonary Disease, University of Colorado Health Sciences Center, Denver, Colorado; The Medical Center of Aurora, Aurora, Colorado

Stephen V. Cantrill, M.D.
Associate Director, Department of Emergency Medicine, Denver Health Medical Center; Assistant Professor, Division of Emergency Medicine, Department of Surgery, University of Colorado Health Sciences Center, Denver, Colorado

Edmund Casper, M.D.
Director, Behavioral Health, and Director of Psychiatry, Denver Health Medical Center; Associate Professor, Department of Psychiatry, University of Colorado School of Medicine, Denver, Colorado

Douglas M. Coldwell, Ph.D., M.D.
Professor, Director of Interventional Radiology, Department of Radiology, Wake Forest University, Winston-Salem, North Carolina

Deborah R. Cook, M.D.
Resident in Internal Medicine, Exempla Saint Joseph Hospital, Denver, Colorado

Elizabeth Cookson, M.D.
Assistant Professor, Department of Psychiatry, University of Colorado School of Medicine; Medical Director of Inpatient Services, Behavioral Health, Denver Health Medical Center, Denver, Colorado

Marc-André Cornier, M.A.
Assistant Professor of Medicine, Division of Endocrinology, Diabetes and Metabolism, University of Colorado Health Sciences Center; Denver Health Medical Center, University of Colorado Hospital, Denver, Colorado

John W. Crommett, M.D., Major, U.S. Air Force
Clinical Assistant Professor, Department of Medicine, Division of Surgical Critical Care, University of Maryland School of Medicine; R.A. Cowley Shock Trauma Center, Baltimore, Maryland

Kristina Crothers, M.D.
Fellow, Pulmonary and Critical Care Medicine, University of California, San Francisco, San Francisco, California

Ira M. Dauber, M.D.
Associate Clinical Professor, Division of Cardiology/Department of Medicine, University of Colorado Health Sciences Center, Denver, Colorado

Maria A. deCastro, M.D.
Attending Anesthesiologist, Cedars-Sinai Medical Center, Los Angeles, California

Gregory J. Dennis, M.D.
Director, Clinical Care and Training, Office of the Clinical Institute of Arthritis, Musculoskeletal and Skin Diseases, National Institutes of Health; Warren G. Magnuson Clinical Center, National Institutes of Health, Bethesda, Maryland

Thomas J. Donnelly, M.D.
Assistant Clinical Professor, Internal Medicine, Wright State University; Miami Valley Hospital, Dayton, Ohio

Christopher R. Dorothy, D.O.
Critical Care Fellow, Department of Medicine, Cooper Health System, Camden, New Jersey

Julia A. Drose, B.A., R.D.M.S., R.D.C.S., R.V.T.
Associate Professor, Ultrasound, University of Colorado Health Sciences Center; University of Colorado Hospital, Denver, Colorado

Erinn Fellner, M.D.
Resident, Department of Psychiatry, University of Vermont, Fletcher Allen Health Care, Burlington, Vermont

Enrique Fernandez, M.D.
Professor of Medicine, University of Colorado; University of Colorado Health Sciences Center, National Jewish Center, Denver Health Hospital, Denver, Colorado

Marilyn G. Foreman, M.D.
Assistant Professor of Clinical Medicine, Pulmonary and Critical Care Section, Department of Medicine, Morehouse School of Medicine; Medical Director, Respiratory Care Services; Co-Director, Medical Intensive Care Unit, Grady Memorial Hospital, Atlanta, Georgia

Mark W. Geraci, M.D.
Associate Professor of Medicine and Pharmacology, Assistant Chief of Medicine, University of Colorado Health Sciences Center, Denver, Colorado

Carlos E. Girod, M.D.
Associate Professor, Department of Internal Medicine, Division of Pulmonary and Critical Care Medicine, University of Texas Southwestern Medical Center; Parkland Memorial Hospital and Zale-Lipshy University Hospital, Dallas, Texas

Mark T. Grabovac, M.D.
Clinical Instructor in Anesthesiology and Critical Care Medicine, Department of Anesthesiology and Perioperative Care, University of California, San Francsico, San Francisco, California

Mary Chri Gray, M.D.
Associate Professor, General Internal Medicine, University of Colorado Health Sciences Center; Denver Health and Hospitals, Denver, Colorado

Michael A. Gropper, M.D., Ph.D.
Associate Professor of Anesthesia, Director, Critical Care Medicine, Departments of Anesthesia and Physiology, University of California, San Francisco; Moffitt-Long Hospital, San Francisco, California

James B. Haenel, R.R.T.
Clinical Instructor, Department of Surgery, University of Colorado Health Sciences Center; Critical Care Specialist, Denver Health Medical Center, Denver, Colorado

Kevin D. Halow, M.D.
Attending Surgeon, Department of Surgery, David Grant Medical Center, Travis Air Force Base, California

Julie Hambleton, M.D.
Associate Professor of Clinical Medicine, Departments of Medicine, Hematology/Oncology, University of California, San Francisco, San Francisco, California

Michael E. Hanley, M.D.
Associate Professor of Medicine, Pulmonary and Critical Care Medicine, University of Colorado School of Medicine; Denver Health Medical Center, Denver, Colorado

Kathryn L. Hassell, M.D.
Associate Professor of Medicine, Division of Hematology, University of Colorado Health Sciences Center; University of Colorado Hospital, Denver, Colorado

John E. Heffner, M.D.
Professor of Medicine, Executive Medical Director, Department of Medicine, Medical University of South Carolina, Charleston, South Carolina

Laurence Huang, M.D.
Associate Professor of Medicine, University of California, San Francisco; Medical Director, Inpatient AIDS Unit, Chief, AIDS Chest Clinic, San Francisco General Hospital, San Francisco, California

Colleen Hubbard, R.T., R.D.M.S., R.D.C.S.
Thornton, Colorado

James L. Jacobson, M.D.
Assistant Clinical Professor of Psychiatry, University of Colorado School of Medicine; Associate Medical Director, The Alternatives Program of Colorado Psychiatric Hospital, Denver, Colorado

Adrian A. Jarquin-Valdivia, M.D.
Clinical Instructor in Neurology, Neurocritical Care Program, University of California, San Francisco, San Francisco, California

James C. Jeng, M.D., F.A.C.S.
Clinical Assistant Professor of Surgery, Uniformed Services University of the Health Sciences, Bethesda, Maryland; Associate Director, The Burn Center, Washington, DC

David A. Kaminsky, M.D.
Associate Professor of Medicine, Pulmonary Disease and Critical Care Medicine, University of Vermont College of Medicine; Fletcher Allen Health Care, Burlington, Vermont

Leoncio Lee Kaw, Jr., M.D.
Clinical Fellow, Trauma and Surgical Critical Care, Division of Trauma, University of California, San Diego, San Diego, California; Research Instructor, Surgery, Uniformed Services University of the Health Sciences, Bethesda, Maryland

Brian J. Kelly, M.D.
Assistant Professor, Department of Neurology, Uniformed Services University of the Health Sciences; Department of Critical Care Medicine, National Naval Medical Center, Bethesda, Maryland

Joyce S. Kobayashi, M.D.
Associate Professor, Department of Psychiatry, University of Colorado Health Sciences Center; Director of Acute Crisis Service, Denver Health Medical Center, Denver, Colorado

Rosemary A. Kozar, M.D.
Assistant Professor, Surgery, University of Texas-Houston; Memorial Herman Hospital, Houston, Texas

Ken Kulig, M.D.
Associate Clinical Professor, Division of Emergency Medicine and Trauma, Department of Surgery, University of Colorado Health Sciences Center, Denver, Colorado

Stephen E. Lapinsky, M.B., B.Ch., M.Sc., F.R.C.P.C.
Associate Professor of Medicine, Division of Respirology, Department of Medicine, University of Toronto; Associate Director, Intensive Care Unit, Mount Sinai Hospital, Toronto, Ontario, Canada

Catherine M. Lee, M.D.
Senior Fellow, Pulmonary and Critical Care Medicine, Harborview Medical Center, University of Washington, Seattle, Washington

William Eng Lee, M.D.
Northwest Hematology-Oncology, Thornton, Colorado; Assistant Clinical Professor, Division of Medical Oncology, University of Colorado Health Sciences Center, Denver, Colorado

David W. Lehman, M.D., Ph.D.
Assistant Professor of Medicine, Division of General Internal Medicine, University of Colorado School of Medicine; Denver Health Medical Center, Denver, Colorado

Ludwig H. Lin, M.D.
Assistant Clinical Professor, Department of Anesthesia and Perioperative Care, University of California, San Francisco; Moffitt-Long and San Francisco General Hospital, San Francisco, California

Morgan Zaw Naing Lin, M.D.
Consultant Attending Cardiologist, Department of Cardiology, Valley Care Hospital, Pleasanton, California

Stuart L. Linas, M.D.
Professor, Department of Medicine, University of Colorado Health Sciences Center and Denver Health; University of Colorado Hospital and Denver Health Medical Center, Denver, Colorado

Kathleen D. Liu, M.D., Ph.D.
Clinical Fellow, Critical Care/Nephrology, University of California, San Francisco, San Francisco, California

Linda Liu, M.D.
Assistant Clinical Professor, Department of Anesthesia and Perioperative Care, University of California, San Francisco; UCSF Medical Center, San Francisco, California

Theodore W. Marcy, M.D., M.P.H.
Associate Professor of Medicine, Department of Medicine, University of Vermont College of Medicine; Fletcher Allen Health Care, Burlington, Vermont

Vincent J. Markovchick, M.D.
Director, Emergency Medical Services, Denver Health; Professor of Surgery, Division of Emergency Medicine, University of Colorado, Denver, Colorado

John A. Marx, M.D.
Chair, Department of Emergency Medicine, Carolinas Medical Center, Charlotte, North Carolina; Clinical Professor of Emergency Medicine, University of North Carolina at Chapel Hill, Chapel Hill, North Carolina

Michael T. McDermott, M.D.
Professor of Medicine, Division of Endocrinology, Metabolism and Diabetes, University of Colorado Health Sciences Center; University of Colorado Hospital, Denver, Colorado

Philip S. Mehler, M.D.
Chief of Internal Medicine, Denver Health; Professor of Medicine, Internal Medicine, University of Colorado Health Sciences Center, Denver, Colorado

John C. Messenger, M.D.
Assistant Professor of Medicine, Division of Cardiology, Department of Medicine, University of Colorado Health Sciences Center; Denver Veterans Affairs Medical Center and University of Colorado Hospital, Denver, Colorado

York E. Miller, M.D.
Professor, Department of Medicine, University of Colorado School of Medicine; Denver Veterans Affairs Medical Center, Denver, Colorado

Wanda C. Miller-Hance, M.D.
Associate Professor of Anesthesiology and Pediatrics, Departments of Anesthesiology and Pediatrics, Baylor College of Medicine; Texas Children's Hospital, Houston, Texas

Benoit Misset, M.D.
Medical/Surgical Intensive Care Unit, Hopital Saint-Joseph, Paris, France

Ernest E. Moore, M.D.
Chief of Surgery, Denver Health Medical Center; Professor and Vice-Chairman, Department of Surgery, University of Colorado Health Sciences Center, Denver, Colorado

Frederick A. Moore, M.D.
James H. "Red" Duke, Jr., Professor and Vice Chairman; Chief, General Surgery and Trauma and Critical Care, University of Texas-Houston Medical School; Medical Director, Trauma Services, Memorial Hermann Hospital, Houston, Texas

Marc Moss, M.D.
Associate Professor of Medicine, Division of Pulmonary and Critical Care, Emory University School of Medicine, Atlanta, Georgia

S. Patrick Nana-Sinkam, M.D.
Fellow, Division of Pulmonary Sciences and Critical Care Medicine, University of Colorado Health Sciences Center, Denver, Colorado

Claus W. Niemann, M.D.
Assistant Professor of Medicine, Anesthesia and Perioperative Care, University of California, San Francisco, San Francisco, California

David Palestrant, M.D.
Clinical Instructor in Neurology, Neurocritical Care Program, University of California, San Francisco, San Francisco, California

Manuel Pardo, Jr., M.D.
Assistant Clinical Professor, Anesthesia and Perioperative Care, University of California, San Francisco; UCSF Medical Center, San Francisco, California

Polly E. Parsons, M.D.
Professor, Department of Medicine, University of Vermont College of Medicine; Director, Pulmonary and Critical Care Medicine, Chief of Critical Care Services, Fletcher Allen Health Care, Burlington, Vermont

Randall M. Patten, M.D.
Professor of Radiology, Department of Radiology, University of Colorado School of Medicine; Denver Health Medical Center, Denver, Colorado

Jon Perlstein, M.D.
Assistant Professor of Surgery (Uniformed Services University of the Health Sciences), Department of Surgery, David Grant Medical Center, Travis Air Force Base, California

Jean-Francois Pittet, M.D.
Associate Professor in Residence, Department of Anesthesia and Perioperative Care, University of California, San Francisco; University of California, San Francisco, and San Francisco General Hospital, San Francisco, California

Peter T. Pons, M.D.
Professor of Emergency Medicine, Division of Emergency Medicine, Department of Surgery, University of Colorado Health Sciences Center; Attending Emergency Physician, Denver Health Medical Center, Denver, Colorado

Jill A. Rebuck, Pharm.D., B.C.P.S.
Clinical Assistant Professor, Department of Surgery, Trauma/Critical Care Division, Fletcher Allen Health Care, Burlington, Vermont

Rita F. Redberg, M.D., M.Sc.
Associate Professor of Medicine, Department of Medicine, Division of Cardiology, University of California, San Francisco, San Francisco, California

Thomas F. Rehring, M.D., F.A.C.S.
Clinical Assistant Professor, Department of Surgery, Vascular Surgery Section, University of Colorado Health Sciences Center; Attending Surgeon, St. Joseph Hospital, Denver, Colorado

Randall Rockne Reves, M.D., M.Sc.
Associate Professor, Infectious Disease Division, Department of Medicine, University of Colorado Health Sciences Center; Denver Health and Hospitals, Denver Public Health Department, Denver, Colorado

Kim F. Rhoads, M.D.
Resident, Surgery, University of California, San Francisco, San Francisco, California

Anand Rhuindran, M.D.
Fellow, Nephrology, Medical College of Ohio, Toledo, Ohio

Jonathan E. Rosenberg, M.D.
Fellow, Department of Medicine, Division of Hematology/Oncology, University of California, San Francisco, San Francisco, California

Jeanne M. Rozwadowski, M.D.
Clinical Instructor, Department of General Internal Medicine, University of Colorado Health Sciences Center, Denver, Colorado

Richard H. Savel, M.D.
Clinical Fellow, Division of Critical Care, Departments of Anesthesia and Medicine, University of California, San Francisco; Clinical Fellow, Moffitt Hospital, San Francisco, California

Lynn M. Schnapp, M.D.
Associate Professor, Pulmonary and Critical Care Medicine, University of Washington; Harborview Medical Center, Seattle, Washington

Martina Schulte, M.D.
Assistant Professor of Medicine, Department of General Medicine, University of Colorado Health Sciences Center; Denver Health, Denver, Colorado

David E. Schwartz, M.D.
Professor of Anesthesiology, Section Critical Care Medicine, University of Illinois at Chicago, Chicago, Illinois

Marvin I. Schwarz, M.D.
The James C. Campbell Professor of Pulmonary Medicine, Head, Division of Pulmonary Sciences and Critical Care Medicine, University of Colorado Health Sciences Center, Denver, Colorado

Stuart I. Senkfor, M.D.
Chief of Nephrology, St. Joseph's Hospital, Denver, Colorado

Joseph I. Shapiro, M.D.
Professor of Medicine and Pharmacology, Department of Medicine, Medical College of Ohio; Chairman, Department of Medicine, Medical College of Ohio, Toledo, Ohio

Thomas E. Shaughnessy, M.D.
Associate Clinical Professor, Anesthesia and Perioperative Care, University of California, San Francisco, San Francisco, California; Attending Physician, Mills-Penninsula Medical Center, Burlingame, California

David W. Shimabukuro, M.D.C.M.
Assistant Professor, Anesthesia and Perioperative Care, University of California, San Francisco, San Francisco, California

Marshall R. Thomas, M.D.
Assistant Professor of Psychiatry, University of Colorado Health Sciences Center; Medical Director and Assistant Professor, Colorado Psychiatric Hospital, Denver, Colorado

Mohamed Turki, M.D.
Clinical Instructor, Department of Medicine, University of Vermont College of Medicine; Fellow, Fletcher Allen Health Care, Burlington, Vermont

Madhulika G. Varma, M.D.
Assistant Professor, Surgery, University of California, San Francisco, San Francisco, California

Fernando Velayos, M.D.
Fellow in Gastroenterology, Division of Gastroenterology, Department of Medicine, University of California, San Francisco, San Francisco, California

Teresa Elizabeth Wagner, M.D.
Fellow, Pulmonary and Critical Care Medicine, University of Washington; University of Washington Medical Center and Affiliated Hospitals, Seattle, Washington

Carolyn H. Welsh, M.D.
Denver Veterans Affairs Medical Center; Pulmonary Sciences and Critical Care Medicine, University of Colorado Health Sciences Center, Denver, Colorado

Timothy Ralph White, M.D., Ph.D.
Assistant Professor, Department of Anesthesiology, University of Illinois, Chicago, Illinois

Jason B. Widrich, M.D.
Resident, Department of Anesthesia, University of California, San Francisco; Moffitt-Long Hospital, San Francisco, California

James E. Wiedeman, M.D.
Associate Professor of Surgery, Department of Surgery, Uniformed Services University of the Health Sciences, Bethesda, Maryland; David Grant Medical Center, Travis Air Force Base, California

Jeanine P. Wiener-Kronish, M.D.
Professor of Anesthesia and Medicine; Vice-Chairman, Department of Anesthesia and Perioperative Care; Investigator, Cardiovascular Research Institute, University of California, San Francisco, San Francisco, California

Danny Claude Williams, M.D., F.R.C.P.C., F.A.C.P., F.A.C.R.
Formerly Assistant Professor of Medicine, Division of Rheumatology, University of Colorado Health Sciences Center, Denver, Colorado

Eugene E. Wolfel, M.D.
Professor of Medicine, Department of Medicine, Division of Cardiology, University of Colorado Health Sciences Center, Denver, Colorado

Michael J. Yanakakis, M.D.
Assistant Professor of Anesthesia and Perioperative Care, and Critical Care Medicine, University of California, San Francisco, San Francisco, California

Michael P. Young, M.D.
Assistant Professor of Medicine, Medical Director of Medical Intensive Care Unit, Division of Pulmonary and Critical Care, University of Vermont College of Medicine; Fletcher Allen Health Care, Burlington, Vermont

Martin R. Zamora, M.D.
Associate Professor of Medicine, Division of Pulmonary Sciences and Critical Care Medicine, University of Colorado Health Sciences Center, Denver, Colorado

Leslie H. Zimmerman, MD
Associate Professor of Clinical Medicine, Pulmonary and Critical Care Medicine, University of California, San Francisco; Medical Director of Intensive Care Unit, San Francisco Veterans Affairs Medical Center; San Francisco Veterans Hospital, San Francisco, California

PREFACE

Over the course of three editions of *Critical Care Secrets*, critical care medicine has become an increasingly important and complex subspecialty, encompassing internal medicine, surgery, anesthesia, and emergency medicine. Now more than ever, the fundamentals and clinical skills required to care for critically ill patients transcend the various subspecialties.

In preparing this third edition, we focused on updating and expanding the original topics and extending the text to incorporate additional areas of critical care. Among the new areas covered are bioterrorism, defibrillators, renal replacement therapy, and ICU scoring systems.

Critical Care Secrets, 3rd edition, is designed for house officers and medical students who are learning to care for the critically ill—whether the patients are in an intensive care unit (medical, surgical, neurosurgical, coronary), the operating room, the recovery room, or the emergency department.

Like the other books in The Secrets Series®, this book is not intended to be a traditional textbook. Rather, its format consists of questions and answers designed both to provide factual information for the reader and to stimulate discussion.

We would like to sincerely thank all of the authors who contributed their time and expertise to this endeavor.

Polly E. Parsons, M.D.
Jeanine P. Wiener-Kronish, M.D.

DEDICATION

To our husbands, Jim and Daniel, and our children, Alec, Chandler, Jessica, and Samuel, for their patience and support, and for allowing us to take the time to complete this edition.

I. Basic Life Support

1. GENERAL APPROACH TO THE CRITICALLY ILL PATIENT

Manuel Pardo, Jr., M.D., and Michael A. Gropper, Ph.D., M.D.

This book deals with many different aspects of critical care. Each disorder has specific diagnostic and management issues. However, when initially evaluating a patient, one must have a conceptual framework for the patterns of organ system dysfunction that are common to many types of critical illness. Furthermore, in the patient with multiple organ failure, resuscitation or "stabilization" is often more important than establishing an immediate, specific diagnosis.

1. Which organ systems are most commonly involved in the critically ill patient?
The respiratory system, the cardiovascular system, the internal or metabolic environment, the central nervous system, and the gastrointestinal tract.

2. What system should be evaluated first?
The first few minutes of evaluation should address life-threatening physiologic abnormalities, usually involving the airway, the respiratory system, or the cardiovascular system. Then the evaluation should expand to include all organ systems.

3. Which should be performed first, diagnostic maneuvers or therapeutic maneuvers?
The management of the critically ill patient differs from the "traditional" history and physical exam followed by diagnostic tests and therapeutic plans. The pace of assessment and therapy is quicker, and simultaneous evaluation and treatment are necessary to prevent further physiologic deterioration. For example, if a patient has a tension pneumothorax, the immediate placement of a chest tube may be lifesaving. Extra time should not be taken to transport the patient to a monitored setting. If there are no obvious life-threatening abnormalities, it may be appropriate to transfer the patient to the intensive care unit (ICU) for further evaluation. Many patients are admitted to the ICU solely for continuous electrocardiogram (ECG) monitoring and more frequent nursing care.

RESPIRATORY SYSTEM

4. How do you evaluate the respiratory system?
The most important function of the lungs is to facilitate oxygenation and ventilation. Physical examination may reveal evidence of airway obstruction or respiratory failure. These signs include cyanosis, tachypnea, apnea, accessory muscle use, gasping respirations, and "paradoxical" respirations. Auscultation may reveal rales, rhonchi, wheezing, or asymmetric breath sounds.

5. Define "paradoxical" respirations and "accessory muscle use." What is their significance?
Normal breathing involves simultaneous rise and fall of the abdomen and chest wall. The patient with paradoxical respirations has asynchrony of abdominal and chest wall movement. With inspiration, the chest wall rises as the abdomen falls. The opposite occurs with expiration. Accessory muscle use refers to the contraction of the sternocleidomastoid and scalene muscles with inspiration.

1

Patients with accessory muscle use or paradoxical respirations have elevated "work of breathing," which is the amount of energy the body consumes for the work of the respiratory muscles. Most patients use accessory muscles before they develop paradoxical respirations. Without support from a mechanical ventilator, patients with paradoxical respirations will eventually develop respiratory muscle fatigue, hypoxemia, and hypoventilation.

6. What supplemental tests are useful in evaluating the respiratory system?

Although all tests should be individualized to the particular clinical situation, arterial blood gas (ABG) analysis, pulse oximetry, and chest radiography frequently provide useful information at a relatively low cost-benefit ratio.

7. What therapy should be considered immediately in the patient with obvious respiratory failure?

Mechanical ventilation may be an immediate life-sustaining therapy in the patient with obvious or impending respiratory failure. Mechanical ventilation can be carried out "invasively" or "noninvasively." Invasive ventilation is carried out via endotracheal intubation or tracheotomy. Noninvasive ventilation is instituted with a nasal mask or a full face mask.

Even if the patient does not have obvious respiratory distress, supplemental oxygen should be administered until the oxygen saturation is measured. The risk of developing oxygen-induced hypercarbia is extremely rare in the patient without an acute exacerbation of chronic obstructive pulmonary disease (COPD).

CARDIOVASCULAR SYSTEM

8. How do you evaluate the cardiovascular system?

The most important function of the cardiovascular system is the delivery of oxygen to the body's vital organs. The determinants of oxygen delivery are cardiac output and arterial blood oxygen content. The blood oxygen content, in turn, is determined primarily by the hemoglobin concentration and the oxygen saturation. It is difficult to determine the hemoglobin concentration and the oxygen saturation by physical examination alone. Therefore, the initial evaluation of the cardiovascular system focuses on evidence of vital organ perfusion.

9. How is vital organ perfusion assessed?

The measurement of heart rate and blood pressure is the first step. If the systolic blood pressure is below 80 mmHg or the mean blood pressure is below 50 mmHg, the chances of inadequate vital organ perfusion are greater. However, because blood pressure is determined by cardiac output and peripheral vascular resistance, it is not possible to estimate cardiac output from blood pressure alone. The presence of orthostatic hypotension may indicate hypovolemia. However, if the blood pressure is already low, orthostatic blood pressure should not be measured, because the patient may lose consciousness. The vital organs and their method of initial evaluation are as follows:

- **Skin:** assess warmth, capillary refill in all extremities
- **Central nervous system:** assess level of consciousness and orientation
- **Heart:** measure blood pressure and heart rate, ask for symptoms of myocardial ischemia (e.g., chest pain)
- **Kidneys:** measure urine output
- **Lungs:** (see questions 4–7)

10. What supplemental tests are useful in the initial evaluation of the cardiovascular system?

ECG is a potentially useful diagnostic test with a low cost-benefit ratio. Other tests, which may entail more risk and cost, should be determined after the initial evaluation. This may include cardiac enzyme tests, echocardiography, right heart catheterization, or coronary angiography.

11. What therapies should be considered immediately in the patient with hypotension and evidence of inadequate vital organ function?

Fluid and vasopressor therapy can rapidly restore vital organ perfusion, depending on the cause of the deterioration. In most patients, a fluid challenge is well tolerated, although it is possible to precipitate heart failure and pulmonary edema in a volume-overloaded patient. Other therapies that may be immediately lifesaving include thrombolysis or coronary angioplasty for an acute myocardial infarction.

METABOLIC ENVIRONMENT

12. How do you evaluate the metabolic environment?

It is nearly impossible to evaluate the metabolic environment by physical examination alone. The clinical laboratory is required for most metabolic tests.

13. Why are metabolic changes important to detect in a critically ill patient?

Metabolic abnormalities such as acid-base, fluid, and electrolyte disturbances are common in critical illness. These disorders may compound the underlying illness and require specific treatment themselves. They may also reflect the severity of the underlying disease. Metabolic disorders such as hyperkalemia and hypoglycemia can be life-threatening. Prompt testing and treatment may reduce morbidity and improve patient outcome.

14. Which laboratory tests should be performed in the initial evaluation of the metabolic environment?

The selected tests should have a rapid reporting time, be widely available, and be likely to produce a change in management. Tests that fit these criteria include white blood cell count, hemoglobin, hematocrit, electrolytes, anion gap, blood urea nitrogen (BUN), creatinine, and pH. Some of these tests may be unnecessary in a particular patient, and supplemental testing may be useful in others.

CENTRAL NERVOUS SYSTEM

15. How do you evaluate the central nervous system (CNS)?

A neurologic examination is the first step in evaluating the CNS. The examination should include assessment of mental status: level of consciousness, orientation, attention, and higher cortical function. CNS disturbances in critical illness can be subtle. Common changes include fluctuations in mental status, changes in the sleep-wake cycle, or abnormal behavior. The remainder of the neurologic examination includes assessment of respiratory pattern, cranial nerves, sensation, motor function, and reflexes.

16. What diagnostic tests and therapies should be immediately considered in the patient with altered mental status?

Oxygen therapy may be useful in the patient with altered mental status from hypoxemia. Pulse oximetry or ABG analysis should be done to evaluate this. Intravenous dextrose may be lifesaving in the patient with hypoglycemia. Additional diagnostic tests may be indicated depending on the clinical situation. Lumbar puncture, head CT scan, electroencephalography (EEG), and metabolic testing may be useful in directing specific therapies.

GASTROINTESTINAL TRACT

17. How do you evaluate the gastrointestinal (GI) tract?

History and abdominal and rectal examination are the first steps in initial evaluation of the GI tract. Abdominal catastrophes such as bowel obstruction and bowel perforation are common inciting events leading to multiple organ failure. In addition, abdominal distention can reduce the compliance of the respiratory system, leading to progressive atelectasis and hypoxemia. Further diagnostic tests such as chest radiography, plain radiography of the abdomen, or abdominal computed tomography (CT) scan may be useful in certain patients. For example, the finding of "free air" in the abdomen may lead to surgery for correction of bowel perforation.

OTHER ISSUES

18. Besides the information about current organ system function, what else should one learn about the patient in the initial evaluation?

After assessing current medical status, one should develop a sense for the "physiologic reserve" of the patient, as well as the potential for further deterioration. This information may often be gained by observing the patient's response to initial therapeutic maneuvers. It is also important to realize that patients may not desire cardiopulmonary resuscitation or other life-support therapies. If the patient has completed an advance directive, such as a durable power of attorney for health care, these should be followed or discussed further with the patient.

19. What measures can be taken to reduce patient morbidity in the ICU?

The prevention of complications in the ICU is an increasingly important patient safety issue. The following actions should be considered: antimicrobial-coated central venous catheters, elevation of the head of the bed in mechnically ventilated patients, deep venous thrombosis prophylaxis, and stress ulcer prophylaxis. In addition, institutional policies to reduce indiscriminant antibiotic therapy may reduce the incidence of multidrug-resistant nosocomial infections.

BIBLIOGRAPHY

1. Franklin C: 100 thoughts for the critical care practitioner in the new millenium. Crit Care Med 28: 3050–3052, 2000.
2. Grenvik A, et al (eds): Textbook of Critical Care, 4th ed. Philadelphia, W.B. Saunders, 2000.

2. CARDIOPULMONARY RESUSCITATION

David Shimabukuro, M.D.C.M.

Most of the information in this chapter can be reviewed in greater detail by referring to specific guidelines published by the American Heart Association (AHA) in conjunction with the International Liaison Committee on Resuscitation (ILCOR) and the American College of Surgeons (ACS).

1. What is meant by cardiopulmonary resuscitation (CPR)?

To most people, CPR refers to basic life support (BLS), which encompasses rescue breathing and closed-chest compressions. For the health provider, the term is much broader and includes advanced cardiac life support (ACLS), pediatric advanced life support (PALS), and advanced trauma life support (ATLS). Thus, it is important for the physician to be specific in discussing resuscitation with patients and families.

2. When is CPR indicated?

CPR should be performed on all patients who want to be resuscitated, provided that there is a reasonable chance of meaningful recovery. When the patient's wishes are unclear, CPR needs to be initiated; support can be withdrawn at a later date.

3. How common is iatrogenic cardiopulmonary arrest?

It probably occurs much too often than it should. Without a doubt, errors of omission and commission contribute to the incidence and poor outcome of in-hospital cardiopulmonary arrests. In a study by Bedell and Fulton of 562 in-hospital arrests, a major unsuspected diagnosis was present (and proved by autopsy) in 14% of cases. The two most common missed diagnoses were pulmonary embolus and bowel infarction, which together accounted for 89% of all missed conditions. Retrospective reviews indicate that as many as 15% of in-hospital arrests are probably avoidable. These cases can be attributed to respiratory insufficiency and hemorrhage that are often undetected or diagnosed too late; aberrations in vital signs and patient complaints (especially dyspnea) are frequently ignored.

Direct iatrogenesis also contributes to in-hospital cardiopulmonary arrests. Almost every procedure, including esophagogastroduodenoscopy (EGD), bronchoscopy, central venous line placement, and abdominal computed tomography (CT) scan with contrast, has been associated, on occasion, with an arrest. The injudicious use of lidocaine, sedative-hypnotics, and opiates is primarily responsible for such arrests throughout the hospital. Careful hemodynamic monitoring, especially pulse oximetry, by a dedicated provider can reduce the occurrence of this easily avoidable complication.

4. What are the ABCs of resuscitation?

Airway, breathing, and circulation.

5. How is BLS performed?

The ABCs should guide, streamline, and organize the resuscitation of all patients who are unconscious or in cardiopulmonary extremis:

Airway. The patient's airway is opened by performing a head tilt-chin lift or a jaw thrust. These maneuvers displace the mandible anteriorly, thereby lifting the tongue and epiglottis away from the glottic opening. To help improve airway patency, the mouth and oropharynx are suctioned (if suction is available), followed by the insertion of a plastic oropharyngeal or nasopharyngeal airway.

Breathing. Once the airway has been opened, the adequacy of respirations needs to be determined. Look at the chest to see if it is rising; listen and feel for air movement. If necessary, assist respirations by performing mouth-to-mouth, mouth-to-mask, or bag-valve-mask breathing. For the apneic patient, give two breaths. The technique depends on the clinical setting, the available equipment, and the rescuer's skill and training. In addition, to avoid insufflation of the stomach with consequent emesis and aspiration, one should deliver slow, even breaths, allowing for full exhalation. Furthermore, keeping peak inspiratory pressures low and using Sellick's maneuver (application of digital pressure to the cricoid cartilage) may reduce the risk of this hazard.

Circulation. After opening the airway and assessing breathing, check for spontaneous circulation by palpating the carotid pulse. If the patient is pulseless, begin chest compressions. Place the heels of the hands, one atop the other, on the lower half of the sternum, two fingerbreadths cephalad of the xiphoid process. Be careful to avoid the ribs and the xiphoid process, because a fracture of either can be highly deleterious. Compress the chest smoothly and forcefully, approximately 100 times per minute. The force used should be enough to depress the chest by 4–5 cm. If only one rescuer is available, the recommended sequence is 15 compressions followed by 2 breaths, repeated continually until help arrives. If there are two rescuers, a breath is given after every five chest compressions, repeated continually until more help arrives.

Once it is established that an adult patient is unconscious, the emergency medical system (EMS) should be activated before continuing with the ABCs if one is alone in the community. In the hospital setting, help should be called for immediately. Of note, CPR ideally should be performed only by people who have been certified by the American Heart Association (AHA). Certification is easily obtained by attending 1 or 2 classes taught by qualified instructors. Most communities offer these classes to the general public.

6. Are there any exceptions to the rule of the ABCs?

No. Depending on the clinical situation, one's approach may be more cautious or the options may be more limited, but the ABCs form the basis of CPR. For example, when a patient in a monitored setting experiences sudden pulseless ventricular tachycardia or ventricular fibrillation, the first priority is electrical defibrillation. While waiting for the defibrillator, bag-valve-mask ventilation (airway, breathing) and chest compressions (circulation) must be initiated and performed. However, one should never delay defibrillation to perform endotracheal intubation or intravenous line placement. Even in ATLS, the airway and breathing are assessed and secured by any technique (not necessarily intubation) before problems with circulation are addressed. Accordingly, in a traumatic cardiac arrest, closed-chest CPR and ACLS are performed while the cause of the arrest is quickly determined and treated.

7. How does blood flow during closed-chest compressions?

Two basic models derived from animal studies explain the movement of blood during closed-chest compressions. In the **cardiac pump model**, the heart is squeezed between the sternum and spine. Systole occurs when the heart is compressed; the atrioventricular (AV) valves close and the pulmonary and aortic valves open, ensuring ejection of blood with unidirectional, antegrade flow. Diastole occurs with the release of the squeezed heart, resulting in a fall in intracardiac pressures; the AV valves open while the pulmonary and aortic valves close. Blood is subsequently drawn into the heart from the vena cavae and lungs.

In the **thoracic pump model**, the heart is considered a passive conduit. Closed-chest compression results in uniformly increased pressures throughout the thoracic cavity. Forward flow of blood occurs with each squeeze of the heart and thorax because of the relative noncompliance of the arterial system (i.e., arteries resist collapse) and the one-way valves preventing retrograde flow in the venous system. Both models probably contribute to blood flow during CPR.

8. What is the main determinant of a successful resuscitation?

Two principal factors can highly influence the outcome of a resuscitation. The first factor is access to defibrillation. For most adults, the primary cause of sudden, nontraumatic cardiac arrest is ventricular tachycardia (VT) or ventricular fibrillation (VF), for which the recommended treatment is electrical defibrillation. The second factor is time or, more specifically, time to defibrillation. Survival from a VF arrest decreases by 7–10% for each minute of delay. Defibrillation at the earliest possible moment is vital in facilitating a successful resuscitation. Of interest, only 15% of patients who suffer an out-of-hospital arrest survive to discharge; the percentage is even lower for patients who have an in-hospital event.

9. What is the role of pharmacologic therapy during ACLS?

The immediate goals of pharmacologic therapy are to improve myocardial blood flow, increase ventricular inotropy, and terminate life-threatening arrhythmias, thereby restoring or maintaining spontaneous circulation. Combined alpha- and beta-adrenergic agonists, such as epinephrine, and smooth muscle V1 agonists, such as vasopressin, augment the mean aortic-to-ventricular end-diastolic pressure gradient (coronary perfusion pressure) by increasing arterial vascular tone. Although primarily alpha-adrenergic agonists, phenylephrine and norepinephrine, also increase arterial pressure and myocardial blood flow, but neither has been shown to be superior to epinephrine. Of note, recent data (both animal and human) have shown that vasopressin may be superior to epinephrine when survival to hospital discharge and residual neurologic deficits are compared.

In addition to improving or maintaining myocardial blood flow, pharmacologic therapy during ACLS is also aimed at terminating or preventing arrhythmias, which can further damage an already severely ischemic heart. VT and VF markedly increase myocardial oxygen consumption at a time when oxygen supply is tenuous because of poor delivery. Intracellular acidosis only causes the myocardium to be more dysfunctional and irritable, making the heart more vulnerable to arrhythmias. Amiodarone, a class III antiarrhythmic agent, has become the drug of choice for the treatment of most life-threatening arrhythmias.

10. Is sodium bicarbonate indicated in routine management of cardiopulmonary arrest?

No. The primary treatment of metabolic acidosis due to tissue hypoperfusion and hypoxia during cardiac arrest is adequate ventilation or even hyperventilation. The metabolic acidosis is usually unimportant in the first 15–18 minutes of resuscitation. If adequate ventilation can be maintained, the arterial pH usually remains above 7.2. However, some experts argue that during CPR ventilation is at best suboptimal, leading to a combined metabolic and respiratory acidosis and, consequently, dropping the pH well below 7.2. Studies have shown that severe acidosis leads to depression of myocardial contractile function, ventricular irritability, and a lowered threshold for ventricular fibrillation. In addition, a markedly low pH interferes with the vascular and myocardial responses to adrenergic drugs and endogenous catecholamines, reducing cardiac chronotropy and inotropy. Although it is appealing to administer sodium bicarbonate in this setting, the clinician must keep in mind that the bicarbonate ion, after combining with a hydrogen ion, generates new carbon dioxide. Cell membranes are highly permeable to carbon dioxide (more so than bicarbonate); therefore, administration of sodium bicarbonate causes a paradoxical intracellular acidosis. The resultant intramyocardial hypercapnia leads to a profound decline in cardiac contractile function and failure of resuscitation. The generated carbon dioxide also needs to be eliminated to prevent worsening of an already present respiratory acidosis. Given the poor cardiac output during CPR and probable suboptimal ventilation, this goal may be quite difficult.

Because the optimal acid-base status for resuscitation has not been established and no buffer therapy is needed in the first 15 minutes, the routine administration of sodium bicarbonate for acidosis secondary to cardiac arrest is not recommended. Only restoration of the spontaneous circulation with adequate tissue perfusion and oxygen delivery can reverse this on-going process.

11. Which arrhythmias are associated with most cardiopulmonary arrests?

Most sudden, nontraumatic cardiopulmonary arrests in adults are caused by ventricular fibrillation (VF) or ventricular tachycardia (VT) due to myocardial ischemia or infarct secondary to coronary artery disease. Electrolyte disturbances (hypokalemia or hypomagnesemia), prolonged hypoxemia, and drug toxicity can also be important inciting factors in patients with multiple medical problems. Also not uncommon are bradyasystolic arrests (as many as 50% of in-hospital arrests). One cause of this arrhythmia may be unrecognized hypoxemia or acidemia. Other causes include heightened vagal tone precipitated by medications, an inferoposterior myocardial infarction (Bezold-Jarisch reflex), or invasive procedures. A third common arrest rhythm seen is pulseless electrical activity (PEA). A common cause of this arrhythmia is prolonged arrest itself. Typically, after 8 minutes or more of VF, electrical defibrillation induces a slow, wide-complex PEA that tends to be terminal and is known as a pulseless idioventricular rhythm. On most occasions of an unsuccessful resuscitation, VF degrades to pulseless idioventricular rhythm before the patient becomes asystolic. The rhythm of PEA can also be narrow and fast; it accompanies other reversible life-threatening conditions rather than simply representing a terminal rhythm. Examples are cardiac tamponade, hypovolemia, pulmonary embolus, or tension pneumothorax (see below).

12. What are the most common immediately reversible causes of cardiopulmonary arrest?

The alert clinician should recognize at the bedside the treatable causes of cardiopulmonary arrest represented by the five Hs and five Ts.

13. List the five Hs.

1. **Hypovolemia** should be suspected in all cases of arrest associated with rapid blood loss. This "absolute" hypovolemia occurs in settings such as trauma (pelvic fractures), gastrointestinal hemorrhage, or rupture of an abdominal aortic aneurysm. "Relative" hypovolemia can occur with sepsis or anaphylaxis secondary to extensive capillary leak. Regardless of the type, a large amount of fluid (crystalloid, colloid, blood) should be rapidly administered and the cause of the hypovolemia corrected (e.g, take the patient to the operating room, administer antibiotics).

2. **Hypoxia** from a variety of etiologies can lead to a cardiac arrest. Tracheal intubation with the delivery of a high concentration of oxygen is the treatment of choice, while the cause of the hypoxia is determined and definitive management instituted.

3. **Hydrogen ions** (acidosis) can lead to myocardial failure, resulting in cardiogenic shock and arrest. The high hydrogen ion concentration also increases myocardial irritability and arrhythmia formation. Severe acidosis can be partially compensated by hyperventilation, but sodium bicarbonate may still need to be administered. The underlying cause of the acidosis should be diagnosed and corrected.

4. **Hyperkalemia** is encountered in patients with renal insufficiency, diabetes, and profound acidosis. Peaked T-waves and a widening of the QRS complex herald hyperkalemia; the electrical activity eventually deteriorates to a sinus-wave pattern. Treatment includes calcium chloride, sodium bicarbonate, insulin, and glucose. Hypokalemia and other electrolyte disturbances leading to a cardiac arrest are much less common. Treating the abnormality should help restore spontaneous circulation.

5. **Hypothermia** should be easily detected on examination of the patient. The electrocardiogram may reveal Osborne waves that are pathognomonic. All resuscitation efforts should be continued until the patient is euthermic.

14. List the five Ts.

1. **Tablets or toxins** should be considered in patients with out-of-hospital cardiac arrest. Some of the more common intoxications include carbon monoxide poisoning after prolonged exposure to smoke or exhaust fumes from incomplete combustion, cyanide poisoning during fires involving synthetic materials, and drug overdoses (intentional or unintentional). High-flow, high-concentration, and, if possible, hyperbaric oxygen, along with the management of acidosis, is the cornerstone of treatment for carbon monoxide and cyanide poisonings. In addition, intravenous sodium nitrite and sodium thiosulfate can be used to help remove cyanide from the circulation. Tricyclic antidepressant drugs act as a type IA antiarrhythmic agent and cause slowing of cardiac conduction, ventricular arrhythmias, hypotension, and seizures. Aggressive alkalinization of blood and urine, in addition to seizure control, should aid in controlling toxicity. An opiate overdose causes hypoxia from hypoventilation, and an overdose of cocaine can lead to myocardial ischemia. Nalaxone reverses the effects of opioids and should be administered immediately if an opioid overdose is suspected.

2. **Cardiac tamponade** presents with hypotension, a narrowed pulse pressure, elevated jugular venous pressure, distant and muffled heart sounds, and low-voltage QRS complexes on the electrocardiogram. Trauma victims and patients with malignancies are at greatest risk. Pericardiocentesis or subxiphoid pericardiorrhaphy can be lifesaving.

3. **Tension pneumothorax** must be recognized immediately. Most often it occurs in trauma patients or patients receiving positive-pressure ventilation. The signs of a tension pneumothorax are rapid-onset hypotension, hypoxia, and an increase in airway pressures. Subcutaneous emphysema and reduced breath sounds on the affected side with tracheal deviation toward the unaffected side are commonly noted. The placement of a 14-gauge or 16-gauge IV catheter into the second intercostal space at the midclavicular line or into the fifth intercostal space at the anterior axillary line for immediate decompression is imperative for restoration of circulation. A chest tube can be placed after the tension pneumothorax is converted to a simple pneumothorax.

4. **Thrombosis of a coronary artery** can lead to myocardial ischemia and infarct. Reperfusion is a vital determinant for eventual outcome. Cardiac catheterization is the primary choice, if it is immediately available; thrombolysis is a good alternative.

5. **Thrombosis of the pulmonary artery** can be devastating. Some patients may present with dyspnea and chest pain, similar to acute coronary syndromes, but those who present in cardiac arrest have a minimal chance of survival. Therapy includes immediate thrombolysis to unload the right ventricle while restoring pulmonary blood flow.

15. How should ventricular fibrillation (VF) be treated?

Early defibrillation with an initial energy of 200 joules for a monophasic waveform (MPW) defibrillator is recommended to minimize myocardial damage and to prevent the development of post-countershock pulseless brady or tachyarrhythmias. The delivered energy is increased to 300 joules, then to 360 joules, where it is kept on subsequent shocks if the patient remains in VF. If a biphasic waveform (BPW) defibrillator is used, 150 joules (or the level recommended by the manufacturer) is the currently recommended energy level.

If three countershocks are not successful in terminating the VF, according to ACLS protocols, epinephrine or vasopressin should be administered while the airway and breathing are more definitively secured via tracheal intubation. If venous access is not yet available, BLS should be continued until intubation, at which time epinephrine may be given via the endotracheal tube. The next step is another attempt at defibrillation with 360 joules (MPW) or 150 joules (BPW). If defibrillation is still unsuccessful, an antiarrhythmic agent—amiodarone, lidocaine, magnesium, or procainamide (*not* bretylium)—should be administered through an intravenous line. The remaining sequence always includes administration of drug followed by defibrillation (if the patient remains in a "shockable" rhythm). Of note, however, neither amiodarone nor any other drug (including magnesium) has been proved to be efficacious in improving survival to hospital discharge.

16. Is pulseless idioventricular rhythm treatable?

Delayed electrical countershock or prolonged VF frequently results in a pulseless idioventricular rhythm or asystole. In most cases, the idioventricular rhythm is not amenable to treatment and results in death. In animal experiments, high-dose epinephrine (0.1–0.2 mg/kg) has helped to restore cardiac contractility and pacemaker activity; however, several clinical studies have shown no benefit in long-term survival or neurologic outcome.

17. How is asystole treated?

1. Rapidly determine whether any evidence indicates that resuscitation should not be attempted.

2. Perform primary and secondary ABCD surveys, including confirmation of the absence of electrical cardiac activity (a flat-line in an electrocardiogram may be due to technical mistakes). Rotate the monitoring leads 90°, and maximize the amplitude to detect fine VF (in which case, defibrillation should be performed immediately). Verify the absence of pulses at the carotid or femoral artery.

3. If transcutaneous pacing is considered, it should be initiated without delay.

4. Every 5 minutes, administer atropine, 1 mg (up to 0.04 mg/kg), to counter vagal activity and epinephrine, 1 mg, to increase myocardial perfusion.

5. Always consider stopping resuscitative efforts.

18. What are the appropriate routes of administration of drugs during resuscitation?

The preferred choice is the intravenous route. If a central venous catheter is in place, it is preferred over a peripheral venous line. Administration of drugs through a peripheral venous line results in a slightly delayed onset of action, although the peak drug effect is similar to that via the central route. Drugs administered peripherally should be followed with at least 20 ml of normal saline to ensure central delivery. Intracardiac administration should not be performed.

A number of drugs (e.g., epinephrine, atropine, lidocaine) are absorbed systemically after endotracheal administration. Although pulmonary blood flow and hence systemic absorption are minimal during CPR, recent animal studies suggest that comparable hemodynamic responses can occur. At this time, standard IV doses are recommended for the endotracheal route.

Virtually every resuscitation drug can be administered in conventional doses via the intraosseous route. This method is preferred in pediatric patients, in whom an intravenous line cannot be established rapidly.

19. What is the usual outcome of in-hospital CPR?

Most patients who receive CPR in the hospital do not survive. In fact, only 5–20% of patients live to be discharged home. Furthermore, many patients who survive have severe impairments of independence and cognition. Unfortunately, it is not yet possible to predict with confidence the outcome of in-hospital resuscitation.

20. What is a do-not-resuscitate (DNR) order?

The DNR order, signed by a physician, is an accepted reason to withhold all efforts or to limit the extent of resuscitation in the event of cardiopulmonary arrest or near arrest.

21. Who is ultimately responsible for determining a patient's DNR status?

The decision to withhold resuscitation attempts from a patient in cardiopulmonary arrest ideally should be a collaborative one, determined by the patient, the patient's family, and the primary physician. However, the attending physician can make a unilateral decision to withhold resuscitative efforts if he or she considers it inappropriate, as when the expectation of a successful resuscitation is nonexistent. If the physician makes a unilateral decision, he or she should immediately meet with the patient and the family to discuss all issues, including alternatives, and to inform them of the decision. On most occasions, the objective medical opinion of the attending physician is the determining factor in a patient's and family's decision not to resuscitate. A DNR order must be signed by a physician; all other signatures, if required, are legally irrelevant. A DNR order is not synonymous with an order to withhold standard medical care.

BIBLIOGRAPHY

1. American Heart Association: Guidelines 2000 for Cardiopulmonary Resuscitation (CPR) and Emergency Cardiovascular Care. Circulation 102:I-1–I-384, 2000.
2. Bedell SE, Fulton EJ: Unexpected findings and complications at autopsy after cardiopulmonary resuscitation (CPR). Arch Intern Med 146:1725–1728, 1986.
3. Brown CG, Martin DR, Pepe PE, et al: A comparison of standard-dose and high-dose epinephrine in cardiac arrest outside the hospital. N Engl J Med 327:1051–1055, 1992.
4. Charlop S, Kahlam S, Lichstein E, Frishman W: Electromechanical dissociation: Diagnosis, pathophysiology, and management. Am Heart J 118:355–360, 1989.
5. Kudenchuk PJ, Cobb LA, Copass MK, et al: Amiodarone for resuscitation after out-of-hospital cardiac arrest due to ventricular fibrillation. Circulation 341:871–878, 1999.
6. Linder KH, Dirks B, Strohmenger HU, et al: Randomized comparison of epinephrine and vasopressin in patients with out-of-hospital ventricular fibrillation. Lancet 349:535–537, 1997.
7. Lowenstein SR: Cardiopulmonary resuscitation for non-injured patients. In Wilmore DW, Brennan MF, Harken AH, et al (eds): Care of the Surgical Patient. New York, Scientific American, 1990, pp 1–24.
8. Ornato JP, Paradis N, Bircher N, et al: Future directions for resuscitation research. III: External cardiopulmonary resuscitation advanced life support. Resuscitation 32(2):139, 1996.
9. Paradis NA, Martin GB, Rivers EP, et al: Coronary perfusion pressure and the return of spontaneous circulation in human cardiopulmonary resuscitation. JAMA 263:1106–1113, 1990.

3. PULSE OXIMETRY AND CAPNOGRAPHY

Philip E. Bickler, M.D., and Thomas E. Shaughnessy, M.D.

1. What is pulse oximetry?

Pulse oximetry is a continuous noninvasive estimation of arterial hemoglobin oxygen saturation. It is a routine monitor of oxygenation in diverse clinical settings, including the operating room, emergency ward, and intensive care unit (ICU). Clinical use of pulse oximeters falls into two main categories: (1) as a screening or warning system of arterial hemoglobin/oxygen desaturation and (2) as an end-point for titration of therapeutic interventions. Because the instruments detect pulsatile blood flow, they also serve as heart rate monitors.

2. How does a pulse oximeter determine arterial oxygen saturation?

Pulse oximetry is based on the spectrophotometric measurement of the degree of oxygen binding to hemoglobin at a point in time when the signal represents the arterial blood. In other words, saturation is determined at the moment of the peak blood pulse, when oxygen removal by the tissues has not been significant and when the contribution to the signal of unsaturated blood in the tissue is minimal. Hemoglobin-oxygen binding is measured by the degree of absorbance of red light, and the timing of the arterial pulse is detected by an infrared light. Spectrophotometry is based on the Beer-Lambert law, which holds that optical absorbance is proportional to the concentration of the substance and the thickness of the medium. Using this principle, two wavelengths of light are used to measure both the absorption of oxyhemoglobin (O_2Hb) and reduced hemoglobin (Hb).

Pulse oximeters function by transmitting light from two light-emitting diodes (LEDs) through tissue containing pulsatile blood flow. Light is transmitted through the tissue at two wavelengths, 660 nm (red, principally absorbed by O_2Hb) and 940 nm (infrared, primarily absorbed by Hb), thus allowing differentiation of oxyhemoglobin from reduced hemoglobin. The infrared signal serves an additional critical function: it detects the timing of the blood pulse through the tissue. The arterial saturation is related to the ratio of the 660/940 ratios at peak pulse; thus, the calculation is based on a ratio of the two absorbance ratios. This approach is the key to pulse oximetry and represents a quantum leap from previous attempts to measure blood oxygen noninvasively. The measurement of saturation based on these ratios cancels out differences in factors such as tissue geometry, tissue and skin color, and venous blood content. The microprocessor algorithm used to calculate the arterial saturation includes empirical factors necessary to produce accurate readings for a particular instrument. Several recently introduced pulse oximeter instruments include noise/artiface rejection.

3. How accurate are pulse oximeters?

In published reports, pulse oximetry has an accuracy within 2–3% of the oxyhemoglobin levels measured in vitro with multiwavelength oximeters. The Food and Drug Administration requires manufacturers to demonstrate that their instruments conform to this degree of accuracy in humans with 70–100% oxygen saturation. Because the principle of measurement is based on a ratio of absorbance ratios, no calibration of the instrument by the user is needed or possible.

4. Where are pulse oximetry measurements taken?

Pulse oximeter probes may be applied to any site that allows orientation of the LED and photodetector opposite one another across a vascular bed. If the tissue is too thick, the signal is attenuated before reaching the detector and the oximeter cannot function. Oximeters may be applied to fingers, toes, earlobes, lips, cheeks, and the bridge of the nose. Several manufacturers offer reflectance oximeter probes that may be applied to flat tissue surfaces such as the forehead.

5. What factors affect pulse oximetry measurements?

Several factors can greatly affect the accuracy and reliability of pulse oximetry. Most errors in oximetry measurement are the result of poor signal quality (i.e., hypoperfusion, vasoconstriction) or excessive noise (i.e., motion artifact). Optical interference may be produced by extraneous lights (especially fluorescent sources). Intravenous dyes as well as nail polishes (especially green, blue, or black) absorb at the wavelengths used by the oximeter and produce artificially low measurements. Contamination from venous pulsations caused by dependent venous pooling or valvular insufficiency may also cause low readings. For a similar reason, the simultaneous nature of arterial and venous pulsation during cardiopulmonary resuscitation makes oximeter data unreliable. Extreme hyperbilirubinemia has been reported to have variable effects on functional oxygen saturation (SpO_2) values. The presence of dysfunctional hemoglobins can alter the ability of oximetry to reflect the true oxygen saturation.

6. Describe the effects of dyshemoglobinemia on pulse oximetry.

Because pulse oximeters measure two wavelengths of light, they are capable of differentiating only two types of hemoglobin, Hb and O_2Hb. Given that abnormal species such as carboxyhemoglobin (CoHb) or methemoglobin (MetHb) also absorb red and infrared light at these same wavelengths, their presence affects the SpO_2 measurement, and their quantitative contribution cannot be determined. The pulse oximeter assumes that only "functional" hemoglobin is present (O_2Hb or Hb), and the oxygen saturation is calculated based on these amounts.

$$\text{Functional oxygen saturation (\%)} \quad SpO_2 = \frac{OxyHb}{OxyHb + Hb}$$

A multiwavelength CO-oximeter determines oxygen saturation (SaO_2) more accurately in the presence of significant dyshemoglobinemias because it possesses wavelengths of light that can be used to detect the presence of carboxyhemoglobin and methemoglobin.

$$\text{Fractional oxygen saturation (\%)} \quad SaO_2 = \frac{OxyHb}{OxyHb + Hb + [HbCO + HbMet, \text{etc.}]}$$

For example, carboxyhemoglobin (HBCO), which is scarlet red, is interpreted by the limited wavelength analysis of a pulse oximeter as O_2Hb, which falsely elevates the SpO_2 reading. The absorption pattern of methemoglobin (HbMet) is interpreted by the pulse oximeter as 85% saturation; thus, progressively higher levels of methemoglobin cause the SpO_2 value to converge on 85% regardless of the actual SaO_2. When the presence of significant amounts of dysfunctional hemoglobin is suspected, a CO-oximeter should be used to determine Hb-O_2 saturation. The presence of fetal hemoglobin has not been shown to affect significantly the accuracy of SpO_2 measurements because its light absorption properties are simlar to those of adult hemoglobin.

7. Can pulse oximetry detect an increase in intrapulmonary shunting?

Pulse oximetry can only differentiate hemoglobin oxygen saturation from desaturation. At higher levels of oxygenation, it offers little resolution because the hemoglobin is already nearly 100% saturated with oxygen. An increase in shunting sufficient to cause a decrease in PaO_2 from 200 to 100 mmHg thus would not be detectable by pulse oximetry. However, shunting or any other cause of hypoxia significant enough to cause a drop in oxygenation below approximately 60 mmHg would yield a significant drop in SpO_2 because the oxyhemoglobin dissociation curve begins to have a strong association with oxygen partial pressure at these levels. Thus the pulse oximeter is a useful monitor of changes in oxygenation and ventilation in patients breathing room air and patients whose PaO_2 is approaching the threshold requiring acute clinical intervention.

8. What are the complications of pulse oximetry?

Pulse oximetry is noninvasive and relatively safe. Complications are most commonly caused by errors in data interpretation that lead to inappropriate treatment. The response to decreased saturation should include verifying that the photoplethysmogram is free of artifacts and that an ECG-derived heart rate matches that of the pulse oximeter. If the oximeter cannot detect arterial pulsations, the SaO_2 reading will not be accurate. The sensors contain electronic circuitry that potentially may malfunction. There have been infrequent reports of thermal burns resulting from defective LED probes. Standard pulse oximeter probes cannot be used for patients undergoing magnetic resonance imaging (MRI) for two reasons: (1) the high radiofrequency and magnetic fields can induce probe or wire heating that may cause thermal burns and (2) the wiring may produce artifacts in the MR images. Pressure necrosis, which may result from prolonged placement in one position, occurs most often with spring-loaded sensors and in patients with impaired peripheral perfusion.

9. How can pulse oximetry measurements be obtained in patients with severe vasoconstriction?

The cause of vasoconstriction should be addressed. The patient with hypoperfusion should receive adequate volume therapy and inotropic support, if necessary. The hypothermic patient should receive therapy that addresses both core and peripheral warming. Heating the hand with warm blankets often can increase perfusion significantly and improve the function of the oximeter. In selected cases, a digital nerve block using 1% lidocaine without epinephrine often restores sufficient pulsatile flow to enable SpO_2 monitoring.

10. What is capnography? How does it work?

Capnography is a graphic display of the continuous measurement of exhaled carbon dioxide (CO_2) over time. It provides a noninvasive method to monitor both ventilation and perfusion. Most commonly, infrared spectrophotometry is used to determine the CO_2 concentration of a continuous sample of airway gas. Sampling usually occurs in one of two ways. In a mainstream capnograph, CO_2 trends are measured with a sensor (light source and detector) placed directly in-line with the patient's breathing circuit. Alternatively, sidestream capnographs continuously divert a sample of gas away from the patient's breathing circuit to the capnograph for analysis and display. The mainstream method has a very brief response time, but because the sensor must be placed near the patient, long-term monitoring may prove cumbersome. The sidestream method is lighter and allows greater flexibility, but because transit time is unavoidable, a slower response time (approximately 1.5 seconds) results. Because of mixing of gases in the sample stream, the absolute values of the plateau and baseline also may be slightly attenuated. The sidestream device also can be used with a modified nasal cannula to monitor CO_2 concentrations in the airway of nonintubated patients.

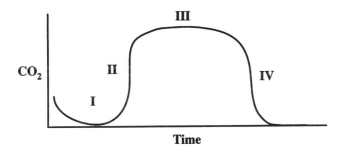

A capnogram is a plot of airway CO_2 versus time. **Phase I** (inspiratory baseline): inspired gas devoid of CO_2. **Phase II** (beginning expiration): represents expiration of anatomic dead space followed by gas from respiratory bronchioles and alveoli. **Phase III** (alveolar plateau): corresponds to exhalation of alveolar gas. The last portion of the plateau is termed end-tidal ($PETCO_2$). **Phase IV** (inspiratory downslope): the beginning of the next inspiration.

11. What other methods are used to measure CO_2 in respiratory gases?

The most commonly used method for measuring carbon dioxide in expired gases is infrared light absorbance. In addition, technologies such as raman spectrometry and mass spectrometry are relatively reliable, accurate, and responsive. Although generally more expensive, they also detect a variety of other gases and anesthetic vapors. Colorimetric detectors that attach to endotracheal tubes are available to help assess endotracheal tube placement. The colorimetric detector uses a pH-sensitive indicator strip for semiquantitative detection of exhaled CO_2. Although portable and convenient, these devices are often more difficult to interpret than conventional capnographs and can be used only once.

12. Why is measurement of end-tidal carbon dioxide important?

A capnograph provides a continuous display of the CO_2 concentration of gases in the airways. The CO_2 partial pressure at the end of normal exhalation (end-tidal CO_2, $PETCO_2$) is a reflection of gas leaving the alveoli and an estimate of the alveolar CO_2 concentration ($PACO_2$). When ventilation and perfusion are well-matched, the $PACO_2$ closely approximates the $PaCO_2$, and thus $PaCO_2 \approx PACO_2 \approx PETCO_2$. The presence of cyclical exhaled CO_2 is useful in confirming airway patency and verifying endotracheal tube placement as well as adequacy of pulmonary ventilation. In addition, decreases in cardiac output caused by hypovolemia or cardiac dysfunction result in decreased pulmonary perfusion. This causes an increased alveolar dead space, which dilutes $PETCO_2$. The resulting depression of end-tidal CO_2 may be monitored by capnography. Animal studies show that a 20% decrease in cardiac output causes a 15% decrease in $P_{ET}CO_2$.

13. What can the capnogram reveal about the patient's condition?

Alterations in the shape of the capnogram in the intubated, ventilated patient often provide clues to alterations in pulmonary pathology and malfunction of ventilation equipment. For example, a staircase pattern in phase II may indicate sequential emptying of the lung, which may occur in mainstem partial bronchial obstruction. An upward sloping plateau in phase III is a classic indication of late emptying of poorly ventilated alveolar spaces with elevated PCO_2, which may occur with expiratory obstruction at the level of smaller airways, as seen in chronic obstructive pulmonary disease (COPD), bronchospasm, and other forms of ventilation-perfusion mismatching. Pulmonary embolus also causes a decrease in end-tidal CO_2.

14. What factors affect the arterial-end tidal CO_2 gradient?

The gradient between $PaCO_2$ and $P_{ET}CO_2$, represented as $P(a\text{-}ET)CO_2$, is normally less than 6 mmHg. The gradient between $PaCO_2$ and $P_{ET}CO_2$ increases when pulmonary perfusion is reduced or ventilation is maldistributed. This occurs with the development of high ventilation/perfusion alveolar units (increased dead-space ventilation). The results are an increase in $P(a\text{-}ET)CO_2$ and a decrease in $P_{ET}CO_2$. Examples of this state are COPD, pulmonary hypoperfusion, and pulmonary emboli. Technical failures such as accidental extubation and endotracheal tube cuff leak also may cause a decrease in $P_{ET}CO_2$.

15. Is it possible to see an expired CO_2 waveform after esophageal intubation?

The stomach may contain some exogenous CO_2 or carbonated solutions before intubation. In addition, aggressive positive-pressure ventilation may force previously exhaled gas from the pharynx into the stomach. Initially, this may produce a normal capnogram tracing, but because CO_2 is not continuously generated, the expired concentration will fall toward zero as sequential breaths dilute the existing gases. Esophageal intubation should be suspected if the capnogram tracing begins to "fall off" after 5 or 6 breaths.

16. What physiologic parameters affect the measurement of end-tidal CO_2 ($ETCO_2$)?

$ETCO_2$ may be altered by changes in CO_2 production and elimination. $ETCO_2$ may be expected to increase during hypermetabolism, as during hyperthermia or sepsis, and decrease with hypothermia or hypometabolism. More often, however, changes in the pulmonary system affect CO_2 elimination. Hypoventilation and rebreathing result in increased $ETCO_2$, whereas hyperventilation and ventilation/perfusion mismatching produce decreased $ETCO_2$. Only in circumstances that result from ventilation/perfusion mismatching (e.g., hypoperfusion, embolism, impaired diffusion) does the $P_{ET}CO_2$ fail to reflect accurately the state of arterial carbon dioxide levels ($PaCO_2$). Because the gradient between end-tidal and arterial CO_2 reflects a greater degree of inefficient ventilation, the respiratory system must compensate for this inefficiency by increasing the minute ventilation (via increased tidal volume or respiratory rate) to maintain clearance of the body's CO_2 production.

17. How does capnography assist in cardiopulmonary resuscitation (CPR) efforts?

In the course of CPR, capnography not only helps to verify tracheal intubation but also can monitor the adequacy of circulatory assistance. The presence of exhaled CO_2 during CPR is useful in that it provides evidence of enough circulation to produce CO_2 transport from tissues to the lungs. Thus, assuming a constant minute ventilation and CO_2 production, changes in $P_{ET}CO_2$ reflect the status of overall circulation. Some investigators have suggested that if the $P_{ET}CO_2$ is > 15 mmHg at the beginning of CPR, it may predict successful resuscitation. Failure to achieve any recovery of $P_{ET}CO_2$ should prompt consideration of a diagnosis of inadequate cardiac filling, which may be caused by hypovolemia, tamponade, pneumothorax, or pulmonary embolism. Low $P_{ET}CO_2$ also may be caused by alveolar hyperventilation or may indicate ineffective CPR. The return of spontaneous circulation is heralded with a profound increase in $P_{ET}CO_2$, primarily because of increased flow of hypercarbic blood to the lungs.

CONTROVERSY

18. Is pulse oximetry cost-effective?

The effectiveness of pulse oximetry in the ICU must be extrapolated from studies of its use in the operating/recovery room. These reports suggest that the enhanced early detection of arterial oxygen desaturation afforded by pulse oximetry may lead to improved outcomes, such as a decreased incidence of perioperative myocardial ischemia. However, its benefit in terms of decreasing the incidence of respiratory complications has been difficult to demonstrate, even in large populations.

Few published data permit direct, outcome-based conclusions about either the clinical impact or cost-benefit ratio of pulse oximetry. One study demonstrated a decrease in total cost of care associated with the introduction of pulse oximetry and capnography. The savings realized were a result of a reduced need for arterial blood gas measurements and associated operating costs. Pulse oximetry and capnography also may aid in the weaning of ventilatory support by decreasing the need for arterial blood gas sampling. In a consensus statement, the Technology Assessment Task Force of the Society of Critical Care Medicine asserted that routine use of pulse oximetry in the critically ill results in cost savings because of the positive impact on patient outcomes, but it also acknowledged the need for more detailed study of the subject.

BIBLIOGRAPHY

1. Ely EW, Baker AM, Evans GW, Haponik EF: The distribution of costs of care in mechanically ventilated patients with chronic obstructive pulmonary disease. Crit Care Med 28:408–413, 2000.
2. Gravenstein N, Good ML: Noninvasive assessment of cardiopulmonary function. In Civetta JM, Taylor RW, Kirby RR (eds): Critical Care, 2nd ed. Philadelphia, J.B. Lippincott, 1992, pp 291–312.
3. Lampotang S, Gravenstein JS, Euliano TY, et al: Influence of pulse oximetry and capnography on time to-diagnosis of critical incidents in anesthesia: A pilot study using a full-scale patient stimulator. J Clin Monit 14:313–321, 1998.
4. Maccioli GA, Calkins JM, Collins VJ: Monitoring the anesthetized patient. In Collin VJ (ed): Principles of Anesthesiology, 3rd ed. Philadelphia, Lea & Febiger, 1993, pp 67–99.
5. Marini J, Truwit S: Monitoring the respiratory system. In Hall JB, Schmidt GA, Wood LDH (eds): Principles of Critical Care, 2nd ed. New York, McGraw-Hill, 1998, pp 131–154.
6. Moller JT, et al: Randomized evaluation of pulse oximetry in 20,802 patients. II. Anesthesiology 78:445–453, 1993.
7. Niehoff J, DelGuercio C, LaMorte W, et al: Efficacy of pulse oximetry and capnometry in postoperative ventilatory weaning. Crit Care Med 16:701–705, 1988.
8. Roizen MF, et al: Pulse oximetry, capnography, and blood gas measurements: Reducing cost and improving the quality of care with technology. J Clin Monit 9:237–240, 1993.
9. Technology Assessment Task Force of The Society of Critical Care Medicine: A model for technology assessment applied to pulse oximetry. Crit Care Med 21:615–624, 1993.

4. INVASIVE HEMODYNAMIC MONITORING

Mark W. Bowyer, M.D.

1. What tools are available for invasively monitoring the hemodynamic status of critically ill patients?

Arterial catheters, central venous pressure monitors, and pulmonary artery or Swan-Ganz catheters.

2. What data can be obtained with an arterial catheter?

Arterial catheters are used for moment-to-moment recording of blood pressure and to derive the mean arterial pressure (MAP), which is frequently used in the calculation of several derived hemodynamic variables.

3. How is the MAP calculated?

The MAP is calculated by adding the value for the diastolic pressure to the value obtained by subtracting the diastolic pressure from the systolic pressure, and dividing this sum by three.

4. What are the preferred sites for insertion of arterial catheters?

The radial artery is most commonly used because of its superficial location and its collateral anastomoses with the ulnar artery. Other sites, in order of decreasing frequency, are the dorsalis pedis, femoral, brachial, and axillary arteries.

5. What are the complications of radial arterial catheter monitoring? How common are they?

Thrombosis is the most common complication (up to 50% by angiography), the risk of which increases with increased size of the catheter and longer duration of catheterization. Other complications that occur much less frequently are embolization (0–23%), hematoma (0–10%), infection, median nerve neuropathy, pseudoaneurysm of the artery, and ischemic necrosis.

6. What steps can be taken to minimize arterial line thrombosis?

The incidence of arterial line thrombosis can be minimized by using nontapered Teflon catheters of small diameter, avoiding multiple attempts at the same artery, and using a continfuous flush device.

7. What information is obtained with central venous pressure (CVP) monitoring?

CVP is a numerical value that represents the right atrial pressure or right ventricular filling pressure. In simplistic terms, CVP is an indication of fluid status and right cardiac function. In normal people, changes in CVP correlate with changes in left ventricular filling pressure.

8. How are CVP monitors placed?

A catheter is placed into the central venous system (superior vena cava or, less commonly, inferior vena cava or right atrium), usually via the subclavian or internal jugular veins. The patient is placed in a head-down (Trendelenburg) position, and the catheter is inserted using the Seldinger technique. This technique involves placing a soft, flexible wire through the needle that has been placed in the vein, removing the needle, inserting the catheter over the wire, and removing the wire. The catheter is secured with suture, and its position is confirmed with a chest radiograph.

9. Who is credited with performing the first right-heart catheterization in a human?

In 1929 Werner Forssmann, a 25-year-old surgery student in Berlin, performed the first true human cardiac catheterization *on himself.* Using a mirror and fluoroscopic guidance, he passed a urologic catheter through one of the veins in his arm into his right atrium.

10. What is a normal CVP? What factors may affect it?

In healthy persons, a CVP of 0–4 mmHg provides adequate filling of the right ventricle. For acutely ill patients, 10–12 mmHg is commonly considered the upper limit of normal. Several factors affect this value, including cardiac performance, blood volume, vascular tone, increased intra-abdominal or intrathoracic pressures, and vasopressor therapy.

11. What is a Swan-Ganz catheter?

The Swan-Ganz or pulmonary artery catheter was introduced in 1970 by cardiologists Harold James C. Swan, M.D., and William Ganz, M.D., both cardiologists. It is a multilumen catheter with a balloon on the tip that allows it to be flow directed through central venous access into the right side of the heart and then into the pulmonary artery.

12. What values can be measured with the pulmonary artery catheter?

The catheter allows direct measurement of the pulmonary artery (systolic, diastolic, and mean) pressures, the pulmonary artery wedge pressure, the cardiac output, and the mixed venous blood parameters.

13. In what clinical situations might you consider using a Swan-Ganz catheter?

The Swan-Ganz or pulmonary artery (PA) catheter is usually reserved for critically ill patients in which cardiac or fluid status is difficult to determine by physical exam alone. Examples of patient groups in which PA catheters are often used include the following:

1. Patients with complicated myocardial infarction, during complex general and cardiac surgery.
2. Patients with severe cardiopulmonary disease.
3. Critically ill patients with extensive multisystem falure, shock states, or major trauma.
4. Other situations in which hemodynamic status is difficult to assess adequately.

The risks must be weighed against the benefits in each case. Use of this catheter should imply that the information obtained will affect decisions regarding therapy. Appropriate use of hemodynamic data acquired via the PA catheter requires accurate measurement, analysis, and interpretation of hemodynamic pressure waveforms.

14. What is pulmonary artery wedge pressure (PAWP)?

PAWP is a reasonably accurate measurement of the mean left atrial pressure, which closely parallels the left ventricular end-diastolic pressure (provided that left ventricular compliance and the mitral valve are normal). PAWP, therefore, is considered an accurate reflection of left ventricular diastolic dynamics and thus left ventricular function.

15. How is PAWP measured?

PAWP is obtained by inflating the balloon at the tip of the Swan-Ganz catheter, which has been inserted into the pulmonary artery. When the balloon fills the lumen of the vessel, the transducer measures the pressure transmitted across the pulmonary vasculature from the left atrium. The measurement is obtained at end expiration, when this value is least affected by the transmitted pleural pressure. When the balloon is inflated, a characteristic waveform is seen.

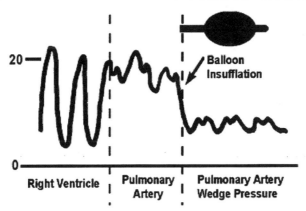

Characteristic Swan-Ganz catheter waveforms from the right ventricle and pulmonary artery. A characteristic waveform also is seen when the balloon is inflated (wedged).

16. How is cardiac output usually measured?

Cardiac output is measured with the Swan-Ganz catheter using a thermodilution technique. The thermodilution technique involves injecting a solution that is colder than blood through the right atrial port of the catheter and measuring the temperature change distally with a thermistor located 4 cm from the catheter tip. The area under the thermodilution curve (by computer) and the volume and temperature of the indicator injection allow calculation of the thermodilution cardiac output. Cardiac output varies, depending at what point during the respiratory cycle the solution is injected; therefore, by convention, cardiac output is measured at end-expiration.

17. What is a mixed venous blood sample? How is it helpful?

Mixed venous blood is obtained by drawing blood from the end of the Swan-Ganz catheter and represents blood from all the organs of the body. The oxygen content of mixed venous blood is a sensitive indicator of the adequacy of the oxygen delivery to the tissues. Serial determinations of mixed venous oxygen can be used to guide efforts to improve oxygen delivery to the tissues.

18. Which hemodynamic values can be derived from Swan-Ganz measurements? How are they calculated?

1. **Cardiac index (CI)** = cardiac output ÷ body surface area

This measurement allows standardization of the cardiac output to account for differences in body size when comparing patients.

2. **Vascular resistance** represents the afterload against which the left and right ventricles must work. Pressure is a function of flow times resistance; therefore, resistance equals pressure divided by flow.

    a. The afterload to the left ventricle is the **systemic vascular resistance (SVR)**, which is calculated as follows:

$$SVR = \frac{\text{mean arterial pressure} - \text{central venous pressure}}{\text{cardiac output}} \times \text{factor (80)}$$

    b. The afterload to the right ventricle is the **pulmonary vascular resistance (PVR)**, calculated by:

$$PVR = \frac{\text{mean pulmonary artery pressure (MPAP)} - \text{PAWP}}{\text{cardiac output}} \times \text{factor (80)}$$

3. **Stroke volume** is a measure of the volume of blood ejected by the heart with each beat and is calculated by dividing the cardiac output by the heart rate.

4. **Oxygen transport** is the amount of oxygen delivered to the heart by the tissues.

5. **Oxygen return** is the amount of oxygen returning to the heart.

6. **Oxygen consumption** reflects the overall ability of the peripheral tissues to extract oxygen.

    O_2 consumption = CI (O_2 content arterial blood − mixed venous O_2 content).

7. **Oxygen delivery** reflects the ability of the body to supply oxygen to the tissues. It must increase as the tissue demand increases with injury or illness.

Oxygen delivery = arterial O_2 content × cardiac output

where O_2 content = PO_2 × 0.0031 + [Hgb] × SaO_2 × 1.34
0.0031 = the solubility coefficient of oxygen
1.34 = the milliliters of oxygen bound to Hgb when it is fully saturated

19. What are considered normal hemodynamic values?

Central venous pressure	= 0–6 mmHg
Right atrial pressure	= 0–6 mmHg
Right ventricular pressure	= 25/0–6 mmHg
Pulmonary artery pressure	= 25/6–12 mmHg
Pulmonary artery wedge pressure	= 6–12 mmHg
Mean arterial pressure	= 85–95 mmHg
Aortic pressure	= 130/80 mmHg
Cardiac index	= ≥ 2.8–3.6 (L/min/m^2)
Systemic vascular resistance	= 770–1500 (dynes/sec/cm^5)
Pulmonary vascular resistance	= 20–120 (dynes/sec/cm^5)
Mixed venous oxygen content	= 15 ml/dl
Mixed venous oxygen tension	= 35–45 torr
Mixed venous oxygen saturation	= 70–75%
Oxygen delivery	= 600 ml/min/m^2
Oxygen consumption	= 150 ml/min/m^2

20. Which hemodynamic derangements would you expect to see with cardiogenic shock?

Cardiogenic shock arises from a primary cardiac cause and leads to ineffective pumping of blood. This status is reflected hemodynamically by a decreased cardiac index, increased pulmonary artery wedge pressure, increased systemic vascular resistance, and inadequate delivery of oxygen to the tissues.

21. Which hemodynamic derangements would you expect to see with hypovolemic or traumatic shock?

Hypovolemic or traumatic shock results in depletion of vascular volume causing a decreased cardiac index, decreased pulmonary artery wedge pressure, increased systemic vascular resistance, and inadequate delivery of oxygen to the tissues.

22. Which hemodynamic derangements would you expect to see with septic shock?

Classic septic shock results in a profound state of vasomotor collapse, which includes vasodilatation with tissue hypoxemia and leakage of intravascular fluid into the tissues. Hemodynamically, this state is manifested by an early increase in cardiac index (hyperdynamic state), a profound decrease in the systemic vascular resistance, and a decrease in the wedge pressure. Oxygen delivery is adequate, but the peripheral tissues are unable to use this oxygen; therefore, oxygen consumption is low. As the sepsis continues, toxic factors released from infected tissues lead to further hypovolemia and cardiac depression.

23. Which hemodynamic derangements would you expect to see with neurogenic shock?

Neurogenic shock may result from spinal cord injuries, spinal anesthesia, or drug overdoses. It results from loss of venous adrenergic tone with pooling of blood in the periphery. This leads to inadequate ventricular filling, decreased wedge pressures, and decreased cardiac index. The loss of adrenergic tone also results in a profound decrease in the systemic vascular resistance.

24. Compare the classic hemodynamic findings for various forms of shock.

Type of Shock	Cardiac Index	Wedge Pressure	Sytemic Vascular Resistance
Cardiogenic	Decreased	Increased	Increased
Hypovolemic or traumatic	Decreased	Decreased	Increased
Septic	Increased	Decreased	Decreased
Neurogenic	Decreased	Decreased	Decreased

25. What are the complications of Swan-Ganz catheterization?

Insertion of the Swan-Ganz catheter shares all of the complications associated with central venous catheter placement: pneumothoraces, hemothoraces, inadvertent arterial punctures, infections, venous air embolism, arrhythmias, airway injuries, nerve injuries, and chylothoraces. Complications unique to Swan-Ganz catheters include ventricular rupture, valvular damage, pulmonary artery rupture, pulmonary artery aneurysm, pulmonary artery thrombosis or infarction, bundle-branch blocks, ventricular arrhythmias, endocardial damage, balloon rupture, and knotting of the catheter.

26. How should pulmonary artery rupture be treated?

Pulmonary artery rupture as a complication of pulmonary artery catheterization is an infrequent but life-threatening complication. Most patients do not die as a result of exsanguination, but rather from causes secondary to aspiration and asphyxia; therefore, the initial management should focus on airway management, oxygenation, fluid replacement, and control of bleeding. Endotracheal intubation using a double-lumen tube is recommended, with positioning of the patient in a lateral decubitus position with the side of the injury down. Fluid resuscitation, reversal of anticoagulation, and lowering of pulmonary hypertension are useful adjuncts to control the bleeding. Thoracotomy and pulmonary resection are rarely required because of frequent spontaneous cessation but should be done promptly if all other measures fail.

27. What noninvasive methods for determining cardiac output are under study?
Several noninvasive techniques are being studied to measure cardiac output in critically ill patients, including:
1. **Thoracic electrical bioimpedance.** This technique has shown good correlation with invasive methods in spontaneously breathing patients; however, the results with this technique and invasive techniques vary when patients are on mechanical ventilation and PEEP.
2. **Two-beam pulsed Doppler.** This technique takes advantage of recent advances in Doppler technology; one probe can simultaneously measure aortic blood velocity and the cross-sectional area of the aorta. These measurements allow calculation of the cardiac output from a single suprasternal reading. Correlation with thermodilution is good, but results are highly operator-dependent and the technique may be difficult in some ICU scenarios.
3. **Thoracocardiography.** This technique estimates changes in cardiac output by recording ventricular volume curves from an inductive plethysmographic transducer placed around the chest near the xiphoid process. Absolute values of cardiac output are not obtained but relative changes in cardiac output are detected, making this a potentially promising technique.
4. **Fast Fourier transform analysis.** This technique relies on fast Fourier transform analysis of pulses measured externally at the carotid and femoral pressure points. A transfer function of the aorta is computed from these pressure measurements, and a tapered model of the aorta is parametrically adapted such that cardiac output can be measured. This technology is currently under investigation.
5. **Transesophageal echocardiography (TEE).** TEE can establish a hemodynamic profile by careful interpretation of anatomic appearance and Doppler flow. Detailed imaging of the chambers, intra-atrial septum, and great veins combined with Doppler imaging of pulmonary veins, pulmonary artery, mitral inflow, tricupsic regurgitation, and hepatic and great veins is necessary to obtain accurate results. This approach allows qualitative but not quantitative determination of cardiac and hemodynamic function.
The ultimate role of noninvasive hemodynamic monitoring remains to be determined, but as these techniques improve, they will no doubt become more widely used.

CONTROVERSY

28. Do Swan-Ganz catheters contribute to improved patient outcome?
Since the introduction of the Swan-Ganz catheter in 1970, a small but vocal minority has expressed concerns that PA catheterization is performed too frequently and that the data obtained may not be optimally used. This controversy recently was rekindled by Connors et al. in an article indicating that critically ill patients in whom the catheter was used had a higher mortality rate than patients managed without a PA catheter. In an editorial accompanying the article, two respected critical care specialists suggested a moratorium on the continued use of PA catheters until a prospective trial is undertaken to investigate their efficacy and safety. In response, the American College of Chest Physicians and the American Thoracic Society released the following recommendations about the use of PA flotation catheters:
1. There is no indication at present for a moratorium.
2. Prospective, randomized, controlled trials of the PA catheter are indicated, ethical, and appropriate. (The Canadian Critical Care Trials Group is currently undertaking such a study.)
3. The decision to insert a PA catheter should be based on specific clinical circumstances with weiging of risk vs. benefit by the patient's physician.
4. Informed consent should be obtained whenever possible, and physicians should be prepared to discuss recent articles with patients and/or surrogates.

5. Physicians should be knowledgeable about the proper placement and use of a PA catheter and the proper collection, documentation, interpretation, and use of data generated by the PA catheter. (This principle is underscored by a recent article reporting uniformly poor performance on a multiple-choice test on all aspects of PA catheterization, given to 535 critical care physicians.)

6. Physicians should know the potential complications associated with the insertion and prolonged use of PA catheters. At present PA catheters continue to be widely used in the care of critically ill patients. The critical care community awaits the results of the first prospective, randomized, controlled trial and any subsequent trials for guidance.

BIBLIOGRAPHY

1. Bowyer MW, Bonar JP: Non-infectious complications of invasive hemodynamic monitoring in the intensive care unit. In Matthay MA, Schwartz DE (eds): Complications in the Intensive Care Unit. Chapman and Hall, 1997, pp 92–122.
2. Chernow B: Pulmonary artery flotation catheters. A statement by the American College of Chest Physicians and the American Thoracic Society. Chest 111:261, 1997.
3. Clark VL, Kruse JA: Arterial catheterization. Crit Care Clin 8:687–689, 1992.
4. Conners AF Jr, Speroff T, Dawson N, et al: The effectiveness of right heart catheterization in the initial care of critically ill patients. JAMA 276:889–897, 1996.
5. Coulter TD: Complications of hemodynamic monitoring. Clin Chest Med 20:249–267, 1999.
6. Gracias VH, McGonigal MD: Monitoring organ function: Heart, liver, and kidney. Surg Clin North Am 80:911–919, 2000.
7. Ivanov R: The incidence of major morbidity in critically ill patients managed with pulmonary artery catheters: A meta-analysis. Crit Care Med 28:615–619, 2000.
8. Kohli-Seth R, Oropello JM: The future of bedside monitoring. Crit Care Clin 16:557–578, 2000.
9. Ott K, Johnson K, Aherns T: New technologies in the assessment of hemodynamic parameters. J Cardiovasc Nurs 15:41–45, 2001.
10. Prentice D, Aherns T: Controversies in the use of the pulmonary artery catheter. J Cardiovasc Nurs 15:1–5, 2001.
11. Shoemaker WC, Woo CCJ, Chan L, et al: Outcome prediction of emergency patients by noninvasive hemodynamic monitoring. Chest 120:526–537, 2001.
12. Schiller NB: Transesophageal echocardiography: Hemodynamics derived from transesophageal echocardiography (TEE). Cardiol Clin 18:699–709, 2000.

5. INTERPRETATION OF ARTERIAL BLOOD GASES

E. Michael Canham, M.D.

1. What do arterial blood gas (ABG) instruments measure?

The current ABG instruments measure pH, PCO_2, and PO_2 using three separate electrodes. The blood gas samples are placed through an inlet into a temperature-controlled chamber (usually 37°C) where the blood is exposed to these three electrode tips.

2. When should ABGs be analyzed?

Analysis of ABGs is used extensively in the critical care setting to evaluate both acid-base status and oxygen and carbon dioxide gas exchange. Analysis of ABGs is indicated in virtually all cardiopulmonary conditions.

3. What are the problems associated with obtaining ABGs?

The arterial puncture may result in acute hyperventilation, which is often minimized by good technique, by use of a small needle, or by instillation of a local anesthetic. After the sample is obtained, all air bubbles should be expelled and the syringe capped. Air bubbles that are mixed or agitated into the sample will equilibrate with the blood, possibly altering the PO_2 toward room air and lowering the PCO_2. The sample should be placed on ice unless the analysis is performed within 15 minutes. Plastic syringes may allow greater diffusion of gases than glass syringes and so should also be run promptly. In the absence of extreme leukocytosis, an iced, glass ABG syringe will maintain the PO_2 value for up to 3 hours.

4. What does extreme leukocytosis ("leukocyte larceny") do to the ABG analysis?

The presence of large numbers of leukocytes or platelets will reduce the PO_2 value, giving a false impression of hypoxemia. This drop in PO_2 is negligible if the sample is stored in ice and analyzed within 1 hour. Presumably the ongoing metabolism of the cellular elements of blood consume oxygen, reducing PO_2.

5. How long after starting or stopping supplemental oxygen should one wait before ABGs can be drawn and reflect baseline or plateau values?

In patients with severe obstructive lung disease and air trapping, 25 minutes may be required; however, in the absence of significant lung disease, 5–7 minutes would be adequate.

6. What is the alveolar gas equation?

The alveolar gas equation is a formula used to approximate the partial pressure of oxygen in the alveolus (PAO_2).

$$PAO_2 = (PB - PH_2O) \ FiO_2 - \frac{PaCO_2}{R}$$

where PB is the barometric pressure, PH_2O is the water vapor pressure (usually 47 mmHg), FiO_2 is the fractional concentration of inspired oxygen, and R is the gas exchange ratio. (The rate of CO_2 production to O_2 utilization is usually around 0.8 at rest.) For example, at sea level:

$$PAO_2 = (760 - 47).21 - \frac{40}{0.8} = 100 \ mmHg$$

7. What is the alveolar-arterial PO2 difference, or "A-a gradient" (AaO_2 gradient)?

After calculation of the PAO_2 from the alveolar gas equation, the AaO_2 gradient can be obtained by subtracting the PaO_2 measured from the ABGs. For example, at sea level (with $PCO_2 – 40$, $PO_2 – 92$):

$$PAO_2 - PaO_2 = AaO_2 \ gradient$$
$$100 \ mmHg - 92 \ mmHg = 8 \ mmHg$$

The normal AaO_2 gradient is dependent on age, body position, and nutritional status. The AaO_2 gradient is widened under normal conditions by age, obesity, fasting, supine position, and heavy exercise. One predictive equation for estimating PO_2 (at PB = 760 mmHg) in relation to age is as follows: $PO_2 = 109 – .43 \times age$ (in years).

8. How is the AaO_2 gradient useful?

The AaO_2 gradient may be widened by any significant cardiopulmonary condition that results in hypoxemia and/or hypocarbia. Hypoxemia caused by simple alveolar hypoventilation will not widen the AaO_2 gradient. Most pulmonary emboli, on the other hand, will widen the AaO_2 gradient, because even if hypoxemia does not occur, hypocarbia is very common.

9. What is the difference between a calculated versus a measured oxygen saturation?

The calculated oxyhemoglobin saturation is calculated from the measured values of PaO_2 and pH by the Severinghaus slide rule, by a nomogram, or by the blood gas instrument microprocessor. The measured oxyhemoglobin saturation is obtained with a co-oximeter (a spectrophotometer), which measures reduced hemoglobin, oxyhemoglobin, carboxyhemoglobin, and methemoglobin. Errors in the calculation of oxygen saturation may occur if carboxyhemoglobin is present, which is commonly seen in cigarette smokers. Carbon monoxide does not affect oxygen tension (PaO_2) but does bind and displace oxygen from hemoglobin. Consequently, the calculated oxygen saturation is falsely elevated.

The calculated oxygen saturation may also be in error if the oxyhemoglobin dissociation curve is displaced by changes in 2,3-diphosphoglycerate (2,3-DPG). The binding of 2,3-DPG to hemoglobin reduces the affinity of hemoglobin for oxygen, facilitating the unloading of oxygen at the tissue level. The binding of 2,3-DPG to hemoglobin shifts the oxyhemoglobin dissociation curve to the right. A common example of 2,3-DPG depletion occurs in the storage of blood. Consequently, a patient receiving multiple units of stored blood, with a leftward shift of the oxyhemoglobin dissociation curve, will have a calculated oxygen saturation less than the measured oxygen saturation.

Hemoglobinopathies will also cause a discrepancy between the measured and calculated oxygen saturation, depending on which way they shift the oxyhemoglobin dissociation curve.

10. How do continuous intra-arterial blood gas monitors (CIABGM) work?

Most of the CIABGMs in development or in current use utilize optical fiber sensors (optodes), which quantify photochemical reactions from light absorption, light reflection, or fluorescence. The optical fibers transmit a light signal down the fiber where it interacts with a dye. Changes in the concentration of the measured substance (i.e., CO_2, O_2) within the dye complex causes an alteration of the light signal by absorption, reflection, or fluorescence. The CIABGM probe generally consists of three fiberoptic fibers with specific dyes for measuring pH, PCO_2, and PO_2. Additionally, a thermocouple is included for continuous temperature measurement of blood. The role of CIABGM is unclear until outcome and cost-benefit studies are completed.

11. What are point-of-care (POC) ABGs?

Current technology allows measurement of ABGs at the bedside with hand-held blood gas analysis devices that use disposable cartridges. Several commercially available devices provide different test options to measure in addition to routine ABG values. Consequently, the reliability of each measured parameter may differ from one device to another.

12. How do POC ABGs work? What are their advanges and disadvantages?

The herparinized ABG specimen is placed into the POC cartridge, where the blood flows to different sites-sensors for analysis. The pH and pCO_2 are measured by direct potentiometry, and the pO_2 is measured amperometrically. The values for HCO_3, total CO_2, base excess, and oxygen saturation are calculated. POC testing can be performed by nurses, physicians, and respiratory therapists, and the ABG results are obtained more rapidly and may influence critical decisions. The major disadvantages include cost per cartridge and lack of preanalysis calibrations to ensure accuracy.

13. Given that oximetry is so readily available, painless, and accurate, why is ABG analysis necessary?

Oximetry and the newer technology that made it more accessible, affordable, and accurate have decreased the need for ABG analysis in monitoring oxygen saturation. In fact, in many hospitals the number of ABGs done has decreased with the influx of oximeters into virtually every department within a hospital. However, relying on oximetry alone can lead to misdiagnosis, increased cost, and potentially fatal respiratory arrest. Consider the following examples of pitfalls of using oximetry alone that have been observed in practice.

1. A patient was noted to have oxygen desaturation via oximetry during a routine check after minor orthopedic surgery. The physicians evaluated this oximetric abnormality by ordering a chest x-ray, pulmonary function tests, and a ventilation-perfusion lung scan, all of which were normal. Finally, ABG analysis was done and revealed alveolar hypoventilation alone with a normal AaO_2 gradient. The oxygen desaturation was simply the result of an increased PCO_2 from hypoventilation in a patient receiving narcotics.

2. Following an episode of smoke inhalation, a patient came to the emergency room for headache and nausea. The oxygen saturation by oximetry was normal, and the patient was nearly dismissed after symptomatic treatment alone. Fortunately, recognizing the limitation of oximetry in differentiating oxygenated hemoglobin from carboxyhemoglobin, the physician drew an ABG sample, which revealed profound carbon monoxide poisoning. The patient was treated appropriately with 100% oxygen and close monitoring.

3. Another example involved a house officer who was asked to see a febrile, septic patient with a respiratory rate of 40 and a chest x-ray revealing early alveolar infiltrates bilaterally. Oxygen was initiated, and with the use of oximetry, the oxygen saturation was titrated to 90%. The patient required FiO_2 of 100% by non-rebreather mask to achieve the 90% oxygen saturation. Unfortunately, the house officer did not draw an ABG sample and failed to realize that with marked hyperventilation and respiratory alkalosis, the oxyhemoglobin dissociation curve is shifted to the left, thereby causing a much higher oxygen saturation for a given PaO_2. Had ABG analysis been done at that time, it would have revealed pH 7.58, $PACO_2$ 22, PAO_2 50, and O_2 sat 90%, all clearly indicating intubation and assisted ventilation with PEEP. Later that evening, the patient suffered a near-fatal respiratory arrest.

4. A patient is intubated for respiratory failure and has a vigorous cough against the endotracheal tube (ETT). Lidocaine solution is given through the ETT to anesthetize the airways and reduce the cough. Oxygen saturation as measured by oximetry drops to 70%. A POC ABG reveals that the pO_2 is 250 mmHg, but the blood specimen appears brownish. A second ABG sent to the lab reveals a methemoglobin level of 28%. Lidocaine-induced methemoglobinemia is diagnosed and resolves with intravenous instillation of methylene blue.

BIBLIOGRAPHY

1. Asmussen E, Nielsen M: Alveolo-arterial gas exchange at rest and during work at different O_2 tensions. Acta Physiol Scand 50:153–160, 1960.
2. Cissik JH, Salustro J, Patton OL, Louden JA: The effects of sodium heparin on arterial blood gas analysis. Cardiovasc Pulm 5:17–21, 1977.
3. Cugell DW: How long should you wait? (editorial). Chest 67:253, 1975.
4. Cvitanic O, Marino PL: Improved use of arterial blood gas analysis in suspected pulmonary emboli. Chest 95:48–51, 1989.
5. Hansen JE: Arterial blood gases. In Mahler DA (ed): Pulmonary Function Testing. Clin Chest Med 5:277–237, 1989.
6. Hansen JE, Simmons DH: A systematic error in the determination of blood PCO_2. Am Rev Respir Dis 115:1061–1063, 1977.
7. Hess CE, Nichols AB, Hunt WB, Suratt PM: Pseudohypoxemia secondary to leukemia and thrombocytosis. N Engl J Med 301:361–363, 1979.
8. Raffin TA: Indications for arterial blood gas analysis. In Sox HC Jr (ed): Common Diagnostic Tests, 2nd ed. Philadelphia, American College of Physicians, 1990, pp 100–119.
9. Severinghaus JW: Blood gas calculator. J Appl Physiol 21:1108–1116, 1966.
10. Severinghaus JW, Astraup P, Murray JF: Blood gas analysis and critical care medicine. Am J Respir Crit Care Med 157:S114–S122, 1998.
11. Sorbini CA, Grassi V, Solinas E, Muiesan G: Arterial oxygen tension in relation to age in healthy subjects. Respiration 25:3–13, 1968.
12. Venkatesh B, Hendry SP: Continuous intra-arterial blood gas monitoring. Intensive Care Med 22:818–828, 1996.

6. FLUID THERAPY

James E. Wiedeman, M.D., and Mark W. Bowyer, M.D.

1. How is water distributed throughout the body?

Total body water comprises 60% of body weight in the male and 50% of body weight in the female. The distribution of this water is 40% in intracellular space (30% in females) and 20% in extracellular space. The extracellular fluid is broken down into 15% interstitial and 5% plasma.

2. What governs the distribution of fluid in the body?

The membranes between the fluid compartments are semipermeable, allowing rapid equilibration of free water and low-molecular-weight solutes. Particles and solutes unable to cross the membrane create oncotic pressure. The relative difference in oncotic pressure between various compartments governs the distribution of fluid.

3. How are maintenance fluid requirements calculated?

For a 70-kg patient, obligatory fluid losses that must be replaced include insensible losses from skin and lungs (about 800 ml), fecal losses (200 ml), and sweat. In addition, enough urine must be produced to excrete a solute load of 600 mOsm produced each day by the body (for healthy people, this amounts to 500 ml of urine; for critically ill patients with decreased renal concentrating abilities, this amounts to 900 ml). These sensible and insensible losses account for 2000–2500 ml per day, giving a 24-hour fluid requirement of 30–35 ml/kg to maintain a normal fluid balance.

4. What are fluid maintenance requirements for children?

Twenty-four–hour fluid requirements for children have been formulated based on weight:
0–10 kg = 100 ml/kg
11–20 kg = 1000 ml + 50 ml/kg for every kg above 10 kg
> 20 kg = 1500 ml + 20 ml/kg for every kg above 20 kg

5. Describe the clinical features of volume deficit and volume excess.

Patients with a **volume deficit** may exhibit altered mentation, hypotension, tachycardia, decreased skin turgor, and hypothermia.

Volume excess leads to distended neck veins, S3 gallop, basilar rates, and peripheral edema. Volume deficit and volume excess are clinical diagnoses, independent of changes in concentration (sodium) or composition (potassium, calcium, magnesium, or bicarbonate) that may be detected on laboratory tests.

6. What are the classes of hemorrhagic shock?

The percentage of blood loss in each class is the same as the score in a tennis game: 15–30–40–game over:
Class I: up to 15%   Class III: 30–40%
Class II: 15–30%   Class IV: over 40%
Hypotension first occurs in class III shock.

7. What are the common sources, volumes, and compositions of GI fluid losses?

Common Sources, Volumes, and Compositions of GI Fluid Losses

	COMPOSITION (MEQ / L)				
SOURCE	Na	K	CL	HCO$_3$	VOLUME
Gastric (NG tubes, vomiting)	60	10	130	—	100–400 ml
Duodenum (fistulas)	140	5	80	—	100–2000 ml
Bile (T tubes, fistulas)	145	5	100	35	50–800 ml
Pancreas (fistulas)	140	5	75	115	100–800 ml
Ileum (ileostomies, fistulas)	140	5	104	30	100–9000 ml
Colon (diarrhea)	60	30	40	20	

8. What empiric replacement fluids can be used for GI losses?

Sweat   D4 ¼ normal saline with 5 KCL/L
Gastric   D5 ½ normal saline with 30 KCL/L
Duodenum   Normal saline with 10 KCL/L
Bile, pancreas, small bowel   Lactated Ringer's solution
Colon   D5 ½ normal saline with 30 KCL/L
Third space   Lactated Ringer's solution

9. What is the difference between crystalloids and colloids? Give examples of each.

Crystalloids are mixtures of sodium chloride and other physiologically active solutes. The distribution of sodium determines the distribution of the infused crystalloid. Examples are normal saline, Ringer's lactate, and hypertonic saline.

Colloids are high-molecular-weight substances that stay in the vascular space and exert an osmotic force. Examples are albumin, Hetastarch, Dextran, and blood.

10. What is the 3:1 rule in fluid therapy after acute blood loss?

Three milliliters of crystalloid are required for each one ml of blood loss to compensate for administered fluid that is lost into the interstitial and intracelluar spaces.

11. Describe the electrolyte composition of normal saline and lactated Ringer's solution. Which should be used for acute resuscitation?

Normal saline contains 154 mEq sodium (Na^+) and 154 mEq chloride (Cl^-) per liter. Lactated Ringer's solution contains 130 mEq Na^+, 109 mEq Cl^-, 4 mEq potassium (K^+), 3 mEq Ca^{2+}, and 28 mEq lactate per liter. Lactated Ringer's solution is preferred for acute volume replacement because normal saline can result in hyperchloremic metabolic acidosis.

CONTROVERSY

12. What is the best fluid to give in hypovolemic shock due to trauma?

1. **No fluid**

    For: Hypotension decreases blood loss in penetrating torso injuries.

    Against: Withholding fluid is harmful in patients with multisystem blunt trauma. Decreased perfusion pressure in head trauma can lead to secondary brain injury.

2. **Lactated Ringer's solution**

    For: Inexpensive. Because electrolyte content approaches that of interstitial fluid, it is the ideal replacement for intracellular shifts.

    Against: The 3:1 rule demands excessive volume administration, which leads to interstitial and intracellular edema as well as dilution of hematocrit and clotting factors. Restoration of blood pressure dislodges soft clots and increases blood loss before definitive surgical control.

3. **Hypertonic saline**

    For: Improves survival rates in patients with traumatic brain injury and hypotension. Smaller volumes are easy to store and transport.

    Against: Rapid expansion of plasma space may lead to ongoing hemorrhage due to clot disruption. Administration can cause sodium overload.

4. **Albumin or Hespan**

    For: Increased oncotic pressure leads to fluid retention in intravascular space.

    Against: Expensive. Albumin causes reperfusion injury, contributing to acute respiratory-distress syndrome and other organ failure. Hespan leads to coagulopathy.

5. **Blood or blood substitutes**

    For: Facilitates oxygen delivery in low-flow states while maintaining potential benefits of hypotensive resuscitation (limits blood loss).

    Against: Blood has storage and infectious risks. Substitutes seem to be promising alternatives but are still in preclinical trials.

BIBLIOGRAPHY

1. Bickell WH, Matthew JW, Pepe PE, et al: Immediate versus delayed fluid resuscitation for hypotensive patients with penetrating torso injuries.N Engl J Med 331(17):1105–1109, 1994.
2. Gould SA, Rosen B, Rosen AL, et al: Hemorrhage and resuscitation. In Rippe JM, et al (eds): Intensive Care Medicine, 3rd ed. Boston, Little, Brown, 1996, pp 1878–1886.
3. McNeil JD, Smith DL, Jenkins DL, et al: Hypotensive resuscitation using a polymerized bovine hemoglobin-based oxygen-carrying solution (HBOC-201) leads to reversal of anaerobic metabolism. J Trauma 50:1063–1075, 2001.

4. Noone RB: Fluid and electrolytes and acid-base management. In Clary BM, Milano CA (eds): The Handbook of Surgical Intensive Care, 5th ed. St. Louis, Mosby, 2000, pp 17–38.
5. Tremblay LN, Rizoli SB, Brenneman FD: Advances in fluid resuscitation of hemorrhagic shock. Can J Surg 44(3):172–179, 2001.
6. Wade CE, Grady JJ, Kramer GC, et al: Individual patient cohort analysis of the efficacy of hypertonic saline/Dextran in patients with traumatic brain injury and hypotension. J Trauma 42:S61–S65, 1997.

7. NUTRITION IN CRITICALLY ILL PATIENTS

Mark T. Grabovac, M.D.

1. Describe the metabolic changes that occur during critical illness.

Critical illness is frequently accompanied by starvation and malnutrition. Metabolic changes associated with critical illness include a shift to a hypermetabolic and hypercatabolic state characterized by the release of catecholamines, glucocorticoids, inflammatory mediators, and cytokines. Consequences of these changes include anorexia, weight loss, loss of lean body mass, alterations in immune function, and impaired wound healing. Specific changes in the metabolism of glucose, protein, and fats occur during critical illness. For glucose these changes are characterized by hyperglycemia due to both insulin resistance and increased glucose synthesis. For protein metabolism the changes include increased proteolysis of skeletal muscle with resultant gluconeogenesis and production of a host of acute-phase reactants and cytokines. Changes in fat metabolism include an increase in lypolysis and replacement of glucose with fatty acids as the preferred oxidative fuel for most tissues.

2. What are the daily nutritional requirements for critically ill patients?

Calories. Caloric requirements are estimated as approximately 25 kilocalories/kg of body weight/day. The number of required calories is increased by burns, fever, or other hypercatabolic states, whereas for other conditions, such as chronic obstructive pulmonary disease (COPD), the number of required calories may be reduced.

Glucose. Thirty to 70% of total calories should be administered as dextrose (generally about 2–5 gm of glucose/kg/day). Conditions such as COPD or inability to wean from mechanical ventilation can decrease the requirement for carbohydrates. This decision frequently can be guided by calculation of the respiratory quotient (see below).

Protein. Fifteen to 20% of total calories per day should be administered as proteins or amino acids. Therapy is generally initiated with 1.2–1.5 gm/kg/day and adjusted after measuring nitrogen retention and other clinical indicators of protein catabolism. Considerations that may warrant a decrease in protein administration include worsening encephalopathy with a rising blood ammonia level or renal failure with a rising blood urea nitrogen level.

The nutritional requirements for many micronutrients, such as vitamins, minerals, and trace elements, are not well established. Electrolytes such as sodium, potassium, magnesium, and phosphate should be supplied, and serum levels should be checked.

3. Discuss the nutritional assessment of critically ill patients and the clinical indicators of malnutrition.

Many patients enter the intensive care unit (ICU) malnourished, and their nutritional status tends to decline with length of stay in the hospital. Adequate nutritional assessment is critical to formulation of a nutritional care plan. Assessment of nutritional status begins with a history and physical examination. Indicators of malnutrition include recent involuntary weight loss (which can be masked by fluid retention), changes in appetite or bowel habits, presence of persistent gastrointestinal (GI) symptoms, muscle wasting, and signs of specific micronutrient deficiencies such as glossitis or anemia.

Many tests are available to assess nutritional status, each with specific applications and limitations. Examples include anthropometry (e.g., body mass index [BMI]), measurement of hepatic secretory proteins (e.g., albumin, transferrin), estimation of lean body mass (using creatinine height index derived from measurement of a 24-hour urine collection), cutaneous testing of cellular immunity, muscle function testing, and multiparameter nutritional indexes.

4. What are the goals of nutritional support in critically ill patients?

The goals of nutritional support in critically ill patients include the preservation and repletion of lean body mass, prevention of macronutrient and micronutrient deficiencies, reduction in overall morbidity and mortality, improvement in patient outcomes, and avoidance of complications related to the delivery of nutritional support. Examples of goals of more specialized nutritional support include improvement of immune function or wound healing and support of hepatic protein synthesis.

5. How can energy requirements be estimated in critically ill patients?

Resting energy expenditure (REE) can be estimated by using the Harris-Benedict equation. For males:

$$REE = 66.5 + 13.75 \times (\text{weight in kg}) + 5 \times (\text{height in cm}) - 6.76 \times (\text{age in years})$$

For females:

$$REE = 655 + 9.56 \times (\text{weight in kg}) + 1.86 \times (\text{height in cm}) - 4.68 \times (\text{age in years}).$$

A major limitation of the Harris-Benedict equation is that it was derived from data in normal volunteers. Stress factors ranging from 1.2 to 2.1 can be used to correct for disease states and can be multiplied by the REE to estimate more accurately the true energy expenditure of critically ill patients.

Indirect calorimetry provides a more accurate estimate of energy expenditure in the ICU by measurement of respiratory gas exchange. Bedside devices (metabolic cart) measure oxygen consumption (VO_2), carbon dioxide production (VCO_2), and minute ventilation (VE). These values are then used in the Weir equation to determine energy expenditure. A major limitation to the use of indirect calorimetry in the ICU is that the measurements become unreliable when the inspired oxygen concentration is greater than 50%. The Weir equation is as follows:

$$\text{Energy expenditure} = [(VO_2) \times (3.941) + (VCO_2) \times (1.11)] \times 1440$$

6. How is the respiratory quotient defined? How can it be used clinically?

The respiratory quotient (RQ) is the ratio of carbon dioxide production (VCO_2) to oxygen consumption (VO_2). These values are obtained by a metabolic cart at the patient's bedside. The RQ is helpful in planning of nutritional therapy. The physiologic range for RQ values (0.7–1.2) is influenced by the relative contributions from fat, protein, and carbohydrate. RQ values for fat, protein, and carbohydrate are 0.7, 0.8 and 1.0, respectively. Thus, an RQ > 1.0 may suggest the feeding of excessive carbohydrate or calories, which may result in increased CO_2 production and cause difficulty in weaning from mechanical ventilation.

7. How can protein requirements be assessed in critically ill patients? Explain nitrogen balance and its significance.

Nitrogen balance is defined as nitrogen intake minus nitrogen losses from urine, skin, and feces:

$$\text{Nitrogen balance (gm)} = (\text{protein intake}/6.25) - (\text{urinary urea nitrogen} + 2\text{–}4)$$

Nitrogen balance determines the quantity of protein required to maintain equilibrium between nitrogen intake and losses. Positive nitrogen balance is associated with improved outcomes and is the best single marker of the effectiveness of nutritional intervention. Because of the catabolic state associated with critical illness, a positive nitrogen balance is frequently difficult to achieve. Liver failure renders nitrogen balance calculations inaccurate because of decreased urea nitrogen production, whereas excessive diarrhea, high ostomy output, serous drainage from wounds, or other fluid losses make the calculations difficult because of excessive unmeasured losses. Nitrogen balance cannot be interpreted in the presence of renal dysfunction (creatinine clearance < 50 ml/min).

8. Discuss the specific nutritional considerations for ventilator-dependent patients.

Patients who require ventilatory support can suffer from multiple comorbidities that affect their ability to be weaned from the ventilator. These comorbidities can be influenced by nutritional support. Nutritional depletion can affect the immune system and predispose to infection, weaken the respiratory muscles, and exacerbate respiratory failure. Malnutrition also causes hypoalbuminemia, thereby potentially accelerating the formation of pulmonary edema fluid. Electrolyte abnormalities such as hypophosphatemia or hypermagnesemia can worsen the function of already weak respiratory muscles. Overfeeding with calories or carbohydrates can lead to excessive CO_2 production and exacerbate respiratory failure.

9. List two other clinical conditions that have implications for nutritional support. How do these conditions affect formula selection and nutritional requirements?

Renal failure. Administration of excessive protein to patients in renal failure can promote azotemia and, over a long period, accelerate the progression of chronic renal failure. Less than 1 gm/kg/day of protein is sufficient for patients with chronic renal insufficiency. Fluid and potassium restriction also may be necessary in patients with renal insufficiency.

Liver disease. In patients with hepatic insufficiency, hepatic encephalopathy is frequently exacerbated or initiated by excessive protein administration. Reducing the total protein and increasing the amount of branched-chain amino acids administered has been demonstrated to improve mental status in such patients.

10. What are enteral and parenteral nutrition?

Enteral nutrition is the administration of nutrients via the existing gastrointestinal tract, whereas **parenteral nutrition** is the aministration of nutrients via peripheral or central venous routes.

11. When should enteral nutrition be instituted after admission to the ICU? Describe some of the potential benefits to early enteral nutrition.

Current research supports the administration of supplemental enteral nutrition to critically ill patients unable to meet nutritional requirements through oral intake as soon as possible after admission to the ICU. The presence of bowel sounds and the passage of flatus are not necessary before the institution of enteral nutrition. Potential benefits to early enteral nutrition include attenuation of the stress response, lessening of gut atrophy, and decrease in abnormal gut permeability associated with starvation.

12. Describe the routes of administration and the preferred method of delivery for enteral nutrition.

Enteral nutrition is generally administered nasoenterically via gastric or small bowel feeding tubes. Intragastric feedings require adequate motility and increase the risk of aspiration but do not require the placement of a nasoenteric tube into the small bowel, which can be technically more challenging and may even require fluoroscopic guidance. Transpyloric (small bowel) feedings are better tolerated, have fewer complications, and can be used even in the presence of gastric and colonic ileus.

Enteral nutrition can be delivered via bolus, intermittent, or continuous feeding. Bolus feeding involves the delivery of a large volume of formula over a short period and carries a greater risk of aspiration, diarrhea, nausea, vomiting, and distention. Intermittent feeding delivers a defined volume of formula over 1–12 hours. Continuous feedings deliver a small amount of formula continuously over 24 hours via a mechanical pump. In the setting of critical illness, continuous feedings delivered into the small bowel are far better tolerated than the other two methods and are associated with a lower incidence of aspiration, stress uleration, and diarrhea.

13. Describe the physiologic role of the gut in critically ill patients.

In health the GI tract acts to digest food, to absorb nutrients, and to maintain a barrier against bacterial flora and toxic substances. The ability of the gut to perform these functions depends on contact of the GI tissues with intraluminal nutrients, maintenance of normal intestinal flora, and presence of gut-associated lymphoid tissue (GALT) as well as many nonspecific defenses such as peristalsis, gastric acid production, and bile salts. Many of these conditions for normal function are directly or indirectly affected during critical illness. Critical illness frequently is associated with atrophy of intestinal mucosa and GALT, disruption of normal intestinal flora by antibiotics, ileus induced by a variety of drugs, and decreased production of gastric acid caused by proton pump inhibitors. All of these factors can lead to barrier dysfunction in the gut. This breakdown in intestinal structure and barrier function can lead to malabsorption and bacterial translocation. The term *bacterial translocation* describes the migration of bacteria from the gut lumen to the lymph tissue or blood stream and has been implicated in the pathogenesis of sepsis and the septic inflammatory response syndrome (SIRS).

14. What are pharmaconutrients? Give some examples.

Pharmaconutrients are specific nutrients that are provided in addition to (or in larger amounts than) the usual macro- and micronutrients to produce specific effects on certain organs or metabolic functions. Examples of pharmaconutrients include:

Glutamine. Glutamine is an abundant amino acid and a major gut fuel. Supplementation of enteral nutrition formulas with glutamine has been shown to maintain normal GALT size and function, decrease bacterial translocation, and increase the thickness of GI mucosa.

Omega-3 fatty acid. Older enteral nutrition formulas were high in omega-6 fatty acids, which have been shown to be immunosuppressive. Newer formulas are higher in omega-3 fatty acids,which are less immunosuppressive and may provide an anti-inflammatory effect.

Branched-chain amino acids (BCAA). BCAAs (leucine, isoleucine, and valine) are essential amino acids that improve nitrogen retention and protein synthetic function.

Arginine. Arginine is an amino acid that may enhance immune function, wound healing, and nitrogen balance when supplied in enteral nutrition formulas.

Many other substances, including growth hormone, antioxidants, and nucleic acids, are currently under investigation. Although many of these pharmaconutrients show promise, their precise role in routine clinical care and in improving outcomes remains uncertain.

15. What types of enteral nutrition solutions are available? How is the right solution selected for a given patient?

There is tremendous variety in the commercially available enteral nutritional formulas. Formulas are frequently classified as polymeric, elemental or semielemental/peptide-based, and modular. **Polymeric** formulas contain intact nutrients and require a fully functional GI tract. **Elemental and semielemental** formulas contain partially digested nutrients and have applications in patients with compromised GI function. **Modular** formulas consist of different macronutrient modules that can be combined to meet specific nutritional needs of a particular patient.

Formulas should be selected with consideration of the patient's digestive function, absorptive capacity, nutrient requirements, fluid requirements, intolerances, and allergies. High-osmolality or hypertonic formulas are often poorly tolerated and frequently require initial dilution to half-strength for patients who have had to avoid oral ingestion (NPO) for long periods or who have underlying malabsorption due to intestinal resection or diarrhea.

There has been a tremendous proliferation in disease-specific formulas, which frequently contain specific pharmaconutrients, immunomodulatory substances, or specific combinations of macro- and micronutrients. These formulas are generally expensive, and few data support improved outcome or efficacy; they should be selected with care.

16. What clinical conditions provide newer applications for enteral nutrition?

Acute pancreatitis. Patients with acute pancreatitis were previously kept NPO and fed parenterally. Recently, jejunal feedings,that bypass the cephalic and gastric phases of digestion and thus decrease stimulation for exocrine pancreatic secretion have come to be viewed as a safe and efficacious way to provide nutrition for patients with acute pancreatitis

Enterocutaneous fistula. Enteral feedings are used with increasing frequency in the management of enterocutaneous fistulas. The enteral feeding must be infused 40 cm distal to the fistula to prevent reflux.

Short gut syndrome. A combination of enteral and parenteral nutritional support can be used to manage short gut syndrome. The enteral nutrition is infused at a very low continuous rate to promote intestinal adaptation and to sustain the gut-associated lymphoid tissue.

17. What complications may be associated with enteral nutrition? How can they be minimized?

Complications of enteral nutrition can be classified as mechanical, gastrointestinal, and metabolic. **Mechanical complications** include obstruction of the tube with medications or pills; irritation of or erosion into nasal or gastric tissue with the associated risk of bleeding, infection, or perforation; pulmonary injury during placement;and displacement of the tube with the associated risk of aspiration. To minimize these complications, tubes should be flushed frequently with water; they should be soft and well lubricated for insertion; and tube position should be verified before use.

GI complications include diarrhea, nausea, vomiting, constipation, and aspiration. To minimize diarrhea, enteral feedings are usually instituted with an elemental formula with low fat content, at half strength, and at a low rate until tolerance is determined. Nausea and vomiting are frequently caused by large volume gastric residuals or drugs and sometimes can be improved by postpyloric placement of the feeding tube and delivery by continuous infusion. Ileus is often associated with narcotic drug administration and can be treated with small doses of oral naloxone with little change in systemic analgesic effect of the opioid. The risk of aspiration is decreased by proper postpyloric tube placement, elevation of the head of the bed, use of smaller feeding tubes, elimination of drugs that decrease lower esophageal sphincter tone, and frequent checks of gastric residuals.

Metabolic complications are similar to those for parenteral nutrition but are usually less severe. Examples include hyperglycemia, electrolyte imbalances, and dehydration or overhydration. Frequent monitoring of blood glucose and urine output and judicious use of blood and urine testing can detect these disorders and lead to appropriate alterations in feedings for preventioin or treatment as they arise.

18. What are the contraindications to enteral feedings?

Critically ill patients who do not have adequate GI function should not receive enteral feedings. Conditions that may lead to a nonfunctioning GI tract include short gut syndrome, ischemic bowel, intestinal obstruction, severe malabsorption, or high-output fistulas. High-volume diarrhea or severe distention while receiving tube feeds requires evaluation and perhaps discontinuation of tube feeds. Pancreatitis, enterocutaneous fistulas, and recent GI surgery are not necessarily contraindications to enteral feeds.

19. What are the indications for parenteral nutrition in critically ill patients?

Parenteral nutrition is indicated when patients are unable to meet nutritional requirements by oral or tube feedings. Examples include patients who meet some of their nutritional requirements by the enteral route but do not tolerate full enteral nutritional support. For many patients a combination of both enteral and parenteral nutrition may be required to meet full requirements.

20. What is the difference between peripheral parenteral nutrition (PPN) and total parenteral nutrition (TPN)?

The primary difference between PPN and TPN is the concentration of dextrose. A central line is required to infuse parenteral nutrition solutions containing more than 10% dextrose (TPN), whereas parenteral solutions containing less than 10% dextrose can be infused through a peripheral vein. Because of the constraints of concentration, the volume of PPN required to provide full nutritional support is frequently so large that full nutritional support via PPN is not feasible.

21. What are some of the complications of parenteral nutrition?

Complications of parenteral nutrition can be classified as mechanical, metabolic, infectious, and hepatobiliary.

Mechanical complications include those related to the catheters used for delivery of parenteral nutrition. Examples are pneumothorax associated with placement of a central venous catheter, thrombus formation and embolization, and air embolus.

The most common **metabolic complication** is hyperglycemia. Insulin may be added to the TPN solution or administered separately to control hyperglycemia. New evidence suggests that better control of blood sugar in critically ill patients results in decreased morbidity and mortality. Other metabolic complications include refeeding syndrome, excessive carbon dioxide production, and electrolyte abnormalities. Refeeding syndrome occurs when feedings are started rapidly in patients with severe malnutrition. The syndrome is characterized by hypophosphatemia, hypokalemia, volume overload, and congestive heart failure.

Infectious complications are generally related to the central venous access catheters used for the delivery of TPN. Catheter-related sepsis is an example.

Hepatobiliary complications include elevation in transaminases, alkaline phosphatase, and bilirubin; steatosis (fatty liver); and acalculous cholecystitis.

22. Which electrolytes are usually added to PN solutions? How does acid-base status affect the choice of electrolytes and their concentration in the PN solution?

Sodium chloride, potassium chloride, sodium acetate, potassium acetate, calcium gluconate, and magnesium sulfate are the usual electrolytes added to TPN solutions. Acetate is metabolized to bicarbonate. For patients without significant acid-base abnormalities, the ratio of chloride to acetate is generally kept at 1:1. For patients with metabolic alkalosis, the acetate can be minimized to decrease the amount of bicarbonate produced. For patients with metabolic acidosis, the acetate in the PN solution should be maximized to increase the amount of bicarbonate produced.

23. Describe the basic composition of TPN solutions.

TPN formulas may contain water, carbohydrates, amino acids, vitamins, minerals, electrolytes, and fats. The usual concentration of carbohydrate, in the form of dextrose, is 20–30%. The usual concentration of amino acids ranges from 3% to 15%. Intravenous fat emulsions contain soybean or safflower oil, egg yolk phospholipid, and glycerin. These are available in emulsions of 10%, 20%, or 30%. Multivitamins and certain medications are often added to TPN formulas.

24. What vitamins and minerals should be supplemented with parenteral nutrition? What vitamins and minerals are not supplied with the usual multivitamin preparations?

The following vitamins and minerals are suggested as supplements for parenteral nutrition: vitamin A, vitamin D, vitamin E, folic acid, niacin, riboflavin, thiamine, pyridoxine (vitamin B_6), vitamin B_{12}, pantothenic acid, biotin, zinc, copper, chromium, and manganese. Multivitamin preparations do not contain vitamin K or iron because of concern about possible allergic reactions. These nutrients may require additional supplementation, if indicated.

25. How should TPN be initiated?

TPN therapy should begin at a slow rate and be advanced as the patient's glucose tolerance permits. The initial rate should be 30–40 ml/hour; the rate is increased by 20 ml every 24 hours until the goal rate is achieved. During this period frequent glucose monitoring is required until the infusion rate has been stabilized.

26. How should critically ill patients receiving parenteral nutrition be monitored?

Baseline values of electrolytes (sodium, potassium, bicarbonate, magnesium, phosphate, and calcium), blood urea nitrogen, creatinine, glucose, albumin, triglycerides, complete blood count, and liver function tests (transaminases, alkaline phosphatase. and bilirubin) should be checked before therapy is initiated. After the initiation of therapy, blood glucose monitoring should be performed every 4–6 hours until the infusion is stabilized. Serum triglycerides should be checked about 6 hours after completing the infusion of IV fat to ensure that the patient is able to clear the lipids adequately. Serum triglycerides should be less than or equal to 500 mg/dl. Electrolytes should be checked every day until the infusion is stabilized and then every 3–4 days, along with blood urea nitrogen and creatinine. Liver function tests and albumin should be checked weekly.

27. How can the administration of propofol potentially influence the nutritional support provided to critically ill patients?
Propofol is a sedative commonly used in the ICU. It is supplied as a 10% lipid emulsion and provides 1.1 kcal/ml. When propofol is administered for long periods or in large doses, intravenous fat supplementation with TPN may need to be decreased or eliminated to avoid excessive administration of fat or calories. In patients receiving large doses of propofol, serum triglyceride levels should be checked to prevent hypertriglyceridemia. Hypertryglyceridemia due to propofol has been implicated as a cause of pancreatitis.

BIBLIOGRAPHY

1. Beale RJ, Bryg DJ, Bihari DJ: Immunonutrition in the critically ill: A systematic review of clinical outcome. Crit Care Med 27:2799–2805, 1999.
2. Cerra FB, Benitez MR, Blackburn GL, et al: Applied nutrition in ICU patients: A consensus statement of the American College of Chest Physicians. Chest 111:769–778, 1997.
3. Chan S, McCowen KC, Blackburn GL: Nutrition management in the ICU. Chest 115(5):145–148, 1999.
4. DeWitt RC, Kudsk: The gut's role in metabolism, mucosal barrier function, and gut immunology. Infect Dis Clin North Am 13:465–481, 1999
5. Jeejeebhoy KN: Total parenteral nutrition: Potion or poison? Am J Clin Nutr 74:160–163, 2001.
6. Montejo JC, for the Nutrition and Metabolic Working Group of the Spanish Society of Intensive Care Medicine and Coronary Units: Enteral nutrition-related gastrointestinal complications in critically ill patients: A multicenter study. Crit Care Med 27:1447–1453, 1999.
7. Thompson JS: The intestinal response to critical illness. Am J Gastroenterol 90:190–200, 1995.
8. Schloerb PR, Hehning JF: Patterns and problems of adult total parenteral nutrition use in U.S. academic medical centers. Arch Surg 133:7–12, 1998.
9. Stralovich-Romani A, Mahutte CK, et al: Administrative, nutritional, and ethical principles for the management of critically ill patients. In George RB, Light RW, et al (eds): Chest Medicine: Essentials of Pulmonary and Critical Care Medicine, 4th ed. Philadelphia, Lippincott William & Wilkins, 2000, pp 517–538.
10. Van Den Berghe G, Wouters P, et al: Intensive insulin therapy in critically ill patients. N Engl J Med 345:1359–1367, 2001.

8. NONINVASIVE VENTILATION

Manuel Pardo, Jr., M.D.

1. What is noninvasive ventilation?
Noninvasive ventilation is mechanical ventilation without the use of an endotracheal tube or tracheotomy.

2. What are the main types of noninvasive ventilation?
The two main types are positive-pressure and negative-pressure noninvasive ventilation. With positive-pressure ventilation, positive pressure is applied to the airway to inflate the lungs directly. With negative-pressure ventilation, negative pressure is applied to the abdomen and thorax to draw air into the lungs through the upper airway. This chapter deals mainly with positive-pressure ventilation, the most commonly used noninvasive ventilator mode in the ICU.

3. When was noninvasive ventilation first described?
The first "tank respirator" was described in 1832 by Scottish physician John Dalziel. The apparatus was an airtight box with the patient seated inside. The head and neck were placed outside the box, and a bellows and piston were used to create negative pressure inside the box.

4. When did noninvasive ventilation first become widely used? For what disease?
Noninvasive ventilation became widely used during the polio epidemics of the 1920s through the 1950s. The ventilators used included the rocking bed, various types of tank respirators or "iron lungs," and body-wrapping "cuirass" respirators. Patients with chronic respiratory failure after polio could be supported for years with these forms of negative-pressure noninvasive ventilation.

5. Why did the use of noninvasive ventilation decrease in the 1950s and 1960s?
The success of the polio vaccines led to the control of the epidemic. In addition, the use of positive-pressure ventilation became more widely used. The success of this form of "invasive" positive-pressure ventilation was described during the Copenhagen polio epidemic of 1952. At the start of the epidemic, the Blegdam Hospital had only seven ventilators, yet up to 70 patients required ventilatory support simultaneously. Lassen and Ibsen developed the technique of tracheotomy and manual intermittent positive-pressure ventilation and described their success in 1953.

6. Why has the use of noninvasive positive-pressure ventilation (NIPPV) increased in the past few years?
Several developments have led to its increased use. The use of continuous positive airway pressure for obstructive sleep apnea was described in the early 1980s. The development of a more comfortable nasal mask was important to the success of this therapy. These masks became widely available in the 1980s and were found to be effective in delivering noninvasive positive-pressure ventilation. Recently, inexpensive portable ventilators have been developed specifically for noninvasive positive-pressure ventilation (see figures, top of next page). As physicians gained experience with this mode of ventilation, it has been used in many different forms of acute and chronic respiratory failure.

7. What are the advantages of NIPPV compared with conventional mechanical ventilation with an endotracheal tube?
The main advantage is the avoidance of artificial airway complications. These complications include infections (e.g., nosocomial pneumonia, sinusitis), laryngeal injury, and tracheal injury. In addition, conventional ventilation usually requires the administration of sedative agents.

8. What are the disadvantages?
Patient selection is more important to ensuring success with noninvasive ventilation. Patients who are uncooperative, need immediate intubation, have upper airway pathology, are hemodynamically unstable, or have excessive secretions are not likely to succeed. In addition, there are limitations to the amount of oxygen that can be delivered with noninvasive ventilators.

9. Has noninvasive ventilation been used for chronic respiratory failure? For what disorders?
As described above for the polio epidemics, negative-pressure ventilation has a long history of success for chronic respiratory failure. Similar benefits have also been shown in uncontrolled studies for NIPPV. The disorders for which it has been used include thoracic restrictive diseases (e.g., kyphoscoliosis, chestwall deformities), central hypoventilatory disorders, and slowly progressive neuromuscular diseases (e.g., amyotrophic lateral sclerosis, muscular dystrophy). If the patient is able to maintain only brief periods of spontaneous breathing, tracheotomy along with positive-pressure ventilation is usually a better option. Otherwise, intermittent (usually nocturnal) noninvasive ventilation may be successful in controlling hypercarbia and promoting daytime independence.

The results of NIPPV for severe chronic obstructive pulmonary disease (COPD) are controversial, but most trials have shown no survival advantage. NIPPV may have a role in improving exercise tolerance during pulmonary rehabilitation.

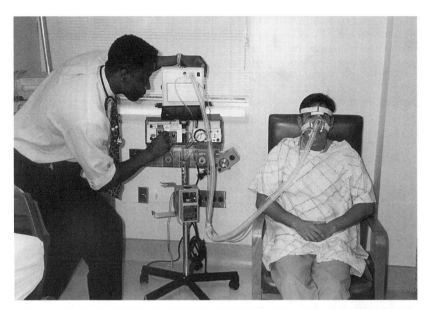

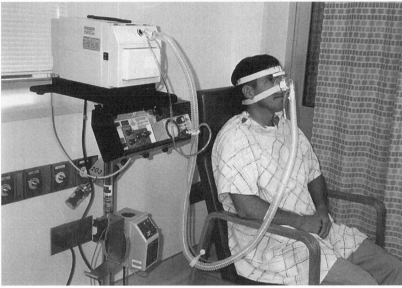

A demonstration of noninvasive positive pressure ventilation with a nasal mask. The respiratory therapist is adjusting the inspiratory pressure support level and checking for proper mask fit. The nasal mask is less claustrophobic than the full face mask. Both types of masks must be fitted properly to achieve minimal air-leak and minimal pressure on the skin.

10. Can noninvasive ventilation be used for acute respiratory failure? For what disorders?

Noninvasive ventilation has been used for acute respiratory failure of diverse causes. Most clinical trials have studied patients with acute exacerbations of COPD. NIPPV has been shown to improve vital signs and dyspnea and to reduce the need for intubation. Evidence also suggests an improvement in mortality rates. Of note, most studies exclude patients with the need for immediate intubation (e.g., patients with apnea).

Because of its success in patients with acute exacerbations of COPD, NIPPV has been tried with numerous other patiens in acute respiratory failure. Examples include acute asthma, cystic fibrosis, hypoxemic respiratory failure, immune compromise, and extubation failure. Although the evidence supporting benefit in such patients is not as strong, NIPPV may help to reduce the need for tracehal intubation.

11. What is the role of NIPPV in the management of acute respiratory failure? Which patients with acute respiratory failure should be started on noninvasive ventilation?

Clearly NIPPV has a role in the management of patients with acute respiratory failure, especially when it is due to COPD exacerbation. However, it is important to remember that most controlled studies showing benefits of NIPPV have excluded patients with the need for immediate intubation. NIPPV can be viewed as a tool to delay the need for intubation while other therapies are instituted. In general, patients should meet the following criteria:
- Respiratory failure without the need for immediate intubation
- Motivated and cooperative attitude
- Hemodynamically stable without cardiac arrhythmias or ischemia
- Minimal secretions or adequate cough
- Normal upper airway
- Admission to a closely monitored bed

12. What are the complications of noninvasive ventilation?

The main complication of negative-pressure ventilation is development of upper airway obstruction and hypoxemia during sleep. This complication may be caused by changes in the upper airway muscle activation when exposed to ventilator breaths.

Complications of NIPPV include pressure necrosis of the skin, aerophagia, and intolerance of the mask. The incidence of mask intolerance can be as high as 25%.

13. What ventilator settings are used for NIPPV?

A variety of ventilator settings have been used. The actual settings depend on patient requirements and the capabilities of the particular ventilator. Most ventilators use inspiratory pressure support ventilation. In this form of pressure-limited ventilation, the patient must trigger all breaths. When an inspiratory effort is sensed, the ventilator delivers enough flow to reach the desired peak inspiratory pressure. On expiration, the ventilator delivers enough flow to maintain the desired expiratory pressure. A typical setting for a patient with acute exacerbation of COPD is inspiratory pressure of 10–20 cmH$_2$O and expiratory pressure of 0–2 cmH$_2$O. Some ventilators incorporate a backup ventilator rate so that patients are given a mandatory breath if their respiratory rate is less than the desired rate. The pressure level is adjusted by subjective comfort or by measurement of the exhaled tidal volume. An exhaled tidal volume of 7–10 cc/kg is appropriate for most patients. The method of oxygen enrichment depends on the specific ventilator. Some ventilators are limited in the amount of supplemental oxygen they can deliver.

BIBLIOGRAPHY

1. Hill NS: Noninvasive ventilation. Does it work, for whom, and how? Am Rev Respir Dis 147:1050–1055, 1993.
2. Keenan SP, Kernerman PD, Cook DJ, et al: Effect of noninvasive positive pressure ventilation on mortality in patients admitted with acute respiratory failure: A meta-analysis. Crit Care Med 25:1685–1692, 1997.
3. Mehta S, Hill N: State of the art: Noninvasive ventilation. Am J Respir Crit Care Med 163:540–577, 2001.
4. Woollam CH: The development of apparatus for intermittent negative pressure respiration. (2) 1919-1976, with special reference to the development and uses of cuirass respirators. Anaesthesia 31:666–685, 1976.
5. Woollam CH: The development of apparatus for intermittent negative pressure respiration. Anaesthesia 31:537–547, 1976.

9. MECHANICAL VENTILATION

Carolyn H. Welsh, M.D.

1. What are the indications for mechanical ventilation?

The majority (75%) of patients requiring mechanical ventilation have **ventilatory failure** with an inability to exchange air and adequately expire carbon dioxide (CO_2). This results in a high blood PCO_2 and low pH. Causes of this type of respiratory failure include sedation from medications, general anesthesia, drug overdose, neuromuscular disease, chest wall deformity, and airway diseases such as chronic obstructive lung disease and asthma.

In general, patients with **acute ventilatory failure** require intubation and ventilation if they hypoventilate to a PCO_2 greater than 50 mmHg with a pH less than 7.30. Patients with acute ventilatory failure superimposed on chronic ventilatory failure may have a much higher PCO_2, up to 80 mmHg, before requiring intubation, since they frequently develop a compensatory metabolic alkalosis.

A smaller number of patients require ventilation for **hypoxemia**, because they fail to oxygenate their blood, even with supplemental oxygen. Such patients are often able to ventilate well, as demonstrated by a low arterial PCO_2. Causes of hypoxemic respiratory failure include pneumonia, aspiration, acute respiratory distress syndrome (ARDS), and pulmonary emboli. Hypoxemic patients usually require mechanical ventilation for a PO_2 less than 50 mmHg on a 100% oxygen nonrebreather mask.

2. How are ventilator settings determined?

Ventilator settings are chosen to optimize both oxygen exchange and acid-base status. Most clinicians choose to start patients with a fraction of inspired oxygen (FiO_2) of 1.00 (100% oxygen). If the PO_2 is high on arterial blood gas analysis, the FiO_2 is decreased incrementally to give a PO_2 of 60–90 torr. When possible, a fraction of inspired oxygen of 0.4–0.5 is selected to avoid oxygen toxicity.

As a general estimate, a tidal volume of 6–8 ml/kg is chosen, which is approximately 450 ml for a 70-kg person. This change in practice is based on recent randomized clinical trials in which survival was improved in patients with acute lung injury who received lower tidal volumes (6 ml/gk) compared with higher tidal volumes (12 ml/kg). For routine postoperative care, somewhat larger tidal volumes are still used. Peak airway pressures are assessed to fine-tune tidal volumes, targeting pressures less than 35–40 mmHg for most patients. Respiratory rate is set to achieve adequate ventilation and may vary from 10–25 breaths per minute as an initial selection.

3. What parameters are followed to see if a patient is receiving adequate ventilation?

The simplest method to assess adequacy of ventilation is observation of the patient for comfort, synchrony of chest and abdominal movement with delivered ventilator breaths, absence of cyanosis, and symmetry of chest movement. Observation can detect major problems. For example, if the right mainstem bronchus rather than the trachea is intubated, the right chest will move but the left will be stationary, and breath sound asymmetry can be auscultated to confirm this. Twenty to thirty minutes after initiation of ventilation or after ventilator changes, an arterial blood gas is drawn to check for adequacy of oxygenation (PO_2 = 60 mmHg) and ventilation (PCO_2 = 30–45 mmHg, pH = 7.33–7.49). Once acceptable acid-base status is achieved, further decreases in FiO_2 are often monitored by noninvasive oximetry.

Important parameters to follow also include the peak and static airway pressures, which are recorded on a pressure manometer dial or digital printout. **Peak pressures** are the highest pressures measured in the airways during end inspiration. High peak pressures may indicate bronchospasm, inappropriate selection of ventilator settings, or pneumothorax. **Static pressures** reflect underlying properties of lung tissue and are measured during the last second of expiration by adding an inspiratory pause to the next breath. Static pressures will be increased with processes that stiffen the lung such as ARDS, pulmonary edema, pneumonia, or fibrosis. Static pressures may be decreased with emphysema, reflecting the loss of lung parenchyma characteristic of this disease.

4. How can static pressures be normalized for changes in ventilator tidal volume?

During mechanical ventilation, static pressures may rise because of increases in the tidal volume settings as well as increases in lung stiffness. Thus, a decreased pressure may reflect a lower tidal volume rather than a change in the lung itself. We calculate static compliance as follows:

$$\frac{\text{tidal volume}}{(\text{static pressure-PEEP})}$$

where PEEP = positive end-expiratory pressure, and normal static compliance is 60–100 ml/cmH$_2$O.

By calculating compliance, we can compare information on lung stiffness across changes in the tidal volume settings. Compliance decreases with processes that stiffen the lung, such as ARDS, pulmonary edema, pneumonia, and fibrosis, and can be followed serially to assess patient improvement or deterioration over time.

5. What is oxygen delivery?

$$\text{Oxygen delivery} = \text{cardiac output} \times \text{oxygen content}$$
$$\text{Oxygen content} = (1.38 \times \text{Hgb} \times \text{SaO}_2) + (\text{PaO}_2 \times 0.003)$$

where Hgb = hemoglobin concentration, SaO$_2$ = arterial oxygen saturation, 1.38 = affinity constant of oxygen for hemoglobin, and 0.003 reflects the solubility of oxygen in plasma.

Delivery of oxygen to tissues is a more sensitive measure of dysfunction than a single PO$_2$ reading, since oxygen delivery incorporates PO$_2$, cardiac output, and hemoglobin concentration, all of which affect tissue utilization of oxygen. Oxygen delivery may be impaired when PO$_2$ is in the normal range. It is frequently compromised in the settings of cardiogenic shock, anemia, ARDS, and sepsis.

6. Do mechanical ventilators affect the cardiovascular system?

Positive-pressure ventilation decreases cardiac output and may lead to hypotension. The most common mechanism is via positive pressure in the thorax diminishing venous return to the heart by compression of the inferior vena cava, thus creating a low cardiac output state. Decreased cardiac output will ultimately result in poor tissue delivery of oxygen. In patients with cardiogenic pulmonary edema, the lowering of venous return to the heart during mechanical ventilation may lessen edema and actually improve oxygenation. The proposed mechanism is by the lesser intravascular volume allowing for shortening of cardiac muscle fiber length and subsequent improved contractility of the heart muscle (see figure on following page).

7. What is the most common complication of mechanical ventilation? Why? What are other common complications?

Barotrauma. High airway pressures may damage airway epithelium, leading to ventilator-induced lung injury. In addition, high airway pressures may induce rupture of the alveolar wall at its weakest point, leading to egress of air into the bronchovascular sheath. If air remains in the sheath, it tracks to the mediastinum and pleura, leading to pneumomediastinum, pneumothorax, pneumoperitoneum, and subcutaneous emphysema. If air enters the pulmonary vessels, the devastating air emboli syndrome characterized by livedo reticularis, cardiac arrhythmias, and unexplained altered mental status or stroke may ensue.

Other common complications of positive-pressure mechanical ventilation include increased intracranial pressure, fluid retention, renal failure, hyponatremia, local trauma to the nares and mouth, tracheal necrosis and hemorrhage from high endotracheal tube cuff pressures, and nosocomial infections such as sinusitis and pneumonia.

8. What is ventilator-induced lung injury?

Ventilator-induced lung injury is thought to be caused by alveolar overdistension, alveolar rupture, and epithelial injury in the setting of high positive airway pressures. Positive-pressure ventilation,

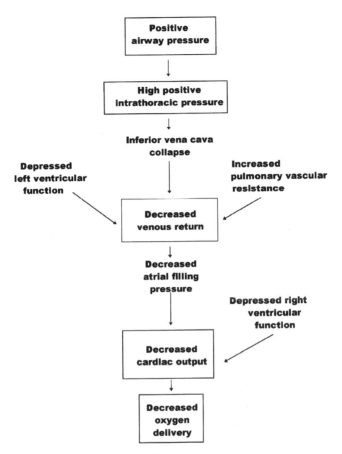

Three pathophysiologic mechanisms of decreased cardiac output and oxygen delivery during mechanical ventilation. Clinically, decreased venous return due to compression of the inferior vena cava appears to be most important.

particularly in the setting of ARDS, may worsen outcome by causing this type of damage. In a recent controlled trial in patients with ARDS, low tidal volumes improved mortality by 22%. Other strategies to avoid ventilator-induced lung injury include limitation of peak airway pressures and use of **permissive hypercapnia**, in which achieving ideal acid-base status takes a back seat to limiting peak pressure and changes in pressure (transalveolar cycling pressure) in the airways and alveoli.

In general, ventilator management has changed from prioritizing normalization of acid-base status and avoidance of oxygen toxicity to maintenance of low airway pressures. This **pressure-protective strategy** encompasses lowering of peak airway pressures, use of smaller tidal volumes, permissive hypercapnia, and changes in ventilator airway pressure waveforms. The clinical trials showing beneficial results are limited to patients with acute lung injury, but this strategy also is used for ventilator management in many other patients.

9. How significant is nosocomial pneumonia in ventilated patients?

In ventilated patients, it is frequently difficult to distinguish clinical bronchitis or pneumonia from tracheal colonization with bacteria. Bronchitis or tracheitis is defined as fever, change in character of the sputum, rise in the white blood cell count, a Gram stain showing bacteria and more than 25 neutrophils per field in the absence of epithelial cells, and a positive bacterial culture. Pneumonia is defined as the above but also includes infiltrates on chest radiograph. Colonization is characterized by a positive Gram stain or culture without the clinical changes of infection and white blood cell rise. Pneumonia clearly warrants treatment, whereas colonization does not. Ventilator-associated pneumonia is defined as pneumonia occurring more than 48 hours after ventilation is started.

Variable but often large numbers of patients (6–69%) requiring mechanical ventilation for longer than 48 hours develop nosocomial pneumonia. Mortality rates increase in such patients, and as many as 30% may die. The rate of pneumonia is highest during the first 10 days of ventilation. Mechanical disruption of mucociliary clearance by endotracheal tubes and suction catheters increases bacterial colonization and predisposes to infection. In addition, increased infection risk is attributable to bacteremia from intravenous line contamination or altered host immune function due to immunocompromising diseases and treatment. Use of cuffed endotracheal tubes, the semirecumbent position, and early extubation are successful measures to minimize ventilator-associated pneumonia. Newly described subglottic catheters that continuously aspirate secretions also lower rates of pneumonia, although their use is not widespread.

10. What are the common modes of ventilation?

On microprocessor computer ventilators, volume-cycled ventilation using assist control or intermittent mandatory ventilation and pressure-cycled ventilation using presssure support ventilation are the most common choices. These strategies deliver positive pressure in the airways with inspiration, whereas in normal breathing inspiratory pressure is negative. For volume-cycled modes, the breath is limited by a preset volume. For pressure-cycled modes, including pressure support ventilation, the volume of the breath is limited by a preset pressure.

11. How do assist control and intermittent mandatory ventilation (IMV) differ?

Assist control (continuous mandatory ventilation) and IMV are commonly used ventilator modes of positive-pressure ventilation available on most commercial ventilators. Both modes share several common features and are standards of care. Both deliver a preset volume such that if set at a tidal volume of 500 ml and a rate of 15, both will deliver at least an 7.5-liter minute ventilation. To improve patient comfort and synchrony, both modes are designed to accommodate additional patient-initiated breaths.

These types of ventilation differ in that assist control delivers each initiated breath to the full preset tidal volume, whereas IMV delivers each initiated breath to only as much volume as pressure from the patient's muscles generates and also intermittently delivers the full preset tidal volume at the preset rate. Modern ventilators synchronize breath delivery to patient-initiated breathing, frequently referred to as **synchronized intermittent mandatory ventilation** (SIMV). (See figure on next page.)

To initiate an IMV breath on many ventilators, the patient must generate enough force to pop open both a demand valve for inspiration and a second valve for exhalation. Thus, IMV increases the work of breathing by the amount of work required to overcome the valve pressures. The effort required for this can be considerable, and has been measured as high as 6 cm H_2O pressure. Due to this increased work of breathing, IMV may hasten fatigue and compromise weaning in patients with neuromuscular weakness, severe COPD, or high minute ventilation needs. For these patients, the assist control mode is preferable.

12. What is the role of pressure support ventilation mode in ventilating patients?

This alternative positive-pressure mode available on microprocessor ventilators is pressure- rather than volume-limited. It is used primarily for weaning but also can be used as a primary ventilatory support mode. Airflow is limited by pressure rather than preset volume,and is patient-triggered. Pressure is delivered only during inspiration. It is thought to improve patient ventilator synchrony and patient comfort and, in some settings, appears to reduce work of breathing by as much as 30%. It is not an ideal choice when ventilatory drive is blunted from disease or sedative medications, because sufficient ventilation may not be achieved. Some physicians routinely add 5 cm pressure of pressure support ventilation (PSV) to all ventilated patients to overcome the resistance in the endotracheal tube and ventilator circuit. PSV may be advantageous in asthmatic exacerbations to avoid high peak airway pressures; however, no

AIRWAY PRESSURE WAVEFORMS

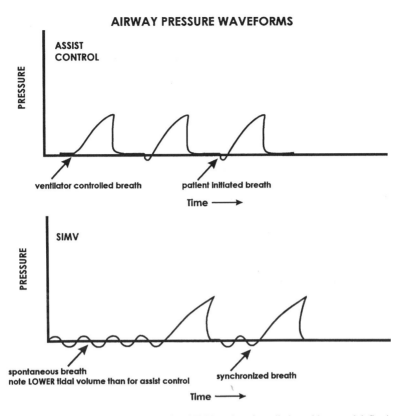

Pressure = airway pressure during assist control and IMV modes of ventilation with upward deflections positive in pressure and downward negative. In contrast to normal breathing, both phases of respiration are positive in pressure with ventilator-delivered breaths.

outcome studies suggest its superiority except for a weaning trial which found that it shortened weaning duration for difficult-to-wean patients. To use with weaning, start PSV at 18–20 cmH$_2$O and check the delivered tidal volume to see if ventilation is adequate. If tidal volumes are maintained, pressure support is dropped by 2–4 cm increments as tolerated.

13. What do you do if a patient on the ventilator is agitated or the ventilator alarm sounds?
Agitation is a clue to machine malfunction or a change in the patient's medical status. Remove the patient from the ventilator and ventilate with a resuscitation bag while evaluating the problem.

Common ventilator problems include (1) inadvertent disconnection of the patient from the ventilator, and (2) use of inappropriate ventilator settings such as low trigger sensitivity, low flow rates, or ventilator response delay. Poor synchrony of the patient with the ventilator can lead to development of auto-PEEP (see below). Always check the ventilator for problems with settings and connections, which are easily correctable.

Changes in the patient's medical condition that may affect ventilation include both airway and neurologic problems: mucous plugs and copious secretions, bronchospasm, pneumothorax, pulmonary edema, sepsis, carbon dioxide retention, hypoxemia, lobar collapse, pulmonary emboli, pain, hallucinations, and awakening from sedation.

14. What is PEEP?
Positive end-expiratory pressure (PEEP) is application of positive pressure to the expiration circuit. In effect, PEEP works by increasing the functional residual capacity of the lung, prevent-

ing collapse of some alveoli while overdistending others. This strategy usually leads to improved ventilation-perfusion matching in the pulmonary circulation.

15. What are the indications for PEEP? How do you monitor its effects?

PEEP is used primarily to improve arterial oxygenation in severely hypoxemic patients or to decrease the fraction of inspired oxygen to avoid pulmonary oxygen toxicity. PEEP is part of the pressure-protective strategy to avoid lung injury and is thought to work by maintaining oxygenation through ventilation-perfusion matching while minimizing transalveolar cycling pressures. PEEP has also been advocated to decrease mediastinal bleeding immediately after open heart surgery, although this remains controversial. A large number of studies show no efficacy of PEEP in this regard, and recommend avoiding PEEP because of its potential for decreasing cardiac output. PEEP can be monitored with a "best PEEP" trial:

1. Use stepwise increments of 3–5 cm H_2O PEEP, starting at 0 cm.

2. Minimize the time interval between changes (20–30 minutes is ideal) to increase the likelihood that a response is due to PEEP itself rather than a change in the patient's condition.

3. Note and evaluate the response to each change with blood pressure measurements, an arterial blood gas sample, cardiac output, and oxygen delivery calculations. The best PEEP is that achieved when the inspired oxygen decreases to a minimal level without compromising oxygen delivery.

16. What is auto-PEEP?

Auto-PEEP, or intrinsic PEEP, is the inadvertent development of PEEP due to the ventilator delivery of a positive-pressure breath prior to complete exhalation of the previous breath. Thus it is seen in patients with high minute ventilation, as in ARDS, and in diseases of airflow limitation, such as asthma and chronic obstructive lung disease. Since the ventilator manometer dial does not reflect auto-PEEP, detection involves occlusion of the expiratory port at end exhalation, allowing equilibration of airway and circuit pressure. The complications of auto-PEEP are similar to those of applied PEEP: diminished cardiac output and hypotension, barotrauma, and inaccurate pulmonary artery catheter measurements leading to inappropriate fluid and pressor administration or diuresis.

17. How can auto-PEEP be remedied?

Primary treatment for auto-PEEP is treatment of the underlying bronchospasm. Other treatment approaches include raising inspiratory flow rates to maximize expiratory time, increasing endotracheal tube size, and lowering minute ventilation by decreasing respiratory rate or tidal volume. If this dangerous problem persists, the patient should be sedated and perhaps paralyzed. Although some practitioners treat auto-PEEP by applying PEEP in centimeters equivalent to the original auto-PEEP, others think this enhances the risk of barotrauma and should be avoided.

18. What is noninvasive positive-pressure ventilation (NIPPV)? When should it be used?

NIPPV is the use of a standard ventilator to deliver positive-pressure breaths via a mask rather than an endotracheal tube. A bilevel pressure machine also may be used. Both inspiratory and expiratory pressures are selected, a respiratory rate is sometimes set. In general, inspiratory positive airway pressure (I-PAP) is increased for hypoventilation and expiratory positive airway pressure (E-PAP) for hypoxemia. In acute respiratory failure due to chronic obstructive pulmonary disease (COPD), for example, settings of 10 cm I-PAP and 3 cm E-PAP are often used as a starting point. For hypoxemic respiratory failure, 10 cm I-PAP and 5–8 cm E-PAP are selected initially. For some patients, NIPPV by mask has reduced the need for endotracheal intubation, lowered the frequency of infectious complications, and shortened ICU or hospital stay. A mortality benefit has been shown in patients with exacerbations of COPD. Sound data support the use of NIPPV in such patients and in selected patients with hypoxemic respiratory failure. In addition, NIPPV can be a useful bridging tool to early extubation in patients with COPD and marginal weaning parameters.

19. Are there other options for ventilation in patients with respiratory failure?

Although mechanical ventilation saves lives, it clearly has complications and limitations. For patients with acute bronchospasm in whom positive-pressure ventilation poses a risk for pneumothorax, vigorous pharmacologic treatment of the underlying disease may abolish the need for mechanical ventilation. Occasionally, intermittent positive pressure breathing (IPPB) delivery of inhalation treatments may be used for patients with acute exacerbations of chronic obstructive lung disease to avoid long-term mechanical ventilation. Negative-pressure ventilators are used for pediatric patients and may be used for adults with normally compliant lungs as in neuromuscular disease. For patients with respiratory failure due to an exacerbation of COPD, **noninvasive positive airway pressure ventilation** by mask has reduced the need for endotracheal intubation, lowered the frequency of complications, and shortened hospital stay. Patients with ARDS who remain hypoxic despite 100% FiO_2 and PEEP are sometimes given a trial of **inhaled nitric oxide therapy**, despite the lack of positive outcome studies. Placement in a **prone position** improves oxygenation in approximately 70% of patients, probably because of better ventilation distribution. In a recent randomized clinical trial, prone positioning offered no survival benefit but significantly improved oxygen saturation. Although the effects on survival were disappointing, the study was underpowered to show a survival advantage and use of prone positioning was limited to only 7 hours/day. Because prone positioning is logistically difficult, it has been slow to gain acceptance in the ICU; nonetheless, it remains a promising treatment.

Other modes of ventilation such as airway pressure release or pressure control ventilation may offer improvement in oxygenation beyond that achieved with the standard modes. Severely hypoxemic patients are also occasionally treated with extracorporeal membrane oxygenation (ECMO), bypassing the diseased lungs to better oxygenate blood and tissue. This technqiue, however, remains unproved and may worsen survival rates.

BIBLIOGRAPHY

1. Acute Respiratory Distress Syndrome Network: Ventilation with lower tidal volumes as compared with traditional tidal volumes for acute lung injury and the acute respiratory distress syndrome. N Engl J Med 342:1301–1308, 2000.
2. Antonelli M, Conti G, Rocco M, et al: A comparison of noninvasive positive-pressure ventilation and conventional mechanical ventilation in patients with acute respiratory failure. N Engl J Med 339:429–435, 1998.
3. Ashbaugh DG, Petty TL: Positive end-expiratory pressure: Physiology, indications, and contraindications. J Thorac Cardiovasc Surg 65:165–170, 1973.
4. Bowton DL: Nosocomial pneumonia in the ICU—Year 2000 and beyond. Chest 115:28s–33s, 1999.
5. Brochard L, Mancebo J, Wysocki M, et al: Noninvasive ventilation for acute exacerbations of chronic obstructive pulmonary disease. New Engl J Med 333:817–822, 1995.
6. Brochard L, Rauss A, Benito S, et al: Comparison of three methods of gradual withdrawal from ventilatory support during weaning from mechanical ventilation. Am J Respir Crit Care Med 150:896–903, 1994.
7. Dekel B, Segal E, Perel A: Pressure support ventilation. Arch Intern Med 156:369–373, 1996.
8. Gammon RB, Shin MS, Buchalter SE: Pulmonary barotrauma in mechanical ventilation. Patterns and risk factors. Chest 102:568–572, 1992.
9. Gattinoni I, Tognoni G, Presenti A, et al: Effect of prone positioning on the survival of patients with acute respiratory failure. N Engl J Med 345:568–573, 2001.
10. Hudson LD, Hurlow RS, Craig KC, Pierson DJ: Does intermittent mandatory ventilation correct respiratory alkalosis in patients receiving assisted mechanical ventilation? Am Rev Respir Dis 132:1071–1074, 1985.
11. Keenan SP, Brake D: An evidence-based approach to noninvasive ventilation in acute respiratory failure. Crit Care Clin 14:359–372, 1998.
12. Nava S, Ambrosino N, Clini E, et al: Noninvasive mechanical ventilation in the weaning of patients with respiratory failure due to chronic obstructive pulmonary disease: A randomized clinical trial. Ann Intern Med 128:721–728, 1998.
13. Nourdine K, Combes P, Carton MHJ, et al: Does noninvasive ventilation reduce the ICU nosocomial infection risk? A prospective clinical survey. Intens Care Med 25:567–573, 1999.
14. Qanta A, Ahmed A, Niederman MS: Respiratory infection in the chronically critically ill patients: Ventilator-assisted pneumonia and tracheobronchitis. Clin Chest Med 22:71–85, 2001.
15. Tobin MJ: Advances in mechanical ventilation and weaning. N Engl J Med 344:1986–1996, 2001.

10. WEANING FROM MECHANICAL VENTILATION

Theodore W. Marcy, M.D., M.P.H.

1. What proportion of patients can be readily removed from mechanical ventilation?

The vast majority (80–90%) of patients on ventilatory support can resume spontaneous ventilation once their underlying illness resolves or improves. The precise method of withdrawing ventilator support is not critical and does not determine success or failure. Instead, the clinician's primary task is to assess whether the patient is ready to be extubated.

2. When should removal of the patient from mechanical ventilation be considered?

Deciding when to liberate a patient from mechanical ventilation can be one of the more challenging problems in critical care medicine. On the one hand, continuing mechanical ventilation beyond the time that is necessary exposes the patient to continuing risks of nosocomial infection and barotrauma. On the other hand, prematurely removing a patient from ventilatory support can lead to severe stress from respiratory and cardiovascular decompensation and exposes the patient to the risks associated with reintubation.

3. What is the first step in deciding whether the patient is ready for extubation?

Assess the patient's clinical status:
• Have the causes of respiratory failure been effectively treated or reversed?
• Is the patient medically stable in terms of both the inciting illness and any intervening complications (e.g., infections, electrolyte imbalance, arrhythmias) or other problems?
• Is the patient alert enough to protect his or her airway and participate in pulmonary toilet?
• Does the patient have a cough effective enough to clear secretions, and are the secretions neither copious nor tenacious? This assessment requires talking to the nursing and respiratory care personnel who actually perform the suctioning.

4. What is the second step?

Assess the capability of the two respiratory "systems": the gas-exchange organ (lung) and the ventilatory pump (rigid thoracic cage, respiratory muscles, and nerves and central nervous system centers that innervate and coordinate ventilation). Both systems must function adequately if the patient is to resume spontaneous ventilation successfully. The following parameters have been used:

Gas exchange organ assessment
• Partial arterial oxygen tension (PaO_2) > 60 mmHg or oxygen saturation > 90% on ≤ 0.50 fractional concentration of oxygen in inspired gas (FiO_2)
• PaO_2/FiO_2 ratio > 200
• Partial arterial carbon dioxide tension ($PaCO_2$) < 45 mmHg (except in patients with chronic hypercapnia)

Ventilatory pump assessment
• Rapid shallow breathing index: the frequency (f) in breaths per minute divided by the average tidal volume (V_t) in liters during a 1-minute T-piece trial (no ventilatory support). An f/Vt < 105 predicts successful extubation; an f/V_t > 105 predicts failure.
• Spontaneous breathing trials or pressure support ventilation trials (5 cmH_2O) for 30–120 minutes. The patient is considered to have failed the trial if any of the following occur: respiratory rate > 35 breaths/minute for 5 minutes or longer, oxygen saturation < 90%, sustained changes in heart rate > 20% in either direction, blood pressure > 180 or < 90 mmHg, or evidence of patient distress (anxiety or diaphoresis).

Traditional weaning parameters, such as maximal inspiratory pressure (Pi_{max}), minute volume, vital capacity, maximum voluntary ventilation, thoracic compliance, and respiratory resistance do not discriminate very well between patients who will succeed and those who will fail following extubation, although they may help determine the reason(s) why patients fail spontaneous breathing trials. For instance, Pi_{max}—the pressure generated by having a patient make a voluntary inspiratory effort at functional residual capacity—may identify patients with reversible respiratory muscle weakness.

More sophisticated measures, such as airway occlusion pressure (P 0.1), inspiratory pressure-time product, gastric mucosal PCO_2, and the ratio of electromyographic power in high and low bands are not practical because of the need for specialized equipment; in addition, they still require validation in clinical settings.

5. Has any systematic method of assessing patients for extubation been demonstrated to improve outcomes?

Yes. Physicians do not accurately predict whether ventilatory support can be discontinued successfully when using clinical judgment alone. Evidence indicates that systematic daily assessments for extubation improve patient outcomes. One randomized controlled trial performed in patients in medical and coronary intensive care units on mechanical ventilation for less than 2 weeks demonstrated that the patients who had daily screens, followed by a spontaneous breathing trial if they passed the screen, had shorter durations on mechanical ventilation, fewer complications, and lower intensive care costs than patients who had standard care. The screening followed these steps:

Step 1: Is the patient eligible for evaluation protocol?
- ❏ Patient has been on ventilator less than 2 weeks
- ❏ Patient has had *no* life-threatening complications (e.g., arrhythmias, large gastrointestinal bleed) during the past 12 hours

Step 2: If both answers are checked, proceed to the initial screening:
1. Is the patient's PaO_2/FiO_2 ratio > 200 or oxygen saturation > 90% on $FiO_2 \leq 0.50$?   ❏ Yes
2. Is the positive end-expiratory pressure (PEEP) ≤ 5 cmH_2O?   ❏ Yes
3. Does the patient have an adequate cough during suctioning?   ❏ Yes
4. The patient is *not* taking vasopressors (dopamine at 5 µg/min is acceptable) or continuous sedative infusions?   ❏ Yes
5. The ratio of f/V_t (breaths/liter tidal volume) ≤ 105?   ❏ Yes
   (Performed on continuous positive airway pressure [CPAP]; no pressure-support ventilation [PSV]. Measure VE and f at 1 minute: $V_t = VE/f$)   _____ f/V_t

Step 3: If all five answers are yes, proceed to 2-hour spontaneous breathing trial on CPAP 5 cm, PSV 5 cmH_2O, maintaining same FiO_2.

Terminate trial if any of the following develops:
- a. Respiratory rate > 35 breaths/min for more than 5 minutes   ❏ Occurred
- b. Oxygen saturation < 90%   ❏ Occurred
- c. Heart rate (HR) > 140 beats/min or sustained 20% changes in HR   ❏ Occurred
- d. Systolic blood pressure > 180 mmHg or < 90 mmHg   ❏ Occurred
- e. Increased anxiety or diaphoresis   ❏ Occurred

Arterial blood gases at end of trial: pH ___ $PaCO_2$ ___ PaO_2 ___ FiO_2 ___

Step 4: Inform patient's physician or house staff.
- ❏ Your patient has successfully completed a 2-hour trial of spontaneous breathing and could be considered a candidate for immediate extubation.
- ❏ Unsuccessful because _____ did not pass screen, or _____ failed 2-hour trial.

Another randomized controlled trial demonstrated that protocol-driven weaning performed by nurses or respiratory therapists resulted in more rapid liberation from mechanical ventilation as well as lower hospital costs, with no change in mortality, in comparison with the usual care of physician-directed weaning.

6. What about patients who have been on mechanical ventilation for longer than 2 weeks?

Approximately 10% of patients placed on mechanical ventilation require prolonged ventilatory assistance. A number of factors contribute to ventilator dependence, including hemodynamic instability, persistent lung disease, unresolved medical problems, malnutrition, and psychological dependency (see list below). Often there is an imbalance between the patient's ventilatory capability and the demand imposed by both minute ventilation requirement and the elastic and resistive load on the respiratory muscles. Patients with COPD who have respiratory failure are particularly challenging to withdraw from mechanical ventilation.

If patients have been on ventilatory support for an extended period , they may not tolerate an abrupt conversion to spontaneous ventilation; instead, they may require a gradual withdrawal of ventilatory support. No definite evidence indicates that gradual withdrawal of support itself facilitates physiologic improvement. Nonetheless, there may be no other way of determining whether the patient has recovered sufficiently to resume spontaneous ventilation.

7. What are the options for gradual withdrawal of ventilatory support?

With microprocessor-equipped ventilators, the clinician has a bewildering array of ventilator modes from which to choose a strategy for gradual withdrawal of ventilatory support. Most of the newer modes have not been evaluated for efficacy or effectiveness. This discussion describes the common modes that have been subjected to randomized controlled trials: pressure support ventilation (PSV), synchronized intermittent mandatory ventilation (SIMV), and intermittent spontaneous trials with T-piece, low-level PSV, or continuous positive airway pressure (CPAP). These trials have not determined which mode is best, in part because the protocols for using the different modes were probably not optimal. However, a protocol approach to weaning, regardless of the mode, may be better than clinical judgment alone. In addition, individual patients may tolerate one mode better than another. Regardless of the mode used, the clinicians should continue efforts to identify and correct physiologic reasons for the patient's inability to resume spontaneous ventilation (see below).

8. How is PSV used for gradual weaning?

During PSV, the ventilator provides a rapid flow of gas to the airway opening when the patient initiates an inspiratory effort until the pressure support level is reached. The gas flow necessary to maintain that pressure continues until the flow rate falls below a certain threshold, at which point the flow is shut off. The clinician selects the pressure support level, and the patient controls the respiratory rate. The PSV level, the patient's efforts, and respiratory system impedance determine the delivered tidal volume. Progressively lower pressure support levels are used during weaning attempts until the patient is breathing spontaneously at minimal levels of PSV or shows signs of distress or intolerance (e.g., a respiratory rate $\geq$ 25 breaths/minute). The appropriate minimal level of PSV has not been determined but usually is defined as 5–8 cmH$_2$O.

9. Describe the use of SIMV for gradual weaning.

During SIMV, a clinician-selected number of mandatory machine breaths is interspersed each minute among unsupported (or PSV-supported) spontaneous breaths. The clinician gradually reduces the SIMV rate at intervals, as tolerated. Unlike PSV, the set SIMV rate provides a minimal minute ventilation in the event that the patient makes no inspiratory efforts. In controlled trials of different weaning modes, SIMV was associated with a longer duration of ventilation. However, the protocol for reducing the SIMV rate may have resulted in inappropriately delayed reductions in levels of support.

10. How is weaning achieved with intermittent spontaneous breathing trials with T-piece, low-level PSV, or CPAP?

A T-piece consists of a circuit with a constant flow of oxygen and a downstream extension past the endotracheal tube to prevent entrainment of room air. A problem with this approach is that the patient is not connected to the ventilator's alarm systems, which monitor for apnea or tachypnea. Low levels of PSV (5 cmH$_2$O) have been used to compensate for the added resistance of the endotracheal tube. However, the endotracheal tube in fact may contribute less resistance than that of an edematous upper airway after extubation. Therefore, patient tolerance of low-level PSV may be falsely reassuring. CPAP has been used to reduce the threshold inspiratory load on the inspiratory muscles due to air-trapping in patients with COPD. Air-trapping reflects a positive residual pressure within the lung that must be counteracted by the inspiratory muscles before gas can enter the lung. CPAP has been demonstrated to reduce the work of breathing in patients with COPD and hyperinflation.

11. How should the patient be monitored during withdrawal of ventilatory support?

During trials of reduced ventilatory support, the patient should be monitored for clinical signs of impending failure, at which point full support modes of ventilation should be reinitiated. These signs include the following:

- Tachycardia
- Tachypnea
- Hypertension or hypotension`
- Mental status changes
- Anxiety, diaphoresis, or other signs of subjective intolerance

Ventilatory support should be withdrawn gradually during the day, allowing rest and sleep on full support modes at night. Once the patient tolerates spontaneous ventilation throughout the day, withdrawal of nocturnal ventilation often proceeds relatively quickly.

12. What potentially reversible factors may contribute to continued dependence on mechanical ventilation?

To sustain spontaneous ventilation successfully, the patient must have an intact respiratory center drive, adequate neuromuscular function, and relief of excessive loads on the respiratory muscles. The following outline provides one method of systematically reviewing possible causes of failure during trials of decreased ventilatory support based on the patient's response to a spontaneous breathing trial. Patients often have more than one cause for failure to wean, and correction of these factors may require multiple interventions.

1. The patient has an increasing $PaCO_2$ without increases in respiratory effort or rate
   (a) Inadequate respiratory center drive due to narcotics, sedatives, hypothyroidism, or brain injury
   (b) Appropriate compensation for metabolic alkalosis due to excessive diuresis or nasogastric suctioning
   (c) Return to a chronic hypercapnic state after inappropriate overventilation in patients with COPD or sleep apnea
2. The patient has tachypnea, tachycardia, or distress
   (a) Impaired neuromuscular function
      - Fatigue due to prolonged high loads, inadequate rest, or ventilator dyssynchrony
      - Hypothyroidism
      - Electrolyte deficiencies: hypokalemia, hypophosphatemia, hypomagnesemia
      - Critical illness myopathy/polyneuropathy
      - Steroid myopathy
      - Effects of drugs: aminoglycosides, neuromuscular antagonists
      - Sepsis
      - Diaphramatic paresis or paralysis due to phrenic nerve injury secondary to cold cardioplegia or thoracic or neck surgery
      - Prolonged malnutrition
   (b) Excessive respiratory load
      - Increased airway resistance (asthma, COPD, excessive secretions, small endotracheal tube)
      - Air-trapping and increased threshold load due to positive residual pressures (particularly in patients with COPD)
      - Decreased respiratory system compliance (pulmonary edema or fibrosis, pneumonia, abdominal distention, thoracic cage abnormalities, pleural effusions)

- High minute ventilation requirements (fever, sepsis, metabolic acidosis, high physiologic deadspace, excessive caloric intake, pulmonary embolism)

(c) Impaired left ventricular function: increased inspiratory efforts (and decreased intrathoracic pressures) increase left ventricular afterload by reducing juxtacardiac pressures. Patients with poorly compensated heart failure may decompensate further, exacerbating pulmonary edema.

(d) Psychological dependence:a diagnosis of exclusion, but not rare in patients confined to intensive care units.

In summary, the clinician should minimize the duration of mechanical ventilation by identifying and treating underlying causes of respiratory failure while systematically monitoring the patient daily for evidence that the patient can be liberated from the ventilator.

BIBLIOGRAPHY

1. Butler R, Keenan S, Inman K, et al: Is there a preferred technique for weaning the difficult-to-wean patient? A systematic review of the literature. Crit Care Med 27:2331–2336, 1999.
2. Ely E, Baker A, Dunagan D, Burke H, et al: Effect on the duration of mechanical ventilation of identifying patients capable of breathing spontaneously. N Engl J Med 335:1864–1869, 1996.
3. Hill N: Following protocol: weaning difficult-to-wean patients with chronic obstructive pulmonary disease. Am J Respir Crit Care Med 164:186–187, 2001.
4. Kollef M, Shapiro S, Silver P, et al: A randomized, controlled trial of protocol-directed versus physician-directed weaning from mechanical ventilation. Crit Care Med 25:567–574, 1997.
5. Manthous C, Schmidt G, Hall J: Liberation from mechanical ventilation: A decade of progress. Chest 114:886–901, 1998.
6. Petrof B, Legare M, Goldberg P, et al: Continuous positive airway pressure reduces work of breathing and dyspnea during weaning from mechanical ventilation in severe chronic obstructive pulmonary disease. Am Rev Respir Dis 141:281–289, 1990.
7. Strauss C, Louis B, Isabey D, et al: Contribution of the endotracheal tube and the upper airway to breathing workload. Am J Respir Crit Care Med 157:23–30, 1998.
8. Tobin M: Weaning from mechanical ventilation: What have we learned? Respir Care 45:417–431, 2000.
9. Tobin M: Advances in mechanical ventilation. N Engl J Med 344:1986–1996, 2001.
10. Yang K, Tobin M: A prospective study of indexes predicting the outcome of trials of weaning from mechanical ventilation. N Engl J Med 324:1445–1450, 1991.

II. Procedures

11. TRACHEAL INTUBATION AND AIRWAY MANAGEMENT

Manuel Pardo, Jr., M.D.

1. What is the airway?
The airway is the conduit through which air and oxygen must pass before reaching the lungs. It includes the anatomic structures extending from the nose and mouth to the larynx and trachea.

2. What is airway management?
Airway management is making sure that the airway remains patent. It is the first step in the ABCs of basic resuscitation (B = breathing, C = circulation).

3. Why does airway management precede management of breathing and circulation?
If the airway is completely obstructed, no oxygen can reach the lungs and no carbon dioxide can leave the lungs. If oxygen does not reach the lungs, the heart and circulation will have no oxygen to distribute to the body's vital organs.

4. Name the ways to manage the airway.
The airway may remain patent without any intervention and can be managed with or without tracheal intubation. Airway management without intubation can involve a variety of maneuvers. In unconscious patients, the tongue commonly obstructs the airway. Maneuvers to open the airway include the head tilt/chin lift maneuver and the jaw thrust maneuver. Placement of oral or nasal airways may also help to maintain a patent airway. The use of a face mask with a bag-valve device (e.g., ambu-bag) is the usual next step in airway management. In the vast majority of patients, it is possible to maintain a patent airway without tracheal intubation. If tracheal intubation is required, it can be accomplished through surgical or nonsurgical techniques.

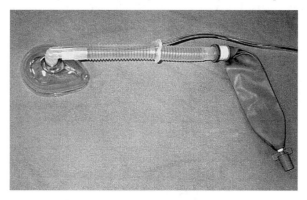

Mask and breathing circuit used for delivering positive pressure ventilation. Oxygen is administered through the small plastic tubing to inflate the reservoir bag. With proper mask application, squeezing the bag results in lung inflation. Oral or nasal airways can be used to help maintain a patent airway.

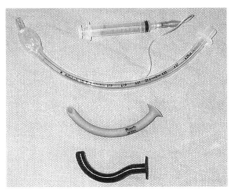

Other airway equipment. Top: size 7.5 cuffed endo-tracheal tube. The size represents the internal diameter of the tube in millimeters. A 10-ml syringe is used to inflate the cuff and provide a seal in the trachea. Most cuffs are now high-volume low pressure cuffs, which have a lower incidence of tracheal damage. Middle: nasal airway. After it is lubricated, it is inserted in the nostril. The tip of the airway creates space between the tongue and posterior oropharynx, which helps to open the airway. Bottom: oral airway. A tongue blade can be used to place the oral airway in the mouth. Like the nasal airway, it is designed to create space between the tongue and the oropharynx.

5. What are the indications for tracheal intubation?

There are five main indications: airway obstruction, inadequate oxygenation, inadequate ventilation, elevated work of breathing, and "airway protection."

1. **Airway obstruction.** If the airway is obstructed and cannot be opened with the maneuvers described above, the trachea must be intubated.

2. **Inadequate oxygenation.** If the patient's oxygen saturation is less than 90% despite the use of high-flow oxygen delivered through a face mask, tracheal intubation should be considered. 100% oxygen can be delivered reliably only with an endotracheal tube. Other factors to consider are the adequacy of cardiac output, blood hemoglobin concentration, presence of chronic hypoxemia, and reason for the hypoxemia. For example, patients with hypoxemia due to intracardiac right-to-left shunts may have chronic hypoxemia. The body usually adjusts by increasing the blood hemoglobin concentration. Because of the intracardiac shunt, the administration of 100% oxygen with an endotracheal tube may not be effective in raising the oxygen saturation.

3. **Inadequate ventilation.** With hypoventilation, the blood pCO_2 progressively rises, which also lowers the blood pH level (respiratory acidosis). With increasing CO_2 levels, patients eventually become unconscious (CO_2 narcosis). Low systemic pH may be associated with abnormal myocardial irritability and contractility. If these events occur, the patient may need to undergo tracheal intubation and mechanical ventilation. Assisted ventilation can also be accomplished without intubation, but in most patients this goal is easier to accomplish with intubation. The exact level of pH or pCO_2 that requires assisted ventilation must be determined for each patient. Important factors include the cause of the hypoventilation and its chronicity. Chronic respiratory acidosis (e.g., in a patient with severe COPD) is usually better tolerated than acute respiratory acidosis. Myocardial ischemia, congestive heart failure, and increased intracranial pressure are several factors that favor earlier use of mechanical ventilation.

4. **Elevated work of breathing.** Normally, the respiratory muscles account for less than 5% of the total body oxygen consumption. In patients with respiratory failure, this can increase to as high as 40%. It can be difficult to assess the work of breathing by clinical examination. However, patients who have rapid, shallow breathing, use of accessory respiratory muscles, or paradoxical respirations have a predictably high work of breathing. The arterial blood gas (pH, pCO_2, and PO_2) may be initially normal in such patients. Eventually, the respiratory muscles fatigue and fail, causing inadequate oxygenation and ventilation. Tracheal intubation and mechanical ventilation are necessary to reduce the work of breathing. Mechanical ventilation can sometimes be done without tracheal intubation (see chapter on noninvasive ventilation) but is more reliably accomplished with intubation.

5. **Airway protection.** In the awake patient, protective airway reflexes normally prevent the pulmonary aspiration of gastric contents. Patients with altered mental status from a variety of causes may lose these protective reflexes. The loss of airway reflexes places them at increased risk of aspiration pneumonia, which is associated with increased morbidity and mortality.

Tracheal intubation with a cuffed tube can decrease the risk of aspiration. It cannot totally prevent aspiration, however, because liquids can still leak around the endotracheal tube cuff.

6. What are the surgical techniques for tracheal intubation?

Surgical techniques include cricothyroidotomy or tracheotomy, which involve placing an endotracheal tube directly into the trachea through the cricothyroid membrane or between two tracheal rings.

7. What are the nonsurgical techniques for tracheal intubation?

Nonsurgical techniques can be divided into techniques that incorporate direct vision and "blind" techniques.

The most commonly used direct vision intubation technique is direct laryngoscopy. The laryngoscope is placed in the mouth and manipulated to expose the larynx. An endotracheal tube is then placed through the larynx into the trachea.

Another direct vision technique uses the flexible fiberoptic bronchoscope. An endotracheal tube is loaded onto the bronchoscope, which is advanced through the larynx via the nose or mouth. Once the bronchoscope is in the trachea, the endotracheal tube is advanced into position. Intubation with the fiberoptic bronchoscope requires more time and patient preparation.

Blind intubation can be accomplished through the nose or the mouth. In general, blind nasal intubation is easier to accomplish than blind oral intubation because the nasopharynx guides the endotracheal tube toward the larynx. Blind intubation can also be accomplished by "retrograde" intubation, in which a wire is inserted through the cricothyroid membrane and passed through the mouth. This wire is then used as a guide for passing an endotracheal tube into the trachea.

8. What drugs can be given to facilitate intubation?

When direct laryngoscopy is used, two types of drugs can be given to facilitate intubation: sedatives or analgesics and muscle relaxants. Sedatives or analgesics are given to reduce the discomfort of laryngoscopy and to blunt the hemodynamic response. Muscle relaxants can make direct laryngoscopy easier to perform.

9. What are the risks of these drugs?

The main risks of sedative or analgesic drugs in this setting are hypotension and respiratory depression. The muscle relaxants cause paralysis of all skeletal muscle, including the respiratory muscles. If the trachea cannot be intubated, the patient may not resume spontaneous breathing if sedatives, analgesics, or muscle relaxants have been given. Critically ill patients are more likely to develop hypotension and respiratory depression from these drugs.

10. What equipment should be prepared before direct laryngoscopy is attempted?

Before attempting laryngoscopy, all equipment should be checked for proper function. This equipment includes laryngoscope blades, laryngoscope handle, suction source, suction catheter, oxygen source, self-inflating bag or breathing circuit, face mask, oral airways, nasal airways, sedative agents, muscle relaxants, functioning IV, and patient monitors.

11. How is direct laryngoscopy accomplished?

The technique varies slightly depending on the type of blade used (see figures, top of next page). First, the head is placed in the "sniffing" position with cervical spine flexion and atlanto-occipital joint extension. The blade is inserted into the right side of the mouth. Then the tongue is moved to the left. With a curved (Macintosh) blade, the tip is inserted between the base of the tongue and the superior surface of the epiglottis, an area called the vallecula. If a straight (Miller or Wisconsin) blade is used, the tip is manipulated to lift the epiglottis. With both blade types, once the tip is in position, the blade is moved forward and upward to expose the larynx. An endotracheal tube is then inserted into the trachea. Gentle downward pressure on the thyroid cartilage may help to improve the view of the larynx.

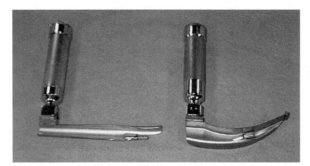

Two types of commonly used laryngoscope blades. The straight blade on the left is a size 3 Wisconsin blade. The one on the right is a size 3 Macintosh blade.

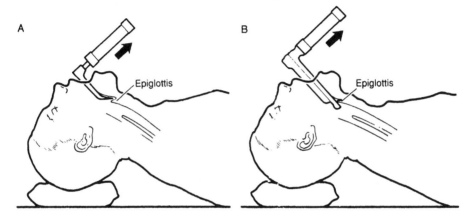

Procedure for direct laryngoscopy. *A,* a curved laryngoscope blade is placed in the vallecula. Lifting the blade forward and upward exposes the larynx. *B,* a straight blade is used to lift the epiglottis directly and expose the larynx. (From Stone DH, Gal TJ: Airway management. In Miller RD (ed): Anesthesia. New York, Churchill Livingstone, 1994, p 1418, with permission.)

12. What anatomic features are necessary for easy direct laryngoscopy and intubation?

Four anatomic features are necessary to do direct laryngoscopy and view the vocal cords: mouth opening, pharyngeal space, neck extension at the atlanto-occipital joint, and submandibular compliance.

Mouth opening. Because the laryngoscope blade is placed orally, mouth opening must be adequate.

Pharyngeal space. To see the larynx, there must not be an excess of pharyngeal tissue. Excess tissue, which may be caused by various conditions (e.g., pharyngeal edema), can block the view of the larynx and can make intubation difficult.

Neck extension. To align the axes of the mouth, pharynx, and larynx, there must be adequate extension of the atlanto-occipital joint.

Adequate submandibular compliance. With laryngoscopy, the submandibular tissue is displaced anteriorly to expose the larynx. The term *compliance* refers to the change in volume for a given change in pressure. The laryngoscope is used to apply pressure and reduce the volume of tissue obstructing the view of the larynx. If submandibular compliance is low (e.g., neck irradiation, submandibular abscess), it may be impossible to apply enough force to expose the larynx.

13. What is a "difficult airway"? What is a difficult intubation?

The difficult airway is a clinical situation in which an anesthesiologist or other specially trained clinician has difficulty with mask ventilation or tracheal intubation. Difficult intubation may be defined as one requiring more than three attempts at laryngoscopy or more than 10 minutes of laryngoscopy. Although the definitions are arbitrary, the inability to maintain a patent airway (with or without intubation) may be associated with anoxic brain injury and death.

14. How do you evaluate the airway for potential difficulty?
The history should address the ease of prior tracheal intubations. Patients who have general anesthesia for surgery frequently undergo tracheal intubation. The anesthetic record for the procedure should document the ease of intubation and the equipment used. On examination, one must evaluate the four anatomic features mentioned above.

1. **Mouth opening.** In the adult, a mouth opening of 2–3 finger-breadths is usually adequate.

2. **Pharyngeal space.** One measure of pharyngeal space is the Mallampati class (see figure below). Patients are asked to sit upright with the head in a neutral position. Then they are asked to open their mouth as widely as possible and protrude their tongue as far as possible. The classification is based on the pharyngeal structures seen:

Class I: soft palate, fauces, entire uvula, tonsillar pillars
Class II: soft palate, fauces, part of uvula
Class III: soft palate, base of uvula
Class IV: soft palate not visible at all

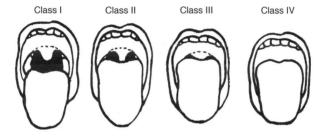

The Mallampati classification to evaluate pharyngeal space. See text for details. (From Samsoon GL, Young JR: Difficult tracheal intubation: A retrospective study. Anaesthesia, Blackwell Science, Ltd., 42:487–490, 1987, with permission.)

Patients with class I airways are generally easier to intubate than patients with class IV airways. However, this test addresses only one of the four anatomic features required for easy direct laryngoscopy. When used alone, the Mallampati class should not be considered adequate to predict a difficult intubation.

3. **Neck extension.** A normal adult has approximately 35° of extension at the atlanto-occipital joint. A decrease in extension may make it impossible to view the larynx with direct laryngoscopy.

4. **Adequate submandibular compliance.** It can be difficult to assess the submandibular compliance by physical exam. Assessment of the mandibular space can be attempted by measuring the distance from the chin to the thyroid cartilage, the "thyromental distance." An adult with less than 6.5 cm of thyromental distance may have a greater chance of difficult intubation than one with greater than 6.5 cm.

One abnormality does not necessarily predict a difficult intubation. The presence of several mild abnormalities may produce a difficult intubation. Combining the various tests improves the ability to predict a difficult intubation, but no combination is foolproof.

15. How do you manage a potentially difficult intubation?
Three types of plans must be made when managing a difficult airway.

The first is the primary approach to the intubation. The second is the plan for an emergency nonsurgical airway. Finally, there should be a plan for an emergency surgical airway. Many factors affect the management plan for a potentially difficult airway. These factors include the indication for intubation, the urgency of the intubation, the availability of skilled personnel, and the availability of special equipment. The primary approach to intubation should include consideration of the following questions:

- How cooperative is the patient?
- Is mask ventilation likely to be difficult?
- Should the initial approach to secure the airway be surgical or nonsurgical?
- Should the intubation be done with the patient awake or asleep?
- Should the patient be allowed to breathe spontaneously during the intubation?

Because an awake, cooperative, spontaneously breathing patient normally has a patent airway, an awake intubation is usually the safest. When a patient is sedated or given muscle relaxants, the respiratory drive is decreased and pharyngeal muscle tone is lost. If intubation or mask ventilation is unsuccessful, the patient may be unable to breathe spontaneously and anoxic brain damage may occur.

16. What is an awake intubation?

An awake intubation is tracheal intubation done when the patient is awake. This term is used because most intubations performed before surgery are done with the patient asleep under general anesthesia. All of the techniques described above can be accomplished in the awake patient. Topical local anesthetics can be used to decrease airway sensation and patient discomfort.

17. What are the ways to provide an emergency nonsurgical airway?

If tracheal intubation and mask ventilation are not possible and the airway is not patent, an emergency airway must be provided. The options for providing an emergency nonsurgical airway include laryngeal mask ventilation, transtracheal jet ventilation, or esophageal-tracheal combitube ventilation. These options require time and special training to perform properly. Equipment should be prepared in advance if it is available.

The laryngeal mask is probably the most widely available of the three options. It is inserted into the posterior pharynx and lies opposite the larynx (see figures). In elective situations, it has a success rate of over 90%. It is less successful in emergencies, but its availability and relatively low price make it a valuable option in managing the difficult airway. Special versions of the laryngeal mask incorporate features designed to facilitate blind passage of an endotracheal tube into the trachea.

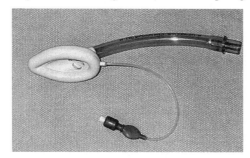

Laryngeal mask airway. This airway device can be inserted without using laryngoscopy or muscle relaxants. The cuff provides a gentle seal around the larynx.

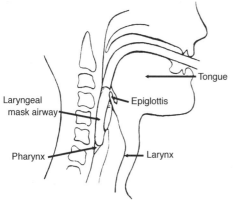

Diagram of a properly placed laryngeal mask airway (LMA). The larynx is opposite the distal opening of the LMA. The device does not prevent gastric acid aspiration. (From Stone DH, Gal TJ: Airway management. In Miller RD (ed): Anesthesia. New York, Churchill Livingstone, 1994, p 1412. Reproduced with permission.)

18. What are the ways to provide an emergency surgical airway?

A surgical airway can be provided by crycothyroidotomy or tracheotomy. These procedures also require special training and equipment to perform. The necessary equipment should be prepared in advance if a surgical airway is anticipated. A physician skilled in these procedures should be immediately available if a difficult airway is anticipated.

19. What do you do if a patient has an unsuspected difficult airway?

The patient with an unsuspected difficult airway usually presents after sedatives, anesthetics, or muscle relaxants have been given. These agents pose a problem because they remove the patient's ability to breathe spontaneously. Depending on the patient's lung function and previous oxygen therapy, the oxygen saturation may drop in less than one minute. If cerebral hypoxia is sustained for more than a few minutes, the chances of anoxic brain injury increase.

If attempts at intubation are unsuccessful, mask ventilation should be attempted. At this stage you should consider calling for help, awakening the patient, or allowing spontaneous ventilation to return. If mask ventilation is successful, alternative nonsurgical or surgical airways can be attempted. Mask ventilation can allow time for the patient to awaken. At this point an awake intubation can be done. If mask ventilation is not successful, then an emergency airway is necessary. The fastest nonsurgical or surgical airway should be established.

20. How is tracheal intubation confirmed?

There are many ways to confirm tracheal intubation. It is important to understand that each method has its limitations. If there is doubt about proper placement, another method should be used for confirmation.

Auscultation for bilateral breath sounds and absence of stomach inflation are done after each intubation attempt. The chest should rise symmetrically. With an esophageal intubation, however, these signs may still be present.

Another way is to view the endotracheal tube passing through the vocal cords during laryngoscopy. If an experienced clinician clearly sees the tube between the cords, this is a definitive confirmation. However, this view cannot be obtained in many instances. The endotracheal tube itself commonly blocks sight of the vocal cords, and inexperienced clinicians may insert the tube in the esophagus despite having a good view of the larynx.

Other ways to assess proper placement are carbon dioxide capnography and fiberoptic bronchoscopy. Carbon dioxide can be measured as it is exhaled by the patient (end-tidal capnography). The presence of continuous end-tidal carbon dioxide is considered definitive proof of tracheal intubation. Fiberoptic bronchoscopy may reveal tracheal rings and bronchi. This is also a definitive sign of proper tube placement. However, the equipment is expensive and must be readily available. Blood and secretions can make it difficult to identify the trachea.

The pulse oximeter is not a reliable way to confirm intubation. With an esophageal intubation, the oxygen saturation will eventually fall, but this can take several minutes. Portable chest radiography is an unreliable method of confirmation because only two dimensions are seen. An endotracheal tube in the esophagus may appear to be in the trachea on an anterior-posterior film.

21. What are the immediate, short-term complications of tracheal intubation?

Immediate complications of intubation include dental injury, cervical spine injury, pharyngeal trauma, laryngeal injury, aspiration of gastric contents, and tracheal rupture. Nosebleed is a risk with nasal intubations. The most common injuries are minor lip trauma and tooth damage.

22. What are the long-term complications of tracheal intubation?

Potential problems include endotracheal tube obstruction, cuff leak, tube displacement, and laryngeal injury. The incidence of tracheal stenosis has decreased with the widespread use of high-volume, low-pressure endotracheal tube cuffs. Tracheoesophageal fistula is a rare complication. With nasal intubation, sinusitis is a particular risk, although this complication can occur with oral intubation as well.

BIBLIOGRAPHY

1. Practice guidelines for management of the difficult airway. A report by the American Society of Anesthesiologists Task Force on Management of the Difficult Airway. Anesthesiology 78:597–602, 1993.
2. Blosser SA , Stauffer JL: Intubation of critically ill patients. Clin Chest Med 17:355–378, 1996.
3. Mallampati SR, Gatt SP, Gugino LD, et al: A clinical sign to predict difficult tracheal intubation: A prospective study. Can J Anaesth 32:429–434, 1985.
4. McCulloch TM, Bishop MJ: Complications of translaryngeal intubation. Clin Chest Med 12:507–521, 1991.
5. Stone DH, Gal TJ: Airway management. In Miller RD (ed): Anesthesia. New York, Churchill Livingstone, 2000, pp 1414–1451.

12. TRACHEOTOMY

John E. Heffner, M.D., F.C.C.P.

1. What are the different techniques for obtaining tracheal access in critically ill patients?

A **standard tracheotomy** is a surgical procedure wherein a standard tracheostomy tube is inserted through an incisional tracheostoma. The tube enters the trachea between cartilaginous rings. The rings can be divided for passage of the tube by various surgical techniques, including incision and dilation of the inter-ring membranes, vertical incisions through rings, removal of portions of the anterior tracheal wall including ring segments, or formation of an anterior tracheal tissue flap.

The term **percutaneous tracheotomy** refers to various procedures that share in common a modified Seldinger technique for placing a standard or modified tracheostomy tube. After performance of a cutaneous incision, a needle, guidewire, and introducer are placed percutaneously below the first or second tracheal ring. Progressively larger dilators or a single horn-shaped dilator is introduced through the tract into the trachea over the introducer. A tracheostomy tube loaded onto a stylet is then placed through the dilated tissue structures, followed by removal of the stylet.

A **cricothyroidotomy** is a surgical technique for placement of an airway into the trachea through the cricothyroid space. The superficial location of anatomic landmarks at the level of the cricothyroid membrane offers simplicity of technique, which makes cricothyroidotomy the preferred technique for placement of a surgical airway in emergency settings.

A **minitracheotomy** allows the percutaneous placement of a 7-French cannula through the tracheal rings for patients with difficulty in clearing airway secretions. The minitracheotomy tube is just large enough to allow passage of a suction catheter for frequent removal of secretions.

2. Should all tracheotomies in critically ill patients be performed in the operating room?

Not necessarily. Tracheotomy in intubated patients undergoing mechanical ventilation can be done efficiently and safely in the intensive care unit (ICU), thereby avoiding patient transport and operating room (OR) scheduling delays. The patient's critical care room must be transformed, however, to an OR environment, with adequate instrumentation, sterile fields, lighting, and suction. At present, however, most standard surgical tracheotomies are performed in the OR. Most intensivists who perform percutaneous tracheotomies prefer the ICU setting for the procedure; the ability to perform percutaneous tracheotomies in the ICU safely and quickly is seen as one of the advantages of the procedure. Percutaneous dilational tracheotomies can be performed in the ICU at a lower cost than standard tracheotomies in the OR. This cost advantage no longer applies when both procedures are performed in the ICU.

3. Is percutaneous dilational tracheotomy performed as a blind technique with dilator insertion directed by neck and airway palpation?

Percutaneous dilational tracheotomy was first described as a blind technique in which the operator directed the needle and guidewire into the airway guided by careful palpation of the neck. Reports of extraluminal insertion of tracheostomy tubes and lacerations of the posterior tracheal wall by needles and guidewires promoted the performance of percutaneous dilational tracheotomy under direct bronchoscopic visualization. A bronchoscope with video imaging is inserted through the endotracheal tube, which is pulled back into the subglottic region of the airway to allow visualization of the tracheotomy site. The operator then can observe the needle and guidewire enter the trachea to ensure proper placement of the introducer and dilator.

4. Is emergency tracheotomy the surgical procedure of choice in apneic patients with acute upper airway obstruction?

No. Tracheotomy is acceptably safe when performed electively in an OR environment under controlled clinical conditions. Risks of surgical complications increase five-fold, however, when tracheotomy is applied in the emergency situation. An emergency cricothyroidotomy provides the greatest likelihood of successful airway placement with the lowest risks for complications in patients with acute upper airway obstruction who cannot undergo translaryngeal intubation.

5. What is the most lethal complication of tracheotomy in the perioperative period?

Inadvertent decannulation of a tracheostomy tube during the first 3–5 days after its placement represents a potentially lethal clinical event. It may take several days for a tracheostomy incision to form a stomal tract that allows blind replacement of a decannulated tracheostomy tube. Before this time, attempts to reinsert a tracheostomy tube will most likely create a false tissue tract in the pretracheal space. Subsequent attempts to ventilate the patient with positive pressure through a misplaced tube result in profound cervical emphysema and external compression of the trachea, leading to asphyxia.

A general rule dictates that only surgeons experienced with the patient's cervical anatomy should attempt replacement of a decannulated tube within the first 5 days after surgery. In the absence of a skilled surgeon, patients who require urgent airway control can undergo translaryngeal intubation and replacement of the tracheostomy tube under a controlled setting after they stabilize. If the patient cannot be intubated through the nose or mouth because of upper airway obstruction, a narrow-caliber, cuffless endotracheal tube can be inserted through the surgical incision into the trachea with the assistance of a lighted laryngoscope blade. In some patients, the trachea may require initial intubation with a flexible endotracheal stylet ("tube changer") or nasogastric tube over which an airway can be guided into place.

6. How is a cricothyroidotomy performed?

The cricothyroid membrane is located approximately 2–3 cm below the thyroid notch. The membrane, which is typically 1 cm in height, lies below the vocal cords but within the subglottic larynx. A surgical scalpel is used to incise the overlying skin and stab the membrane. The resultant opening into the airway is enlarged with a spreader, allowing placement of a tracheostomy tube. Commercially available instruments designed for the emergency situation allow puncture of the membrane and introduction of an airway cannula in one maneuver.

7. Can mechanically ventilated patients with a tracheostomy speak?

Several techniques promote speech in mechanically ventilated patients with a tracheostomy tube in place. Patients with low-to-moderate minute ventilation requirements can whisper intelligibly if the tracheostomy tube cuff is deflated to allow a small "cuff leak" during the ventilatory inspiratory cycle. Addition of a small amount of positive end-expiratory pressure (PEEP) creates a leak throughout inspiration and expiration and promotes more continuous and spontaneous speech. A "speaking tracheostomy tube" provides an external cannula that directs compressed gas to exit the tube below the vocal cords, allowing some patients to communicate in whispered tones. An "electrolarynx" placed against the neck near the laryngeal cartilage generates a vibratory tone that can be articulated with practice into intelligible speech. If patients have limited ventilatory requirements, a one-way valve can be placed in-line between a fenestrated tracheostomy tube with a deflated cuff and the ventilator tubing, allowing expiration through the native airway and promoting intelligible speech.

8. What precautions should be exercised in patients with a cuffed tracheostomy tube who undergo general anesthesia?

Some volatile anesthetics, such as nitrous oxide, diffuse more rapidly into a tracheostomy tube cuff than oxygen or nitrogen can diffuse out and thereby increase intracuff pressures. During a 2-hour operation, cuff pressures may increase from 15 mmHg to over 80 mmHg, which can cause ischemic injury to the tracheal mucosa. Appropriate precautions include frequent monitoring of cuff pressures in the OR or inflation of the tube cuff at the outset of the surgical procedure with the anesthetic gas mixture administered to the airway.

9. What is the ideal size of tracheostomy tube for a patient?

No one size is best for all patients because tracheal caliber and clinical situations vary. Small-caliber tubes may decrease the incidence of tracheal stenosis at the stoma site because of the smaller tracheal incision required. Unfortunately, small tubes present difficulties in airway suctioning, spontaneous ventilation, and fiberoptic bronchoscopy. Furthermore, small tubes have small cuffs that may damage the tracheal mucosa because they require high intracuff pressures to overdistend in order to seal the airway. Overly large tubes require wide stomas and prohibit adequate cuff inflation to cushion the rigid tube from the tracheal mucosa and to effectively prevent aspiration. The best approximation of ideal size requires the surgeon to select a tube with an outer diameter two-thirds the inner caliber of the patient's trachea at the point of insertion.

10. Should tracheostomy tube cuff pressures be checked periodically in patients undergoing mechanical ventilation?

Frequent monitoring of cuff pressure provides the best measure to prevent tracheal injury at the cuff site. Cuff pressures in excess of mucosal capillary perfusion pressures (usually 25 mmHg) can rapidly cause mucosal ischemia and resultant tracheal stenosis. Reliance on minimal leak technique to inflate cuffs without actually measuring cuff pressures may prevent detection of patients with high cuff pressure requirements. A linear relationship exists between the intracuff pressure required to seal the airway (minimal leak cuff pressure) and the peak inspiratory pressure generated by positive pressure ventilation. Patients with peak inspiratory pressures above 48 cmH_2O will usually require cuff inflations pressures above 25 mmHg.

Recent data suggest that if a tracheotomy tube is underinflated (< 18 mmHg) in a patient undergoing mechanical ventilation, the risks for aspiration and nosocomial pneumonia increase. Therefore, most experts recommend maintaining cuff pressure between 18 and 25 mmHg. Clinicians should notice the units of measurement of cuff pressures and make the appropriate conversion from cmH_2O to mmHg to allow adherence to cuff pressure standards (cuff pressure in mmHg = measured cuff pressure in $cmH_2O/1.36$).

11. What should the clinician consider in any patient with airway hemorrhage after the first 48 hours of insertion of a tracheostomy tube?

Bleeding within the first 48 hours of tracheotomy is usually a result of hemorrhage from the incisional wound. Any bleeding that develops longer than 48 hours after surgery, however, should suggest the possibility of a tracheoinnominate fistula. This life-threatening complication requires immediate evaluation by a thoracic surgeon capable of performing an emergency sternotomy for ligation of the innominate artery, because massive hemorrhage often develops after an initial "herald" episode of mild-to-moderate bleeding.

12. How should a patient be evaluated who continues to have cough and shortness of breath 2 months after removal of a tracheostomy tube?

Although these symptoms often accompany underlying lung disease, they also occasionally represent the only clinical manifestations of a tracheoesophageal fistula. A tracheoesophageal fistula related to pressure necrosis by the tube cuff or catheter tip occurs as a complication of tracheostomy in less than 1% of patients. Risk factors include excessive tube movement, high ventilator inflation pressures, overinflated cuffs, prolonged intubation, diabetes mellitus, and the presence of a nasogastric tube.

Suspicion of a tracheoesophageal fistula should be pursued with contrast imaging studies, such as a cine-esophagram. Endoscopic evaluation either by bronchoscopy or esophagoscopy may fail to identify the fistula tract.

13. What are the indications for tracheotomy in critically ill patients?

Common indications include removal of airway secretions, relief of upper airway obstruction, provision of airway access for long-term mechanical ventilation, and prevention of aspiration.

14. Do ventilator-dependent patients wean faster from the ventilator if an "early" tracheotomy is performed?

Several prospective, randomized studies that enrolled ventilator-dependent, critically ill patients have examined potential benefits of performing early tracheotomy (after 3–7 days of intubation) compared with delayed tracheotomy (8 days or longer after intubation). Some of these studies demonstrated lower rates of hospital-acquired pneumonia and shorter duration of mechanical ventilation among patients undergoing early tracheotomy. Unfortunately, design flaws in these studies prevent widespread acceptance of their findings. Evidence-based guidelines for weaning patients from ventilatory support, recently published by the American College of Chest Physicians, reported no high-grade evidence that routine performance of early tracheotomy promotes earlier weaning.

15. Describe the role of a fenestrated tracheostomy tube in the ICU.

Newer fenestrated tracheostomy tubes with multiple small holes in their greater curvature assist speech and weaning from tracheostomy in spontaneously breathing patients without stimulating growth of granulation tissue. After removal of an inner cannula (if present) and deflation of the cuff, patients can breathe around the cuff and through the fenestrations in addition to the stoma to decrease airway resistance. Placement of a one-way valve, such as the Passy-Muir valve, on the tracheostomy tube allows patients to inhale through the tube and exhale out their native upper airways, thereby promoting speech.

Some physicians recommend placement of a fenestrated tracheostomy tube to facilitate gradual weaning toward decannulation. Others prefer use of a stomal button, arguing that placement of a fenestrated tube interferes with spontaneous clearing of secretions through the native airway and delays decannulation.

16. What is a tracheal button?

Tracheal buttons, such as the Olympic tracheal button and the Montgomery tracheal button, assist weaning from a tracheostomy tube. Designed as a straight, rigid, or flexible plastic or Silastic tube, tracheal buttons fit through the stoma to maintain its patency in case patients need suctioning or reinsertion of a tracheostomy tube through the tract. The button is ideal for patients with borderline ventilatory status, because the distal end abuts the anterior tracheal wall and does not protrude into the airway to impede respiration or clearance of secretions by coughing.

17. Why do patients aspirate after removal of a tracheostomy tube?

Scarring at the stoma site may interfere with the rostrocaudal excursion of the larynx during swallowing, which is necessary for glottic closure. In addition, prolonged diversion of ventilation away from the glottis causes attenuation of the vocal cord adductor response that is important in aspiration prevention.

CONTROVERSIES

18. What is the appropriate time to convert an intubated patient undergoing mechanical ventilation to a tracheotomy?

No study or accumulation of data from combined investigations has determined the ideal time to perform a tracheotomy in patients who require long-term mechanical ventilation. Recent consensus, however, is that the decision should be individualized, with a tracheotomy being performed when a patient appears likely to benefit from the procedure. The potential benefits of tracheotomy over prolonged translaryngeal intubation include improved comfort, enhanced ability to communicate, greater mobility, and diminished risk for direct laryngeal injury.

Consensus further emphasizes that the decision for a tracheotomy in ventilator-dependent patients should be determined by a patient's anticipated likelihood of requiring prolonged mechanical ventilation rather than by the arbitrary duration of ventilator dependency that has already transpired. As an example, patients with respiratory failure should be evaluated within 7 days of treatment with a translaryngeal endotracheal tube for the probability of successful extubation within the first 10–14 days of intubation. Patients determined unlikely to improve rapidly on the basis of severity of disease should undergo tracheotomy at an early and convenient opportunity rather than waiting for an arbitrary and obligate 1–2 weeks of mechanical ventilation.

19. What is the preferred technique for performing a tracheotomy for long-term airway access in a critically ill patient undergoing mechanical ventilation?

Considerable discussion has focused on the comparable value of standard open tracheotomy compared with the percutaneous technique. Recent systematic reviews and meta-analyses of the literature indicate that both procedures can be performed safely with similar perioperative risk in suitable patients. Some authors suggest that percutaneous dilational tracheotomy is the preferred procedure because of a lower incidence of wound infections and stomal postoperative bleeding and a shorter operative time. The clinical importance and degree of these differences, however, are marginal. The preferred procedure in any specific institution is the one that can be performed with available physician expertise and resources. Fewer data address the comparative differences between the two procedures in long-term airway complications, such as tracheal stenosis. Accumulating experience indicates that standard and percutaneous tracheotomies involve similar and acceptable long-term risk.

Patients must be selected carefully for percutaneous dilational tracheotomy, however, to maintain complications at an acceptable level. Patients with tracheas that lie deep in the neck are at increased risk and should be referred for standard tracheotomy. Obesity, cervical and airway abnormalities, previous tracheostomy, and anatomic variation in the neck warrant consideration of standard rather than percutaneous tracheotomy. Some physicians perform portable ultrasound, magnetic resonance imaging, or other imaging studies of the neck to identify clinically occult airway abnormalities before proceeding to percutaneous dilational tracheotomy.

BIBLIOGRAPHY

1. Albarran JW: A review of communication with intubated patients and those with tracheostomies within an intensive care environment. Intensive Care Nurs 7:179–186, 1991.
2. Berenholz LP, Vail S, Berlet A: Management of tracheocutaneous fistula. Arch Otolaryngol Head Neck Surg 118:869–871, 1992.
3. Boyd SW, Benzel EC: The role of early tracheotomy in the management of the neurosurgical patient. Laryngoscope 102:559–562, 1992.
4. Ciaglia P, Graniero KD: Percutaneous dilational tracheostomy. Results and long-term follow-up. Chest 101:464–467, 1992.
5. Cowan T, Op't-Holt TB, Gegenheimer C, et al: Effect of inner cannula removal on the work of breathing imposed by tracheostomy tubes: A bench study. Respir Care 46:460–465, 2001.
6. Curtis JJ, Clark NC, McKenney CA, et al: Tracheostomy: A risk factor for mediastinitis after cardiac operation. Ann Thorac Surg 72:731–734, 2001.
7. Davis K, Campbell RS, Johannigman JA, et al: Changes in respiratory mechanics after tracheostomy. Arch Surg 134:59–62, 1999.
8. Diehl J-L, Atrous SE, Touchard D, et al: Changes in the work of breathing induced by tracheotomy in ventilator-dependent patients. Chest 159:383–388, 1999.
9. Freeman BD, Isabella K, Cobb P, et al: A prospective, randomized study comparing percutaneous with surgical tracheotomy in critically ill patients. Crit Care Med 29:926–930, 2001.
10. Freeman BD, Isabella K, Lin N, Buchanan TG: A meta-analysis of prospective trials comparing percutaneous and surgical tracheostomy in critically ill patients. Chest 118:1412–1418, 1994.
11. Gelman JJ, Aro M, Weiss SM: Tracheo-innominate artery fistula. J Am Coll Surg 179:626–634, 1994.
12. Godwin JE, Heffner JE: Special critical care considerations in tracheostomy management. Clin Chest Med 12:573–583, 1992.

13. Guyton DG, Barlow MR, Besselievre TR: Influence of airway pressure on minimum occlusive endotracheal tube cuff pressure. Crit Care Med 25:91–94, 1997.
14. Heffner JE: Medical indications for tracheotomy. Chest 96:186–190, 1989.
15. Heffner JE (ed): Airway management in the critically ill patient. Clin Chest Med 12:415–630, 1991.
16. Heffner JE: Tracheotomy: Indications and timing. Respir Care 44:807–819, 1999.
17. Heffner JE: The role of tracheotomy in weaning. Chest 120:477S–481S, 2001.
18. Heffner JE, Casey K, Hoffman C: Care of the mechanically ventilated patient with a tracheotomy. In Tobin MJ (ed): Principles and Practice of Mechanical Ventilation. New York, McGraw-Hill, 1994, pp 749–774.
19. Heffner JE, Hess D: Tracheostomy management in the chronically ventilated patient. Clin Chest Med 22:55–69, 2001.
20. Heikkinen M, Aarnio P, Hannukainen J: Percutaneous dilational tracheostomy or conventional surgical tracheostomy? Crit Care Med 28:1399–1402, 2000.
21. Issa MM, Healy DM, Maghur HA, et al: Prophylactic minitracheotomy in lung resections. J Thorac Cardiovasc Surg 101:895–900, 1991.
22. Isaacs JH Jr, Pedersen AD: Emergency cricothyroidotomy. Am Surg 63:346–349, 1997.
23. Johnson JL, Cheatham ML, Sagraves SG, et al: Percutaneous dilational tracheostomy: A comparison of single- versus multiple-dilator techniques. Crit Care Med 29:1251–1254, 2001.
24. Kollig E, Heydenreich U, Roteman B, et al: Ultrasound and bronchoscopic controlled percutaneous tracheostomy on trauma ICU injury. Injury 31:663–668, 2000.
25. Leder SB: Prognostic indicators for successful use of "talking" tracheostomy tubes. Perceptual Motor Skills 73:441–442, 1991.
26. Leonard RC, Lewis RH, Singh B, von Heeerden PV: Late outcome from percutaneous tracheostomy using the Portex kit. Chest 115:1070–1075, 1999.
27. Massick DD, Yao S, Powell DM, et al: Bedside tracheostomy in the intensive care unit: A prospective randomized trial comparing open surgical tracheostomy with endoscopically guided percutaneous dilational tracheotomy. Laryngoscope 111:494–500, 2001.
28. Maziak DE, Meade MO, Todd TRJ: The timing of tracheotomy: A systematic review. Chest 114:605–609, 1998.
29. McGeehin WH, Scoma R, Igidbashian L, et al: Tracheostomy versus endotracheal intubation: The ICU nurse's perspective. Crit Care Med 18:S224, 1990.
30. Muhammad JK, Major E, Patton DW: Evaluating the neck for percutaneous dilational tracheostomy. J Maxillofac Surg 28:336–342, 2000.
31. Myers EN, Carrau RL: Early complications of tracheotomy. Incidence and management. Clin Chest Med 12:589–595, 1991.
32. Nash M: Swallowing problems in tracheotomized patient. Otolaryngol Clin North Am 21:701–709, 1988.
33. Norwood S, Vallina VL, Short K, et al: Incidence of tracheal stenosis and other late complications after percutaneous tracheostomy. Ann Surg 232:233–241, 2000.
34. Stock MC, Woodward CG, Shapiro BA, et al: Perioperative complications of elective tracheostomy in critically ill patients. Crit Care Med 14:81–863, 1986.
35. Streitz JM Jr, Shapshay SM: Airway injury after tracheotomy and endotracheal intubation. Surg Clin North Am 71:1211–1230, 1991.
36. van Heurn Lw: When and how should we do a tracheostomy? Curr Opin Crit Care 6:267–270, 2000.
37. Wright CD: Management of tracheoinnominate artery fistula. Chest Surg Clin North Am 6:865–973, 1996.

13. CHEST TUBES

Kevin D. Halow, M.D., and Mark W. Bowyer, M.D.

1. What is the purpose of a chest tube?

A chest tube is placed to evacuate fluid and air from the pleural space and to reestablish negative intrapleural pressure so that the lung may reexpand.

2. What type of tubes are available?

Many different types of tubes are available for pleural drainage. The tube most often used is a standard thoracostomy drainage tube. These tubes come in sizes ranging from 10 to 36 French.

They are inserted at bedside and can be used to drain air or fluid. Smaller catheters (including pigtail catheters) inserted under radiologic guidance can also be used to drain the chest. They are more effective for air than fluid but can be used in both situations. A thoracic vent, a device consisting of a small urethane catheter that is connected to a plastic collection chamber with a one-way valve (similar to a Heimlich valve), can also be used alone or connected to suction. This tube should be used for evacuation of air only.

3. How does a chest tube work?

The suction system for chest tubes is based on a three-bottle system. The first bottle is connected directly to the patient's chest tube for fluid collection. The second bottle is connected to the first bottle and is used to create a water seal. The third bottle connects the first two bottles to wall suction and is used to control the amount of suction applied to the system (see figure below). Modern systems have the same three compartments as the original three-bottle system, but they are contained together in one sealed plastic container. One need only inject 10–15 ml of sterile water into the water seal chamber and the system is ready to connect to the chest tube in the patient. The amount of suction applied to the system is controlled by opening or closing a system valve.

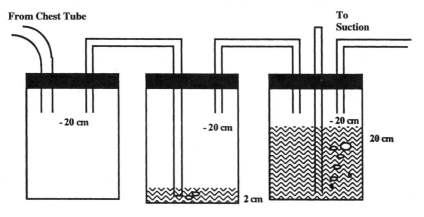

The three-bottle collection system.

4. How much suction is applied to the chest tube?

Under most circumstances, about –20 cmH$_2$O is applied to the chest tube via the collection system. This amount of suction is usually adequate to keep the pleural space evacuated but does not damage the lung. The highest pressure ever routinely used is –40 cmH$_2$O.

5. Where are chest tubes placed?

Chest tubes are generally placed in the fourth or fifth intercostal space just anterior to the mid-axillary line and directed apically in the chest cavity. In men the nipple line generally is used to estimante the fifth intercostal space, whereas in women the inframmamary fold or crease is used for the same purpose (see figure on following page). Chest tubes should rarely, if ever, be placed posterior to the posterior axillary line because this is an uncomfortable location for the patient. In addition, a chest tube in a posterior position can become compressed and nonfunctional. Occasionally, chest tubes can be placed anteriorly through the second intercostal space in the midclavicular line for treatment of a pneumothorax. Chest tubes placed exclusively for drainage of fluid should be placed in the axillary location and directed posteriorly.

6. How does one select an appropriate size for a chest tube?

The size should be tailored to the specific need. Large chest tubes (36 French) should be used to drain a hemothorax. Smaller tubes can become obstructed with blood clots, requiring

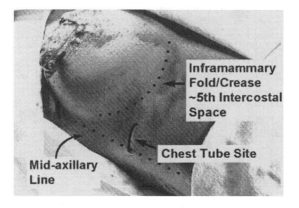

The inframammary fold is used to estimate the site for chest tube insertion just anterior to the mid-axillary line in this woman with a gunshot wound to the right chest.

Inframammary Fold/Crease ~5th Intercostal Space

Chest Tube Site

Mid-axillary Line

repeat tube placement. Small chest tubes (10–14 French) should be used exclusively for treatment of a simple pneumothorax. In the ICU, the most commonly used tube size is 28 French. This size allowsdrainage of both air and pleural fluid. The tube can continue to function even in the presence of a large pulmonary air leak in the patient on positive-pressure mechanical ventilation.

7. How is a chest tube placed?

Chest tubes are generally placed with the patient in the decubitus position, allowing better access to the lateral chest wall. This position allows better access to the lateral chest wall for proper placement It also helps to direct the chest tube to the appropriate intrathoracic location (apically for a pneumothorax or posteriorly for drainage). In the ICU, the physician may not be able to turn the patient because of the use of positive-pressure ventilation, hemodynamic instability, multiple intravenous and monitoring lines, or the need for rapid chest tube insertion. In this setting or for placement into the second intercostal space, the patient can be left in a supine position. For comfort and sedation, intravenous morphine and benzodiazepines are used.

After the area is prepared and draped, local anesthesia using 1% lidocaine is administered. A small incision is made below the planned interspace, and a tract for insertion is made by bluntly spreading the muscle with either a Kelley clamp (Fig. A below) or Mayo scissors. For a pneumothorax, the pleura should be entered over the rib. This approach helps provide a seal for the chest tube tract. For drainage only, a more direct tract between the interspaces can be used. After entering the pleura, a digital exam of the chest cavity should be done to ensure proper position and to lyse any local adhesive bands that may prevent insertion of the tube (Fig. B on following page). The tube then can be inserted using a blunt-tip clamp and directed to the

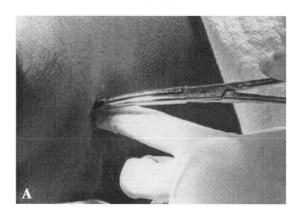

A, After making a skin incision, a Kelley clamp is advanced up and over the next rib, spreading muscle and entering the chest.

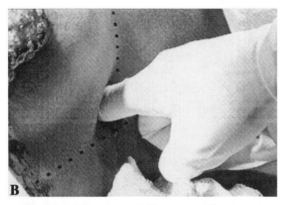

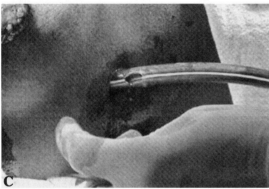

B, A gloved finger is placed into the chest to ensure proper position and to lyse any adhesions that may prevent tube placement. *C,* The chest tube is inserted toward the apex and advanced until the last hole is in the chest. The tube is then sewn in place and attached to an underwater suction device.

appropriate location in the chest (Fig. C on following page). In pediatric patients, digital examination of the inside of the chest may not be possible. A hemostat inserted through the last hole in the chest tube and directed toward the tip of the tube may help to stent the chest tube and ease its insertion through the chest wall. The chest tube should be sewn in place with a single silk suture and connected to the drainage system.

8. What are the complications of chest tube placement? How are they avoided?

Common complications of chest tube placement include mechanical failure, infection, and bleeding. Mechanical failures may result from obstruction of the chest tube by blood clots, kinks in the tube, or improper placement (e.g., into a lung fissure). Tubes inadvertently can be placed outsidethe pleural space (i.e., subcutaneously), subdiaphragmatically, or not far enough into the chest. These complications can be avoided by using the appropriately sized tube and by meticulous attention to detail during the insertion. Any problem noted on the follow-up chest x-ray should be corrected immediately. Diagnosis of a malpositioned tube is sometimes difficult to establish on a chest x-ray. Recent reports suggest that computed tomography (CT) can be helpful in establishing the exact position of the tube and may be indicated in some cases.

Empyemas can complicate tube thoracostomy. To avoid this complication, chest tubes should be placed under sterile conditions. The use of prophylactic antibiotics is controversial. Evidence suggests that they decrease the infectious complications of pneumonia and empyema when chest tubes are placed for traumatic hemopneumothoraces, but no evidence supports their use when the chest tube is placed for a simple pneumothorax.

Bleeding after chest tube placement is rare. When it occurs, usually it is due to the laceration of an intercostal vessel. This complication can be avoided by placing the tube over the top of the rib, avoiding the vessels that run along the inferior aspect of the rib.

9. What is reexpansion pulmonary edema?

Reexpansion pulmonary edema is a rare event resulting in unilateral pulmonary edema after rapid evacuation of a pleural effusion or rapid reexpansion of the lung in patients with a pneumothorax. A mortality rate as high as 20% has been noted in recognized cases. The pathophysiologic mechanism is not entirely clear but is thought to be related to mechanical stresses on the pulmonary vasculature during reexpansion, which may result in increased vascular permeability. Most reported cases have occurred after drainage of large collections of fluid (i.e., > 2 L) that have been present for more than 3 days. Efforts to decrease the likelihood of this complication include (1) initial drainage of a large pleural effusion or initial reexpansion of a large chronic pneumothorax using water seal only and (2) clamping the chest tube for several hours after draining the initial 2 L of a large, chronic pleural effusion.

10. How do you monitor the patient with a chest tube?

The amount and character of fluid output should be monitored throughout the day. The presence or absence of an air leak should be noted by looking for bubbles in the water seal chamber during inspiration or coughing. When a continued air leak is noted, it is important to ensure that the leak is not within the system itself. The system can be checked by sequentially clamping the tube before each connection and looking for an air leak. If there is a leak from the system, the system must be replaced. It is also important to ensure that there is no leak at the point where the tube enters the chest and to check the chest x-ray to ensure that the last hole in the chest tube is within the chest.

11. How much blood draining from a hemothorax should prompt operative intervention?

Most intrathoracic hemorrhages will cease when pleural apposition is achieved with the use of chest tube suction. Acute drainage of $\geq$ 1500 ml of blood from a hemothorax, which represents approximately 40% of the circulating blood volume, should raise serious concerns that the hemorrhage may require operative intervention. If bleeding ceases at this point, thorocotomy probably is not indicated. If bleeding continues, the patient should undergo surgical exploration. Postoperatively, the amount of pleural drainage that should prompt a return to the operating room may vary according the procedure, coagulation status of the patient, and the amount of irrigation that was left in the chest prior to surgical closure. In general, more than 800 ml of blood in 1 hour, 400 ml/hr for 2 consecutive hours, 200 ml/hr for 4 consecutive hours, or 800 ml over 8 hours should prompt consideration of operative intervention.

12. Should chest tubes be clamped during transport of patients?

No. When suction is unavailable, the patient should be transported on water seal, and the water seal chamber should be kept at least 20 cmH$_2$O below the level of the patient to prevent reflux of fluid up the tube with any high negative intrathoracic pressures that may occur. Clamping the chest tube during transport can result in a tension pneumothorax if a significant air leak from the lung is present.

13. What is chest tube stripping?

Stripping is the practice of compressing the chest tube (or the drainage tubing coming from it) with either the thumb and forefingers or with a mechanical stripper and pulling away from the chest wall while continuing to compress the tube. The objective is to generate a negative pressure in order to dislodge any clots within the tube and promote pleural drainage. No evidence suggests that stripping the tube actually accomplishes this goal. Routine use of this procedure probably should be abandoned.

14. What is a Heimlich valve? How is it used?

A Heimlich valve is a simple one-way flutter valve. It is made of a soft rubber tube (similar to a Penrose drain) that is held open at the proximal (patient end) by a rigid ring and is allowed to collapse at the distal end. Air that is moving from the pleural space can exit the valve, but air cannot enter because the distal end collapses with inspiration. It is usually used in an outpatient setting or during patient transport to prevent a pneumothorax. It is usually not used in critically ill patients.

15. When are chest tubes removed?

Chest tubes can be pulled when no air leak is noted on water seal for 24 hours, the drainage falls below 100 ml/day, and the chest x-ray demonstrates complete expansion of the lung. Mechanical ventilation should not be a deterrent to removal of the chest tube, because the risk of recurrent pneumothorax following chest tube removal in such patients is low. An exception to the above rule is the patient in whom the tube was placed for an empyema. Pulling a chest tube that is draining an empyema cavity may result in reaccumulation of an abscess cavity. In this setting, when no fluctuation occurs in the water seal chamber with respiration, the tube may be cut off and converted to an open drain that is slowly removed as the drainage decreases. The chest tube can also be replaced with successively smaller tubes as it is withdrawn to allow the space to close down from the inside to the outside.

16. How is a chest tube removed?

After taking down the dressing, carefully cut the sutures holding the tube in place. Place a greased gauze pad on a 4×4 dressing and hold it over the chest tube exit site. Instruct the patient to take a large breath and perform a Valsalva maneuver; then rapidly pull the chest tube while covering the exit site with the greased gauze dressing. The objective is to create positive pressure in the pleural space in order to prevent a pneumothorax during tube removal. If great care is not taken during this maneuver, a pneumothorax may occur, requiring replacement of the chest tube. The patient should have a follow-up chest x-ray after tube removal.

17. Should a chest tube be removed at end-inspiration or end-expiration?

As described above, the classic approach is to remove the chest tube at end-inspiration. This conventional wisdom recently was challenged by a randomized study that found no difference in the rate of pneumothorax after removal at end-inspiration or end-expiration.

18. Does removal of a chest tube mandate a follow-up chest radiograph?

According to conventional wisdom, yes. But at least two recent studies suggest that chest x-rays should not be routinely performed after removal of chest tubes. The decision should be based on sound clinical judgment.

BIBLIOGRAPHY

1. Bell RL, Ovadia P, Abdullah F, et al: Chest tube removal: End-inspiration or end-expiration? J Trauma 50:674–677, 2001
2. Gayer G, Rozenman J, Hoffmann C, et al: CT diagnosis of malpositioned chest tubes. Br J Radiol 73:786–790, 2000.
3. Gilbert TB, McGrath BJ, Soberman M: Chest tubes: Indications, placement, management, and complications. Intensive Care Med 8:73–86, 1993.
4. Pacanowski JP, D, Kopelman AE: Chest tube insertion: A simplified technique. Pediatrics 83:784–785, 1989.
5. Palesty JA, McKelvey AA, Dudrick SJ: The efficacy of x-rays after chest tube removal. Am J Surg 179:13–16, 2000.
6. Parry GW, Morgan WE, Salama FD: Management of haemothorax. Ann R Coll Surg Engl 78:325–326, 1996.
7. Ray RJ, Alexander CM, Williams J, Marshall BE: Influence of the method of re-expansion of atelectatic lung upon the development of pulmonary edema in dogs. Crit Care Med 12:364, 1984.
8. Schoenenberger RA, Haefeli WE, Weiss P, Ritz R: Evaluation of conventional chest tube therapy for iatrogenic pneumothorax. Chest 104:1170–1172, 1993.
9. Timby J, Reed C, Zeilender S, Glauser FL: "Mechanical" causes of pulmonary edema. Chest 98:973, 1990.
10. Wilkerson PD, Keegan J, Davies SW, et al: Changes in pulmonary microvascular permeability accompanying re-expansion oedema: Evidence from dual isotope scintigraphy. Thorax 45:456, 1990.

14. BRONCHOSCOPY

Catherine M. Lee, M.D., and Lynn M. Schnapp, M.D.

1. What is flexible bronchoscopy?

Bronchoscopy literally means "to see the airways" and provides a means to visualize the upper airways, trachea, and bronchi. Flexible bronchoscopy uses a small-caliber fiberoptic scope, which is passed either through the nose or mouth or through a tracheostomy or endotracheal tube. The bronchoscope is then directed down the trachea to the main carina and the regions of interest. In most patients, the airways can be well visualized to the segmental bronchi,and often a few generations beyond.

2. How is flexible bronchoscopy performed?

Flexible bronchoscopy can be performed either at the bedside or in a specialized suite with the assistance of a nurse and a respiratory therapist. The preparation for the procedure involves (1) numbing of the nose, pharynx, and upper airways with topical lidocaine; (2) monitoring of cardiac rhythm, blood pressure, and oxygenation and set-up of suction; (3) further control of cough, gag, and anxiety using small doses of short-acting narcotic and benzodiazepines; (4) addition of supplemental oxygen; and (5) lubrication of the bronchoscope. Anesthesia of the posterior pharynx and vocal cords is important, because passing the bronchoscope through the glottis is the least tolerated part of the procedure.

A spontaneously breathing patient scheduled to undergo flexible bronchoscopy without an artificial airway or mechanical ventilation should be cooperative, without violent coughing, and without risk for upper airway obstruction or hypoxic or hypercarbic respiratory failure. In all cases, equipment for endotracheal intubation should be easily accessible, although it is rarely needed.

3. How is bronchoscopy different for patients receiving mechanical ventilation?

Fiberoptic bronchoscopy can be performed through an endotracheal tube ≥ 7.5 mm by using a special adapter. Topical anesthesia is limited to 1–2 ml of lidocaine through the endotracheal tube. A silicone-based lubricant applied to the bronchoscope facilitates passage through the endotracheal tube. The bronchoscope will partially obstruct the endotracheal tube, leading to increased airway pressure and potentially to air trapping. The respiratory therapist should set the ventilator on a volume mode with increased peak airway pressure limits to ensure that the patient receives adequate minute ventilation. The fractional concentration of oxygen in inspired gas (FiO_2) should be increased (usually to 1.0) because short-lived hypoxia may result from bronchoscopy and lavage.

4. What is rigid bronchoscopy?

Rigid bronchoscopy is performed through a rigid hollow tube that provides a large working channel, direct illumination, and an attachment to allow mechanical ventilation during the procedure. This technique is preferable to flexible bronchoscopy when more suction is required (as in the workup of hemoptysis); in the removal of tenacious or copious secretions or foreign bodies; in the surgical or laser removal of endobronchial lesions; and in the placement of endobronchial stents. The procedure is performed under general anesthesia in the operating room by thoracic surgeons or interventional pulmonologists and requires a stable cervical spine and manipulation of the mandible.

5. What are the usual indications for bronchoscopy in the intensive care unit (ICU)?

Bronchoscopy allows inspection of the airways, collection of samples from the lower airways, and performance of various interventions.

	Indication	Goal
Inspection	Hemoptysis	Localization of bleeding
		Search for endobronchial lesion
	Infection	Evidence of inflammation or pus
	Aspiration	Look for foreign bodies
	Mass	Look for endobronchial masses
	Chest trauma	Evidence of airway injury
	Inhalational injury	Evicence of airway injury
Sample collection	Pulmonary infiltrates (infectious)	Samples for Gram stain, silver stain, bacterial cultures, viral and fungal studies
	Pulmonary infiltrates (noninfectious)	Alevolar hemorrhage
		Eosinophilia (cell differential and count)
	Mass or adenopathy	Transbronchial biopsy for cytology/pathology
Interventions	Hemoptysis	Control bleeding
	Bronchial obstruction	Removal ormucus or foreign bodies
		Laser removal of masses
		Stent placement
	Alveolar proteinosis	Lavage
	Intubation	Visualization of anatomy for tube placement

6. List the absolute and relative contraindications for bronchoscopy.

Absolute contraindications include inability to maintain a patent airway during the procedure (such as upper airway obstruction, laryngospasm, or intubation with a small endotracheal tube); inability to oxygenate or ventilate adequately during bronchoscopy; active cardiac ischemia; malignant arrhythmias; and severe hemodynamic instability.

Relative contraindications include poor patient cooperation, elevated intracranial pressure, presence of lung abscess, and severe coagulopathy. Patients with impending respiratory failure or laryngeal edema may undergo bronchoscopy more safely if the airway is secured by elective endotracheal intubation before the procedure.

7. What are the potential complications of bronchoscopy?

Flexible bronchoscopy is generally a safe procedure. However, complications do occur, with an incidence in observational studies of 0.1% for death and 2–5% for major complications. Sources of complication include the bronchoscopy itself, bronchoscopic procedures, and anesthetic/sedative medications.

Intervention	Potential Complication	Prevention
Passing bronchoscope through nose	Epistaxis, nasal discomfort	Topical anesthesia and vasoconstriction
Passing bronchoscope through pharynx	Gagging, emesis, aspiration	Topical anesthesia, benzodiazepines
Passing bronchoscope into trachea	Laryngospasm, laryngeal trauma	Topical anesthesia
	Bronchospasm	Pretreatment with beta agonists
Bronchoalveolar lavage	Postoperative fever	Minimize lung contamination by oral secretions
	Hypoxemia	Supplemental oxgen; good wedge technique
Cytology brush	Endobronchial hemorrhage	Avoid vascular lesions
Transbronchial biopsy	Hemorrhage	Avoid vascular lesions
	Pneumothorax	Avoid distal biopsies; consider fluoroscopy

Continued on following page

Topical lidocaine administration	Arrhythmias, seizures	Use < 7 mg/kg (< 25 ml of 2% lidocaine)
Conscious sedation	Hypotension	IV access, prehydration in hypovolemic patients
	Respiratory depression	Avoid oversedation, stimulate patient

8. What kinds of samples can be collected by bronchoscopy?

Bronchoscopy allows collection of samples by wash, brush, biopsy, or aspiration. The most common samples collected in the ICU are **bronchoalveolar lavage (BAL)** and **protected specimen brush**. In BAL the tip of the bronchoscope is wedged into a distal airway (e.g., subsegmental bronchus) while 5- to 30-ml aliquots of saline are injected and aspirated into sterile traps. This technique allows collection of alveolar cells while preventing flooding of other regions of the lung and is used most commonly in the diagnosis of infection. With the protected specimen brush technique, a sterile brush with a gelatin cap is inserted into a potentially infected area, then removed an placed in 1 mm of sterile saline and sent for culture. Other sample collections include:

Cytology brush: an abrasive brush that is agitated against potentially malignant tissue and then sent for cytologic analysis.

Transbronchial biopsy: biopsy forceps are pushed past distal airways outward into the pulmonary parenchyma to obtain lung tissue samples. This technique may be used to diagnose infection (i.e., miliary tuberculosis), other granulomatous diseases (e.g., sarcoidosis, hypersensitivity pneumonitis), or malignancy.

Wang needle aspiration: a short, rigid needle is thrust through the airway, usually near the main carina, to sample subcarinal or paratracheal lymph nodes. Suction is then applied to attempt to aspirate cells. This technique can be used in diagnosis and staging of cancer.

9. Can BAL be safely performed in patients with the acute respiratory distress syndrome (ARDS)?

Yes—if the partial arterial oxygen tension (PaO$_2$) is at least 80 mmHg (with an FiO$_2$ as high as 1.0) and if the patient has no other absolute contraindications for bronchoscopy. A study of 110 patients with ARDS who met these criteria found no significant morbidity or mortality associated with bronchoscopy and BAL. The protocol included sedation to improve patient cooperation and to minimize coughing during the procedure. The investigators found a nonsustained decrease in oxygen saturation (to < 90%) in 4.5% of patients. Mild, self-limited bleeding followed the procedure in 34% of patient.

10. Discuss the role of bronchoscopy in the management of hemoptysis in the ICU.

Hemoptysis that warrants admission to the ICU is generally massive, defined as expectoration of ≥ 100 ml of blood within 24 hours. Initial management of hemoptysis includes airway protection (because the danger of hemoptysis is suffocation, not exsanguination), localization of the site of bleeding, and interventions to prevent further bleeding and contamination of the remaining lung.

Bronchoscopy can plan a role both in localization of the bleeding source and in aiding cessation of hemorrhage. Although a chest radiograph may suggest the location of hemorrhage, aspirated blood to other parts of the lung may limit the specificity of plain films. Bronchoscopy within the first 48 hours may reveal the bleeding source and, in certain cases (such as bronchitis), the cause.

When bleeding is brisk, the small suction channel of the flexible bronchoscope may be overwhelmed; in such cases, rigid bronchoscopy may be preferable. For patients unable to expectorate the blood adequately, endotracheal intubation and mechanical ventilation may be needed, followed by either fiberoptic or rigid bronchoscopy.

If the site of bleeding is identified by bronchoscopy, several maneuvers may lead to cessation of bleeding. Local injection of cold saline, epinephrine, vasopressin, and fibrin as well as laser or electrocautery can be performed via the bronchoscope. Methods of tamponade also have been described, using the tip of the bronchoscope or a Fogerty balloon placed through the suction channel of the bronchoscope. In patients with continued bleeding, interventional radiology (IR) may help better localize the bleed, and either IR embolization or surgical resection may be warranted.

Bronchoscopy is particularly useful early in the management of patients with less vigorous hemoptysis and normal chest radiographs when the possibility of an endobronchial malignancy or foreign body aspiration exists. Such cases rarely present to the ICU.

11. Describe the role of bronchoscopy in potential lung donors.

Bronchoscopy is routinely performed on potential lung donors before the decision is made to perform lung explantation. The purpose of this examination is threefold. First, the anatomy of the airways is assessed. Second, the operator searches for evidence of airway trauma, infection, or previous aspiration; it is likely that the lungs will be rejected if any of these is found. Third, samples are taken and sent for culture so that the microbiologic flora (if present) can be known before transplantation and covered in the recipient, who soon will be heavily immunosuppressed.

12. Is bronchoscopy indicated for management of patients with acute lobar atelectasis?

Probably not. A randomized, controlled trial revealed that therapeutic bronchoscopy combined with vigorous respiratory therapy was no better than the respiratory therapy alone. The therapy consisted of 3 minutes of 1- to 2-liter inflations, provoked cough, and percussive chest physiotherapy, all performed every 4 hours. The authors concluded that bronchoscopy was not routinely indicated in patients with acute lobar atelectasis. However, certain cases may benefit from bronchoscopic intervention, such as removal of retained, inspissated secretions or the possibility of a covert foreign body.

13. When is bronchoscopy required in the evaluation of pneumonia?

Community-acquired pneumonia in an immunocompetent host does not require microbiologic confirmation and is typically treated with empirical antibiotics. However, the diagnosis of pneumonia becomes more complicated in patients with preexisting lung disease or critical illness, and the microbiologic flora involved become more varied and less predictable. In addition, for patients failing conventional treatment for community-acquired pneumonia, BAL with or without biopsies may provide information about bacterial resistance, atypical organisms, or the presence of noninfectious pneumonitis.

Pulmonary infiltrates in an immunosuppressed host generally cannot be treated empirically, because the differential diagnosis is broad and includes a long list of infectious and noninfectious etiologies. Bronchoscopy is used to diagnose many infectious agents by collecting samples that are analyzed by culture, special stains, and serologies. These methods are useful in the diagnosis of *Pneumocystis carinii*, atypical bacteria, viruses (e.g., cytomegalovirus, respiratory syncytial virus, adenovirus), fungal pathogens, and mycobacteria. In addition, bronchoscopy and cytology may reveal alveolar hemorrhage, malignancy, or other noninfectious sources.

14. Discuss the role of bronchoscopy in the diagnosis and management of ventilator-associated pneumonia (VAP).

The clinical diagnosis of VAP is made when an intubated patient develops a fever or leukocytosis, a new infiltrate on chest radiograph, and purulent tracheal secretions. However, this presumptive diagnosis is more sensitive than specific; many patients in ICUs meet these three criteria without having pneumonia.

A recent study compared the clinical diagnosis of VAP with an invasive strategy, in which bronchoscopy and either a protected specimen brush (PSB) or BAL was performed. The samples were then sent for quantitative cultures. PSB with at least 10^3 colonies of bacteria, or BAL with at least 10^4 colonies of bacteria was considered diagnostic for VAP. The cut-offs were based on previous studies that compared culture results with warm autopsy specimens and found that these colony counts correlated with histologic evidence of pneumonia. In the invasive arm, only the patients with positive bronchoscopy results were treated for VAP, with antibiotics tailored according to microbiologic results. Negative bronchoscopy led to discontinuation of empirical antibiotics and search for nonpulmonary sites of infection. The investigators found that the invasive arm was associated with less antibiotic use and lower 14-day mortality rate than the noninvasive, empirical approach.

Thus, bronchoscopic diagnosis of VAP and adjustment of antibiotics (or search for cause of infection elsewhere) is becoming standard of care in many medical centers.

15. Should transbronchial biopsy be performed in patients receiving mechanical ventilation?
Mechanical ventilation increases the risk of bleeding and pneumothorax associated with transbronchial biopsy. A report of 15 mechanically ventilated patients who underwent bronchoscopy with transbronchial biopsies under fluoroscopy revealed that 3 patients had self-limited endobronchial bleeding and 1 patient had a tension pneumothorax. Important information was obtained in over half of the cases. Mechanical ventilation, therefore, is not an absolute complication to transbronchial biopsy, which may provide a less morbid alternative to surgical lung biopsy in selected cases. In light of the complication rate, the bronchoscopist should be prepared to manage potential hemorrhage and pneumothorax.

BIBLIOGRAPHY

1. Fagon JY, Chastre J, Wolff M, et al: Invasive and noninvasive strategies for management of sduspected ventilator-associated pneumonia. Ann Intern Med 132:621–630, 2000.
2. Hertz MI, Woodward ME, Gross CR, et al: Safety of bronchoalveolar lavage in the critically ill mechanically ventilated patient. Crit Care Med 19:1526–1532, 1991.
3. Marini JJ, Pierson DJ, Hudson LD: Acute lobar atelectasis: A prospective comparison of fiberoptic bronchoscopy and respiratory therapy. Am Rev Respir Dis 119:971–978, 1979.
4. Pisani RJ, Wright AJ: Clinical utility of bronchoalveolar lavage in immunocompromised hosts. Mayo Clin Proc 67:221–227, 1992.
5. Seijo LM and Sterman DH: Interventional Pulmonology. N Engl J Med 344:740–749, 2001.
6. Steinberg KP Mitchell DR, Maunder RJ, et al: Safety of bronchoalveolar lavage in patients with acute respiratory distress syndrome. Am Rev Respir Dis 148:556–561, 1993.
7. Wang KP, Mehta AC (eds): Flexible Bronchoscopy. Cambridge, Blackwell Scientific, 1995.

15. PACEMAKERS AND DEFIBRILLATORS

Linda Liu, M.D.

1. What is the NASPE/BPEG Generic (NBG) Pacemaker Code?
In 1987 the North American Society of Pacing and Electrophysiology (NASPE) together with the British Pacing and Electrophysiology Group (BPEG) developed a pacemaker code that replaced the older 3- and 5-letter codes and incorporated the newer characteristics of the modern pacemaker.

The NASPE/BPEG Generic (NBG) Pacemaker Code

POSITION	I	II	III	IV	V
Category	Chamber(s) paced	Chamber(s) sensed	Response to sensing	Programmability, rate modulation	Antiarrhythmia function(s)
Letters:	O = none	O = none	O = none	O = none	O = none
	A = atrium	A = atrium	T = triggered	P = simple programmable	P = pacing (anti-tachyarrhythmia)
	V = ventricle	V = ventricle	I = inhibited	M = multiprogrammable	
	D = dual (A+V)	D = dual (A+V)	D = dual (T+I)	C = communicating	S = shock
				R = rate modulation	D = dual (P+S)

For example, a VVIMD pacemaker is a multiprogrammable ventricular pacemaker, inhibited by ventricular sensing, with defibrillation (or cardioversion) and antiarrhythmia-pacing capabilities.

2. What are the major indications for cardiac pacing?
- Acquired atrioventicular (AV) block
- AV block associated with myocardial infarction
- Bifascicular and trifascicular block
- Sick sinus syndrome
- Hypersensitive carotid sinus syndrome

In recent years several new indications for permanent pacemakers have evolved, including hypertropic cardiomyopathy, dilated cardiomyopathy, orthostatic hypotension, long Q-T interval, atrial fibrillation, syncope and bradyarrythmias after orthotopic heart transplant, postoperative block that is not expected to resolve, and neuromuscular diseases with AV block.

3. What are the contraindications to temporary pacing?
Cardiac pacing is contraindicated in the presence of profound hypothermia. Under these conditions, refractory fibrillation can be induced. Relative contraindications include digitalis toxicity with recurrent ventricular tachycardia, impassable tricuspid valve prosthesis, and a bleeding diathesis.

4. Which access sites can be used for transvenous pacing?
The preferred sites are the right internal jugular and left subclavian veins, although the external jugular, brachial, cephalic, and femoral sites also can be used.

5. What is the advantage of dual-chamber pacing vs. ventricular pacing?
The advantage of dual-chamber pacing is its ability to maintain AV synchrony. The atria are responsible for 25–30% of ventricular filling. The loss of "atrial kick" can cause hypotension and decreased cardiac output in some patients.

6. What is the pacing threshold? How is it determined?
The threshold is the amount of energy needed to capture the atrium and/or ventricle. The level is determined by gradually decreasing the output in milliamperes (mA) until 1:1 capture is lost. The threshold should then be set at 2–3 times the current at which capture is lost.

7. Describe pacemaker-mediated tachycardia.
In dual-chamber pacemakers, the atrial lead may sense a retrograde P wave conducted from a premature ventricular contraction or paced ventricular beat, which triggers a ventricular depolarization after the programmed atrioventricular delay. The paced beat may conduct retrograde again and set off a sustained tachycardia. This complication is rare in the more recent pacemakers with programmable atrial refractoriness.

8. List complications associated with temporary cardiac pacing.
- Pericardial friction rub
- Abdominal twitchings or hiccups
- Dysrhythmia
- Perforation of the ventricular wall or septum
- Local infection and phlebitis
- Inadvertent arterial puncture
- Pneumothorax
- Cardiac tamponade

9. Should a temporary pacemaker be placed during pulmonary artery (PA) line placement in a patient with preexisting left bundle-branch block (LBBB)?
In the past, pacing was recommended in patients with preexisting LBBB as a prophylactic measure against PA catheter-induced right bundle-branch block (RBBB). However, this precaution probably is not necessary. A recent retrospective study found no incidence of complete heart block during PA line placement in 38 patients with LBBB that was chronic (> 1 month) or of indeterminate age. Ready access to transthoracic pacing is an adequate precaution.

10. Describe the benefits of rate-adaptive pacemakers.

Rate-adaptive pacemakers have sensors that can increase the pacing rate with exercise and demand. They are identifiable by the letter R in the fourth position of the NASPE/BPEG Generic (NBG) pacemaker code (e.g., DDDR vs. DDD). Many studies have shown that rate-adaptive pacing modes lead to subjective improvement in energy level, objective improvement in exercise tolerance, and measurable improvement in cardiac output and other hemodynamic variables.

11. What determines the probability of successful defibrillation for a patient in ventricular fibrillation (VF)?

The probability of successful defibrillation is related directly to the time interval to delivery of the first shock. The earlier defibrillation is performed, the higher the rate of survival. After 10 minutes, the success rate of defibrillation is almost 0%.

12. Why is it important to select an appropriate energy level for defibrillation?

An energy level that is too low will not terminate the arrhythmia, whereas cardiac damage may result if the energy level is too high. The appropriate current also reduces the required number of repetitive shocks and reduces the amount of damage to the heart. Unfortunately, there is no absolute relationship between adult body sizes and energy requirements because transthoracic impedance plays an important role.

13. What determines the defibrillation threshold?

The defibrillation threshold varies markedly among patients for many reasons. Variation in transthoracic impedance is affected by interelectrode distance, electrode size, electrode–chest wall contact pressure, use of conductive paste, and respiratory phase. Impedance also decreases after repeated shocks, partly because of hyperemia and edema in the current pathway. Factors other than impedance include drugs. For example, lidocaine can increase the defibrillation threshold by as much as 50%, whereas beta agonists and aminophylline lower the defibrillation threshold.

14. Where should the defibrillator electrodes be placed?

The goal in electrode placement is to maximize current flow through the myocardium. The standard placement is to the right of the upper sternal border below the clavicle and to the left of the nipple with the electrode on the midaxillary line. An anterior/posterior position is also acceptable (one electrode over the precordium and the second electrode posterior to the heart in the right infrascapular location).

15. Compare monophasic waveform and biphasic waveform defibrillators.

Monophasic waveforms deliver current in one direction. Biphasic waveforms deliver current that flows in a positive direction and then reverses in the negative direction for the remainder of the electrical discharge. Recent studies indicate that low-energy biphasic waveforms achieve equivalent clinical outcomes compared with monophasic waveforms using much higher energy levels. Modern defibrillators are beginning to use biphasic waveforms.

16. What is an AED?

Automated external defibrillators (AEDs) are computerized, portable devices that allow lay rescuers to provide defibrillation during cardiac arrest with minimal training. AEDs are placed in airports, airplanes, casinos, office buildings, and other public locations. They analyze multiple features of the electrocardiogram and advise shock for ventricular fibrillation and monomorphic or polymorphic ventricular tachycardia.

17. Decribe the recommended use of AEDS in children.

Cardiac arrest is less common in children than adults, and most arrests are caused by sudden infant death syndrome or respiratory disease. When pediatric cardiac arrest rhythms are reported, estimates of VF range from 7% to 15%. Currently available AEDs deliver charges that exceed the recommended dose of 2–4 J/kg, and human pediatric data related to sensitivity, specificity, safety, and efficacy are extremely limited. For these reasons, use of AEDs in infants and children younger than 8 years or weighing less than 25 kg is not recommended.

18. List the components of an implantable cardiac defibrillator system.
• Power source (lithium iodide battery)
• Lead system (usually placed transvenously)
• Bradycarida pacing (device paces at a faster rate in the event of bradycardia to prevent symptomatic bradyarrhythmias)
• Antitachycardia pacing (various pacing algorithms or a shock can be used for ventricular tachycardia)
• Memory (used to assess efficacy of therapy or to trouble-shoot the system)

19. What complications are associated with implantable cardiac defibrillators?
• Pocket problems (infection, hematoma, erosion into other structures, migration)
• Sensing problems (failure to sense intrinsic cardiac potentials due to loose wires or sensing of artifacts due to myopotentials from the chest wall or diaphragm)
• Increased defibrillator thresholds (due to worsening heart function, ischemia, or drugs such as amiodarone or mexiletine, which alter the threshold)
• Increased pacing thresholds (due to drugs or lead dislodgment)

20. Define synchronized cardioversion.
Energy delivered during the refractory period of the cardiac cycle can induce VF. In synchronized cardioversion, the energy is delivered during the QRS complex to reduce the possibility of inducing VF. Synchronization is recommended for all hemodynamically stable wide complex tachycardias requiring cardioversion, superventricular tachycardia, atrial fibrillation, and atrial flutter. Patients in ventricular tachycardia may be difficult to synchronize, and if symptoms of low perfusion are present, patients should receive unsynchronized shocks to avoid delay.

BIBLIOGRAPHY

1. American Heart Association: The automated external defibrillator: Key link in the chain of survival. Guidelines 2000 for cardiopulmonary resuscitation and emergency cardiovascular care. Circulation 102(Suppl I):I-60–I-76, 2000.
2. American Heart Association: Defibrillation. Guidelines 2000 for cardiopulmonary resuscitation and emergency cardiovascular care. Circulation 102(Suppl I):I-90–I-94, 2000.
3. Glikson M, Hayes DL: Cardiac pacingd: A review. Med Clin North Am 85:369–422, 2001.
4. Gollob MH, Seger JJ: Current status of the implantable cardioverter-defibrillator. Chest 119:1210–1221, 2001.
5. Gregoratos G, Cheitlin MD, Conill A, et al: ACC/AHA guidelines for implantation of cardiac pacemakers and antiarrhythmia devices: Exectuive summary. A report of the American College of Cardiology/ American Heart Association Task Force on Practice Guidelines (Committee on Pacemaker Implantation). Circulation 97:1325–1335, 1998.
6. Peters RW, Gold MR: Implantable cardiac defibrillators. Med Clin North Am 85:343–368, 2001.

16. CIRCULATORY ASSIST DEVICES

Lundy Campbell, M.D., and David Shimabukuro, M.D.C.M.

1. What is an intra-aortic balloon pump (IABP)?

An IABP consists of a large control module (monitors, software, pump, gas cylinder) attached to a catheter that has an externally mounted balloon. The balloon catheter is placed into the patient while the control module remains outside. Via the control module, the balloon is set to inflate just after the closure of the aortic valve, at the onset of diastole, and to actively deflate just before the opening of the aortic valve (systole). The balloon is normally inflated with 40 ml of helium (low viscosity) or carbon dioxide (high blood solubility).

2. How is an IABP placed into the patient?

In most patients, the balloon catheter is percutaneously introduced into the femoral or iliac artery through a sheath. The catheter is advanced until the tip is just distal to the take-off of the left subclavian artery while also ensuring that the balloon remains above the level of the renal arteries. Fluoroscopic guidance is most often used to achieve proper placement. The catheter can also be properly positioned under direct visualization intraoperatively when a sternotomy or thoracotomy has already been performed. If the femoral and iliac arteries are severely diseased, the IABP catheter can be placed via a transthoracic route by a cardiovascular surgeon.

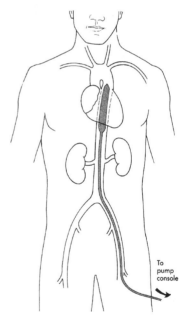

IABP placement: balloon tip is distal to the left subclavian artery and balloon end is proximal ot the renal arteries. (From Flynn J, Bruch N: Introduction to Critical Care Skills. St. Louis, Mosby, 1993, p 262, 262, with permission.)

To pump console

3. What are the goals of intra-aortic balloon counterpulsation?

The primary goal of an IABP is to improve myocardial function by increasing myocardial oxygen supply and decreasing myocardial oxygen demand. Secondary gains include an increase in cardiac output, ejection fraction, and increased coronary perfusion pressure resulting in an improvement in systemic perfusion with a decrease in heart rate, pulmonary capillary wedge pressure, and systemic vascular resistance.

4. How does an IABP accomplish these goals?

Coronary blood flow and myocardial oxygen supply are improved by balloon inflation that leads to augmentation of diastolic pressure and blood flow to the failing heart. The balloon on the catheter is set to inflate at the onset of diastole (at closure of the aortic valve or at the dicrotic notch on an arterial waveform). The inflation of the balloon causes retrograde blood flow and an increase in pressure toward the aortic root, thereby increasing coronary perfusion pressure. This increase in perfusion pressure improves oxygen delivery and can improve cardiac performance in an ischemic myocardium. Ideally, the augmented diastolic pressure should be greater than the patient's unassisted systolic pressure.

Balloon deflation causes unloading during systole, thus decreasing the workload of the left ventricle and decreasing myocardial oxygen demand. Specifically, at the end of diastole and just at the start of systole, the balloon is set to deflate rapidly, leaving an area of markedly decreased volume and pressure. The low pressure in this region decreases the afterload of the left ventricle, resulting in an improvement in cardiac output and end-organ perfusion. This decrease in afterload should be represented as a balloon-assisted end-diastolic pressure that is less than the patient's unassisted end-diastolic pressure.

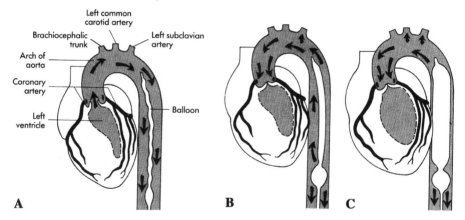

A, Balloon deflation decreases left ventricular afterload. *B* and *C,* Balloon inflation increases coronary perfusion pressure. (From Flynn J, Bruce N: Introduction to Critical Care Skills. St. Louis, Mosby, 1993, p 262, with permission.)

IABP waveform. A, End-disatolic pressure; B, systolic pressure; C, dicrotic notch (balloon inflates); D, augmented diastolic pressure; E, assisted end-diastolic pressure. (From Flynn J, Bruce N: Introduction to Critical Care Skills. St. Louis, Mosby, 1993, p 269, with permission.)

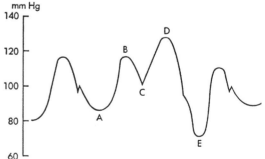

5. What are the indications for placement of an IABP?

The most common indications for the use of an IABP are left ventricular failure, cardiogenic shock, or unstable angina refractory to medical therapy. Other applications include use as a bridge to coronary artery bypass grafting (CABG) after high-risk or failed percutaneous transluminal coronary angioplasty (PTCA) or to cardiac transplant in end-stage heart failure. It is also placed in patients who are unable to wean from cardiopulmonary bypass during cardiac surgery.

6. What are the contraindications to the use of an IABP?

The major absolute contraindications are structural aortic problems, such as dissection or aneurysm, in which IABP use could lead to a worsening of the aortic injury or even rupture. In addition, aortic valvular insufficiency negates the effectiveness of the device and may even worsen cardiac output by increasing the regurgitant fraction. Although severe peripheral vascular disease is not an absolute contraindication to IABP placement, one needs to consider that the catheter can more readily cause lower limb ischemia or infarct. Finally, its use in patients with no hope of recovery should be very carefully evaluated and the benefits clearly defined.

7. How is the IABP controlled?

Proper use of the IABP consists of setting the augmentation frequency ratio as well as adjusting the timing of the start of balloon inflation and deflation. The augmentation frequency ratio refers to how often the balloon inflates with respect to the cardiac cycle. Maximal support occurs when the balloon inflates with each cardiac cycle, also known as a 1:1 ratio. Less support can be obtained by sequentially decreasing the augmentation ratio to 1:2 or 1:3 (i.e., the balloon inflates once every second or third cardiac cycle). As the augmentation ratio is decreased, the risk of forming a thrombus on the balloon significantly increases; thus, a ratio of 1:3 should not be used for a prolonged period.

The triggering of balloon inflation and active deflation can be accomplished by several means: (1) the R-wave on the electrocardiogram (ECG); (2) the arterial waveform; (3) ventricular pacemaker spikes; or (4) a preset rate. Of these, the most common method is the ECG R-wave. Triggering from the R-wave causes balloon inflation to begin in the middle of the T-wave and active balloon deflation to occur just before the start of the QRS complex. Newer IABP devices can trigger appropriately even if the patient is in atrial fibrillation. The exact timing of balloon inflation and deflation can be manually adjusted. If the ECG cannot be used for any reason (i.e., too much artifact during patient transport), most clinicians use the arterial waveform as a second choice.

8. What are the potential complications with IABP use?

Although complications can arise from anywhere within the IABP device secondary to mechanical failure, the most common complications are related to the presence of the intra-aortic balloon catheter itself and the technique used for insertion. The movement of the balloon causes trauma to the formed elements of blood, leading to anemia and thrombocytopenia. There may also be platelet dysfunction or activation of clotting factors, which may result in disseminated intravascular coagulation (DIC), arterial thrombosis, and embolization. Because of the risk of thrombus formation and the possibility of an embolus, patients with an IABP catheter are systemically anticoagulated. Thus, bleeding at the insertion site tends to occur quite frequently. In addition, other complications that may occur at the site of insertion include infection or pseudoaneurysm formation. Furthermore, improper technique with device insertion can result in incorrect positioning with loss of effective diastolic augmentation, possible limb or visceral ischemia, or aortic dissection or perforation, leading to massive hemorrhage. Finally, the balloon can perforate or rupture, causing a gas embolus and device ineffectiveness.

9. How are patients weaned from IABP support?

To be successfully weaned from IABP support, patients must not be in cardiogenic shock. They should have an adequate blood pressure and cardiac output on little or no vasopressor or inotropic support. A mean arterial pressure ≥ 65 mm Hg and a cardiac index > 2 L/min/m^2 are the usual criteria. Weaning is generally accomplished by decreasing the augmentation ratio every 1–6 hours, as tolerated, until a ratio of 1:3 is achieved. The balloon catheter can then be removed when the patient is no longer anticoagulated. An alternative strategy for IABP weaning is to decrease the balloon filling volume by 10 ml every 1–6 hours until a final filling volume of 20 ml is reached.

10. What are the four major types of ventricular assist devices (VADs)?

1. Two types of **extracorporal nonpulsatile VADs** are currently in use. Of the two, the more common is the centrifugal pump. Continuous flow is generated via centrifugal forces created at the base of the pump using a spinning impeller. Roller pumps, although much more familiar, are

not used as frequently, probably because of the effects on red blood cells. Flows of up to 5 L/min can be generated with either device.

2. **Extracorporal pulsatile pumps** are either pneumatic or electric. In pneumatic pumps, compressed gas is "driven" during systole into a pneumatic chamber adjacent to the blood sac, which is then squeezed with resultant ejection of blood. During diastole, the gas is actively removed, causing a vacuum effect that draws blood into the blood sac. Electric pumps operate on the same basic principle but use a piston and plate to compress the blood sac for ejection during systole. Whether the pumps are nonpulsatile or pulsatile, the term *extracorporal* implies that the device chambers and/or pump mechanism remain external.

3. Presently, the **totally implantable pulsatile type** is the most commonly used VAD as a bridge to transplant and as an aid to cardiac recovery. Of these, the most advanced portable left ventricular assist systems (LVAS) are the Thoratec Heartmate and Baxter's Novacor. Both devices can operate in either a fixed mode or, more frequently, an automatic mode that mimics normal physiology. In the automatic mode, the device ejects when the pump is 90% full; it detects a reduction in the rate of filling or senses an increase in native heart rate. Thus, as the patient's workload increases, the pump fills faster and cardiac output correspondingly increases to meet the demand. The cannulas are typically placed through the diaphragm, with the device chambers implanted in the abdomen and the control module with power source remaining external (normally on a belt or shoulder strap carried by the patient).

4. **Total artificial hearts** are not approved by the Food and Drug Association (FDA) for general use, although clinical trials are ongoing.

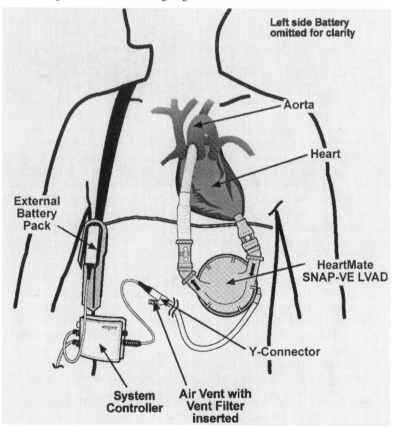

The HeartMate, a totally implantable VAD. (Reprinted with permission from Thoractec Corporation.)

11. How does a VAD work?

VADs can be used to assist the right (RVAD), left (LVAD), or both ventricles (BiVAD). When placed temporarily, the cannulas are normally inserted into the atria with blood returned to the pulmonary artery or aorta. If the device is to be used as a bridge to cardiac transplantation, the cannulas are inserted into the apices of the heart. Regardless of the exact device used, its placement, and its components, VADs are capable of supporting up to 100% of the cardiac output, thereby bypassing the need for any ventricular work or activity.

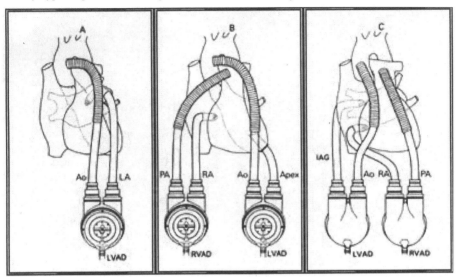

Examples of ventricular assist devices. A, LVAD. B and C, BiVADs with the left inflow cannulas at different locations. (Reprinted with permission from Thoratec Corporation.)

12. What are the indications for the placement of a VAD?

VADs are used in patients as a bridge to cardiac transplantation or as an aid in cardiac recovery. Possible transplant patients include those with chronic heart failure or acute decompensation of chronic heart failure, postcardiotomy failure, or acute myocardial infarction (MI) in an already failing heart. Patients who may benefit from VAD support as an aid in recovery include those with severe myocarditis, severe ventricular arrhythmias unresponsive to pharmacologic therapy, postcardiotomy failure, or acute MI with resulting heart failure.

13. How are patients selected for VAD support?

Once maximal pharmacologic and IABP therapy prove unsuccessful, most clinicians use the following parameters to consider initiation of VAD support:

Cardiac index (CI) < 2 L/min/m^2
Systolic blood pressure (SBP) < 80 mmHg
Mean arterial pressure (MAP) < 65 mmHg
Systemic vascular resistance (SVR) > 2100 dynes/sec/cm^5
Urine output (UOP) < 20 ml/hr
Pulmonary capillary wedge pressure (PCWP) > 20 mmHg

14. What are the contraindications for VAD use?

Contraindications for VAD placement include severe multiorgan system disease or failure from which the patient is not expected to recover. In addition, disease states that cause patients to be too unstable to undergo surgical placement of the device with significant risk of death can be considered as contraindications. Specific examples include (but are not limited to) the following:

• Severe obstructive or restrictive pulmonary disease
• Severe pulmonary hypertension
• Right heart failure or CVP > 20 mmHg
• Prothrombin time (PT) >16 sec from liver failure or DIC
• Dialysis-dependent renal failure
• Sepsis or current infection
• Irreversible severe cerebral injury

Not considered as a contraindication, structural heart defects should be repaired before or at the time of,VAD placement. Intracardiac septal defects need to be repaired to avoid right-to-left shunting from sudden left ventricular unloading after initiation of VAD support. Preexisting mitral stenosis, mitral regurgitation, or aortic insufficiency may require correction before or during VAD implantation, as both significantly reduce cardiac output even with the device.

15. What are the possible complications of VAD placement?

1. **Bleeding.** Hemorrhage is the most prevalent complication associated with VAD placement. Causes of major bleeding include preoperative coagulopathy due to hepatic dysfunction, poor nutritional status, antibiotic therapy, and cardiopulmonary bypass-induced thrombocytopenia and platelet dysfunction. Historically, the risk of major hemorrhage has been reported to be approximately 50%. The current risk has been reduced to 30% with the routine use of the serine protease inhibitor, aprotinin.

2. **Infection.** Postoperative patients are prone to nosocomial and device-related infections. Infection occurs most commonly at the cannula sites. Such infections are managed primarily with antibiotics and local wound care. Clinically important infections occur in approximately 25% of patients and are caused by both gram-positive cocci (*Staphylcoccus aureus, Staphylcoccus epidermidis*) and gram-negative rods (*Pseudomonas aeruginosa*). On rare occasion, the entire VAD must be replaced because of significant infection or sepsis. Prophylactic antimicrobial therapy is initiated at the time of placement but discontinued if there are no signs of infection. Because of the location of the device in the chest cavity, patients are also prone to atelectasis with subsequent development of pneumonia. Therefore, aggressive respiratory therapy is vital.

3. **Thromboembolism.** At the beginning of VAD use, approximately 20% of patients suffered a thromboembolic event. The current rate of major embolic events is reported to be as low as 0.01 per patient-month. This significant decrease is attributed to the use of textured blood-contacting surfaces within the VAD itself, which prevent thrombus formation. Although major embolic events have decreased, asymptomatic cerebral microemboli continue to occur in 34–67% of recipients. Systemic anticoagulation remains controversial at present.

4. **Right ventricular failure.** Historically, severe right heart failure, which required the implantation of an RVAD, occurred in 20% of patients in whom an LVAD was placed. Fortunately, improved perioperative management and use of inhaled nitric oxide have decreased the need for RVAD placement over the past several years. The major risk factor for right heart failure is perioperative hemorrhage necessitating multiple blood transfusions. As a result of severe bleeding, the cytokines interleukin (IL)-1β, IL-6, IL-10, and tumor necrosis factor alpha are released into the circulation. These cytokines, in turn, mediate the release of platelet-activating factor, which causes vasoconstriction of the pulmonary vasculature, thus inducing pulmonary hypertension and subsequent right heart failure.

5. **Device malfunction.** Only anecdotal reports of device malfunction exist. For the extracorporeal devices, manual manipulation allows continuous blood flow (pulsatile or nonpulsatile) if the external pump loses power. All of the reported malfunctions were easily repairable, and none caused hemodynamic instability in the device recipient.

6. **Other end-organ failure.** Patients who receive VADs are at very high-risk for sepsis, acute lung injury, acute respiratory distress syndrome, acute renal failure, or hepatic dysfunction. Some of these complications are directly related to the device itself (infection), but most are due to the underlying disease severity in patients in whom a VAD is placed.

16. How is weaning from a VAD accomplished?

Weaning is attempted only in patients in whom a VAD was placed as a bridge to recovery or the heart has undergone sufficient remodeling so that a transplant is no longer necessary. The patient must be adequately assessed to ensure sufficient recovery of myocardium before weaning can be attempted. Methods to determine recovery include echocardiography, radionucleotide scans, and exercise testing. If the patient is hemodynamically stable, has demonstrated adequate myocardial recovery, and no longer meets the criteria for device placement, weaning trials can begin. Weaning is generally accomplished by sequentially reducing VAD flow rates while cardiac performance (e.g., ejection fraction, cardiac output) is closely monitored. If the patient is able to tolerate a VAD support of only 1–1.5 L/min, the device probably can be discontinued.

BIBLIOGRAPHY

1. DeWood MA, Notske RN, Hensley GR, et al: Intraaortic balloon counterpulsation with and without reperfusion for myocardial infarction shock. Circulation 61:1105–1112, 1980.
2. Goldstein DJ, Oz MC, Rose EA: Implantable left ventricular devices. N Engl J Med 339:1522–1532, 1998.
3. Hensley FA, Jr, Martin DE (eds): A Practical Approach to Cardiac Anesthesia, 2nd ed. New York, Little, Brown, 1995.
4. Kaplan JA, Craver JM, Jones EI, Sumpter R: The role of the intra-aortic balloon in cardiac anesthesia and surgery. Anesthesiology 98:580–586, 1979.
5. Overwalder PJ: Intra-aortic balloon pump (IAPB) counterpulsation. Internet J Thorac Cardiovasc Surg 2(2), 1999.
6. Pennington DG, Smedira NG, Samuels LE, et al: Mechanical circulatory support for acute heart failure. Ann Thorac Surg 71:S56–S59, 2001.
7. Ryan EW, Foster E: Augmentation of coronary blood flow with intra-aortic balloon pump counter-pulsation. Circulation 102:364–365, 2000.
8. Williams MR, Oz MC: Indications and patient selection for mechanical ventricular assistance. Ann Thorac Surg 71: S86–S91, 2001.

III. Pulmonary Medicine

17. ACUTE PNEUMONIA

Marvin I. Schwarz, M.D.

1. What normal defense mechanisms protect against the development of pneumonia?

Normal lung defense mechanisms include (1) filtration and humidification of the inspired air as it passes through the upper airway; (2) an intact cough reflex; (3) mucous secretion and mucociliary transport by the tracheobronchial respiratory epithelium; (4) normal macrophage and lymphocyte function (cellular immunity); (5) adequate function of B-lymphocytes, immunoglobulin, and complement (humeral immunity); and (6) adequate number of functioning neutrophils.

2. In the immunocompetent host, why does acute pneumonia develop?

In a patient with normal defense mechanisms, there is either an overwhelming exposure to an infectious agent or the agent is particularly virulent. Both situations can lead to pneumonia. However, factors known to predispose to acute bacterial pneumonia include a previous viral upper respiratory infection, gastroesophageal reflux, chronic alcohol consumption, cigarette smoking, an alteration in the level of consciousness, anesthesia, tracheobronchial intubation, pre-existing lung disease, diabetes mellitus, and corticosteroid medication.

3. Under what circumstances does community-acquired pneumonia result in respiratory failure and require an ICU admission?

Under ordinary circumstances, most patients with viral, mycoplasmal, or bacterial pneumonias do not require ICU admission. Situations in which admission is required include (1) pneumonia superimposed on preexisting lung disease (e.g., COPD or cystic fibrosis); (2) pneumonia complicated by septicemia and the superimposition of the acute respiratory distress syndrome (ARDS); (3) extensive aspiration pneumonia, usually following an alteration in the level of consciousness; (4) pneumonia in the alcoholic patient; (5) infrequently, viral, mycoplasmal, or bacterial pneumonia that causes diffuse lung injury and leads to respiratory failure; and (6) elderly patients, who in general are predisposed to more severe bacterial pneumonias.

4. Which noninfectious diseases occur acutely and have symptoms, signs, and radiographic findings similar to those of acute diffuse pneumonia?

These include (1) acute respiratory distress syndrome secondary to sepsis, toxic inhalations (chlorine), massive trauma, air embolism, near-drowning, high altitude, neurogenic pulmonary edema, and excessive blood product replacement; (2) acute immunologic pneumonia (systemic lupus erythematosus); (3) hypersensitivity pneumonitis; (4) drug-induced pneumonitis; (5) diffuse alveolar hemorrhage (Goodpasture's syndrome); (6) bronchiolitis obliterans organizing pneumonia; (7) acute (idiopathic) interstitial pneumonia (Hamman-Rich syndrome); and (8) acute eosinophilic pneumonia.

5. What organisms are most likely responsible for acute community-acquired pneumonia in patients less than 60 and without comorbid illness?

Infections due to *Streptococcus pneumoniae* are most frequent, followed by *Mycoplasma pneumoniae*, respiratory viruses, and *Chlamydia pneumoniae*. In cigarette smokers *Haemophilus influenzae* is commonly found. In patients over the age of 60 with comorbid illness (COPD, diabetes mellitus, chronic renal failure, congestive heart failure, chronic liver disease), the bacterial spectrum changes. Aerobic gram-negative bacilli, *Moraxella catarrhalis*, and *Staphylococcus aureus* are more likely to appear.

6. Which clinical information influences the decision to hospitalize a patient with acute community-acquired pneumonia?

Patients with a respiratory rate that exceeds 30 breaths/minute, blood pressure less than 90/60 mmHg, temperature above 101°F, mental confusion, and signs of extrapulmonary spread of infection should be considered for hospitalization. Laboratory results that influence the decision for inpatient treatment include a PO_2 > 50 mmHg, a white blood cell count less than 4000 or greater than 30,000 cells/mm^3, and evidence of renal dysfunction. Obviously, septic patients and those who require mechanical ventilation also require admission.

7. How does the clinical presentation of acute pneumonia differ in the elderly?

A typical presentation of pneumonia includes productive cough, chills, fever, and pleurisy. In the elderly, however, this clinical symptom complex is often absent; fever, altered mental status (confusion), and dehydration are more common in this age group. On the other hand, leukocytosis and a leftward shift of the white blood cell count is to be expected in all patients with bacterial pneumonia. Most hospital admissions for community-acquired pneumonia are in the elderly. The mortality rate is as high as 40%.

8. What is the significance of leukopenia in the immunocompetent patient with acute pneumonia?

The failure to incite leukocytosis in response to a bacterial infection is associated with a very poor prognosis and increased mortality. This situation is more likely in alcoholics at any age and in elderly patients generally.

9. What constitutes an adequate sputum Gram stain?

The sputum Gram stain is the most important diagnostic technique for the identification of the causative agent of an acute pneumonia in the nonintubated patient. An adequate sample is one in which the neutrophil count is ≥ 25 and the epithelial cell count ≤ 10 cells per low power field. Any sample that does not fulfill the above requirements probably represents oropharyngeal secretions and should be discarded.

10. How sensitive is the sputum Gram stain for the diagnosis of a community-acquired bacterial pneumonia?

The finding of gram-positive lancet-shaped diplococci (> 10 high-power field) is 85% specific and 62% sensitive for *S. pneumoniae*. Gram-negative coccobacillary stains typify *H. influenzae*. *S. aureus* are gram-negative organisms that occur in clusters. The sputum Gram stain influences the initial choice of antibiotic; however, the test is rarely done in patients who do not require hospitalization.

11. Which laboratory tests are most definitive for diagnosis of acute bacterial pneumonia?

Because 25–30% of patients with community-acquired pneumonia are bacteremic, a positive blood culture is diagnostic. All hospitalized patients with suspected pneumonia should have a blood culture. The same can be said for bacterial growth from the pleural fluid. Sputum cultures, on the other hand, are notoriously inaccurate in proven cases of pneumonia and often give false-positive results because of oropharyngeal contamination.

12. What is nosocomial pneumonia? What is its significance?

Nosocomial pneumonia is acquired in the hospital and is associated with different organisms that are often more resistant to antibiotic therapy compared with the bacteria responsible for community-acquired pneumonia. The mortality rate for nosocomial pneumonia is significantly higher (20–50% vs. 3–5%).

13. How common are nosocomial pneumonias?

Approximately 2 million nosocomial infections occur annually in the United States. Nosocomial pneumonia accounts for 15% of these, or 300,000 cases yearly.

14. How does the bacteriology of nosocomial pneumonias differ from community-acquired pneumonias?

As opposed to community-acquired pneumonias, nosocomial pneumonias are most often caused by aerobic gram-negative rods (*Klebsiella* sp., *Pseudomonas* sp., *Enterobacter* sp., *Escherichia coli*, *Proteus* sp., *Serratia* sp., enterococci), *S. aureus*, and group B streptococci. Contamination of the hospital water supply can result in *Legionella* sp. pneumonia.

15. Describe the pathogenesis of nosocomial pneumonia.

Nosocomial pneumonia results from colonization of the digestive tract and subsequent repeated small aspirations of oropharyngeal secretions. In addition, retrograde oropharyngeal contamination from the gastrointestinal tract is thought to play an important role. This is particularly significant because of the recent trend toward gastric alkinazation in critically ill ICU patients. Increasing the pH in the stomach allows bacterial overgrowth.

16. What conditions are conducive to nosocomial pneumonia?

The two most important predisposing factors are ICU admission and endotracheal intubation. The pneumonia associated with intubation is often called **ventilator-associated pneumonia**. When these conditions exist, up to 20% of patients develop nosocomial pneumonia. Other factors that contribute significantly include previous use of antibiotics, which allows for preselection of antibiotic-resistant strains, postsurgical state (50% of all nosocomial pneumonias), preexisting chronic lung disease, azotemia, and advanced age.

17. Which clinical criteria suggest the development of nosocomial pneumonia?

This is a difficult problem because oropharyngeal growth on sputum culture and the presence of purulent sputum do not necessarily equate with pneumonia. In addition, the appearance of radiographic infiltrates can have other etiologies. Although the clinical diagnosis of nosocomial pneumonia is far from precise, persistent fever, increasing infiltrates on chest radiograph, purulent airway secretions, and increasing problems with oxygenation raise the suspicion.

18. What other conditions can cause fever and pulmonary infiltrates in an ICU setting?

Besides nosocomial pneumonia, one has to consider atelectasis, pulmonary embolism, pulmonary edema secondary to congestive heart failure or volume overload, and sepsis causing the acute respiratory distress syndrome.

CONTROVERSY

19. Are culture and Gram stain of endotracheal secretions of significant importance in the bacteriologic diagnosis of nosocomial pneumonia?

For:
1. Endotracheal secretions are easily accessible. A change in their amount and color is often the first sign of nosocomial pneumonia and therefore suggests the etiologic agent.
2. Growth of an organism, particularly if supported by a positive blood culture, indicates the diagnosis.

Against:
1. Contamination of suctioned endotracheal secretions occurs frequently and does not reflect the underlying cause of pneumonia.

2. Only 10% of nosocomial pneumonias are associated with bacteremia.
3. Other diagnostic methods are available that bypass the tracheobronchial tree, such as bronchoscopy with bronchoalveolar lavage and the use of a plugged protected brush for culture of secretions from the lower respiratory tract.

BIBLIOGRAPHY

1. American Thoracic Society: Guidelines for the initial management of adults with community acquired pneumonia: Diagnosis, assessment of severity and initial antimicrobial therapy. Am Rev Respir Dis 148:1418–1426, 1993.
2. American Thoracic Society: Hospital acquired pneumonia in adults: Diagnosis, assessment of severity, initial antimicrobial therapy, and prevention strategies: A consensus statement. Am J Respir Crit Care Med 153:1711–1725, 1995.
3. Bergmans CJJ, et al: Prevention of ventilator associated pneumonia by oral decontamination. Am J Respir Care Med 164:382–388, 2001.
4. Faling JL: New advances in diagnosing nosocomial pneumonia in intubated patients. Part I. Am Rev Respir Dis 137:253–255, 1988.
5. Lambert RS, George RB: Diagnosing nosocomial pneumonia in mechanically ventilated patients: Which techniques offer the most reliability and the least risk? J Crit Illness 2(8):57–62, 1987.
6. MacFarlane J, et al: BTS guidelines for the management of community acquired pneumonia in adults. Thorax 56(Suppl 4):1–64, 2001.
8. Morehead RS, Pinto SJ: Ventilator-associated pneumonia. Arch Intern Med 160:1926–1036, 2000.
8. Penn RL: Choosing initial antibiotic therapy in pneumonia patients. J Crit Illness 1(4):57–67, 1986.
9. Perlino CA, Rimland D: Alcoholism, leukopenia, and pneumococcal sepsis. Am Rev Respir Dis 132:757–760, 1985.
10. Rello, et al: International conference on the diagnosis and treatment of ventilator-associated pneumonia. Chest 120:955–970, 2001.
11. Toews GB: Southwestern internal medicine conference: Nosocomial pneumonia. Am J Med Sci 29:355–367, 1986.
12. Torres A, De La Bellacasa JP, Rodriquez-Roisin R, et al: Diagnostic value of telescoping plugged catheters in mechanically ventilated patients with bacterial pneumonia. Using the Metras catheter. Am Rev Respir Dis 138:117–120, 1988.
13. Verghese A, Berk SL, Boelen LJ, et al: Group B streptococcal pneumonia in the elderly. Arch Intern Med 142:1642–1645, 1982.
Rev Respir Dis 148:1418–1426, 1993.
9. Santamauro JT, White DA: Respiratory infections in HIV-negative immunocompromised patients. Curr Opin Pulm Med 2:253–258, 1996.

18. ASTHMA

Gil Allen, M.D., and David A. Kaminsky, M.D.

1. Discuss important elements in the history of patients with acute severe asthma.

First exclude other possible causes of the patient's presentation. A history of heart failure may suggest wheezing and shortness of breath secondary to left ventricular failure and pulmonary edema. A history of allergies or prior anaphylactic reactions, along with a recent exposure to certain foods, new medications, or other known triggers, may be an important warning of potentially imminent upper airway inflammation and closure. Pulmonary embolism also can mimic asthma and should be considered especially in patients with dyspnea, anxiety, and hypoxemia but clear breath sounds. In this case, it is important to elicit any history of deep venous thrombosis or embolism as well as pertinent risk factors. In a patient with dyspnea, anxiety, and inspiratory stridor, vocal cord dysfunction should be considered. A history of anxiety, voice changes, or sudden truncation of vocalizations may be a clue to this disorder. Spirometry can be an especially useful tool for evaluating patients in the emergency department, and flow-volume loops often yield the characteristic truncated or flattened inspiratory loops. The majority of these patients also have true asthma, but they often appear more flow-limited than in fact they are. If peak expiratory flow rate is at baseline and the patient has no signs of fatigue, low doses of benzodiazepines can often break the cycle of paradoxical vocal cord closure.

2. What are the important indicators of a severe asthma attack?

Use of accessory muscles, a limited number of words per breath or monosyllabic utterances, heart rate > 130 beats/min, pulsus paradoxus > 15 mmHg, respiratory rate > 30 breaths/min, an inability to lie down, a silent chest, lethargy, somnolence, advancing fatigue, and normal or elevated partial pressure of carbon dioxide in arterial blood ($PaCO_2$) are suggestive of a severe asthma attack.

3. Which patients are at greatest risk of near-fatal or fatal asthma?

Although it is difficult to identify such patients prospectively, some risk factors have been identified retrospectively. A high degree of bronchial reactivity, a history of poor compliance with therapy and follow-up, and a history of recurrent admissions or previous intubations are believed to be significant risk factors. Both patients who develop sudden, severe attacks and patients with severe, slowly progressive disease are typically at risk. A history of marked diurnal variation in forced expiratory volume in one second (FEV_1) is also believed to be a risk factor, but it may simply be a marker for increased bronchial responsiveness. Patients who are judged to be poor at perceiving the severity of their own attack, as demonstrated by a poor correlation between reported symptoms and peak expiratory flow rate (PEFR) values, are also at increased risk of near-fatal asthma. For such patients, home monitoring of PEFR is strongly indicated. Although not widely identified as a true marker of increased risk, the use of inhaled heroin is also frequently associated with near-fatal or fatal attacks of asthma. It is not known whether the increased risk is due to a direct effect of the inhaled drug (or its diluents) on the degree of airflow limitation or simply to impaired judgment, which delays arrival at the emergency department for the initiation of appropriate care. However, opioids have long been known to cause bronchoconstriction via mast cell degranulation and histamine release. Although most reports of severe asthma attacks following inhaled narcotics have been in known asthmatics, they have also been reported in patients with no history of asthma.

4. How should a severe asthma attack be treated?

Beta agonists are the first-line therapy in acute asthma attacks. Corticosteroids also play a key role. Other options include anticholinergics, aminophylline, and inhaled anesthetic agents.

5. How are beta agonists delivered?

The inhaled forms are superior to the subcutaneous or intravenous route and have fewer side effects. The subcutaneous route is reserved for patients who are so dyspneic that they cannot take deep enough breaths, but such patients usually require intubation. Metered-dose inhalers are equally as effective as aerosolized delivery, provided good technique is used with a spacer device. Nebulized or aerosolized delivery is still used frequently in the emergency department, partly from convention and partly because less instruction and observation are needed to ensure good delivery.

6. Describe the appropriate use of corticosteroids.

The typical dose is 60–125 mg of intravenous solumedrol every 6 hours for the first 24 hours. Solu-Medrol should be delivered as soon as possible because peak onset of action can take several hours. Therapy is typically continued every 6 hours until the attack appears to be breaking and then gradually tapered over days to weeks.

7. What is the role of anticholinergics in the treatment of a severe asthma attack?

Many studies have shown marginal benefits of adding inhaled ipratropium to beta-agonist therapy for acute asthma. A recent meta-analysis showed a significant 10% increase in FEV_1 or PEFR and a significant reduction in hospital admissions from the emergency department when ipratropium is added to standard therapy regimens.

8. Discuss the role of aminophylline.

Oral theophylline is again becoming a popular secondary agent for the chronic management of asthma, in part because of its intrinsic anti-inflammatory properties, even at serum levels lower than those once thought necessary to achieve significant benefit. However, the use of intravenous aminophylline in the treatment of acute asthma remains controversial. Many consensus statements do not recommend its use as a first-line therapy in the acute setting, and several studies have failed to show any benefit when aminophylline is added to other conventional therapies. Other studies, however, indicate that with more aggressively targeted serum levels (15–20 μg/ml), aminophylline can improve measures of PEFR and FEV_1 as well as decrease hospital admission rates. The treating physician must weigh these benefits against the higher level of undesired side effects that may occur at such higher serum levels.

9. How are inhaled anesthetic agents used?

In mechanically ventilated patients with ongoing severe bronchospasm despite aggressive conventional treatment, inhaled anesthetic agents can be used for their intrinsic properties of bronchodilation. Because delivery requires a special apparatus and conventional management is usually more effective, their use is often considered a last resort. Halothane often depresses cardiac function at doses needed for bronchodilation; for this reason, isoflurane is the agent of choice.

10. Does magnesium sulfate offer any benefit in the treatment of status asthmaticus?

Although a small number of controlled trials have yielded mixed results, one controlled study suggests that severe asthmatics treated with magnesium sulfate in the emergency department (FEV_1 < 25% predicted) had a significantly reduced admission rate compared with placebo-treated patients. The overall admission rate for all combined asthmatics was lower in the magnesium sulfate treatment group (25.4% vs. 35.3%), but not significantly so. A more recent meta-analysis did not support these findings. Proposed mechanisms of possible benefit are (1) blockage of calcium channels and reduced calcium entry into smooth muscle cells, leading to bronchodilation; (2) possible inhibition of mast cell degranulation; and (3) improvement of respiratory muscle function by correction of lower baseline serum levels. Because the only reported untoward side effects from a single dose are flushing, mild fatigue, or burning at the IV site, its use in the treatment of severe asthmatics may be warranted because of the potential for lowering admission rates, but this issue remains controversial. Magnesium sulfate is generally delivered intravenously as 2 grams in 50 ml of normal saline over 20 minutes.

11. How can I best decide when to admit a patient and when to discharge home from the emergency department?

All patients who have a poor response to treatment, defined as persistent wheezing, dyspnea, and accessory muscle use at rest despite 3 hours of treatment in the emergency department, should be admitted to the hospital. A recent study suggests that in severe asthmatics (PEFR and FEV_1 < 35% of predicted), PEFR as a percentage of predicted and PEFR change from baseline, measured 30 minutes after initiation of therapy, may be good early predictors of a good or poor response to treatment after 3 hours. Any patient with worsening PEFR, rising $PaCO_2$, or advancing fatigue should, at the very least, be monitored in the intensive care unit and possibly intubated.

12. Which patients need to be intubated?

Any patient with apnea, near apnea, or cardiopulmonary arrest should be intubated. Any patient with progressive lethargy, somnolence, or near exhaustion should be intubated. Any patient with a progressive rise in $PaCO_2$ despite therapy and increasing fatigue probably will require intubation. Other relative indications are coexistent medical conditions that can increase minute ventilation requirements or compromise oxygen delivery, such as sepsis, myocardial infarction, metabolic acidosis, or life-threatening arrhythmias.

13. Is normocapnea or hypercapnea an absolute indication for intubation in asthmatic patients?

Most severe asthmatics present with hypocapnea (decreased $PaCO_2$) due to the hyperventilation associated with dyspnea and hypoxemia. A normal or elevated $PaCO_2$ is usually a sign of fatigue but also may be due to a high ratio of dead space to tidal volume secondary to air-trapping and ineffective ventilation of noncommunicating segments of the lung. In either case, it should be taken seriously and may be a sign of impending respiratory failure. Studies indicate, however, that most patients with normal or elevated $PaCO_2$ on blood gas analysis at initial evaluation improve before mechanical ventilation is required. In most patients, ventilation improves with time in response to conventional therapy. Because mechanical ventilation in severe asthma can be complicated by increased air-trapping and barotrauma, it is advisable not to begin mechanical ventilation merely because of an elevated $PaCO_2$, unless it is associated with somnolence, progressive fatigue, or significant acidosis.

14. Can noninvasive mechanical ventilation be used safely to avoid intubation in asthmatic patients?

Noninvasive positive-pressure ventilation (NPPV) via face mask has been shown to be safe and effective when applied to the patient with severe asthma and hypercapnea that fails to improve with conventional therapy. It can be effective in unloading respiratory muscles, improving dyspnea, lowering respiratory rate, and improving gas exchange. It should not be used in asthmatics with life-threatening hypoxemia, somnolence, or hemodynamic instability, and it should be aborted in the patient who fails to improve or cannot tolerate the mask.

15. Are helium admixtures of any proven benefit in the treatment of severe asthma?

When helium is blended with oxygen in an 80%-to-20% mixture, the gas density becomes approximately one-third that of room air, and airway resistance is significantly reduced in areas of greatest turbulent flow. Helium-oxygen admixtures can reduce the work of breathing needed to meet the same minute ventilation requirement on room air. Because work of breathing is reduced, it seems likely that respiratory fatigue may be delayed until conventional therapy has had time to take effect. Unfortunately, no trials have demonstrated that helium-oxygen admixtures can prevent the need for intubation. However, they have been shown to improve PEFR and reduce the degree of pulsus paradoxus in acute asthma attacks. This effect presumably results from the decrease in airway resistance and generation of lower negative pleural pressures, but it also may be due to improved expiratory flow and less dynamic hyperinflation. Because mixtures typically include only 20–30% oxygen, hypoxemia is a barrier to their use. However, when the patient is not hypoxemic, helium-oxygen admixtures are safe and worthwhile, particularly in patients with fatigue and hypercapnea who are at risk for progressing to the need for mechanical ventilation.

16. Once a patient requires intubation, what is the best management strategy?

Blind nasoendotracheal intubation is often better tolerated in the awake patient, but oral endotracheal intubation is preferred because it permits the use of an endotracheal tube (ETT) with a larger internal diameter. A larger internal diameter leads to lower resistance within the respiratory circuit and allows easier deep suctioning of secretions and potential mucous plugs. The resistance of a tube is indirectly proportional its internal radius (to the fourth power), and the resistance of an 8-mm ETT is roughly one-half that of a 7-mm ETT. Oral intubation is indicated for apneic, cyanotic patients. Because intubation in asthmatic patients is often difficult and may induce laryngospasm or lead to increased bronchospasm, it should be attempted by the most experienced person available. Sedation is usually necessary, and sometimes paralysis may be warranted, although it should be avoided if possible. Barbiturates such as thiopental should be avoided because of their association with histamine release and potential worsening of bronchoconstriction. Although narcotics such as fentanyl are often useful, one should be aware of their potential for bronchoconstriction and laryngospasm.

17. Discuss the potential complications of intubation.

Dynamic hyperinflation (DHI). When airflow limitation is severe, the next ventilated breath may be initiated before the lungs can fully exhale to a normal functional residual capacity (FRC), and air is successively trapped with each breath. This process leads to DHI and elevated end-expiratory alveolar pressures, referred to as intrinsic positive end-expiratory pressure (PEEPi). Measuring PEEPi can be problematic, and it is often underestimated by the brief end-expiratory pause used for estimation on the ventilator. The often heterogeneous distribution of early airway closure can prevent many hyperinflated segments from even communicating their alveolar pressures to the transducer at the airway opening. The key determinants of DHI are minute ventilation, tidal volume, exhalation time, and severity of airflow limitation. DHI can often be predicted by elevated plateau pressures and failure to achieve zero expiratory flow on flow-time curves on the ventilator. DHI can lead to less effective use of respiratory muscles due to less-than-optimal curvature of the diaphragm, which in turn can lead to less effective triggering of the ventilator, especially when negative-pressure triggering mechanisms are used. DHI also can lead to decreased venous return and right ventricular preload, increased right ventricular afterload (via extrinsic compression of the pulmonary vasculature), and decreased left ventricular compliance, all of which can result in diminished cardiac output and hypotension. When DHI is strongly suspected, the best immediate treatment (and test) is brief disconnection of the patient from the ventilator to allow more complete exhalation. The other concern is that the high degree of associated PEEPi can lead to barotrauma.

Barotrauma. High airway pressures may lead to pulmonary interstitial emphysema, subcutaneous emphysema, pneumomediastinum, pneumothorax, and even pneumoperitoneum. Barotrauma correlates directly with the degree of DHI. Plateau pressures are traditionally believed to be a good indicator of the degree of DHI, and a level below 30 cmH_2O is still a widely recommended target for minimizing barotrauma. However, one study has shown that end-inspiratory lung volume (the exhaled volume measured from end-inspiration to FRC during a period of apnea) may be a more reliable predictor of barotrauma than airway pressures. The most feared consequence of barotrauma is a tension pneumothorax, typically characterized by a precipitous rise in airway pressures (peak and plateau), a drop in oxygen saturation, hypotension, tachycardia, unilaterally absent breath sounds and chest excursions, and possibly tracheal deviation. It is a clinical diagnosis and, if strongly suspected in an unstable patient, should be treated immediately with chest tube placement or needle thoracostomy followed by chest tube placement.

18. Describe the proper ventilator settings.

The best mode of ventilation is one that minimizes minute ventilation and allows sufficient exhalation time to minimize DHI. This goal generally can be achieved with low tidal volumes of 6–8 ml/kg, a respiratory rate of 8–10 breaths/min, minimal added PEEP, and moderate inspiratory flow rates of 80–90 L/min. Decelerating flow waveforms may improve overall flow distribution and hence optimize gas exchange. Higher inspiratory flow rates with square waveforms allow a shorter inspiratory time and hence, at the same respiratory rate, a longer expiratory time. The longer expiratory time, rather than simply the inspiratory-to-expiratory (I:E) ratio, is critical. Lowering total minute ventilation is the most crucial goal, because a longer expiratory time and a smaller burden of volume to be exhaled minimize DHI. Intentional hypoventilation with low minute volumes can significantly reduce the risk of DHI and barotrauma and, allowing for a maximum $PaCO_2$ of 80 mmHg or a minimum pH of 7.20, is a safe and acceptable practice when ventilating patients with severe airflow limitation. However, because an elevated $PaCO_2$ can increase cerebral perfusion, permissive hypercapnea should be avoided in patients with intracranial bleeding, edema, or a space-occupying lesion.

19. What is the role of sedation?

Agitation can lead to hyperventilation and asynchrony with the mechanical ventilator and hence result in DHI and unacceptably high airway pressures. Deep anesthesia with benzodiazepines or propofol is often necessary to achieve optimal control, especially when intentional hypoventilation and permissive hypercapnea are used. Paralytics should and often can be avoided by using sufficient levels of sedatives. Patients are at a much higher risk of prolonged weakness when paralytics are administered in combination with corticosteroids.

20. Can added PEEP help reduce air-trapping in mechanically ventilated asthmatic patients?

Some have argued that added PEEP can help minimize air-trapping by "stenting" open peripheral airways. Although this principle may apply to some degree in patients with emphysema and easily collapsible central airways, it is unlikely to be of much benefit in patients with severe asthma. In the classic model of airflow limitation, airway collapse occurs when extraluminal pressure overcomes intraluminal pressures (and any architectural properties of the airway itself). In patients who already have significant PEEPi and in whom distal alveolar pressures (P_{alv}) already exceed extraluminal pressures at end expiration, added PEEP probably will only increase P_{alv} and worsen hyperinflation. DHI can occur even in the absence of airflow limitation if the respiratory rate is high enough; thus, the above strategies are still best for minimizing DHI.

21. Can helium admixtures be used in mechanically ventilated asthmatic patients?

Heliox may improve the delivery of aerosolized medications by minimizing turbulent flow and hence reducing premature deposition of drug within the endotracheal tube and proximal airways. Because heliox offers a three-fold reduction in density and a reduction in airway resistance, it may help to improve ventilation-perfusion matching via improved ventilation of obstructed lung segments and to minimize DHI via improved expiratory flow. Unfortunately, administration of heliox through commonly available ventilators is problematic because its higher specific heat and viscosity cause erroneous flow measurements through hot-wire and screen pneumotachometers. For this reason, its use by inexperienced operators is not recommended.

22. What new pharmacologic strategies are emerging for the treatment of acute asthma?

A recent Cochrane review found that the use of inhaled steroids in the emergency department reduces admission rates in patients with acute asthma, but they seem to benefit only patients who are not already receiving systemic corticosteroids. Inhaled budesonide has been shown to improve markers of airway inflammation and hyperresponsiveness as early as 6 hours after dosing. Another potential therapy for acute asthma is the anti-leukotriene agent montelukast. One study found that intravenous delivery of montelukast improved FEV_1 faster than oral dosages, but both forms ultimately resulted in equivalent degrees of improvement. The use of leukotriene inhibitors for acute asthma warrants further investigation.

BIBLIOGRAPHY

1. Benatar SR: Fatal asthma. N Engl J Med 314:423–429, 1986.
2. Bloch H, Silverman R, Mancherje N, et al: Intravenous magnesium sulfate as an adjunct in the treatment of acute asthma. Chest 107:1576–1581, 1995.
3. Cochrane Review: Early use of inhaled corticosteroids in the emergency department treatment of acute asthma. Cochrane Database Syst Rev 1:CD002308, 2001.
4. Cygan J, Trunsky M, Corbridge T: Inhaled heroin-induced status asthmaticus: Five cases and a review of the literature. Chest 117:272–275, 2000.
5. Dockhorn RJ, Baumgartner RA, Leff JA, et al: Comparison of the effects of intravenous and oral montelukast on airway function: A double-blind, placebo-controlled, three-period, crossover study in asthmatic patients. Thorax 55:260–265, 2000.
6. Jain S, Hanania NA, Guntupalli KK: Ventilation of patients with asthma and obstructive lung disease. Crit Care Clin 14: 685–705, 1998.
7. Kass JE, Terregino CA: The effect of heliox in acute severe asthma: A randomized controlled trial. Chest 116:296–300, 1999.
8. Manthous CA, Hall JB, Melmed A, et al: Heliox improves pulsus paradoxus and peak expiratory flow in nonintubated patients with severe asthma. Am J Respir Crit Care Med 151:310–314, 1995.
9. Makino S: Theophylline in the treatment of asthma. Clin Exp Allergy 26:S47–S54, 1996.
10. Meduri GU, Cook TR, Turner RE, et al: Noninvasive positive pressure ventilation in status asthmaticus. Chest 110:767–774, 1996.
11. Molfino NA, Nannini LJ, Rebuck AS, Slutsky AS: The fatality-prone asthmatic patient: Follow-up study after near-fatal attacks. Chest 101:621–623, 1992.

12. Mountain RD, Sahn SA: Clinical features and outcome in patients with acute asthma presenting with hypercapnea. Am Rev Respir Dis 138:535–539, 1988.
13. Rodrigo G, Rodrigo C, Burschtin O: Efficacy of magnesium sulfate in acute asthma: A meta-analysis of randomized trials. Am J Emerg Med 18: 216–221, 2000.
14. Rodrigo G, Rodrigo C, Burschtin O: A meta-analysis of the effects of ipratropium bromide in adults with acute asthma. Am J Med 107:363–370, 1999.
15. Rodrigo G, Rodrigo C: Early prediction of poor response in acute asthma patients in the emergency department. Chest 114:1016–1021, 1998.
16. Williams TJ, Tuxen DV, Scheinkestel CD, et al: Risk factors for morbidity in mechanically ventilated patients with acute severe asthma. Am Rev Respir Dis 146: 607–615, 1992.

19. CHRONIC OBSTRUCTIVE PULMONARY DISEASE

Enrique Fernandez, M.D.

1. What is COPD?

Chronic obstructive pulmonary disease (COPD) is a disease state characterized by airflow limitation that is not fully reversible. The airflow limitation is usually progressive and associated with an abnormal inflammatory response of the lungs to noxious particles and gases.

The disease state includes three pathologic entities: emphysema, chronic bronchitis, and small airway disease, which can occur alone or in a variable mix. Improved physiologic evaluation often separates the various contributions of these pathologic entities.

Other diseases, such as bronchiectasis, cystic fibrosis, tuberculosis, pneumoconiosis, or asthma, can present with poorly reversible airflow limitation and overlap with COPD, but they are not included in the definition of COPD.

2. What are the criteria for diagnosis of COPD?

A diagnosis of COPD should be considered in any patient who has symptoms of cough, sputum production, dyspnea, and/or a history of exposure to risk factors for the disease. Smoking the main risk factor for COPD, but other risk factors may contribute: exposure to dust, air pollution, childhood respiratory infections, preexisting bronchial hyperreactivity, poor nutrition, and genetic deficiency of alpha$_1$-antitrypsin.

The diagnosis of COPD is confirmed by spirometry. Forced expiratory volume in 1 second (FEV$_1$) and forced vital capacity (FVC) are measured before and after administration of a bronchodilator. Expiratory airflow limitation is the hallmark of the disease. A postbronchodilator FEV$_1$/FVC ≤ 70% confirms the presence of airflow limitation that is not fully reversible. Widespread availability of standardized spirometry should facilitate the early diagnosis of COPD.

3. Describe the pathogenesis of COPD.

COPD is characterized by chronic inflammation of all structures of the lung: airways, parenchyma, and pulmonary vasculature. Macrophages, T lymphocytes (predominantly CD$_8$+), and neutrophils are increased in various parts of the lung. Various mediators, including leukotriene B$_4$ (LTB$_4$), interleukin 8 (IL-8), tumor necrosis factor alpha (TNFα), and others, are released and contribute to the inflammatory process. An imbalance of proteinases and antiproteases in the lung and oxidative stress also contribute to the pathogenesis of COPD.

Of interest, only a small percentage of smokers develop emphysema or chronic bronchitis.

4. What are the major pathologic changes in COPD?

All structures of the lung are subjected to pathologic changes in COPD. In the central airways (trachea, bronchi, and bronchioles with internal diameter > 2–4 mm), inflammatory cells infiltrate the surface epithelilum, edema is present, mucus secreting glands are enlarged, and the number of goblet cells increases with mucus hypersecretion. In the peripheral airways (small bronchi and bronchioles with an internal diameter < 2 mm), chronic inflammation leads to repeated injury and repair of the airway wall.

Destruction of lung parenchyma is seen typically in centrilobular emphysema (in most cases, smoking-related). The destruction of alveolar septa leads to the confluence of adjacent alveoli and enlarged terminal air spaces. The vascular changes, which begin early in the natural history of the disease, are characterized by thickening of the vessel wall, which progressively worsens with a greater amount of smooth muscle, proteoglycans, and collagen deposition.

5. Describe the pathophysiology of COPD.

Pathologic changes in the lungs lead to corresponding physiologic changes characteristic of the disease: mucus hypersecretion and ciliary dysfunction, pulmonary hyperinflation, and gas exchange abnormalities. Later pulmonary hypertension develops, followed by cor pulmonale. Expiratory airflow limitation, best measured by spirometry, is the hallmark physiologic change of COPD and the key to its diagnosis.

6. How is COPD staged in different degrees of severity?

The staging should be regarded only as an educational tool and a general indication of the approach to management. (All FEV_1 values refer to postbronchodilator FEV_1.)

Classification of COPD by Severity

STAGE	CHARACTERISTICS
0: At risk	Normal spirometry Chronic symptoms (cough, sputum production)
I. Mild COPD	$FEV_1/FVC < 70\%$ $FEV_1 \geq 80\%$ predicted With or without chronic symptoms (cough, sputum production)
II. Moderate COPD	$FEV_1/FVC < 70\%$ $30\% \leq FEV_1 < 80\%$ predicted IIA: $50\% \leq FEV_1 < 80\%$ predicted IIB: $30\% \leq FEV_1 < 50\%$ predicted With or without chronic symptoms (cough, sputum production)
III. Severe COPD	$FEV_1/FVC < 70\%$ $FEV_1 < 30\%$ predicted or $FEV_1 < 50\%$ predicted plus respiratory failure* or clinical signs of right-heart failure

FEV_1 = forced expiratory volume in 1 second, FVC = forced vital capacity.
* Respiratory failure is defined as arterial pressure of oxygen (PaO_2) < 8.0 kPa (60 mmHg) with or without arterial partial pressure of carbon dioxide ($PaCO_2$) > 6.7 pKa (50 mmHg) while breathing air at sea level.
From National Institutes of Health: Global Initiative for Chronic Obstructive Lung Disease. Washington, DC, National Institutes of Health.

7. Outline the therapeutic approach to COPD.

In the United States, the mortality rate of COPD is very low among people younger than 45 years but increases with age to become the fourth or fifth leading cause of death among people older than 45 years. COPD cannot be cured but can be alleviated considerably by appropriate treatment. The long-term management of COPD has several objectives:

• Improve and decelerate the decline in lung function
• Relieve symptoms (dyspnea, fatigue, cough)
• Decrease exacerbations
• Decrease hospitalizations
• Improve quality of life
• Increase life expectancy
• Achieve objectives in a cose-effective manner

Smoking cessation is the most important intervention from the epidemiologic point of view. In addition to the modest improvement in FEV_1 seen with smoking cessation, the rate of decline in FEV_1 may be reduced, in some cases even to the rate found in healthy nonsmokers ($\pm$ 30 ml/year).

The pharmacologic measures include anticholinergics, beta-adrenergics, methylxanthines, corticosteroids, antibiotics, expectorants, mucolithics, oxygen, and treatment of respiratory failure.

8. Should bronchodilators be used in the treatment of COPD?

Bronchodilators are the treatment for the reversible component of airway obstruction in patients with COPD. By reducing bronchomotor tone, they decrease airway resistance, which can improve airflow, decreasing the work of breathing and the sensation of dyspnea. The response to bronchodilators should be measured and followed by spirometry. Spirometric changes after bronchodilator therapy may be relatively flat, despite significant clinical benefit, as quantitated by changes in quality-of-life measures and exercise tolerance (6-minute walk).

Anticholinergic agents are the first-line maintenance therapy for COPD. They increase the baseline postbronchodilator FEV_1 value and reduce the rate of COPD exacerbations. Ipratropium is currently the anticholinergic of choice. Delivered via a metered-dose inhaler (MDI) and a spacer device, ipratropium maximizes action in the lungs. Because its duration of action is 6–8 hours, it should be administered on a regular basis (4 times/day) to maintain bronchodilation. A new agent—tiotropium bromide—is more potent and has a longer duration of action than ipratropium, allowing once-daily administration.

Beta$_2$-adrenergic agents. If the outcome of anticholinergic therapy is not optimal, an inhaled short-acting beta$_2$-adrenergic agent, delivered by MDI with a spacer device, should be added. Inhaled, short-acting beta$_2$-adrenergic agents are readily absorbed systemically and can led to numerous systemic side effects, such as tachycardia, tremor, and arrhythmias. They are prescribed at a dose of 2–4 puffs every 3–6 hours, but dosing should be individualized, depending on factors such as the patient's tolerance of systemic side effects and cardiovascular status. The long-acting inhaled beta$_2$-adrenergic, salmeterol, improves health status significantly when administered in doses of 50 mg twice daily. It can be added to ipratropium in patients who frequently require short-acting beta$_2$-adrenergic therapy. It also has therapeutic value in patients with significant nocturnal symptoms.

Theophylline preparations. Only slow-release preparations of theophylline are effective in COPD. In general, methylxanthines are weak bronchodilators, but their action lasts up to 12 hours. They have other actions that may explain their benefit in some patients, including an inotropic effect on diaphragmatic strength and reduced muscle fatigue in vitro and in experimental animals. They also increase mucociliary clearance and central respiratory drive; improve exercise capacity; and reduce nocturnal declines in FEV_1 and early morning respiratory symptoms. Finally, methylxanthines have some anti-inflammatory effects. In a randomized, double-blind, placebo-controlled, crossover trial, Murciano and colleagues evaluated the effects of theophylline in COPD. After 2 months of theophylline therapy, patients had significant improvement in dyspnea, pulmonary gas exchange, partial pressure of arterial carbon dioxide, vital capacity, and FEV_1. Because methylxanthines have a very narrow therapeutic window and serious toxic side effects, their use requires careful supervision. Sleep distrubances, changes in mood, and loss of short-term memory are not uncommon. In patients who benefit from theophylline, a long-acting preparation, taken orally once or twice daily in a dose that keeps the blood level at about 10–12 mg/L, should be used. Theophylline should be continued, in addition to the other medications in the patient's regimen, only if re-evaluation confirms that improvement is evident. Metabolism of methylxanthines varies with the clinical condition of the patient and use of concomitant drugs.

9. What common drugs and diseases may increase serum theophylline concentration?

Drugs

Cimetidine	Oral contraceptives
Troleandomycin	Vaccines: influenza
Erythromycin	BCG: further study required

Calcium channel blockers: single case reports
  Nifedipine
  Verapamil
Diseases
Cirrhosis
Congestive heart failure
Pneumonia

Beta blockers: further study required
Allopurinol: high doses
Vidarasine: single case report

Hypothyroidism
Herpes simplex infection: further study
  required

10. **What common drugs and diseases may decrease serum theophylline concentration?**

Drugs	**Diseases**
Barbiturates	Hyperthyroidism
Carbamazepine	Cystic fibrosis
Isoniazid	Pancreatitis
Rifampin	
Sulfinpyrazone	
Activated charcoal	

11. **Discuss the role of combination bronchodilatory therapy in COPD.**

Combination drugs with different mechanisms and duration of action may increase the degree of bronchodilation with equivalent or fewer side effects. Inclusion of ipratropium in a treatment regimen, either alone or in combination with albuterol sulfate or in an MDI that simultaneously delivers both, produces greater and more sustained improvement in FEV_1 than either drug alone and does not produce evidence of tachyphylaxis over 90 days of treatment. The combination also is associated with lower rates of exacerbations, resulting in lower treatment cost and improved cost-effectiveness.

12. **When should antibiotics be used?**

Older studies evaluating the use of antibiotics produced controversial results. A recent meta-analysis of randomized trials of antibiotic use in acute exacerbations of COPD found a statistically significant clinical improvement in patients treated with antibiotics vs placebo. In exacerbations of COPD related to bacterial infections, the most common pathogens are *Hemophilus influenzae*, *Streptococcus pneumoniae*, and *Moraxella catarrhalis*. Antibiotic therapy with ampicillin, amoxicillin, doxycycline, or the combination of trimethoprim and sulfamethoxazole for 10–20 days is the usual regimen.

13. **Summarize the role and efficacy of mucolytic therapy in the treatment of COPD.**

It is difficult to assess the efficacy of mycolytic therapy because measurements of sputum volume, rheologic tests, and tests for clearance of sputum are difficult to perform and assess. The relevant literature, in general, has not been objective or reliable. A few patients—mainly those with viscous sputum—may benefit from mucolytic agents; however, the benefit seems to be small, and widespread use cannot be recommended on the basis of current evidence.

14. **What other pharmacologic treatments may benefit patients with COPD?**

1. **Alpha₁-antitrypsin replacement.** In the few patients with emphysema related to deficiency of alpha₁-antitrypsin with phenotype PiZ, long-term replacement therapy can be given. A dose of 60 mg/kg body weight, given intravenously on a weekly basis, has been associated with appearance of the enzyme in bronchoalveolar lavage fluid. This treatment, however, is very expensive, and its benefit remains to be proved. In the future, it may prove practical to administer the agent by aerosol. Danazol, 200 mg 3 times/day, also may increase the level of alpha₁-antitrypsin. Neither agent is recommended for patients with COPD unrelated to enzyme deficiency.

2. **Vaccines.** Patients with COPD are at risk for increased morbidity and mortality from respiratory tract infections. Pneumococcal and influenza vaccination, both alone and in combination,

have been shown to reduce hospitalizations and mortality rates. Influenza vaccine containing killed or live inactivated viruses, is recommended yearly (beginning each October). Pneumococcal vaccine, containing 23 virulent serotypes, is given every 5 or 6 years.

3. **Antioxidant agents.** N-acetylcysteine seems to reduce the frequency of exacerbations, but no evidence supports its use in patients with recurrent exacerbations.

Immune regulators, vasodilators, respiratory stimulants, antitussives, and narcotics are not currently recommended for routine therapy

15. Discuss the role of oxygen therapy in COPD.

Chronic arterial hypoxemia is a feature of most advanced chronic lung diseases, almost always because of V/Q maldistribution. Arterial hypoxemia may cause dysfunction in a number of organs, increasing morbidity and mortality. The British Medical Research Council (MRC) Trial and the Nocturnal Oxygen Therapy Trial (NOTT) are two controlled studies that have provided data on which are based the current recommendations and justification for the use of long-term oxygen (LTO$_2$) in hypoxemic patients with COPD. Combining the results from the two studies makes it clear that oxygen therapy has a clear survival advantage over no oxygen therapy and that continuous oxygen therapy (19+ hr/day) results in the greatest benefits in terms of improved survival. The mechanisms by which LTO$_2$ therapy improves survival in patients with COPD is unclear. High pulmonary artery pressure, high pulmonary vascular resistance, and low stroke volumes are associated with increased mortality, and the effects of oxygen on hemodynamics may influence survival. The beneficial effects of oxygen therapy on pulmonary hemodynamics have been confirmed. Beneficial effects have been demonstrated conclusively only in hypoxemic patients.

16. What are the indications for long-term oxygen therapy in COPD patients?

If the patient, when at rest on room air and in stable conditions, has

1. Arterial oxen pressure (PaO$_2$) < 55 mmHg/oxygen saturation in arterial blood (SaO$_2$) < 85% *or* PaO$_2$ = 56–59 mmHg/SaO$_2$ = 86–89% *and*
2. Evidence of one of the following secondary diagnoses:
   • Dependent edema suggesting congestive heart failure or "P" pulmonale on EKG, or erythrocytosis with hematocrit > 56%
   • During sleep:
     PaO$_2$ drops to or below 55 mmHg, or drops more than 10 mmHg, or
     SaO$_2$ drops to or below 85%, or drops more than 5%
   • During exercise:
     PaO$_2$ drops to or below 55 mmHg, or
     SaO$_2$ drops to or below 85%

When the patient fulfills the criteria for continuous oxygen therapy, oxygen should be prescribed in a dose sufficient to raise the PaO$_2$ to 65–80 mmHg at rest during wakefulness. This PaO$_2$ usually is achieved with a 1- to 4-L/min oxygen flow through nasal prongs. The dose of O$_2$ should be increased by 1 L/min during sleep or exercise in order to prevent hypoxemic episodes. Oxygen should be given continuously at least 19 hours/day.

17. What are the reasons for hypoxemia in patients with COPD during sleep?

Sleep depresses ventilation in healthy persons, producing an increase in arterial carbon dioxide pressure (PaCO$_2$) and a decrease in PaO$_2$. Because many patients with severe COPD have reduced alveolar ventilation with hypoxemia and hypercapnia while awake, one would predict that they will have more profound alterations in arterial blood gases than healthy persons during sleep. In fact, these abnormalities occur, and the mechanisms of hypoxemia during sleep in COPD include:

1. Hypoventilation (the most important one)
2. Decrease in functional residual capacity ⎫
3. Ventilation/perfusion imbalance   ⎬ Contributing factors
4. Abnormal ventilatory control   ⎭

18. **What are the consequences of hypoxemia during sleep in COPD patients?**

    Hemodynamics. Hypoxemia at night causes an increase in pulmonary arterial pressure.

    Cardiac dysrhythmias. Patients with COPD have an increased frequency of premature ventricular contractions (PVCs) during sleep, which decreases with supplemental oxygen treatment.

    Polycythemia. Serum erythropoietin values rise at night in patients with COPD and modest hypoxemia.

    Quality of sleep. Patients with COPD sleep poorly compared with matched normal controls. Arousals are common during episodes of desaturation.

    Death during sleep. Death in COPD patients occurs more often at night, and death at night is more common in those with hypoxemia and CO_2 retention.

19. **What are the causes of acute respiratory failure in COPD?**

    Bronchial infection, pulmonary emboli, cardiac failure, pneumonia, pneumothorax, respiratory depression (usually by the injudicious use of sedatives or narcotic analgesic drugs), surgery (especially of chest and upper abdomen), stopping of medications, or occasionally, malnutrition. In general, the criteria for the diagnosis of acute respiratory failure in COPD patients include hypoxemia ($PaO_2 < 60$ mmHg), hypercapnia ($PaCO_2 > 50–70$ mmHg, and respiratory acidosis ($pH < 7.35$) associated with worsening of the patient's respiratory symptoms compared with baseline.

20. **What is the treatment of acute respiratory failure secondary to COPD?**

    - Use a conservative approach if at all possible (i.e., avoid an artificial airway and mechanical ventilation)
    - Apply immediate lifesaving measures (treat hypoxemia and airflow obstruction)
    - Determine and correct the precipitating factors
    - Treat underlying condition
    - Avoid complications
    - Monitor in intensive care unit

    Oxygen therapy is the cornerstone of treatment. Death or irreversible brain damage results within minutes when severe hypoxemia is present, whereas hypercapnia may be well tolerated. The appropriate amount of oxygen is that which satisfies tissue oxygen needs: usually a $PaO_2 > 60$ mmHg, without worsening the respiratory acidosis and/or further depressing sensorium.

21. **Should mechanical ventilation be used in COPD?**

    It seems reasonable to recommend ventilation when conservative aggressive treatment, including controlled oxygen therapy, has failed. This would be indicated by progressive worsening of hypoxia, by acidosis, by increased respiratory muscle fatigue, and by onset of nonarousable somnolence. Still, the need for mechanical ventilation remains a subjective judgment in spite of numerous proposed biologic criteria. Some recommend close monitoring of arterial PaO_2 and pH, and regard controlled oxygen therapy as having failed if PaO_2 could not be maintained over 55 mmHg without the pH falling below 7.26. Intubation should be done with a tube at least 8 mm in internal diameter or greater, because of the frequent need for suctioning thick secretions. Ventilation should be maintained for at least 24–48 hours to allow recovery of fatigued respiratory muscles.

    A frequent result of error in management is hyperventilation: the goal should be to maintain the patient's baseline arterial blood gases. These patients are frequently hypercapnic and have developed renal compensation. Hyperventilation will result in metabolic alkalosis ($pH > 7.50$) with all its side effects—decreased cardiac output, impaired cerebral blood flow, cardiac arrhythmias, decreased ventilatory drive, and prolonged ventilation because of difficulty in weaning.

22. **What is the prognosis for patients with COPD after an episode of acute respiratory failure?**

    Several studies have indicated that respiratory intensive care can have a marked effect on the survival rate of patients with acute respiratory failure. However, the prognosis remains controversial. Hospital mortality has varied from 6–38% and the 2-year survival rate of 25–68%.

The cause of the acute respiratory failure is important in prognosis: mortality in patients presenting with infection (20%) is very different from that of patients presenting with heart failure (40%). The severity of acidosis on admission, expressed as arterial pH, correlates better with survival than does the absolute level of PaO_2; mortality increases markedly if pH is below 7.32.

The influence of mechanical ventilation on outcome remains unclear. Hudson divided several series of COPD patients complicated by acute respiratory failure into two groups: those treated before 1975 had a survival of 72%; those treated after 1975 had a survival of 91%. Thus, most patients with COPD survive an episode of acute respiratory failure, even if the subsequent prognosis for survival is poor and similar to that of other patients with COPD without episodes of acute respiratory failure. However, both are strongly related to the severity of the underlying process.

CONTROVERSIES

23. Are steroids indicated in the emergency treatment of acute exacerbations of COPD?

It is almost a universal practice to use steroids for acute exacerbations of COPD. This comes from the work of Albert and associates, who treated these patients with prednisone, 0.5 mg/kg every 6 hours for 3 days; however, there was only modest improvement in spirometric values after 72 hours of treatment. Emerman and associates used the intravenous administration of methylprednisolone in a randomized, controlled, double-blind study early in the treatment of acute exacerbations of COPD. Ninety-six patients without a history of asthma and all aged 50 years or more were given aminophylline and hourly aerosolized isoetharine. Thirty minutes after arrival in the emergency room, methylprednisolone, 100 mg, or physiologic saline solution was given. There were no better improvements in FEV_1 measured by spirometry initially and after the third and fourth aerosol treatments in patients receiving steroids than in the control group, nor was there a difference between groups in the rate of hospital admissions. So, the use of steroids in this situation is still controversial. However, it is doubtful that steroids are harmful when given only for a few (2–3) days.

24. Are steroids indicated in the chronic treatment of COPD?

Their use is still controversial. The number of "responders" cited varies between 6% and 25%; however, some patients do derive unequivocal benefit from corticosteroids. In general, there is no way to predict who will respond to corticosteroids other than to perform a therapeutic trial. Some experts contend that patients who have a increase in FEV_1 of 15% or more from bronchodilator drugs might respond the best. The steroids are given at a dose equivalent to 40 mg/day of prednisone for 2 weeks, and then FEV_1 is re-measured. Unless the control measurements are markedly reproducible, only increases of FEV_1 greater than 30% are considered to indicate a positive response. In patients who respond, an attempt is made to maintain the response with high doses of inhaled steroids. Unfortunately only a small number of patients can be maintained on inhaled steroids. In patients in need of oral steroids, a dose larger than 20 mg/day of prednisone should be avoided, because complications such as osteoporosis, diabetes, and myopathy, which are disastrous in elderly sick patients, might occur.

BIBLIOGRAPHY

1. Albert RK, Martin TR, Lewis SW: Controlled clinical trial of methylprednisolone in patients with chronic bronchitis and acute respiratory insufficiency. Ann Intern Med 92:735–758, 1980.
2. American Thoracic Society: Standards for the diagnosis and care of patients with chronic obstructive pulmonary disease (COPD) and asthma. Am Rev Respir Dis 136:225–244, 1987.
3. ATS Statement: Standards for the diagnosis and care of patients with chronic obstructive pulmonary disease. Am J Respir Crit Care Med 152(Suppl):5, 1995.
4. Bone RC: Symposium on respiratory failure. Med Clin North Am 67:549–750, 1983.

5. Cherniack RM, Irvin C (eds): Chronic Respiratory Failure. 32nd Annual Aspen Lung Conference. Chest 97(Suppl), 1990.
6. Douglas NJ, Flenley DC: Breathing during sleep in patients with obstructive lung disease. Am Rev Respir Dis 141:1055–1070, 1990.
7. Emerman CL, Connors AF, Lukens TW, et al: A randomized controlled trial of methylprednisolone in the emergency treatment of acute exacerbations of COPD. Chest 95:563–567, 1989.
8. Fernandez E: Beta-adrenergic agonists. Semin Respir Med 8:353–365, 1987.
9. Hubbard RC, Brantley ML, Sellers SE, et al: Anti-neutrophil-elastase defenses of the lower respiratory tract in α_1-antitrypsin deficiency directly augmented with aerosol of α_1-antitrypsin. Ann Intern Med 111:206–212, 1989.
10. Mendella LA, Manfreda J, Warren CPW, Anthonisen NR: Steroid response in stable chronic obstructive pulmonary disease. Ann Intern Med 96:17–21, 1982.
11. Murciano D, Auclair M-H, Pariente R, Aubier M: A randomized, controlled trial of theophylline in patients with severe chronic obstructive pulmonary disease. N Engl J Med 320:1521–1525, 1989.
12. Nocturnal Oxygen Therapy Trial Group: Continuous or nocturnal oxygen therapy in hypoxemic chronic obstructive lung disease: A clinical trial. Ann Intern Med 93:391–398, 1980.
13. Pierson DJ: Acute respiratory failure. In Sahn SA (ed): Pulmonary Emergencies. New York, Churchill Livingstone, 1982.
14. Siafakas NM, Vermeire P, Pride NB, et al: Optimal assessment and management of chronic obstructive pulmonary disease (COPD). Eur Respir J 8:1398–1420, 1995.
15. Watanabe S, Kanner RE, Cutillo AG, et al: Long-term effect of almitrine bismesylate in patients with hypoxemic chronic obstructive lung disease. Am Rev Respir Dis 140:1269–1273, 1989.
16. Ziment T: Pharmacologic therapy of obstructive airway disease. Clin Chest Med 11:461–486, 1990.

20. COR PULMONALE

Enrique Fernandez, M.D., and Michael J. Yanakakis, M.D.

1. What is cor pulmonale?

The causes are multiple, but the unifying process is increased right heart work as a result of pulmonary hypertension. The World Health Organization efines cor pulmonale as "enlargement of the right ventricle (dilation and/or hypertrophy) due to increased right ventricular overload from diseases of the lungs or pulmonary circulation." Right heart failure need not be present. Cor pulmonale is independent of right heart processes that are secondary to left heart failure or congenital heart disease.

2. What are the subtypes of cor pulmonale?

The causes of cor pulmonale can be divided into two subtypes: asphyxial or hypoxic and vascular obliterans. The most common disease process associatesd with the asphyxial or hypoxic subtype is chronic obstructive pulmonary disease (COPD). Common causes of the obliterative subtype are chronic pulmonary thromobemoblic disease and primary pulmonary hypertension.

3. Discuss the prevalence and incidence of right ventricular hypertrophy and edema in COPD.

Cor pulmonale is estimated to be responsible for 7–10% of all diagnoses of heart disease. The prevalence of cor pulmonale increases with worsened airflow limitation in COPD. In fact, any disease state that worsens hypercarbia, hypoxemia, and acidemia can contribute to the further development of cor pulmonale. In the United States, 10–30% of all admissions for congestive heart failure are due to right ventricular hypertrophy and failure.

4. What are the causes of cor pulmonale?

See table on following page.

Classification of Cor Pulmonale According to Causative Factor

CATEGORY	EXAMPLE
Diseases affecting the air passages of the lung and alveoli	Chronic obstructive pulmonary disease
	Cystic fibrosis
	Infiltrative or granulomatous defects
	Idiopathic pulmonary fibrosis
	Sarcoidosis
	Pneumoconiosis
	Scleroderma
	Mixed connective tissue disease
	Systemic lupus erythematosus
	Rheumatoid arthritis
	Polymyositis
	Eosinophilic granulomatosis
	Radiation
	Malignant infiltration
Diseases affecting thoracic cage movement	Kyphoscoliosis
	Thoracoplasty
	Neuromuscular weakness
	Sleep apnea syndrome
	Idiopathic hypoventilation
Diseases affecting the pulmonary vasculature	Primary disease of the arterial wall
	Primary pulmonary hypertension
	Pulmonary arteritis
	Toxin-induced pulmonary hypertension
	Chronic liver disease
	Peripheral pulmonary stenosis
Thrombotic disorders	Sickle cell diseases
	Pulmonary microthrombi
Embolic disorders	Thromboembolism
	Tumor embolism
	Other embolic processes (amniotic fluid, air, fat)
	Schistosomiasis and other parasitic infections
Pressure on pulmonary arteries	Mediastinal tumors
	Aneurysms
	Granulomata
	Fibrosis

Adapted from Rubin LJ (ed): Pulmonary Heart Disease. Boston, Martinus Nijhoff, 1984, p 4.

5. Describe the pathophysiology of cor pulmonale.

The right ventricle pumps against a low-resistance circuit, normally one-tenth the resistance of the systemic arteries. The right ventricle is thin-walled and accommodates considerable changes in volume without large changes in pressure. Increased cardiac output leads to recruitment of underperfused pulmonary vessels and distention of other pulmonary vessels. The initial pathophysiologic event in the production of cor pulmonale is elevation of the pulmonary vascular resistance. As the resistance increases, the pulmonary arterial pressure rises and demands more work from the right ventricle. As the workload increases, right ventricular hypertrophy (thickening and/or dilation) develops.

6. What are the symptoms and signs of cor pulmonale?

The signs and symptoms of cor pulmonale are often subtle unless the disease process becomes far advanced. In addition, clinicians tend to focus on the disease giving rise to cor pulmonale rather than on the cor pulmonale itself. Below are commonly encountered clinical signs of cor pulmonale:

- Accentuated A wave of the jugular venous pulsations
- Prominent jugular V wave, indicating the presence of tricuspid regurgitation
- Palpable left parasternal lift
- Accentuated pulmonic component of the second heart sound
- Right-sided S4
- Murmurs of tricuspid and pulmonic insufficiency
- Dependent peripheral edema and hepatomegaly

7. What are the EKG criteria of right ventricle hypertrophy?

- Right axis deviation or rightward shift in axis
- Right atrial enlargement. An increase in the R atrial potential typically translates into a large P wave, P pulmonale, in the inferior and anterior leads. P pulmonale is present in about 20% of patients with clinical evidence of cor pulmonale. COPD can give rise to P pulmonale without evidence of right ventricular hypertrophy.
- Right ventricular hypertrophy (RVH). The sensitivity of the EKG in diagnosing RVH in patients with chronic cor pulmonale is 60–70% when assessed at autopsy.
- Right bundle-branch block
- Right precordial T-wave inversions
- Delayed intrinsicoid deflection of right precordial leads
- SIQ3T3 pattern
- qR pattern in lead V_1 or V_3R
- An R wave in V_1 or V_3R
- An R/S ratio > 1 in V_1 or < 1 in V_5 or V_6
- An R′ in V_1 or V_3R > 6 mm or an R′s in V1 > 1.0 (QRS duration < 0.10 second)

8. What tests can help determine the diagnosis?

Chest radiograph. Radiographic signs include an enlarged pulmonary artery and/or right ventricle, a distended azygous or other central vein, oligemia of a lung lobe or entire lung (Westermark sign), and a wedge-shaped opacity (Hampton's hump). In addition, the common findings associated with COPD may be seen, including increased anterior-posterior diameter, flattening of the diaphragms, honeycombing, and hyperlucency.

Echocardiography. An adequate examination is reported in up to 65–80% of patients with COPD because of the technical difficulty associated with hyperinflation. A better examination can be obtained with transesophageal echocardiography. Doppler echocardiography has aided in the assessment of pulmonary artery pressures by measuring the flow of regurgitant blood across the tricuspid valve or by measuring right ventricular ejection flow.

Right heart cardiac catheterization. This is the gold standard for thorough evaluation and diagnosis of pulmonary hypertension.

Radionuclide angiography (gated blood pool scan). This test is most useful for measuring right and left ventricular ejection fraction.

Magnetic resonance imaging (MRI). This noninvasive technique yields highly accurate dimensions of the right ventricle.

9. Decribe the treatment options for cor pulmonale.

Oxygen therapy is considered a mainstay of treatment for patients with COPD, and a large controlled trial demonstrated that long-term administration of oxygen improves survival in hypoxemic patients with COPD. Oxygen therapy decreases pulmonary vascular resistance by diminishing pulmonary vasoconstriction and improves right ventricular stroke volume and cardiac output.

Diuretics. This therapy may be needed in congestive cardiac failure to take care of the excessive water that the lungs share and to improve alveolar ventilation and gas exchange. However, the use of diuretics may produce hemodynamic side effects, such as volume depletion, decreased venous return to the right ventricle, and decreased cardiac output. Another complication is the production of hypokalemic metabolic alkalosis, which diminishes the CO_2 stimulus to the respiratory center, decreasing ventilatory drive.

Phlebotomy. In patients with pronounced polycythemia (hematocrit > 60%), phlebotomy may provide symptomatic relief. In resting patients, phlebotomy can effect a mild decrease in pulmonary artery pressure and pulmonary vascular resistance. In general, blood viscosity has less effect than blood volume on pulmonary arterial pressure. Phlebotomy may improve exercise tolerance in patients with polycythemic COPD.

10. Discuss the role of vasodilator therapy in patients with cor pulmonale.
The list of vasodilators is extensive, and their efficacies are unpredictable. They improve cardiac output in many patients with cor pulmnale, but they may be associated with adverse effects, including systemic hypotension that compromises coronary perfusion pressure, blunting of hypoxic pulmonary vasoconstriction, and circulatory collapse. Examples include nonspecific and pulmonary vasodilators as well as inotropes with vasodilatory properties.

  1. **Nonspecific vasodilators**
- **Hydralazine** increases cardiac output in patients with COPD; however, its ablity to decrease pulmonary artery pressure is unpredictable.
- **Nitroprusside** may provide benefit but also runs the risk of systemic hypotension and compromise of adequate coronary perfusion pressure.
- **Calcium channel blockers.** Nifedipine reduces pulmonary vascular resistance and increases cardiac output only for the short term. Verapamil and diltiazem have not proved effective in dilating pulmonary vasculature.

  2. **Pulmonary vasodilators**
- **Prostaglandins** decrease pulmonary artery pressure and increase right ventricular ejection fraction and cardiac output. **Aerosolized prostacyclin** causes pulmonary artery vasodilation and improves cardiac output and arterial oxyhemoglobin saturation in patients with chronic pulmonary hypertension.
- **Nitric oxide** provides the ideal clinical scenario. It reliably decreases pulmonary vascular resistance without causing systemic hypotension and preserves or improves optimal ventilation–perfusion match. Its drawbacks are difficult admininstration, high cost, and a well-documented tachyphylactic effect. Multiple studies have shown that its benefits are most significant for only 1–3 days, especially in patients with ARDS.

  3. **Inotropes with vasodilatory properties**
- **Dobutamine** improves right ventricular function and cardiac output, but its effect on systemic blood pressure is unpredictable. Repeat echocardiography after institution of therapy can help to guide management. However, the effects of dobutamine (and other beta agonists, including isoproterenol and epinephrine) on pulmonary arterial pressure may be minimal and unsustained.
- **Amrinone.** Although few data are available about its action in right heart syndrome, amrinone lowers pulmonary arterial pressure and raises cardiac output and systemic blood pressure.

11. Is left ventricular function impaired in chronic cor pulmonale?
Left ventricular dysfunction has been documented in patients with cor pulmonale. The proposed mechanism is bulging of the ventricular septum toward the left ventricle as a result of ventricular overload. This interplay between right and left ventricles is perhaps best supported by the recovery of left ventricular as well as right ventricular function in patients who have undergone lung transplantation.

12. Should digoxin be used for COPD?
Cardiac output improves in about 10% of patients with primary pulmonary hypertension who receive digoxin. This rate is similar to that in patients with left ventricular dysfunction. Patients who receive digoxin also showed a modest increase in pulmonary pressure, perhaps due to increased cardiac output. Past clinical studies demonstrated a benefit in patients with cor pulmonale only when left ventricular failure was present. Recently digoxin has fallen out of favor in the setting of left ventricular dysfunction; the trend in clinical medicine has been its continued use in rate control.

13. Discuss the considerations for ventilator management of patients with cor pulmonale.

Hypercarbia and acidemia as well as hypoxemia increase pulmonary artery pressure. Therefore, adequate ventilation and oxygenation are critical in the management of patients with cor pulmonale. The effect of positive end-expiratory pressure (PEEP) on right ventricular function is complex and varies from patient to patient; it also depends on the level of PEEP. Clearly, higher levels of PEEP are more likely to impair right ventricular function. It is believed that PEEP used to recruit atelectatic areas of lung, thereby improving the compliance curve, should have no deleterious effects on right ventricular function. However, normal areas of the lung are overdistended, right ventricular function may be compromised.

BIBLIOGRAPHY

1. Braunwald E: Pathophysiology of heart failure. In Braunwald E (ed): Heart Disease. A Textbook of Cardiovascular Medicine, 5th ed. Philadelphia, W.B. Saunders, 1997.
2. Burgess M, Ray S, Mogulkoc N, et al: Doppler echocardiographic index of global right ventricular function. Circulation 101:117, 2000.
3. Chiche J-D, Dhainaut J-FA: Inhaled nitric oxide for right ventricular dysfunction in chronic obstructive pulmonary disease patients: Fall or rise of an idea? Crit Care Med 27:2299–2301, 1999.
4. Chou T: Electrocardiography in Clinical Practice: Adult and Pediatric, 4th ed. Philadelphia, W.B. Saunders, 1996.
5. Klinger JR, Hill NS: Right ventricular dysfunction in chronic obstructive pulmonary disease. Chest 99:715–723, 1991.
6. Kohama A, Tarauchi J, Hori M, et al: Pathologic involvement of the left ventricle in chronic cor pulmonale. Chest 98:794–800, 1990.
7. Olschewski H, Walmrath D, Schermuly R, et al: Aerosolized prostacylin and iloprost in severe pulmonary hypertension. Ann Intern Med 124:820, 1996.
8. Rich S, Seidlitz M, Dodin E, et al: The short-term effects of digoxin in patients with right ventricular dysfunction from pulmonary hypertension. Chest 114:787–792, 1996.
9. Rubin LJ (ed): Pulmonary Heart Disease. Boston, Martin Nijhoff Publishing, 1984.
10. Schmidt GA, Wood LDH: Acute right heart syndrome. In Hall JB, Schmidt GA, Wood LDH (eds): Principles of Critical Care, 2nd ed. New York, McGraw-Hill.
11. Vizza CD, Lynch JP, Ochoa LL, et al: Right and left ventricular dysfunction in patients with severe pulmonary disease. Chest 113:576–583, 1995.
12. Weir EK, Rubin LJ, Ayres SM, et al: The acute administration of vasodilators in primary pulmonary hypertension. Am Rev Respir Dis 140:1623–1630, 1989.
13. World Health Organization: Chronic cor pulmonale. A report of the expert committee. Circulation 27: 594–615, 1963.

21. ACUTE RESPIRATORY FAILURE

Martin R. Zamora, M.D., and Daniel Burkhardt, M.D.

1. Define acute respiratory failure (ARF).

ARF is a physiologically defined condition that may result from a variety of disease processes. It occurs when the respiratory system is unable to adequately absorb oxygen (hypoxemia) and/or excrete carbon dioxide (hypercapnia). It may develop over the course of minutes, hours, or days in patients with previously normal lung function or patients with preexisting disease.

2. How is ARF diagnosed?

Hypoxemia and hypercapnia are difficult to diagnose on physical exam. Noninvasive detection of hypoxemia via pulse oximetry is usually reliable. Noninvasive detection of hypercapnia, however, is not reliable with current technology. Thus, arterial blood gas (ABG) analysis remains the best method of diagnosing ARF. Although no rigid criteria apply for all patients, it is generally accepted that respiratory failure is present when the arterial PO_2 is < 50 mmHg and/or the arterial pH is < 7.30 (usually corresponding to an arterial PCO_2 > 50 mmHg if the bicarbonate level is normal).

3. What are the two primary types of ARF?
ARF may be due to failure of oxygenation (hypoxemia) or failure of ventilation (hypercapnia). Both processes may be present in a given patient, but generally one type predominates.

4. What physiologic mechanisms may cause hypoxemia? What are their responses to supplemental oxygen?
- Alveolar hypoventilation (extreme hypercapnia also occurs)
- Ventilation perfusion mismatch
- Right-to-left shunt ("blood that sees no air")
- Diffusion limitation
- Low inspired oxygen (e.g., high altitude)
- Severe pulmonary venous hypoxia (cardiogenic shock)

The hypoxemia caused by all of these mechanisms responds to supplemental oxygen with the exception of shunt. Because shunted blood by definition bypasses all ventilated lung units, increasing the partial pressure of inspired oxygen has little-to-no effect.

5. What physiologic mechanisms may cause hypercapnic ARF?
ARF occurs only when hypercapnia results in acidemia. The pH, pCO_2, and bicarbonate level have a fixed relationship specified by the Henderson-Hasselbach equation, with bicarbonate as the primary buffer. This holds true regardless of the clinical circumstances. Physiologic mechanisms include the following:
- Central (depressed respiratory drive)
- Neuromuscular (decreased neural transmission or muscular translation of the drive signal)
- Abnormalities of the chest wall (restrictive disease)
- Abnormalities of gas flow in the airways (obstructive disease)
- Increased dead space ("air that sees no blood")
- Increased CO_2 production (rarely a problem without significant underlying lung disease)

6. Which disease processes are associated with each type of ARF? Which are reversible?
The differential diagnosis of hypoxemic ARF can be based on whether hypercapnia or hypoxemia is present and whether the lung fields on chest x-ray are "black"(normal or hyperlucent) or "white" (radiopaque). If the patient is hypoxemic and the chest x-ray is black, pulmonary embolus, circulatory collapse, or right-to-left shunt is likely. If the chest x-ray is diffusely white, acute respiratory distress syndrome (ARDS), cardiogenic pulmonary edema, or pulmonary fibrosis is possible. If the abnormality is localized, the patient may have pneumonia, atelectasis, or pulmonary infarction. If the chest-x-ray is black in patients with hypercapnia, status asthmaticus, chronic obstructive pulmonary disease (COPD), or alveolar hypoventilation secondary to drug overdose, neuromuscular weakness, paralysis, or sleep apnea syndrome is likely. If the chest x-ray is diffusely white, end-stage pulmonary fibrosis or severe ARDS is possible, whereas if the findings are localized, the patient may have pneumonia with underlying COPD or respiratory depression with associated atelectasis. In general, most of the above conditions are reversible. However, severe COPD, sleep apnea syndrome, diseases of the respiratory muscles, cervical fracture leading to paralysis, and kyphoscoliosis may lead to chronic carbon dioxide retention and chronic respiratory failure. In patients with these underlying disorders, ARF due to other causes may occur and should be investigated.

7. What empirical therapy should be used emergently in patients with ARF?
Raising the arterial PO_2 to an adequate level (usually > 50 mmHg) is the first goal of therapy. If the patient is alert and cooperative, supplemental oxygen with a repeat arterial gas within 20–30 minutes and close observation in the ICU may be adequate. If the patient is awake, protecting the airway, and has a reversible condition, noninvasive positive-pressure ventilation (NIPPV) should

be considered. If the patient is stuporous or comatose, has a decreased gag reflex, vomiting, or copious secretions, control of the airway by endotracheal intubation is warranted. In the case of suspected opiate overdose (respiratory depression, pinpoint pupils, and coma), naloxone is indicated.

8. What is the maximal inspired concentration of oxygen (FiO$_2$) that can be delivered noninvasively?

Nasal prongs usually cannot exceed an effective FiO$_2$ of 0.3. Face mask oxygen usually cannot
exceed an FiO$_2$ of 0.5–0.6. Especially with nasal prongs, these techniques deliver a progressively
lower effective FiO$_2$ as the patient develops an increased minute ventilation in response to ARF. (A
fixed flow of oxygen is diluted in a larger and larger total minute ventilation). An FiO$_2$ of 1.0 can be
delivered only via an endotracheal tube or a completely sealed face mask attached to a device that
can deliver 100% oxygen at very high inspiratory flow rates. This approach normally requires a full
ICU ventilator or a sealed nonrebreathing circuit with a large reservoir of 100% oxygen.

9. What are the indications for endotracheal intubation?
- Hypoxemia or hypercapnic acidosis despite maximal noninvasive therapy
- Cardiopulmonary resuscitation with the need for complete control of the airway
- Airway protection from aspiration of gastric contents
- Control of copious airway secretions
- Complete or impending upper airway obstruction
- Significant risk of developing any of the above conditions while in an area where endotra-
  cheal intubation is not immediately available (i.e. during transport)

10. What are the indications for mechanical ventilation?

Mechanical ventilation is required whenever the patient is unable to maintain adequate alveolar ventilation (hypercapnia leading to an arterial pH < 7.30). It is more difficult to determine
when mechanical ventilation is indicated in patients with hypoxemic ARF without hypercapnia.
However, excessive work of breathing to maintain acceptable ABG values may lead to respiratory muscle fatigue and failure, requiring mechanical ventilation. The decision to institute mechanical ventilation must be based on the clinical appearance of the patient and blood gas
analysis and must take into account whether the underlying process is reversible. Mechanical
ventilation may also be used to provide hyperventilation to head trauma patients for transient reduction in intracranial pressure. Mechanical ventilation can be delivered via endotracheal tube,
tracheostomy tube, or (in the awake patient) nasal or full face-mask NIPPV.

11. What is PEEP? When should it be used?

Positive end-expiratory pressure (PEEP) is a technique to mechanically correct hypoxemia. PEEP
increases the end-expiratory pressure, which prevents the patient's airway pressure from falling below
the preset level during the respiratory cycle. This increases the volume of gas in the patient's chest at
end expiration (functional residual capacity) and is thought to prevent alveolar collapse. The treatment, therefore, should be beneficial in patients with diseases such as ARDS or congestive heart
failure, because the hypoxemia in these disorders may be due to alveolar collapse, filling, or both.
Elevated levels of PEEP have been associated with barotrauma (pneumothorax), but the use of high
concentrations of oxygen also has been associated with lung injury. Large trials are currently under
way to determine the relative risks of using high PEEP vs. high FiO$_2$ to avoid hypoxemia.

12. What is the significance of the patient who is "fighting the ventilator"?

The sudden onset of agitation and distress in a patient who previously tolerated mechanical
ventilation is a medical emergency and signifies an acute deterioration in the underlying disease,
malfunction of the ventilator, or obstruction of the airway or endotracheal tube. The patient
should be disconnected from the ventilator and manually ventilated. Vital signs should be obtained, the chest examined, the airway suctioned, and arterial blood gas analysis and chest x-ray
performed. If no cause is found after these measures, the ventilator set-up may be incorrect for

the patient's needs. Changes in the ventilator settings are in order to match the machine more closely with the patient's requirements.

13. When can patients be weaned from mechanical ventilation?

Patients should show clinical improvement, with stabilization and correction of any underlying conditions that may interfere with weaning (electrolyte disturbances, fluid overload, severe anemia, or uncontrolled pain). Patients should be alert, with stable vital signs, and have an intact gag reflex. There are no perfect predictors of successful weaning from mechanical ventilation. Numerous physiologic guidelines exist. Oxygenation is generally adequate when the arterial PO_2 is > 60 mmHg on an FiO_2 ≤ 50% and PEEP = 0–5 cmH_2O. Ventilation is much harder to assess. Factors to consider include respiratory rate (RR) < 20, tidal volume (TV) > 5 ml/kg, RR/TV> ~ 100 L (the rapid shallow breathing index), vital capacity > 10–15 ml/kg, minute ventilation (VE) < 10/Lmin, and negative inspiratory force of at least –25 cmH_2O. Repeated trials of spontaneous breathing have generally proved at least as effective as other weaning strategies.

14. What are some postextubation complications?

• Hoarseness
• Difficulty in swallowing and risk of aspiration
• Severe glottic edema leading to postextubation stridor and obstruction (may be treated with racemic epinephrine (0.5 ml of 2.25% solution in 3 ml saline via nebulized aerosol)

BIBLIOGRAPHY

1. Acute Respiratory Distress Syndrome Network: Ventilation with lower tidal volumes as compared with traditional tidal volumes for acute lung injury and the acute respiratory distress syndrome. N Engl J Med 342:1301–1308, 2000.
2. de Anda GF, Lachmann B: Treatment and prevention of acute respiratory failure: Physiological basis. Arch Med Res 32:91–101, 2001.
3. Epstein DK, Singh N: Respiratory acidosis. Respir Care, 46:366–383, 2001.
4. Evans TW, for the International Consensus Conferences in Intensive Care Medicine: Noninvasive positive pressure ventilation in acute respiratory failure. Am J Respir Crit Care Med 163:283–291, 2001.
5. Greene KE, Peters JL: Pathophysiology of acute respiratory failure. Clin Chest Med 15:1–12, 1994.
6. Irwin RS, French CT, Mike RW: Respiratory adjunct therapy. In Irwin RS, Rippe JM (eds): Irwin and Rippe's Intensive Care Medicine. Philadelphia, Lippincott-Raven, 1999, pp 763–774.
7. MacIntyre NR, et al: Evidence-based guidelines for weaning and discontinuing ventilatory support: A collective task force facilitated by the American College of Chest Physicians; the American Association for Respiratory Care; and the American College of Critical Care Medicine. Chest, 120(6 Suppl):375S–395S, 2001.
8. Tobin MJ: Advances in mechanical ventilation. N Engl J Med 344:1986–1996, 2001.
9. Wood LDH: The pathophysiology and differential diagnosis of acute respiratory failure. In Hall JB, Schmidt GA, Wood LDH (eds): Principles of Critical Care. New York, McGraw-Hill, 1998, pp 499–508.

22. ACUTE RESPIRATORY DISTRESS SYNDROME

Mohamed Turki, M.D., and Polly E. Parsons, M.D.

1. What is acute respiratory distress syndrome (ARDS)?

ARDS, also known as adult respiratory distress syndrome, is a noncardiogenic pulmonary capillary leak syndrome characterized clinically by the development of rapidly progressive hypoxemia, diffuse alveolar infiltrates on chest x-ray, and decreased lung compliance following a known predisposing insult. Pathologically the syndrome is characterized acutely by alveolar and interstitial edema and flooding of the alveoli with a proteinaceous exudate and inflammatory cells, including neutrophils and macrophages, followed by the development of pulmonary fibrosis.

2. What are the diagnostic criteria for ARDS?

The diagnostic criteria for ARDS continue to be refined. Although the pathologic findings are objective and can be agreed on, most patients do not undergo lung biopsy. The diagnosis is made clinically. The following criteria are currently used:

- Bilateral infiltrates on chest x-ray
- Partial arterial oxygen tension (PaO_2)/fractional concentration of oxygen in inspired gas (FiO_2) < 200
- No evidence of left atrial hypertension

These criteria should be applied only to patients with a defined risk factor for ARDS and without evidence of severe chronic pulmonary disease.

3. What is acute lung injury (ALI)?

Traditional definitions of ARDS do not include patients with mild or early evidence of acute lung injury. Accordingly, the following criteria have been established to identify such patients:

- Bilateral infiltrates on chest x-ray
- PaO_2/FiO_2 < 300
- No evidence of left atrial hypertension

Again, these patients should have a defined risk factor and not have severe chronic pulmonary disease. These definitions of ALI and ARDS remain somewhat subjective. Recently it was shown that interobserver variability in radiographic interpretation of bilateral infiltrates is significant. Twenty-one experts were asked to review 28 radiographs and ascertain whether they met criteria for the diagnosis of ALI or ARDS. All of the experts believed that radiograph A was consistent with ALI/ARDS, whereas 52% believed that radiograph B was consistent with the diagnosis.

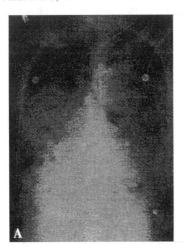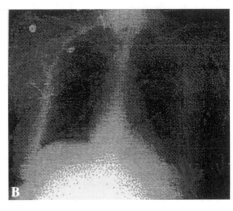

From Rubenfeld GD, Caldwell E, Granton J, et al: Interobserver variability in applying a radiographic definition for ARDS. Chest 116:1347–1353, 1999, with permission.

4. What conditions predispose to the development of ARDS?

Several clinical syndromes, including sepsis, aspiration of gastric contents, trauma, pancreatitis, massive transfusions, and near drowning, have been identified as predisposing risk factors for ALI/ARDS. Sepsis is the most common, with an incidence of ALI/ARDS of approximately 40%.

5. Explain the pathogenesis of ARDS.

The pathogenesis of ALI is complex, and understanding of the process continues to evolve. The hallmark of ARDS is the loss of integrity of the components of the alveolar capillary barrier, the microvascular endothelium, and the alveolar epithelium. Such injury probably results from the systemic release of mediators (e.g., complement fragments, endotoxin, tumor necrosis factor) that activate/stimulate neutrophils and macrophages (and perhaps other cell types) to become sequestered within the pulmonary capillaries and release toxic products such as oxygen metabolites, proteases, and leukotrienes. The inability to delineate clearly the pathogenesis of ARDS has significantly hampered efforts at treatment.

6. Why do patients with ARDS die?

Less than 10% of deaths in patients with ARDS are due to hypoxic respiratory failure. The majority of deaths that occur within 72 hours result from the original precipitating insult, whereas after 72 hours mortality is often related to infection.

7. What is the mortality rate of ARDS?

When ARDS was first described in 1967, the mortality rate was 58% (7/12 patients). In the past decade, the mortality rate has decreased to approximately 40% or less.

8. How fast does ARDS develop?

Very fast: 80% of patients develop ARDS within 24 hours of onset of a predisposing conditions and 95% develop it within 72 hours.

9. Can ARDS be prevented?

No. The precipitating clinical disorder must be prevented.

10. What therapy is available for ARDS?

Currently no specific therapy is effective for ARDS, although several agents, including steroids, prostaglandin E1 (PGE_1), N-acetylcysteine, surfactant replacement, anti-endotoxin antibodies, anti-tumor necrosis factor antibodies, ketoconazole, lisofylline, and nitric oxide have been tried. However, new therapeutic modalities with significant potential continue to be developed.

11. How can pneumonia be diagnosed in patients with ARDS?

This is an area of intense discussion. The clinical diagnosis is generally based on the development of new infiltrates on chest x-ray, purulent sputum, fever, and peripheral leukocytosis. However, an autopsy study of patients with ARDS demonstrated that 80% of patients without pneumonia had fever and leukocytosis and 70% had purulent sputum. Thus, clinical parameters alone do not appear to be adequate. The other tools available include bronchoscopy with lavage, protected brush sampling, transbronchial biopsy, and open lung biopsy. The sensitivity and specificity of these procedures in patients with ARDS are not well defined. The keys to diagnosis are constant surveillance and a low threshold for evaluating and treating the patient.

12. What are the pulmonary sequelae in survivors of ARDS?

Surprisingly, some survivors are virtually unimpaired 1 year after an episode of ARDS despite evidence of pulmonary fibrosis early in the disease course and prolonged mechanical ventilation with high PEEP and FiO_2. The percentage of survivors who return to normal pulmonary function is difficult to ascertain from the literature. Although numerous studies of ARDS survivors have been published, they have been hampered by inconsistent definition of ARDS, different methods of assessing pulmonary function, varying duration of follow-up, and variable attention to pre-ARDS pulmonary status, length of ventilation, severity of ARDS, and in-hospital complications of ARDS. It appears that there is a spectrum of pulmonary impairment. The majority of survivors have mild-to-moderate impairment, a very few patients have severe impairment, and a small but significant group of patients are normal (see figure on following page).

Distribution of pulmonary impairment in survivors of acute respiratory distress syndrome. (From Elliott CG: Pulmonary sequelae in survivors of adult respiratory distress syndrome. Clin Chest Med 11: 789–800, 1990.

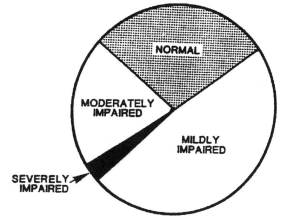

13. Describe the appropriate fluid management for a patient with ARDS.

At present there is no definitive approach to fluid management. A study sponsored by the National Institutes of Health (NIH) to compare two different fluid strategies is ongoing.

14. How should patients with ARDS be ventilated?

The lung injury in ARDS is not homogeneous. Some areas of apparently normal lung are evident on CT scan even when the lungs appear to be diffusely involved on chest x-ray. In animal models, overdistention of normal lung has been associated with the development of inflammation and alveolar flooding. These and other data suggest that patients should be ventilated with low tidal volumes. This approach was recently confirmed by a study performed by the NIH ARDS Network, which compared tidal volumes of 12 ml/kg vs. 6 ml/kg predicted body weight. The mortality rate was 39.8% for the 12-ml group and 31% for the 6-ml group. This study strongly suggests that patients with ALI/ARDS should be ventilated with low tidal volumes. The best level of PEEP is currently under study.

15. What is the effect of prone positioning on the survival of patients with ARDS?

It is not yet clear. A large, recently completed clinical trial compared patients ventilated in a prone or supine position. Prone positioning was associated with an improvement in oxygenation but no improvement in mortality rates. More studies are needed to evaluate the efficacy of prone positioning.

CONTROVERSIES

16. Is there a role for steroids in ARDS?

Steroids clearly do not prevent the development of ARDS when administered to at-risk patients and do not improve mortality rates in patients with early ARDS. The use of steroids to treat persistent ARDS is currently debated.

For: Patients with persistent ARDS, also known as the fibroproliferative phase of ARDS, have ongoing inflammation that responds to steroid therapy. The existence of the fibroproliferative phase of ARDS is relatively well accepted, and clinical studies suggest that the phase is characterized by a persistent inflammatory response (both systemic and pulmonary) and a corresponding fibroproliferative response in the lung. Several small, uncontrolled patient series suggest that the administration of steroids during this fibroproliferative phase improves mortality. A large randomized trial of steroids in late ARDS is currently under way.

Against: The diagnosis of the fibroproliferative phase of ARDS requires careful exclusion of concurrent infection. Because this may be very difficult in patients with ARDS and because the main cause of mortality is sepsis, steroids should not be administered except as part of a controlled clinical trial.

BIBLIOGRAPHY

1. Acute Respiratory Distress Syndrome Network: Ventilation with lower tidal volumes as compared with traditional tidal volumes for acute lung injury and the acute respiratory distress syndrome. N Engl J Med 342:1301–1307, 2000.
2. Artigas A, Bernard GR, et al: The American-European consensus conference on ARDS. Part 2: Ventilatory, pharmacologic, supportive therapy, study design strategies, and issues related to recovery and remodeling. Am J Respir Crit Care Med 157:818–824, 1998.
3. Bernard GR, Artigas A, Brigham K, et al: The American European consensus conference on ARDS: Defintions, mechanisms, relevant outcomes and clinical trial coordination. Am J Respir Crit Care Med 149:818–824, 1994.
4. Elliott CG: Pulmonary sequelae in survivors of adult respiratory distress syndrome. Clin Chest Med 11:789–800, 1990.
5. Gattinoni L, Tognoni G, et al: Effects of prone positioning on the survival patients with acute respiratory distress syndrome. N Engl J Med 345:568–573, 2001.
6. Jantz MA, Sahn SA: Corticosteroids in acute respiratory failure. Am J Respir Crit Care Med 160:1079–1100, 1999.
7. McHugh LG, Milberg JA, Whitcomb ME, et al: Recovery of function in survivors of the acute respiratory distress syndrome. Am J Respir Crit Care Med 150:90–94, 1994.
8. McIntyre RC Jr, Pulido EJ, et al: Thirty years of clinical trials in acute respiratory distress syndrome. Crit Care Med 28:3314–3330, 2000.
9. Milberg JA, Davis DA, Steinberg KP, et al: Improved survival of patients with acute respiratory distress syndrome (ARDS): 1983–1993. JAMA 273:306–309, 1995.
10. Pittet JF, Mackersie RC, Martin TR, Matthay MA: Biological markers of acute lung injury: Prognostic and pathologic significance. Am J Respir Crit Care Med 155:1187–1205, 1997.
11. Rubenfeld GD, Caldwell E, Granton J, et al: Interobserver variability in applying a radiographic definition for ARDS. Chest 116:1347–1353, 1999.
12. Ware BL, Matthay MA: The acute respiratory distress syndrome. N Engl J Med 342:1334–1348, 2000.

23. ASPIRATION

Thomas J. Donnelly, M.D., and York E. Miller, M.D.

1. What is aspiration?

Aspiration is the penetration of foreign material past the vocal cords and into the airways.

2. What are the major consequences of aspiration?

This depends on both the volume and nature of aspirated material. Large volumes of sterile, nonirritating fluid can be introduced into the airways with minor sequelae. Small volumes of oral secretions are universally aspirated during sleep in healthy individuals. Four major groups of clinically significant aspirations are defined by the material aspirated: (1) Foreign bodies or thick particulate fluids can cause airway obstruction. (2) Acidic gastric contents cause a chemical pneumonitis or acute respiratory distress syndrome (ARDS). (3) Aspiration of infected material can result in infectious pneumonia or lung abscess. (4) A syndrome of aspiration occurs in drowning. Overlaps or combinations of these four often occur.

3. Which patients are at risk for aspiration?

Patients with conditions that increase gastric volume, decrease gastric pH, decrease lower esophageal sphincter tone, or lower the normal airway protective mechanisms are at increased risk for aspiration. The risk factors for aspiration may be divided into five categories:

1. **Altered level of consciousness:** alcohol or drug use, cerebrovascular accident, CNS infections or tumors, general anesthesia, hypoxia and metabolic disturbances such as liver failure, sepsis and uremia.

2. **Gastrointestinal diseases:** ascites, esophageal disorders, gastrointestinal bleeding, malignancy and intestinal obstruction.

3. **Mechanical factors:** endotracheal tubes, tracheostomies, upper airway tumors, and nasoenteric tubes.

4. **Neuromuscular diseases:** ALS, botulism, Guillain-Barré syndrome, multiple sclerosis, myasthenia gravis, Parkinson's disease, poliomyelitis, polymyositis, and vocal cord paralysis.

5. **Miscellaneous factors:** obesity, pregnancy, diabetes, and supine patient position.

4. When should airway obstruction by a foreign body be suspected?

Stridor or localized wheezing can occur in this situation. Biphasic stridor over the central airway occurs in partial tracheal obstruction. As the foreign body descends lower in the airway, inspiratory stridor decreases and expiratory stridor becomes more prominent. Cough and localization of wheezing suggest entrapment in a mainstem bronchus. Chest radiographs are helpful to demonstrate radiopaque foreign bodies, such as teeth or bone fragments, or localized areas of atelectasis. CT scan can be helpful. Bronchoscopy (either rigid or fiberoptic) allows the identification and removal of foreign objects and should be performed in all patients in whom aspiration with airway obstruction is suspected. The Heimlich maneuver should be used in critical situations, especially those occurring out of hospital.

5. What is Mendelson's syndrome?

Mendelson originally described cases of large volume gastric aspiration in obstetric patients undergoing general anesthesia. He and other investigators subsequently showed that aspiration of acidic liquids has more severe consequences than aspiration of more neutral pH liquids.

6. What are the results of aspiration of gastric acid?

Aspiration of gastric acid causes immediate and intense injury to the airway and alveolar epithelium. Bronchospasm, pulmonary edema, alveolar collapse due to loss of surfactant, and loss of intravascular fluid volume all occur. ARDS may occur. Although treatment by neutralization of airway fluids has been attempted, acid instilled into the airways is rapidly absorbed and neutralized, rendering these therapies futile. Despite a better understanding of aspiration of acid, mortality is 55–70%.

7. What is lipoid pneumonia?

The aspiration of animal fats, mineral oil or other lipid substances causes an inflammatory response in the lung which is independent of infection. The term "lipoid pneumonia" refers to persistent, alveolar-type infiltrates that occur after aspiration of oil. All patients with a persistent pulmonary infiltrate should be questioned about the use of oral or nasal lubricants (often oily nose drops). Patients who require a nasal emollient (i.e., patients on chronic oxygen therapy by nasal cannula) should be instructed to use only water-based products.

8. What organisms commonly produce infectious complications in aspiration?

The infectious agents depend on the patient population. In normal, healthy individuals who develop aspiration pneumonia, oral anaerobes are usually responsible: *Bacteroides* species, anaerobic streptococci, and *Fusobacterium* species. Hospitalized or debilitated individuals may also have oropharyngeal colonization with *Staphylococcus aureus* or gram-negative organisms. Treatment should be designed to provide anaerobic coverage with high-dose penicillin or clindamycin; additional antibiotics to cover staphylococci or gram-negative organisms should be added in high-risk patients.

9. Does intubation or tracheostomy prevent aspiration?

No. Both intubation and tracheostomy actually breach some of the normal upper airway defenses. Balloon insufflation does not totally protect against fluid entering the airway. In patients with depressed consciousness or neuromuscular disease, however, intubation or tracheostomy may be indicated to decrease the volume of aspiration and to allow suctioning of airway contents.

10. What preventive measures can be used during endotracheal intubation?

Aspiration of gastric contents during intubation can be catastrophic. Several precautions can be taken. Awake intubation, without sedation, can be performed. Fiberoptic intubation may be superior if available. Pressure on the cricoid cartilage (Sellick's maneuver) occludes the esophagus and can prevent aspiration. Excessive assisted ventilation with an Ambu bag prior to intubation often dilates the stomach and predisposes to emesis. Ascertainment of correct placement of the endotracheal tube (both by presence of breath sounds and by absence of gastric sounds during ventilation) should be accomplished rapidly.

Maneuvers designed to decrease gastric pH, increase lower esophageal sphincter tone, and decrease gastric volume (using H_2 blockers, metoclopramide, cisapride) can be considered in high-risk individuals with intubations planned several hours in advance. Particulate antacids can produce pulmonary damage upon aspiration and should be avoided.

11. Should antibiotics be administered prophylactically to hospitalized patients at risk for aspiration?

Prophylactic antibiotics should be avoided in order to decrease the risk of colonization by resistant organisms. In cases of suspected or witnessed aspiration, antibiotic therapy is often initiated because the clinical manifestations of aspiration are similar to those of pneumonia. No data support the use of empirical antibiotics in this setting, however, and they should be discontinued if improvement does not occur in 24–48 hours and no presumptive pathogen is discovered.

12. How should suspected aspiration be evaluated?

The history of choking and coughing with oral intake or the findings of copious salivary secretions with food particles in a patient with a tracheostomy is diagnostic. When in doubt, other tests may be employed to document aspiration. Flexible laryngoscopy can be used to assess the hypopharynx, larynx, and vocal cord function. It can also be used to dynamically visualize swallowing function (videoendoscopic evaluation). Radiographic evaluation may be necessary to identify the type and extent of aspiration in alert patients. Radionuclide scintigraphy records the passage of a radionuclide bolus through the upper digestive tract. Alternatively, a modified barium swallow allows video fluoroscopic assessment of the entire swallowing process with particular emphasis on the oral and pharyngeal phases. Documentation of gastroesophageal reflux may be necessary in some patients. A complete barium upper GI study or esophageal pH monitoring may be employed in this situation.

CONTROVERSIES

13. How does one differentiate between chemical pneumonitis and infectious pneumonitis caused by aspiration?

This can be very difficult. Fever, leukocytosis, purulent sputum, and pulmonary infiltrates occur in both disorders. Gram stain and culture of expectorated sputum are not helpful because of contamination by oropharyngeal flora. If indicated, aerobic and anaerobic cultures of lower airway secretions can be obtained by fiberoptic bronchoscopy and protected brush techniques. Transtracheal aspiration is now rarely performed because of a greater complication rate than that associated with fiberoptic bronchoscopy. Many clinicians prefer to use empiric antibiotics for the treatment of possible infectious aspiration pneumonia.

14. What strategies can be used to prevent aspiration?

All hospitalized patients are candidates for standard aspiration precautions, including elevation of the head of the bed. Patients with intestinal obstruction benefit from nasogastric suction, although nasogastric tubes affect the swallowing mechanism and airway protection.

Several surgical procedures are available in selected patients with recurrent aspiration, including cricopharyngeal myotomy, laryngeal suspension, partial cricoid resection, and vocal cord medialization. In general, these procedures have limited application. In patients with life-threatening, intractable aspiration that is unresponsive to conservative treatment, a variety of definitive surgical procedures can be considered. Definitive procedures include antiaspiration stents, laryngeal diversion/separation, glottic closure, supraglottic closure and total laryngectomy. All of these procedures require the creation and maintenance of a tracheostomy. The use of antiaspiration stents may be the procedure of first choice, especially if the patient's illness is potentially reversible.

15. Does the use of tube feeding prevent aspiration in patients with neurologic diseases?

Although the use of tube feeding in this setting is widespread, there are no data to suggest that tube feeding reduces the risk of aspiration pneumonia. In fact some studies suggest that aspiration may be worse in this setting. It is probably best to attempt feeding by mouth in almost all conscious patients and reserve enteral feeding for those with more severely impaired consciousness.

16. Are corticosteroids indicated in the treatment of gastric acid aspiration?

The use of corticosteroids is attractive because of the theoretical anti-inflammatory effects which may prevent lung injury; however, no clinical studies have demonstrated benefit. Certainly, the administration of corticosteroids for aspiration has little support at present.

BIBLIOGRAPHY

1. Bartlett JG, Gorsbach SL, Finegold SM: The bacteriology of aspiration pneumonia. Am J Med 56:202–207, 1974.
2. Blitzer A: Approaches to the patient with aspiration and swallowing disabilities. Dysphagia 5:129–137, 1990.
3. Dal Santo G: Acid aspiration: Pathophysiologic aspects, prevention, and therapy. Int Anesthesiol Clin 24:31–52, 1986.
4. Finucane TE, Bynum JPW: Use of tube feeding to prevent aspiration pneumonia. Lancet 348:1421–1424, 1996.
5. Gillick MR: Rethinking the role of tube feeding in patients with advanced dementia. N Engl J Med 342:206–210, 2000.

6. Joyce TH: Prophylaxis for pulmonary acid aspiration. Am J Med 83(Suppl 6A):46–52, 1987.
7. LoCicero J: Bronchopulmonary aspiration. Surg Clin North Am 69:71–76, 1989.
8. Lode H: Microbiological and clinical aspects of aspiration pneumonia. J Antimicrobiol Chemother 21 (Suppl C):83–87, 1988.
9. Marlik PE: Aspiration pneumonitis and aspiration pneumonia. N Engl J Med 344:665–671, 2001.
10. Mendelson C: The aspiration of stomach contents into the lungs during obstetric anesthesia. Am J Obstet Gynecol 52:191–205, 1946.
11. Miller FR, Eliachas I: Managing the aspirating patient. Am J Otolaryngol 15(1):1–17, 1994.
12. Pennza PT: Aspiration pneumonia, necrotizing pneumonia and lung abscess. Emerg Med Clin North Am 7:279–307, 1989.
13. Ruffalo RL: Aspiration pneumonitis: Risk factors of the critically ill patient. DICP 24:S12–S16, 1990.
14. Tietjen PA, Kaner RJ, Quinn CE: Aspiration Emergencies. Clin Chest Med 15:117–135, 1994.

24. HEMOPTYSIS

Michael E. Hanley, M.D.

1. What is hemoptysis?

Hemoptysis is expectoration of blood originating from the lower respiratory tract (trachea, bronchi, or lung parenchyma). It is classified as either massive or frank (gross). Massive hemoptysis is expectoration of greater than 600 ml of blood within a 24–48 hour period. Frank or gross hemoptysis is expectoration of less than 600 ml of blood in 24–48 hours but more than blood streaking. True hemoptysis must be differentiated from pseudohemoptysis, which is expectoration of blood originating from a source other than the lower respiratory tract. Pseudohemoptysis may result from either aspiration of blood from the gastrointestinal tract or blood draining into the larynx and trachea from bleeding sites in the oral cavity, nasopharynx, or larynx.

2. What is the differential diagnosis of hemoptysis?

Although hemoptysis may be associated with many conditions (see table below), it results in general from either focal or diffuse pulmonary parenchymal processes or tracheobronchial, cardiovascular, or hematologic disorders. The frequency with which hemoptysis is associated with these conditions is determined by the age of the patient, population being studied (surgical vs. medical, veterans' hospital vs. city/county indigent hospital), and amount of expectorated blood. Lung neoplasms, a common cause of hemoptysis in elderly patients, rarely occur in patients younger than 40 years of age. Scant or frank hemoptysis most commonly results from either bronchitis/bronchiectasis or lung neoplasms. Other common conditions associated with scant or frank hemoptysis include active pulmonary tuberculosis, chronic necrotizing pneumonia, pulmonary infarction, congestive heart failure, and bleeding diatheses.

Causes of Hemoptysis

Tracheobronchial disorders	Localized parenchymal diseases
Acute tracheobronchitis	Nontuberculous pneumonia
Amyloidosis	Actinomycosis
Gastric aspiration	Amebiasis
Bronchial adenoma	Ascariasis
Bronchial endometriosis	Aspergilloma
Bronchial telangiectasia	Bronchopulmonary sequestration
Bronchiectasis	Coccidioidomycosis
Bronchogenic carcinoma	Congenital and acquired cyst
Broncholithiasis	Cryptococcosis

Table continued on following page

Causes of Hemoptysis (Continued)

Tracheobronchial disorders *(cont.)*
Chronic bronchitis
Cystic fibrosis
Endobronchial hamartoma
Endobronchial metastasis
Endobronchial tuberculosis
Foreign body aspiration
Bronchial mucoid impaction
Tracheobronchial trauma
Tracheoesophageal fistula

Cardiovascular disorders
Aortic aneurysm
Congenital heart disease
Congestive heart failure
Fat embolism
Mitral stenosis
Postmyocardial infarction syndrome
Pulmonary arteriovenous malformation
Pulmonary artery aneurysm
Pulmonary embolus
Pulmonary venous varix
Schistosomiasis
Superior vena cava syndrome
Tumor embolization

Hematologic disorders
Anticoagulant therapy
Disseminated intravascular coagulation
Leukemia
Thrombocytopenia

Localized parenchymal diseases *(cont.)*
Lipoid pneumonia
Histoplasmosis
Hydatid mole
Lung abscess
Lung contusion
Metastatic cancer
Mucormycosis
Nocardiosis
Paragonimiasis
Pulmonary endometriosis
Pulmonary tuberculosis
Sporotrichosis

Diffuse parenchymal diseases
Disseminated angiosarcoma
Farmer's lung
Goodpasture's syndrome
Idiopathic pulmonary hemosiderosis
IgA nephropathy
Legionnaires' disease
Mixed connective tissue disease
Mixed cryoglobulinemia
Polyarteritis nodosa
Scleroderma
Systemic lupus erythematosus
Viral pneumonitis
Wegener's granulomatosis

Other
Idiopathic
Iatrogenic

Adapted from Irwin RS, Hubmayr R: Hemoptysis. In Rippe JM, Irwin RS, Alpert JS, Dalen JE (eds): Intensive Care Medicine. Boston, Little, Brown, 1985.

3. What are common causes of massive hemoptysis?

The most common cause of massive hemoptysis in patients who are not intubated when hemoptysis begins is inflammatory lung disease. This category includes tuberculosis (40%), bronchiectasis (30%), necrotizing pneumonitis (10%), lung abscess (5%), and fungal infection (5%). Pulmonary neoplasm and arteriovenous malformation account for only about 10% of cases.

When massive hemoptysis begins after endotracheal intubation, upper airway trauma secondary to the intubation procedure, the endotracheal tube, or from endotracheal suction catheters must also be considered. If hemoptysis begins after a latent period of one or more weeks after intubation, a tracheo-artery fistula may be the source of hemorrhage. This possibility is increased if a tracheostomy tube is present. Pulmonary artery rupture and pulmonary infarction should be considered when hemoptysis occurs in a patient with pulmonary artery catheter. Pulmonary infarctionshould be suspected if a wedge-shaped infiltrate is present distal to the catheter on the chest roentgenogram.

4. What is the significance of massive hemoptysis?

Massive hemoptysis has drastically different implications than smaller amounts of hemoptysis, which are commonly innocuous and self-limited. Massive hemoptysis is generally due to hemorrhaging from the bronchial artery (systemic pressure) circulation as opposed to the low-pressure pulmonary artery circuit and therefore is more capable of generating life-threatening hemorrhage. Mortality from massive hemoptysis in some studies is 75–100%.

5. What tests should be included in the routine evaluation of patients with hemoptysis?

History, physical examination, complete blood counts including platelet count, coagulation studies, urinalysis, chest roentgenogram, and electrocardiogram.

6. What is the initial approach to evaluation of ICU patients with hemoptysis?

Evaluation should begin with the routine tests described above. After the patient has been hemodynamically stabilized, the site, etiology, and extent of bleeding should be determined. Identifying the site of bleeding requires visualization of the airways, including the naso- and oropharynx, and examination of the chest roentgenogram. Pernasal fiberoptic bronchoscopy allows examination of the nasopharynx, larynx, and major airways and may reveal if hemorrhaging is focal or diffuse. Presence of an endotracheal tube may compromise this examination. In this instance, upper airway bleeding may be detected by aspirating the trachea free of blood with a bronchoscope, while the endotracheal balloon is expanded, and then observing fresh blood flow down from above the balloon when it is decompressed. Rigid bronchoscopy may be required if hemorrhaging is massive, such that blood cannot be adequately removed with a flexible bronchoscope.

Examination of the chest roentgenogram often gives clues to both the site and etiology of hemoptysis. Presence of an infiltrate suggests the existence of a pulmonary parenchymal process. However, occasionally an infiltrate may occur after aspiration of blood coming from the upper airway. Similarly, presence of diffuse infiltrates suggests diffuse parenchymal disease, although this roentgenographic pattern may also occur with localized bleeding associated with severe coughing (coughing disperses the blood diffusely).

7. Do all patients with hemoptysis require bronchoscopy?

No. Bronchoscopy may not be indicated if the initial evaluation strongly suggests that hemoptysis is due to a cardiovascular etiology, lower respiratory tract infection, or a single episode of frank hemoptysis due to acute or chronic bronchitis. However, bronchoscopy should be reconsidered in these clinical settings if the patient's hemoptysis does not improve or resolve after 24 hours of empiric therapy. Bronchoscopy is not indicated to make the specific diagnosis of a tracheo-artery fistula.

8. Describe the immediate management of massive hemoptysis.

Goals of immediate management of patients with massive hemoptysis include maintaining airway patency, stopping ongoing hemorrhage, and preventing rebleeding. Maintenance of airway patency is of paramount importance, because death from massive hemoptysis more commonly results from asphyxiation due to major airway obstruction than to exsanguination. Several approaches have been advocated to maintain airway patency. If hemorrhage is occurring from a focal site and the site of hemorrhage is known, the patient should be positioned with the bleeding side dependent to prevent contamination of noninvolved airways. If the site of hemorrhage is unknown or diffuse, the patient should be placed in the Trendelenburg position. Other approaches to protect uninvolved airways include bronchoscopically guided selective intubation of the non-bleeding mainstem bronchus or placement of a double-lumen (Carlen's) endotracheal tube. Carlen's tube should be placed only by physicians experienced in its use.

If the etiology of hemorrhage is known, specific therapy (such as antibiotics for bronchiectasis) should be instituted to stop ongoing hemorrhage. Coagulopathies should be corrected with administration of appropriate blood products. Life-threatening hemorrhage from a focal site may require more aggressive strategies. Surgical resection should be considered in patients with adequate underlying lung function; however, the mortality associated with this approach is high. Focal hemoptysis in patients with severe underlying respiratory disease has been successfully treated by tamponade with Fogarty catheters placed under bronchoscopic guidance and by cautery with bronchoscopic laser photocoagulation. Limited success in stopping parenchymal hemorrhaging has also been achieved by bronchial artery embolization, occlusion of the involved pulmonary artery with a Swan-Ganz catheter, iced normal saline lavage of hemorrhaging lung segments, topical administration of epinephrine, and administration of intravenous vasopressin.

Once active hemorrhaging has been arrested, efforts should be made to prevent rebleeding. They usually include adequate cough suppression with antitussives such as high-dose codeine or morphine and avoidance of chest percussion.

9. Describe the management of a tracheo-artery fistula.

A surgical consultation should be obtained immediately. Bleeding from a tracheo-artery fistula complicating tracheostomy usually occurs at one of three sites: the tracheostomy tube stoma, the tracheostomy tube balloon, or the intratracheal cannula tip. The goals of immediate management are to control bleeding and to maintain a patent airway while preparing the patient for primary surgical correction. Bleeding at the tracheostomy stoma can sometimes be tamponaded by applying forward and downward pressure on the top of the tracheostomy tube. Bleeding at the site of the balloon can be tamponaded by overinflating the balloon. These maneuvers should be performed immediately. However, they will not be helpful if bleeding is occurring at the cannula tip. If the bleeding stops or slows either spontaneously or subsequent to these efforts, an endotracheal tube should be placed distal to the bleeding site. However, the initial tracheostomy tube should not be removed without a surgeon present, as a sudden increase in the rate of hemorrhage may necessitate blunt dissection down the anterior tracheal wall posterior to the sternum to attempt direct finger tamponade of the bleeding site.

10. What is the role of bronchial artery embolization in the management of massive hemoptysis?

Bronchial artery embolization is important in the management of both surgical and nonsurgical causes of massive hemoptysis. It is a temporary measure for surgical lesions, facilitating stabilization of patients while they undergo evaluation and preparation for surgery. It allows surgery to be performed in a more controlled setting. Bronchial artery embolization has become the primary mode of therapy for patients who are considered inoperable because of either diffuse lung disease or poor pulmonary function. Such patients may undergo multiple episodes of embolization over many years if hemoptysis recurs. The success rate of embolization is high. Some studies indicate success rates of 98% in the initial 24-hour period. However, 16–30% of patients rebleed in the first year after embolization. Rebleeding tends to be bimodal in occurrence, with peaks in the first month (generally due to inadequate initial embolization) and at 1–2 years (due to progression of underlying disease).

11. What complications are associated with bronchial artery embolization?

Bronchial artery embolization is associated with low morbidity rates. The most common complications include pleuritic chest pain, fever, leukocytosis, and dysphagia. These symptoms may last for 5–7 days. Other complications are quite rare and related to vascular compromise of organs supplied from vessels that arise downstream from the site of catheter placement. Examples include spinal cord infarction, transverse myelitis, bronchial stenosis, bronchial-esophageal fistula, transient cortical blindness, and cerebrovascular accidents. The risk of these complications has been reduced dramatically by the use of superselective catheterization performed with microcatheters placed deep in the bronchial circulation.

12. When should surgery be considered in the management of massive hemoptysis?

Bronchial artery embolization has largely replaced surgical resection as the intitial therapy in massive hemoptysis. Embolization is associated with much lower morbidity and early mortality rates than emergent surgery. However, because of high rates of recurrence after embolization, surgery should be considered for patients who have hemoptysis due to focal lung lesions and good pulmonary reserve after they had been stabilized with embolization. Surgery is contraindicated in patients with advanced lung disease that results in limited pulmonary reserve, significant comorbidity (especially advanced heart disease), or lung malignancies invading the trachea, mediastinum, heart, great vessels, and parietal pleura. In contrast, it remains the treatment of choice for patients with hemoptysis related to trauma, aortic aneurysm, and bronchial adenomas.

CONTROVERSIES

13. Should antitussives be aggressively administered to patients with massive hemoptysis?
For: Excessive, harassing, violent cough aggravates and stimulates hemorrhage, promoting continued bleeding and rebleeding in patients in whom hemorrhage has stopped.
Against:
1. Excessive administration of narcotic antitussives may result in oversedation and narcosis.
2. An effective cough is required to clear blood from the airways and avoid asphyxiation.
3. Oversuppression of the cough reflex may result in retention of blood in the lungs and/or aspiration, both of which may contribute to development of pneumonia or atelectasis.

14. Does evaluation of massive hemoptysis require rigid bronchsocopy?
For:
1. Higher suctioning capacity of rigid bronchoscopy allows superior clearing of blood from the tracheobronchial tree, permitting better evaluation of airways.
2. Rigid bronchoscopy permits superior maintenance of an adequate airway and alveolar ventilation.
Against:
1. Rigid bronchoscopy is poorly tolerated both subjectively and physiologically in acutely ill patients and allows only limited evaluation of the bronchial tree because only proximal portions of the tree are visualized. This results in insufficient time and maneuverability to permit effective lavage and evaluation of individual lung segments.
2. Increased range of flexible fiberoptic bronchoscopy permits evaluation at the level of segmental and subsegmental bronchi, resulting in increased diagnostic accuracy in both localization and visualization of bleeding site (especially the upper lobes).
3. Flexible fiberoptic bronchoscopy permits selective lavage and selective placement of Fogerty catheters in segmental and subsegmental bronchi.

15. Should fiberoptic bronchoscopy be performed before bronchial artery embolilzation in patients with massive hemoptysis?
For:
1. Fiberoptic bronchoscopy is important in guiding bronchial artery embolization by identifying the site of bleeding.
2. Fiberoptic bronchoscopy is complementary to chest computed tomography in identifying the cause of hemoptysis, allowing institution of specific therapy aimed at the underlying lung pathology.
3. Fiberoptic bronchoscopy facilitates introduction of balloon catheters into the airway to control hemorrhage and protect uninvolved lung parenchyma by isolating actively hemorrhaging segments.
Against:
1. A recent study of 29 patients who underwent bronchial artery embolization to control massive hemoptysis revealed that the site of bleeding could be identified in 80% of patients by chest radiograph alone. Bronchoscopy was essential to localizing the site of hemorrhage in only 10% of patients.
2. The site of embolization is generally identified by angiography at the time of bronchial catheterization.
3. Emergent bronchoscopy results in unnecessary delays before performance of bronchial artery embolization.

4. Endobronchial tamponade with balloon catheters is inferior to embolization as a temporary measure to control hemorrhage before institution of more specific therapy and should be reserved for patients with contraindications to embolization.

BIBLIOGRAPHY

1. Brobowitz ID, Ramakrishna S, Shim YS: Comparison of medical v surgical treatment of major hemoptysis. Arch Intern Med 143:1343–1346, 1983.
2. Conlan AA, Hurwitz SS, Krige L, et al: Massive hemoptysis: Review of 123 cases. J Thorac Cardiovasc Surg 85:120–124, 1983.
3. Corey R, Hla KM: Major and massive hemoptysis: Reassessment of conservative management. Am J Med Sci 294:301–309, 1987.
4. Dweik RA, Stoller JK: Role of bronchoscopy in massive hemoptysis. Clin Chest Med 20:89–105, 1999.
5. Gourin A, Garzon AA: Control of hemorrhage in emergency pulmonary resection for massive hemoptysis. Chest 68:120–121, 1975.
6. Gourin AG, Garzon AA: Operative treatment of massive hemoptysis. Ann Thorac Surg 18:52–60, 1974.
7. Haponiks EF: Managing life-threatening hemoptysis: Has anything really changed? Chest 118:1431–1435, 2000.
8. Hsiao EI, Kirsch CM, Kagawaa FT, et al: Utility of fiberotpic bronchoscopy before bronchial artery emoblization for massive hemoptysis. Am J Roentgenol 177:861–867, 2001.
9. Jean-Baptiste E: Clinical assessment and management of massive hemoptysis. Crit Care Med 28:1642–1647, 2000.
10. Johnston H, Reisz G: Changing spectrum of hemoptysis. Underlying causes in 148 patients undergoing diagnostic flexible fiberoptic bronchoscopy. Arch Intern Med 149:1666–1668, 1989.
11. Mal H, Rullon I, Mellot F, et al: Immediate and long-term results of bronchial artery embolization for life-threatening hemoptysis. Chest 115:996–1001, 1999.
12. McCollum WB, Mattox KL, Guinn GA, Beall AC: Immediate operative treatment for massive hemoptysis. Chest 67:152–155, 1975.
13. Saluja S, Henderson KJ, White RI: Embolotherpy in the bronchial and pulmonary circulation. Radiol Clin North Am 38:525–448, 2000.
14. Schaefer OP, Irwin RS: Tracheo-artery fistula. Intensive Care Med 10:64–75, 1995.

25. VENOUS THROMBOEMBOLISM

Marilyn G. Foreman, M.D., and Marc Moss, M.D.

1. What is the primary source of pulmonary emboli (PE)?

The majority of PEs arise from clots in the deep veins of the legs, particularly the iliac, femoral, and popliteal veins.

2. Are there other sources of PE?

Clots from the pelvic veins commonly occur in women with a history of obstetric difficulties or recent gynecologic surgery. Emboli from the pelvic veins can be septic in nature and create a clinical picture of septicemia with multiple cavitary pulmonary lesions. Other nonhematologic sources of PE include amniotic fluid as a complication of pregnancy, air during the placement of central venous catheters, and foreign bodies such as talc and cotton fibers in intravenous drug users.

3. How common is venous thromboembolism in critically ill patients?

Deep venous thrombosis (DVT) and PE are common and often underdiagnosed problems in critically ill patients. In prospective studies, 33% of medical patients in the intensive care unit (ICU) had DVTs on routine clinical screening, and 18% of trauma patients had proximal DVTs. In a retrospective series of respiratory ICU patients, 27% had pulmonary emboli on autopsy.

4. What are the different pathologic classifications of PE?

Pulmonary emboli have been classified into three categories. The rarest and most serious form of PE is an **acute massive occlusion**, which is defined as an occlusion of more than 50% of the segmental pulmonary vasculature or an equivalent amount of central clot. At autopsy, large clots called saddle emboli are often found in the vicinity of the bifurcation of the main pulmonary artery. The second type is a **pulmonary infarction**, which occurs when the embolism obstructs enough blood flow to a specific area of the lung to cause death of the lung tissue. It occurs in only 10% of all cases of acute PE. The third and most common category is **pulmonary embolism without infarction**. These emboli are the most difficult to diagnose because they manifest no specific symptoms.

5. How do patients with PE present?

The symptoms of PE depend on the severity of the emboli. When there is an acute massive occlusion, patients present with systemic hypotension, with or without syncope, and severe refractory hypoxemia. In patients with underlying cardiac or pulmonary disease, there may be significant hemodynamic compromise with less occlusion of the pulmonary vasculature. Patients with pulmonary infarction present with the acute onset of pleuritic chest pain, tachypnea, and occasionally hemoptysis. On physical exam, one may hear a pleural friction rub. Patients who have a pulmonary embolism without infarction present with nonspecific symptoms of tachypnea, dyspnea, and tachycardia.

6. When should the diagnosis of PE be suspected in a critically ill patient?

Many patients in the ICU are at risk for the development of PE, so the clinician has to have a high index of suspicion for the diagnosis and watch for subtle clues such as:

Acute onset of tachypnea
Tachycardia
Unexplained agitation or anxiety
Changes in chest x-ray (such as atelectasis, basilar infiltrate, or elevated hemidiaphragm)
Hypotension
Nonspecific back or side pain
Unexplained hypoxia
Respiratory alkalosis
Pulmonary hypertension
Asymmetric leg swelling
Unilateral leg pain
Increase in the difference between the pulmonary artery diastolic pressure and the pulmonary capillary wedge pressure.

7. How reliable is the physical exam for diagnosing DVT?

Poor. The classic signs of DVTs are leg swelling, pain to deep pressure over the calf, pain in the calf when the foot is dorsiflexed (Homans' sign), or palpable deep thrombi. Unfortunately, less than 50% of patients with a documented DVT have the classic findings on clinical examination.

8. Are there specific findings on chest radiograph of PE?

No. In many patients the chest x-ray is normal or has subtle abnormalities that are rarely diagnostic. However, many of these radiographic findings have been named. Fleischner lines are linear streaks (areas of platelike atelectasis) that run parallel above an elevated hemidiaphragm. A Westermark sign is an area of lung which is relatively underperfused. Hampton's hump is a pleural-based, wedge-shaped parenchymal density representative of a pulmonary infarct, which usually appears 12–36 hours after the embolism has occurred. An enlarged right descending artery is known as Palla's sign.

9. What are the EKG findings in PE?

The EKG findings are also variable and relatively nonspecific. Sinus tachycardia and nonspecific ST segment and T wave changes occur frequently. The classic EKG findings of S_1, Q_3,

T_3 or right bundle branch block occur in less than 15% of patients. The development of EKG findings of acute pulmonary hypertension (rightward shift of the QRS axis, or peaked P waves in the inferior leads) in a critically ill patient should raise concern about potential PE.

10. Are any laboratory abnormalities helpful in diagnosing PE or DVT?

Routine laboratory studies are not helpful in the diagnostic evaluation of a patient in whom PE is suspected. In fact, a prospective study found that no arterial blood gas or clinical data had adequate specificity, negative predictive value, or likelihoood ratios to exclude PE. Most commonly, hypoxemia and hypocarbia are present, but they are highly nonspecific findings. A normal alveolar-arterial oxygen gradient may be found in 12–15% of patients with PE. The lack of hypoxemia usually is associated with minimal pulmonary vasculature obstruction.

Similarly, an elevated serum D-dimer level is a nonspecific finding in the ICU and may occur in the absence of DVT or PE D-dimers result from the degradation of cross-linked fibrin by plasmin when endogenous fibrinolytic mechanisms are triggered in the setting of active thrombosis. D-dimer levels may be increased by malignancy, sickle cell crisis, congestive heart failure, surgery, myocardial infarction, and disseminated intravascular coagulation. Measurement of D-dimers by enzyme-linked immunosorbent assay is the gold standard test. A level below 500 ng/ml may be more useful in its negative predictive value for eliminating the diagnosis of venous thromboembolism when paired with a negative imaging study.

11. What are some of the risk factors for PE and DVT?

Three general conditions that increase the risk of venous thrombosis are called Virchow's triad: venous stasis, hypercoagulability, and injury to the venous walls. Specific risk factors are listed below.

Hypercoagulability	Venous Stasis	Vessel Wall Injury
Antithrombin III deficiency	Prolonged bed rest	Trauma
Protein C deficiency	Congestive heart failure	
Protein S deficiency	Obesity	
Factor V Leiden mutation	Major surgical procedures	
Cancer	Pregnancy	
Hyperhomocystinemia	Limited mobility	
Antiphospholipid antibodies		
Oral contraceptives		
Hormone replacement therapy		
Nephrotic syndrome		
High levels of factor VIII		

Malignancy: The development of DVT may predate a clinically present malignancy. In one study, 7.6% of patients with idiopathic DVT were diagnosed with a symptomatic malignant disease in the next 18 months. In patients with recurrent venous thrombosis, the incidence of malignancy rose to 17%. The majority of these malignancies were adenocarcinomas.

Hypercoagulability: Protein C is the most powerful endogenous anticoagulant. The factor V Leiden mutation is a point mutation in the gene coding for coagulation factor V. The amino acid substitution makes it more difficult for activated protein C to cleave and inactivate factor V. The functional result is activated protein C resistance. One study found that the relative risk of venous thrombosis in men with the mutation was 2.7. When the mutation is combined with other risk factors, the risk of thromboembolism is increased greatly. For example, the risk of venous thromboembolism in women with the mutation who also use oral contraceptives is estimated to increase 35-fold compared with women without the mutation who do not use oral contraceptives. Elevated levels of factor VIII also have been reported to increase the risk for thrombosis. In a study of the risk of recurrent venous thromobembolism, incremental elevations in the factor VIII level were associated with increasing risk of thrombosis. Overall, patients with levels over the 90th percentile were nearly 7 times more likely to experience recurrent thrombosis.

Trauma: Specific to the hospital environment, central venous catheters are a risk factor for venous thromboembolism. An incidence of thrombus formation as high as 25% is associated with the use of femoral vein catheters. In addition, approximately 15% of patients with catheter-related upper DVT develop PE based on a high-probabilty V/Q scan.

12. Describe the diagnostic work-up for a patient with suspected DVT.

The key is to detect clots in the thigh and pelvis, as it is rare for clots in the calf to produce large or fatal PE. The gold standard test to diagnose DVT is the venogram, which is an uncomfortable and invasive procedure that may be difficult to perform in a critically ill patient. Compression ultrasonography of the femoral and popliteal veins is extremely sensitive (greater than 90%) for diagnosing proximal vein thrombosis in symptomatic patients. Compared with impedance plethysmography, compression ultrasonography had a higher positive predictive value. If compression ultrasonography is abnormal, the patient can be diagnosed with venous thrombosis. If the compression ultrasonography is normal, anticoagulation therapy should not be started and the test should be repeated in seven days. Only 1.5% of patients with repeatedly normal results will develop venous thromboembolism in the subsequent 6-month period.

Venography may be accomplished simultaneously with spiral CT imaging of the pulmonary arteries. Venous phase imaging at the time of spiral CT pulmonary angiography is comparable to ultrasonography in the evaluation of femoropopliteal DVT. In a study evaluating the combined procedure in patients suspected of PE, a sustained number of patients had DVT even when PE was not detected. Therefore, the combined study of spiral CT pulmonary angiography and venography may be an efficient means to evaluate PE as well as the potential source. The conventional study is extended by a few more minutes without the need for additional radiographic contrast.

13. What diagnostic tests are available for a patient with suspected PE?

Five commonly available imaging techniques can be used in the diagnostic evaluation of PE: (1) ventilation-perfusion (V/Q) scanning, (2) spiral CT scanning of the pulmonary arteries, (3) echocardiography, (4) pulmonary angiography, and (5) compression ultrasonography of the lower extremities, which can provide an indirect measure of pulmonary thromboembolic disease. Which of these tests should be performed and their proper diagnostic sequence is at present uncertain (see Controversies).

14. What percentage of patients with DVT without symptoms of PE will have a high-probability V/Q scan?

Approximately 50%.

15. What diseases can cause a false-positive high-probability V/Q scan?

Not all high-probability lung scans are caused by PE. The diseases that cause false-positive V/Q scans include mediastinal/hilar adenopathy, fibrosing mediastinitis, tumor infiltration of a vessel, congenital absence of a pulmonary artery, or ascending aortic aneurysm dissection. One clue that can be helpful in recognizing these other disorders is that most PE are multiple and/or bilateral, and many of the above processes are unilateral.

16. What are the major goals of treatment for PE and DVT? How are they achieved?

The major goals of PE and DVT therapy are to prevent further clot formation, promote resolution of existing clot, and prevent sequelae. Acutely, intravenous heparin should be administered. Warfarin therapy can be started within the first 24 hours of heparin therapy with a target level measured by the international normalized ratio (INR) of 2.0–3.0. It is important to continue the heparin for at least 4 days and until the INR has been therapeutic for at least 2 days. Athough the optimal duration of anticoagulation remains uncertain, warfarin should be continued for a total of 3–6 months for most episodes of DVT or PE. The length of treatment depends on the presence or absence of risk factors and whether thromboembolism recurs.

Low-molecular-weight (LMW) heparin has been found to be safe and effective in the treatment of PE and DVT, but its use in the ICU is presently under investigation. The advantages of LMW heparin include increased bioavailability with a more predictable anticoagulant response, lack of need for phlebotomy to monitor the partial thromboplastin time (PTT), infrequent daily dosing, and subcutaneous administration. In the ICU, the long half-life may complicate plans for invasive procedures, and the absence of documentation of efficacy and safety in critically ill patients limits its usefulness.

17. Which patients with PE should be treated with thrombolytic therapy?

Thrombolytic therapy for PE has been reported to achieve faster clot lysis and improvement in right ventricular function, and may lower the rate of recurrence when compared to heparin therapy alone. However, it is presently unknown whether thrombolytic therapy reduces long-term mortality and morbidity. Based on these findings, thrombolytic therapy is reserved for patients with massive PE and hypotension.

18. When should the placement of an intravenous filter be considered?

When a patient has a documented (i.e., by repeat angiogram) recurrent embolism on "adequate" anticoagulation therapy or when a patient cannot be anticoagulated, a filter can be placed in the inferior vena cava to prevent propagation of clots from the pelvis/lower extremities. Other relative indications for filter placement are: documented free-floating thrombus, poor respiratory reserve or chronic pulmonary hypertension when a subsequent pulmonary emboli could be fatal, and any PE in a patient with cancer due to their persistent hypercoagulable state.

Two recent trials have shed light on the decision to place a vena cava filter. One study found no increase in the development of PE in patients with free-floating proximal DVT treated with anticoagulant therapy alone. The second study reported that in high-risk patients with proximal DVTs, the initial benefit of filter placement for the prevention of PE is offset by an excessive rate of recurrent DVTs.

19. What is the recommended prophylactic therapy for patients at risk for the development of DVT/PE?

Prophylaxis is recommended in all high risk patients, and has been reported to decrease the incidence of DVT by 67%. The most commonly used regimen is low dose heparin, 5000 units subcutaneously every 8–12 hours. Other prophylactic therapies include intermittent pneumatic compression stockings and graded elastic stockings, which also can be used in patients who cannot tolerate anticoagulation. Unfortunately, prophylactic therapy is not always administered to high-risk patients. In a recent study, only 32% of high-risk patients actually received prophylaxis for venous thromboembolism while in the ICU.

Refinements in the perioperative prevention of thromboembolism include the use of fondaparinux, a new synthetic pentasaccharide that selectively inhibits activated factor X. It has been shown to be as safe as and more effective than enoxaparin (an LMW heparin) in preventing thrombosis after hip fracture surgery. A similar study of thrombosis prophylaxis after major elective knee surgery found that fondaparinux is associated with a significantly lower risk of venous thromboembolism and a slightly higher risk of bleeding than enoxaparin.

20. Do some patients actually require higher doses of heparin to maintain adequate anticoagulation? If so, why?

Some patients need larger doses of heparin to achieve therapeutic PTT levels. Patients who require more than 35–40,000 units of heparin per day are arbitrarily defined as "heparin-resistant." These patients appear to have increased plasma concentrations of factor VIII and heparin-binding proteins, resulting in a falsely subtherapeutic PTT while maintaining therapeutic plasma heparin levels. Monitoring such patients with an anti-factor Xa heparin assay is safe and effective and results in less escalation of the heparin dose than when PTT levels are used.

21. What are the potential complications of anticoagulation therapy?

The most common and serious complication of anticoagulation is bleeding. The risk of bleeding correlates with the degree of prolongation of the INR or PTT, age greater than 65 years, a prior history of gastrointestinal bleeding, or concomitant antiplatelet therapy. Immune-mediated thrombocytopenia has been reported in up to 3% of patients receiving heparin. This is often complicated by propagation of the preexisting venous thromboembolism. An often talked about but rare complication of warfarin therapy is skin necrosis caused by preexisting protein C or protein S deficiency. The necrosis is related to blockage of small vessels with thrombi secondary to a transient hypercoagulable state related to an initial decrease in protein C that precedes the reduction in prothrombin, factor IX, and factor X.

22. When should fever in a patient with PE be of concern?

Patients with PE alone may have temperatures > 39° C early in the disease course, and low-grade fevers may persist for 4–6 days. Persistently high fevers should arouse suspicion of super-infection.

CONTROVERSY

23. Is there an algorithm for the diagnosis of PE in the ICU?

At present, no. The diagnosis of PE may be difficult. The patient's hemodynamic status, the availability of diagnostic procedures, and the expertise of local consulting services are crucial considerations in determining the choice and timing of diagnostic procedures. Complications may arise when critically ill patients are transported to the radiology suite for imaging studies. Therefore, the approach to the diagnosis of PE in critically ill patients is highly individualized.

One approach is to order compression ultrasonography as the initial diagnostic procedure for *unstable* patients. This test is noninvasive, and the equipment is portable. Thromboses manifest as intraluminal filling defects or inability to compress the vessel lumen with gentle pressure from the ultrasound transducer. The presence of proximal DVT warrants anticoagulation, and no further testing may be needed. When ultrasonography is inconclusive, V/Q scanning may be the next diagnostic step.

In *stable* patients who can be transported, radionuclide lung scanning may be the initial diagnostic test for PE. Eighty-seven percent of patients with a high-probability scan have documented PEs. If the scan is normal, the diagnosis of PE can be reasonably excluded. Unfortunately, over 50% of scans are nondiagnostic (intermediate or low probability), and further testing is needed. In addition, V/Q scanning may be difficult to interpret if the patient is mechanically ventilated or has preexisting chronic lung disease. When the V/Q scan is inconclusive, compression ultrasonography can be performed as the second diagnostic test.

24. What is the role of spiral CT scanning of the pulmomary arteries in the diagnostic evaluation of PE?

Spiral CT scanning of the pulmonary arteries, also known as helical CT and CT pulmonary angiography, *may* be useful as the first diagnostic step in the evaluation of PE in ICU patients. Several studies have shown that the sensitivity and specificity of spiral CT approach 90% (see table below), exceeding those of V/Q scanning for the diagnosis of segmental or larger clots. Less certain is the ability of spiral CT to diagnose smaller or subsegmental emboli, for which its sensitivity is lower. Among the additional advantages of spiral CT is the ability to obtain diagnostic information from concurrent scanning of the mediastinum, chest wall, and lung parenchyma, which may result in an alternative diagnosis. Another advantage is the ability to scan the legs simultaneously (see question 12). Although spiral CT scanning is a useful noninvasive diagnostic tool, patients with impaired renal function, inability to lie flat, or inability to be transported to the scanner are poor candidates.

Utility of Spiral CT in the Diagnosis of Pulmonary Embolism

STUDY	SENSITIVITY (%)	SPECIFICITY (%)
Remy-Jardin (1992)	100	96
Goodman (1995)	63	89
Remy-Jardin (1996)	91	78
van Rossum (1996)	95	97
Mayo (1997)	87	95
Christiansen (1997)	90	96
Garg (1998)	67	100
Drucker (1998)	53–60	81–97
Kim (1999)	92	96
Qanadi (2000)	90	94

25. What is the role of transthoracic echocardiography is the diagnostic evaluation of PE?

As many as 40% of patients with PE exhibit abnormalities of the right ventricle (RV), including RV dysfunction and thrombus formation (rare). Findings of RV volume and pressure overload include abnormal motion of the interventricular septum, RV dilation, and RV hypokinesis. Echocardiography also may diagnose conditions that simulate PE, such as aortic aneurysm, myocardial infarction, and pericardial tamponade. At present, the exact role of transthoracic echocardiography in the diagnostic evaluation of PE is unknown.

26. What is the role of pulmonary angiography in the diagnostic evaluation of PE?

Pulmonary angiography is considered the gold standard—the most reliable method of diagnosing PE. Although fatal or serious nonfatal complications are uncommon, the majority occur in ICU patients. Because the procedure is invasive, requires transport to a specialized radiology suite, and is not readily available off hours, it should be ordered when other studies are negative or nondiagnostic in the setting of a high degree of clinical suspicion.

BIBLIOGRAPHY

1. Cham MD, Yankelevitz DF, Shaham D, et al: Deep venous thrombosis: Detection by using indirect CT venography. Radiology 216:744–751, 2000.
2. Decousus H, Leizotovicz A, Parent F, et al: A clinical trial of vena caval filters in the prevention of pulmonary embolism in patients with proximal deep-vein thrombosis. N Engl J Med 338:409–415, 1998.
3. Eriksson BI, Bauer KA, Lassen MR, et al: Fondaparinux compared with enoxaparin for the prevention of venous thromboembolism after hip-fracture surgery. N Engl J Med 345:1298–1304, 2001.
4. Ferretti GR, Bosson J-L, Buffaz P-D, et al: Acute pulmonary embolism: Role of helical CT in 164 patients with intermediate probability at ventilation-perfusion scintigraphy and normal results at duplex US of the legs. Radiology 205:453–458, 1997.
5. Goldhaber SZ: Pulmonary embolism. N Engl J Med 339:93–104, 1998.
6. Hirsh DR, Ingenito EP, Goldhaber SZ: Prevalence of deep venous thrombosis among patients in medical intensive care. JAMA 274:335–337, 1995.
7. Kyrle PA, Minar E, Hirschl M, et al: High plasma levels of factor VIII and the risk of recurrent venous thromboembolism. N Engl J Med 343:457–462, 2000.
8. Legere BM, Dweik RA, Arroliga AC: Venous thromboembolism in the intensive care unit. Clin Chest Med 20:367–384, 1999.
9. Levine MN, Hirsh J, Gent M, et al: A randomized trial comparing activated thromboplastin time with heparin assay in patients with acute venous thromboembolism requiring large daily doses of heparin. Arch Intern Med 154:49–56, 1994.
10. Loud PA, Katz DS, Klippenstein DL, et al: Combined CT venography and pulmonary angiography in suspected thromboembolic disease: Diagnostic accuracy for deep venous evaluation. Am J Roentgenol 174:61–65, 2000.

11. Monreal M, Raventos A, Lerma R, et al: Pulmonary embolism in patients with upper extremity DVT associated with venous central lines: A prospective study. Thromb Haemost 72:548–550, 1994.
12. Pacouret G, Alison D, Pottier J-M, et al: Free-floating thrombus and embolic risk in patients with angiographically confirmed proximal deep venous thrombosis: A prospective study. Arch Intern Med 157:305–308, 1997.
13. PIOPED Investigators: Value of the ventilation/perfusion scan in acute pulmonary embolism: Results of the prospective investigation of pulmonary embolism diagnosis. JAMA 263:2753–2759, 1990.
14. Prandoni P, Lensing AWA, Buller HR, et al: Deep-vein thrombosis and the incidence of subsequent symptomatic cancer. N Engl J Med 327:1128–1133, 1992.
15. Rathburn SW, Raskob GE, Whitsett TL: Sensitivity and specificity of helical computed tomography in the diagnosis of pulmonary embolism: A systematic review. Ann Intern Med 132:227–232, 2000.
16. Rodger MA, Carrier M, Jones GN, et al: Diagnostic value of arterial blood gas measurement in suspected pulmonary embolism. Am J Respir Crit Care Med 162:2105–2108, 2000.
17. Shulman S, Granqvist S, Holmstrom M, et al: The duration of oral anticoagulant therapy after a second episode of venous thromboembolism. N Engl J Med 336:393–398, 1997.
18. Trottier SJ, Veremakis C, O'Brien J, Auer AI: Femoral deep vein thrombosis associated with central venous catheterization: Results from a prospective, randomized trial. Crit Care Med 23:52–59, 1995.

IV. Cardiology

26. CHEST PAIN

Morgan Zaw Naing Lin, M.D., and Rita F. Redberg, M.D., M.Sc.

1. Define angina pectoris.

Angina pectoris is a clinical syndrome characterized by a discomfort in the chest or adjacent area associated with myocardial ischemia and typically precipitated by exertion and relieved by rest or sublingual nitroglycerin. Angina means *choking*, not pain. Discomfort is not described as pain at all but rather as an unpleasant sensation: "pressing," "squeezing," "strangling," "constricting," "bursting," and "burning." "A band across the chest" and "a weight in the center of the chest" are other frequent descriptions. Clenching of the fist in front of the chest while describing the sensation (Levine's sign) is a strong indication of an ischemic origin for the pain.

2. What are the precipitating and relieving factors for chronic stable angina?

Angina pectoris occurs characteristically on exertion. Typical scenarios for its occurrence include walking quickly or walking on an incline, walking in the cold or against a wind, and after a heavy meal. Rest and nitroglycerin relieve the discomfort of angina in approximately 1–5 minutes. If more than 10 minutes pass before relief, the diagnosis of chronic stable angina is questionable; instead, the patient may have unstable angina, acute myocardial infarction, or pain unrelated to myocardial ischemia. Discomfort of esophageal spasm and esophagitis also may be relieved by nitroglycerin.

3. What are the important factors determining myocardial oxygen demand and supply?

Myocardial oxygen demand is determined by heart rate, contractility, and the wall tension. It is assessed clinically by the double product or rate-pressure product (heart rate and systolic blood pressure). Physical exertion, emotional stress, and increased metabolic demands (fever, thyrotoxicosis) can increase the double product and hence the myocardial oxygen demand. Myocardial oxygen supply is determined by the oxygen-carrying capacity of the blood and the coronary blood flow, which may be impaired by atherosclerotic narrowing of the coronary arteries, coronary vasoconstriction, or intracoronary thrombi.

4. Compare fixed-threshold angina and variable-threshold angina.

In patients with **fixed-threshold** demand angina, the level of physical activity required to precipitate angina is relatively constant. Characteristically, these patients can predict the amount of physical activity that will precipitate angina (e.g., walking up two flights of stairs at a customary pace). It is due to increased myocardial oxygen demand with insufficient myocardial perfusion beyond the point of a fixed critical coronary obstruction.

In **variable-threshold** angina, dynamic obstruction caused by coronary vasoconstriction plays an important role in causing myocardial ischemia, even though the majority of these patients have some degree of coronary atherosclerosis. The level of physical activity that precipitates angina varies on different days and can vary even in the course of a single day. Mixed angina falls between the two extremes of fixed and variable-threshold angina.

The type of anginal syndrome the patient has determines the kind of antiischemic therapy. Beta blockers are more likely to be effective in patients with fixed demand ischemia, whereas nitrates and calcium channel blockers are preferred to treat episodes primarily due to vasoconstriction.

5. What is typical nonanginal chest pain?

The following characteristics are *not* suggestive of angina:
- Fleeting momentary chest pains described as "needle jabs" or "sticking pains"
- Pain localized to a very small area, e.g., the size of a fingertip
- Pain reproduced by pressure on the chest wall
- Discomfort aggravated by breathing or a single movement of the trunk or arm
- Discomfort relieved within a few seconds of lying horizontally or after one or two swallows of food or water.

6. What is the differential diagnosis of a patient presenting with chest pain?

Condition	Quality of Pain
Cardiac causes	
Aortic stenosis	Angina-like chest pain
Hypertrophic cardiomyopathy	Angina-like chest pain
Syndrome X	Angina-like chest pain
Mitral valve prolapse	Variable character, acute pericarditis, sharper, more left-sided than
Acute pericarditis	central, lasts for hours, aggravated by breathing, turning, and lying; relieved by sitting up and leaning forward
Noncardiac causes	
Aortic dissection	Sudden persistent severe pain radiating to the back
Expanding thoracic aneurysm	Localized severe, boring pain that may be worse at night
Pulmonary embolism	Pleuritic chest pain, pleural rub
Esophageal spasm	Angina-like pain, spontaneous, provoked by cold liquids or exercise, and relieved by nitroglycerin
Esophageal reflux	Substernal and epigastric pain provoked by recumbency, relieved by food and antacids
Peptic ulcer	Epigastric and substernal burning, relieved by antacids and food
Musculoskeletal syndromes	Superficial pain, exacerbated with inspiration, movement or palpation

7. What are angina equivalents?

Angina equivalents are symptoms of myocardial ischemia other than angina, such as dyspnea, faintness, fatigue, and eructation, which commonly occur in the elderly. Patients may describe the midchest as the site of the shortness of breath, whereas true dyspnea is usually not well localized. Other angina equivalents are discomfort limited to areas that are ordinarily sites of secondary radiation, such as the ulnar aspect of the left arm and forearm, lower jaw, teeth, neck, or shoulders, and the development of gas and belching, nausea, "indigestion," dizziness, and diaphoresis. Angina equivalents above the mandible or below the umbilicus are quite uncommon.

8. What is syndrome X?

The syndrome of angina or angina-like chest pain with normal epicardial arteries by angiography is called syndrome X. The cause of syndrome X is not clear. True myocardial ischemia, reflected by myocardial lactate production during exercise or during pacing, is present in some of these patients. It is postulated that microvascular dysfunction or inadequate vasodilator reserve, and abnormal pain perception with sympathovagal imbalance ("sensitive heart syndrome") or esophageal dysmotility may be responsible for this pain. Unlike obstructive CAD, syndrome X is common in premenopaual women and has an excellent prognosis (96% 7-year survival in CASS registry), even though it has a significant impact on the patient's quality of life and on the use of health care resources. In a subset of patients with ischemia diagnosed by noninvasive stress testing, antiischemic therapy with nitrates, calcium channel blockers, and beta blockers is logical, but response is variable. Estrogen replacement therapy should be considered in postmenopausal women, and imipramine (50 mg/day) has been reported to be helpful in some patients with syndrome X.

9. Describe the chest discomfort of mitral valve prolapse.

The chest discomfort of MVP may be similar to angina but more often is atypical in that it is prolonged, not clearly related to exertion, and punctuated by brief attacks of severe stabbing pain at the apex. The discomfort may be secondary to the tension on the papillary muscles, and the pain may be associated with abnormalities of wall motion or indentations of the wall of the left ventricle at the base of these muscles on angiography.

10. What is Da Costa's syndrome?

Da Costa's syndrome (neurocirculatory asthenia) is described as functional or psychogenic chest pain associated with an anxiety state. The pain is typically localized to the area of the cardiac apex and consists of a dull, persistent ache that lasts for hours and is often accentuated by or alternates with attacks or sharp, lancinating stabs of inframammary pain 1 or 2 seconds in duration. The condition may occur with emotional strain and fatigue, bears little relation to exertion, and may be accompanied by precordial tenderness. Attacks are usually associated with palpitation, hyperventilation, numbness and tingling in the extremities, sighing, dizziness, dyspnea, generalized weakness, and a history of panic attacks and other signs of emotional instability or depression.

11. What is Tietze's syndrome?

This syndrome is a type of chest wall pain due to costochondritis; the discomfort is localized in the costochondral and costosternal joints, which are painful on palpation. Chest wall pain due to costochondritis or myositis is common in patients who present with fear of heart disease.

12. What is the role of an exercise ECG in the diagnosis of coronary artery disease?

Exercise testing is most valuable in the diagnosis of CAD in patients with intermediate pretest probability, typically a middle-aged male with atypical chest pain who has a normal ECG at rest. If typical chest pain and > 1 mm horizontal or downsloping ST depression develops during the exercise testing, the predictive value for CAD is > 90%, whereas the likelihood of CAD is only 10% in patients who have a negative exercise test.

Exercise testing adds little in detecting the presence or absence of CAD in patients with a high pretest probability (i.e., history of typical angina with one or more risk factors in men > 40 years of age and postmenopausal women) and in patients with low pretest probability (i.e., history of nonanginal chest pain in a young woman with no family history and no other coronary risk factors.)

13. Discuss the role of electron-beam computed tomography (EBCT) in the diagnosis and prognosis of CAD.

The role of EBCT is currently an important area of investigation. The Multi-Ethnic Study of Atherosclerosis (MESA), a large multicenter trial, was initiated in 1999. Because it has not yet been established that EBCT offers any incremental information to standard office-based risk assessment using the Framingham score, EBCT is not recommended for routine clinical use. Consensus guidelines from the American College of Cardiology/American Heart Association include the following statement:

> [A] positive calcium score might be valuable in determining whether a patient who appears to be at intermediate CHD risk is actually at high risk. Conversely, a low or absent EBCT calcium score may also prove useful in determining a low likelihood of developing CHD. This may be particularly beneficial in elderly asymptomatic patients in whom the management of other risk factors may be modified according to the calcium score. Selected use of coronary calicum scores when a physician is faced with the patient with intermediate coronary disease risk may be appropriate. However, the published literature does not clearly define which asymptomatic people require or will benefit from EBCT. Additional appropriately designed studies of EBCT for this purpose are strongly encouraged. In the setting of this degree of uncertainty, EBCT screening should not be made available to the general public without a physician's request.

14. Summarize the sensitivity and specifity of different noninvasive tests (includng EBCT) for detection of CAD.

Grouping	No. of Studies	Total No. of Patients	Sensitivity (%)	Specificity (%)	Predictive Accuracy (%)
Meta-analysis of standard exercise ECG	147	24,047	68	77	73
Excluding patients with MI	41	11,691	67	74	69
Limiting work-up bias	2	2,350	50	90	69
Meta-analysis of exercise test scores	24	11,788			80
Perfusion scintigraphy	2	28,751	89	80	89
Exercise echocardiography	58	5,000	85	79	83
Nonexercise stress tests					
Pharmacologic stress scintigraphy	11	< 1,000	85	91	87
Dobutamine echocardiography	5	< 1,000	88	84	86
EBCT	16	3,683	91	49	70

15. How does an exercise/stress test help to assess the prognosis of CAD?

The duration of exercise, the symptoms the patient develops, the ischemic ECG changes, and the hemodynamic responses of the patient are very useful in assessing the prognosis of patients with asymptomatic and symptomatic CAD of the patient. In 4083 medically treated patients in the CASS study, a high-risk patient subset was defined as a patient who developed > 1 mm ST depression in Bruce stage 1; this type of patient has an annual mortality > 5% a year, whereas a low-risk patient subset who has normal ECG with > Bruce stage 3 has an annual mortality < 1% per year over 4 years of follow-up. Exercise-induced hypotension correlates with left main or multivessel CAD and indicates a threefold increase in subsequent death or myocardial infarction. Other negative prognostic findings include early-onset ST depression in multiple leads, ST depression for more than 5 minutes during the recovery period, multiple perfusion defects in more than one vascular supply region, and post-exercise LV dilation with increased lung thallium uptake during stress. Patients in the last group should be considered for coronary bypass operations for revascularization.

16. What is the correlation between historical features and coronary angiography?

Middle-aged adults with histories of typical angina, atypical angina, and nonanginal chest pain were found to have angiographic coronary artery disease in 90%, 50%, and 15%, respectively, whereas middle-aged asymptomatic adults had only 3–4% angiographic CAD. However, neither the severity, duration, or nature of the pain nor its precipitating factors correlated with the extent of disease at angiography. For example, patients with advanced obstructive CAD may be asymptomatic with silent ischemia, whereas those with Prinzmetal's angina may have episodes of very severe angina with minimal or no underlying coronary atherosclerosis.

17. What five factors are important in the management of chronic stable angina?

1. Identification and treatment of medical conditions that can precipitate or worsen angina, such as anemia, occult thyrotoxicosis, fever, infections, and tachycardia.

2. Reduction of coronary risk factors, such as dyslipidemia, hypertension, cigarette smoking, and diabetes.

3. Counseling and changes in lifestyle, such as modification of work and leisure activities.

4. Pharmacologic management
   • Only aspirin and lipid-lowering agents have been shown to reduce the morbidity and mortality in chronic stable angina.
   • Nitrates, beta blockers, and calcium antagonists have been shown to improve symptoms and exercise performance, but their effect on survival has not been demonstrated.

5. Revascularization by angioplasty (or other catheter-based techniques) or bypass surgery in patients who have refractory symptoms after taking optimal medical therapy and in patients with high-risk noninvasive tests.

The initial treatment of patients with chronic stable angina should include all of the elements in the mnemonic **ABCDE**:

A = **A**spirin and **a**ntianginal therapy
B = **B**eta blocker and **b**lood pressure
C = **C**igarette smoking and **c**holesterol
D = **D**iet and **d**iabetes
E = **E**ducation and **e**xercise

18. Define unstable angina.

The currently used definition of unstable angina depends on the presence of one or more of the following three historical features:

1. Crescendo angina (more severe, prolonged, or frequent) superimposed on chronic stable angina

2. New-onset angina (within 1 month) brought on by minimal exertion

3. Angina at rest or with minimal exertion. Printzmetal's angina is also characterized by angina at rest and may be considered a form of unstable angina with a pathophysiologically different mechanism. Postmyocardial infarction angina is also considered a form of unstable angina secondary to an active thrombotic process.

19. Describe the underlying pathophysiology in chronic stable angina and unstable angina (acute coronary syndrome).

Chronic stable angina is defined as exertional discomfort in the chest caused by an increase in myocardial oxygen demand with limited coronary flow reserve. Invariably, a fixed coronary artery obstruction is present, which limits the oxygen delivery during times of increased metabolic demands. A normal coronary artery can dilate up to 4–5 times with exercise, while an atherosclerotic coronary artery is unable to dilate with an increased physiologic demand.

Unstable angina (acute coronary syndrome) is caused by a reduction in the myocardial oxygen delivery due to coronary vasoconstriction and/or intracoronary thrombus formation secondary to the rupture of an atherosclerotic plaque.

20. How does the management of chest pain in unstable angina differ from that of chronic stable angina?

Because chronic stable angina is due to an imbalance between myocardial oxygen demand and supply, medical therapy during acute chest pain attempts to decrease the myocardial oxygen demand and to increase coronary perfusion such as rest. These therapies include nitroglycerin, beta blockers, and calcium antagonists.

Unstable angina is associated with an active thrombotic process secondary to the rupture of a plaque and a higher rate of acute MI and sudden death. Intensive antithrombotic management together with antiischemic therapy and close monitoring with telemetry is therefore required. Bedrest, oxygen, nitrates, and beta blockers reduce the episodes of recurrent ischemia and the occurrence of myocardial infarction. Calcium antagonists are effective in relieving symptoms, but they do not prevent myocardial infarction or reduce mortality in this syndrome. Short-acting nifedipine in high doses may be associated with increased risk of myocardial infarction. Aspirin, 160–325 mg, should be started as soon as possible and then continued indefinitely; several randomized trials have shown that aspirin reduces the incidence of MI and death by approximately 50%. Clopidogrel, 300-mg loading dose followed by 75 mg/day (given with aspirin), has been shown to reduce the combined incidence of MI, cerebrovascular accident, and death. Intravenous heparin, 70 units/kg, followed by a continuous infusion of 15 units/kg/hour should be given together with aspirin, because this combination is superior to either drug alone.

BIBLIOGRAPHY

1. American College of Cardiology/American Heart Association: Expert Consensus Document on Electron-beam Computed Tomography for the Diagnosis and Prognosis of Coronary Artery Disease. J Am Coll Cardiol 36:326–340, 2000.

2. Bruanwald E (ed): Heart Disease: A Textbook of Cardiovascular Medicine, 5th ed. Philadelphia, W.B. Saunders, 1997.
3. Cannon RO, Quyyumi AA, Mincemoyer R, et al: Imipramine in patients with chest pain despite normal coronary angiograms. N Engl J Med 330:1411–1417, 1994.
4. Clopidogrel in Unstable Angina to Prevent Events Trial Investigators: Effect of clopidogrel in addition to aspirin in patients with acute coronary syndrome with ST-segment elevation. N Engl J Med 345:494–502, 2001.
5. Diamond GA, Forrester JS: Analysis of probability as an aid in the clinical diagnosis of coronary artery disease. N Engl J Med 300:1350–1358, 1979.
6. Galligan DM, Quyyumi AA, Cannon RO, et al: Effects of physiological levels of estrogen on coronary vasomotor function in postmenopausal women. Circulation 89:2545–2551, 1994.
7. Held PH, Yusuf S, Furberg CD: Calcium channel blockers in acute myocardial infarction and unstable angina: An overview. BMJ 299:1187–1192, 1989.
8. Holdright D, Patel D, Cunningham D, et al: Comparison of the effect of heparin and aspirin versus aspirin alone on transient myocardial ischemia and in-hospital prognosis in patients with unstable angina. J Am Coll Cardiol 24:39–45, 1994.
9. Kemp HG, Kronmal RA, Vlietstra RE, et al: Seven-year survival of patients with normal or near normal coronary angiograms: A CASS registry study. J Am Coll Cardiol 7:479–483, 1986.
10. Lewis HD Jr, Davis JW, Archibald DG, et al: Protective effect of aspirin against acute myocardial infarction and death in men with unstable angina. Results of a Veterans Administration Cooperative Study. N Engl J Med 309:396–403, 1983.

27. ACUTE MYOCARDIAL INFARCTION

Morgan Zaw Naing Lin, M.D., and Rita F. Redberg, M.D., M.Sc.

1. **What are the known risk factors for coronary artery disease?**
Major independent risk factors
1. Cigarette smoking
2. Elevated blood pressure
3. Elevated serum total (and low-density lipoprotein [LDL]) cholesterol
4. Low serum high-density lipoprotein (HDL) cholesterol
5. Diabetes mellitus
6. Advancing age
Other risk factors
Predisposing risk factors
1. Obesity. Body weights are currently defined according to body mass index (BMI) as follows: normal weight = 18.5–24.9 kg/m^2; overweight = 25–29 kg/m^2; obesity = > 30.0 kg/m^2 (obesity class I = 30.0–34.9, class II = 35.9–39.9, class III = ≥ 50 kg/m^2).
2. Abdominal obesity (i.e., waist circumference: men > 102 cm [> 40 in]; women > 88 cm [35 in]).
3. Physical inactivity
4. Family history of premature coronary heart disease
5. Ethnic characteristics
6. Psychosocial factors
Conditional risk factors
1. Elevated serum triglycerides
2. Small LDL particles
3. Elevated serum homocysteine
4. Elevated serum lipoprotein (a)
5. Prothrombotic factors (e.g., fibrinogen)
6. Inflammatory markers (e.g., C-reactive protein)

2. How soon does myocardial ischemia begin after complete coronary occlusion? How soon do myocardial cells die after the onset of ischemia?

The heart has the highest metabolic rate of any organ in the body (6–10 ml 02/100 gm of tissue/minute) and the highest arteriovenous oxygen difference at rest, reflecting near-maximal oxygen extraction. Consequently, the onset of ischemia begins within 60 seconds after complete coronary occlusion. Myocardial cell death occurs within 20–40 minutes in the presence of complete occlusion; however, collateral flow may prolong this period to several hours.

3. What is the sequence of clinical events following myocardial ischemia? What is the correlation between clinical symptoms and left ventricular dysfunction after myocardial infarction?

The earliest abnormality after the onset of myocardial ischemia is a reduction in the diastolic compliance of the heart, followed by local systolic wall motion abnormalities on echocardiography and ST-segment changes on the 12-lead ECG. The patient then has chest discomfort/pain, and serum markers of myocardial infarction (MI) become elevated (myoglobin, cardiac troponin i and t, creatinine kinase isoenzymes).

Diastolic dysfunction > systolic dysfunction > ST changes > chest discomfort > elevated serum markers of infarction.

Rackley et al. have demonstrated a linear relationship between the clinical symptoms and the amount of myocardial loss with the resulting left ventricular (LV) dysfunction after MI.

8% of total LV infarcted = reduced diastolic compliance
> 15% LV infarcted = reduced ejection fraction and elevated LV end-diastolic pressure (LVEDP) and volume (LVEDV)
> 25% of LV infarcted = clinical heart failure
> 40% of LV infarcted = cardiogenic shock

4. What are the acute coronary syndromes? What triggers them?

Acute coronary syndromes are a spectrum of clinical entities, which include unstable angina, non-Q wave infarction, and Q-wave infarction. The rupture of "vulnerable" atherosclerotic plaques is now considered to be the leading cause of acute coronary syndromes. The dynamic process of plaque rupture may evolve to a partially or completely occluded thombus, producing ST segment elevation on the electrocardiogram and ultimately producing necrosis involving full or nearly full-thickness of the ventricular wall in a zone supplied by the affected coronary artery.

	Stable Angina	Unstable Angina	Non–Q-Wave MI	Q-Wave MI
		ACUTE CORONARY SYNDROMES		
Angiographic thrombus		0–1%	75%	> 90%
Acute coronary occlusion		0–1%	10–25%	> 90%
Mortality		1–2%	3–8%	6–15%

5. Describe the mechanism and the process of plaque fissuring and rupture. Compare "vulnerable" plaque with stable plaque.

"Vulnerable" plaque typically has a substantial lipid core and a thin fibrous cap separating thrombogenic macrophages from the blood. In contrast, stable plaque has a relatively thick fibrous cap protecting the lipid core from contact with the blood. Clinical data suggest that stable plaques more often show luminal narrowing on angiography than do vulnerable plaques. Slowly advancing, high-grade stenoses of epicardial coronaries may progess to complete occlusion but do not usually precipitate acute MI, probably because of the development of a rich collateral network. Abrupt and catastrophic rupture of angiographically less significant (< 50% stenosis) "vulnerable" plaques promotes platelet activation and thrombus generation, ultimately leading to myocardial necrosis.

The mechanism for plaque rupture is an area of intense investigation and appears to be multifactorial. A number of key physiologic factors, such as systolic blood presssure, heart rate, blood viscoscity, endogenous tissue plaminogen activator (t-PA) activity, plasma cortisol levels, and plasma epinephrine levels can increase the propensity of plaque rupture with subsequent coronary thrombosis. These factors display a circadian variation that accounts for clustering of acute MI between 6 and 11 AM.

6. What are the nonatherosclerotic causes of acute MI?

1. Coronary artery disease other than atherosclerosis: spasm of coronary arteries, dissection of the coronary arteries, a variety of coronary arteritides associated with systemic diseases, coronary mural thickening secondary to metabolic diseases, and trauma to coronary arteries, including radiation therapy.

2. Embolism to the coronary arteries: infective endocarditis, nonbacterial thrombotic endocarditis, prosthetic valve emboli, cardiac myxoma, mural thrombus from the left atrium or the left ventricle, conditions associated with coronary bypass surgery, and angiography.

3. Myocardial supply-demand disproportion: aortic stenosis, aortic insufficiency, prolonged hypotension.

4. In-situ thrombosis: polycythemia vera, thrombocytosis, disseminated intravascular coagulation (DIC), thrombotic thrombocytopenic purpura (TTP), and hypercoagulable states.

5. Congenital coronary anomalies: anomalous origin of the left coronary artery from pulmonary artery, coronary arteriovenous fistula and aneursyms.

6. Miscellaneous: cocaine abuse, myocardial contusion, complications of cardiac catheterization.

7. Describe the typical signs and symptoms of acute MI.

A prodrome of chest discomfort at rest or with less than usual activity (unstable angina) may precede acute MI together with a feeling of general malaise or frank exhaustion. The classic symptoms of myocardial infarction include dull substernal chest pain, dyspnea, nausea, diaphoresis, palpitations, or sense of impending doom. Chest pain typically lasts at least 15–30 minutes and may radiate to the arms, jaw, or back. The elderly often have atypical presentations, such as dyspnea, confusion, vertigo, syncope, and abdominal pain. Approximately 25% of myocardial infarctions are either asymptomatic or unrecognized (silent).

General examination reveals pallor, diaphoresis, anxiety, and considerable distress. Abnormalities in heart rate, blood pressure, and respiratory rate are variable, depending on the site and the extent of infarction. Low-grade fevers may be present as early as 4–8 hours after the onset of the infarction. Occasionally, rectal temperatures may reach 101–102°F. Jugular venous pressure is markedly elevated in right ventricular infarction and cardiogenic shock. The first heart sound is frequently muffled; paradoxical splitting of the second heart sound may be present when there is ventricular dysfunction and/or left bundle branch block; a fourth heart sound is almost universally audible during sinus rhythm; a third heart sound reflects severe left ventricular dysfunction and is associated with increased mortality. Transient or persistent systolic murmurs may be audible when mitral regurgitation from papillary muscle dysfunction occurs. Pericardial rubs are most commonly heard on the second or third day.

8. What are Killip classes?

In 1967, Killip proposed a prognostic classification of acute MI based on presence and severity of rales:

Class I: no rales; no S3
Class II: rales < 50% of lung fields, may or may not have S3
Class III: rales > 50% of lung fields, with S3 and pulmonary edema present
Class IV: cardiogenic shock

Despite an overall improvement in the mortality of each class compared to the patients in Killips original report, the classification remains useful today in comparing data for treatment of patients with MI.

9. How is the diagnosis of acute myocardial infarction made?
Criteria for acute, evolving, or recent MI
Either one of the following
1. Typical rise and gradual fall (troponin) or more rapid rise and fall (creatine kinase [CK]-MB) of biochemical markers of myocardial necrosis with at least one of the following:
   • Ischemic symptoms
   • Development of pathologic Q waves on ECG
   • ECG changes indicative of ischemia (ST-segment elevation or depression) *or*
   • Coronary artery intervention (e.g., coronary angioplasty)
2. Pathologic findings of an acute MI
Criteria for established MI
Any one of the following:
1. Development of new pathologic Q waves on serial ECGs. The patient may or may not remember previous symptoms. Biochemical markers of myocardial necrosis may have normalized, depending on the length of time since the infarct developed.
2. Pathologic findings of a healed or healing MI

10. What are the ECG criteria for myocardial ischemia and established MI?
ECG changes indicative of myocardial ischemia that may progress to MI
1. New or presumed new ST-segment elevation at the J point in two or more contiguous leads with the cut-off points > 0.2 mV in leads V1, V2, or V3 and ≥ 0.1 mV in other leads (contiguity in the frontal plane is defined by the lead sequence aVL, I, inverted aVR, II, aVF, III).
2. New or presumed new ST-segment depression in two or more contiguous leads.
3. New or presumed new symmetrical inversion of T waves ≥ 1 mm in at least two contiguous leads.
ECG changes in established MI
1. Any Q wave in leads VI through V3 (in two contiguous leads and ≥ 1 mm in depth).
2. Q wave ≥ 30 ms in leads I, II, aVL, aVF, V4, V5, or V6 (in two contiguous leads and ≥ 1 mm in depth).

11. Which currently available cardiac enzymes are useful for the earliest detection of myocardial necrosis? What is the role of cardiac-specific troponins in the diagnosis and the prognosis of tacute coronary syndrome?
Myoglobin is released into the circulation as early as one hour after infarction, and the serum level rapidly falls within 24 hours. Although its measurement has been suggested as a useful index of successful reperfusion, its clinical value in detecting acute MI is limited because of the lack of specificity of its measurement.
Certain isoforms of MM and MB isoenzymes of CK are released into the blood as early as 1 hour after the onset of myocardial infarction. In one study, an absolute level of CK-MB2 isoform > 1.0 U/L or a ratio of CK-MB2/CK-MB1 > 1.5 had a sensitivity for diagnosing acute MI of 59% in 2–4 hours and a sensitivity of 92% at 4–6 hours.
Quantitative assays of cardiac specific antibodies to troponin T and I (cTnT and cTnI) have been recently approved by the Food and Drug Administration (FDA) for clinical use in detecting acute MI. Because cTnT and cTnI are not detectable in peripheral blood under normal conditions, the signal-to-noise ratio is much improved with these markers compared to CK-MB enzymes. Minor degrees of myocardial necrosis can now be detected. cTnT and cTnI begin to rise within 3 hours of chest pain in acute MI, and cTnI remains elevated for 7–10 days; cTnT remains elevated for 10–14 days, permitting diagnosis even in patients who present late after chest pain.
In GUSTO-II, cTnT > 0.1 ng/ml was the most important prognostic indicator for the 30-day mortality in patients with acute myocardial ischemia, compared with a subgroup who had abnormal ECG changes and elevated CK-MB levels. The prognostic value of cTnI in patients with unstable angina or non-Q wave MI in a multicenter study has been demonstrated. cTnI level > 0.4

ng/ml were associated with significantly increased mortalities at 42 days and each increase of 1 ng/ml of cTnI was associated with an increased risk of death.

12. What are the differences between Q-wave and non–Q-wave myocardial infarctions?

Q-wave infarctions (previously called transmural infarctions) account for 60–70% of all acute MIs, whereas non–Q-wave MIs (previously termed subendocardial infarctions) represent 30–40% of all MIs. The presence of Q waves on the ECG does not reliably document transmural vs. a subendocardial infarction (by autopsy data).

Non–Q-Wave Infarction	Q-Wave Infarction
Nonspecific ST changes or ST depression	ST segment elevation
10–25% early total occlusion of infarct-related artery	> 90% total occlusion
Lower CK peaks	Higher CK peaks
Higher ejection fractions	Lower ejection fractions
Lower in-hospital complications and mortality	Higher in-hospital mortality

The 3-year overall mortality rate of patients with both kind of infarcts is the same because of the higher reinfarction rate in patients with non–Q-wave MI. Because up to 60% of patients with non–Q-wave MI have significant two- or three-vessel disease, many physicians recommend early angiography to stratify the risks.

13. How do you risk-stratify patients who present with chest pain in the emergency room, and what is a cost-effective way of managing patients with low risk for complications?

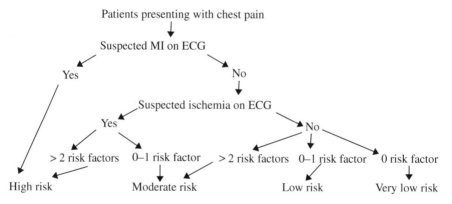

Low-risk patients can be admitted for chest pain evaluation or observation units with rapid "rule-out" MI protocol (enzymes 0, 3, 6, 9 hours) with EKG monitoring and less intensive nursing. They should have a predischarge stress test if cardiac enzymes do not indicate myocardial infarction. There is no significant difference in the complication rate with shorter stays and lower cost.

14. Discuss the principles of initial management for acute MI.

Prehospital care. Most deaths associated with AMI occur within the first hour of its onset and are usually due to ventricular fibrillation. Immediate resuscitation and prompt transport to a hospital are therefore important. Prehospital care should include oxygen, nitroglycerin, and morphine (if hypotension is not present).

Emergency department and hospital care. Immediate assessment of hemodynamic and electrical stability of the patient and eligibility for thrombolytic therapy or emergency angioplasty should be determined. All patients should be given aspirin 160–325 mg as soon as possible unless there is contraindication. The goal for starting thrombolytic therapy after arrival to the emergency department ("door-to-needle time") is < 30 minutes, and the goal for starting angioplasty ("door-to-balloon time") is < 1 hour.

15. What is the recommended management of patients with acute MI with > 0.1 mV ST elevation in more than two contiguous leads?

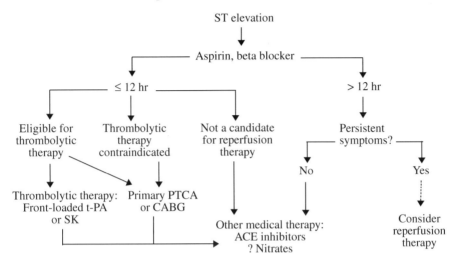

American College of Cardiology/American Heart Association guidelines for the management of patients with acute MI. All patients with ST-segment elevation on ECG should receive aspirin, β-adrenergic blockers (in the absence of contraindications), and an antithrombin (particularly if tissue plasminogen activator [t-PA] is used for thrombolytic therapy). Whether heparin is required in patients receiving streptokinase (SK) remains a matter of controversy; the small additional risk for intracranial hemorrhage may not be offset by the survival benefit afforded by adding heparin to SK therapy. Patients treated within 12 hours who are eligible for thrombolytics should expeditiously receive either front-loaded t-PA or SK or be considered for primary percutaneous transluminal coronary angioplasty (PTCA). Primary PTCA is also to be considered when thrombolytic therapy is absolutely contraindicated. Coronary artery bypass graft (CABG) may be considered if the patient is less than 6 hours from onset of symptoms. Patients treated after 12 hours should receive the intial medical therapy noted above and, on an individual basis, may be candidates for reperfusion therapy or angiotensin-converting enzyme (ACE) inhibitors (particularly if left ventricular function is impaired). Modified from Antman EM: Medical therapy for acute coronary syndromes: An overview. In Califf RM (ed): Atlas of Heart Disorders, vol. VIII. Philadelphia, Current Medicine, 1996.)

16. What is the recommended management for patients with suspected acute MI patients who do not have ST elevation?

See algorithm on following page.

17. Explain the recommendation for thrombolytic therapy.

Thrombolytic therapy is recommended in all patients with suspected acute MI with ST elevation (> 0.1 mV, > two contiguous leads) or new left bundle-branch block if the patient presents within 12 hours of the onset of chest pain. within 4 hours after onset of their chest pain

Comparison of Approved Thrombolytic Agents

	STREPTOKINASE	ANISTREPLASE	ALTEPLASE	RETEPLASE
Dose	1.5 MU in 30–60 min	30 mg in 5 min	100 mg in 90 min	10 U × 2 over 30 min
Bolus administration	No	Yes	No	Yes
Antigenic	Yes	Yes	No	No

Table continued on following page

Comparison of Approved Thrombolytic Agents (Continued)

	STREPTOKINASE	ANISTREPLASE	ALTEPLASE	RETEPLASE
Allergic reactions (hypo-tension most common)	Yes	Yes	No	No
Systemic fibrinogen depletion	Marked	Marked	Mild	Moderate
90-min patency rates (%)	~ 50	~ 65	~ 75	~ 75
TIMI grade 3 flow (%)	32	43	54	60
Mortality rate in most recent comparative trials (%)	7.3	10.5	7.2	7.5
Cost per dose (U.S. dollars)	294	2116	2196	2196

TIMI = Throbolysis in Myocardial Infarction Trial.

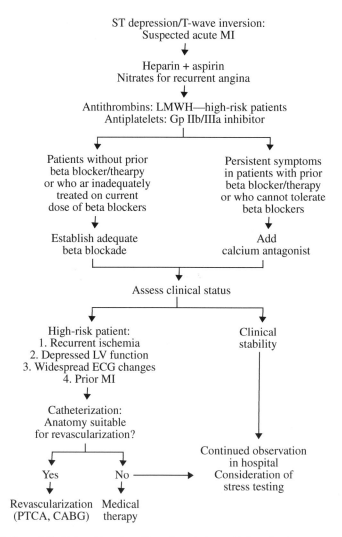

American College of Cardiology/American Heart Association guidelines for the management of patients with acute myocardial infarction.

18. What are the contraindications to thrombolytic therapy?

Absolute contraindications

- Previous hemorrhagic stroke at any time; nonhemorrhagic stroke within 1 year
- Known intracranial neoplasm
- Active internal bleeding (does not include menses)
- Suspected aortic dissection

Relative contraindications/cautions

- Severe uncontrolled hypertension (> 180/110 mmHg) on presentation
- Other intracranial pathology not covered in absolute contraindications
- Recent (within 2–4 weeks) internal bleeding
- Recent trauma (within 2–4 weeks), including head trauma, prolonged traumatic CPR (> 10 minutes), or major surgery within 3 weeks
- Active peptic ulcer
- Current use of anticoagulants with INR > 2–3; known bleeding diathesis
- Non-compressible vascular punctures
- Pregnancy
- For streptokinase/anistreplase: prior exposure (within 5 days to 2 years) or prior allergic reaction
- History of chronic severe hypertension

19. What is the currently recommended role of PTCA in acute MI?

Indications for PTCA in acute MI are rapidly evolving. The newly revised American College of Cardiology/American Heart Association guideline lists the following clinical situations as class I indications:

1. As an alternative to thrombolytic therapy in patients with acute MI and ST-segment elevation or new or presumed new left bundle-branch block (LBBB) who can undergo angioplasty of the infarct-related artery within 12 hours of onset or symptoms or > 12 hours if ischemic symptoms persist and if performed in a timely fashion by persons skilled in the procedure and supported by experienced personnel in an appropriate laboratory environment.

2. In patients who are within 36 hours of an acute ST-elevation/Q-wave or new LBBB MI and who develop cardiogenic shock and are < 75 years of age—if revascularization can be performed within 18 hours of onset of shock.

20. What is the role of bypass surgery in acute MI?

About 10–20% of patients with acute MI are referred to the bypass operation for the following reasons:

1. Persistent or recurrent chest pain despite thrombolysis or PTCA
2. High-risk coronary anatomy (left main stenosis) discovered at catheterization
3. Complications of acute MI, including ventricular septal rupture or severe mitral regurgitation due to papillary muscle dysfunction

21. How do you risk-stratify patients with acute MI before discharge from hospital?

Both short- and long-term survival rates after acute MI depend on three factors:

1. Resting left ventricular function (the most important prognostic factor)
2. Residual ischemic myocardium
3. Susceptibility to serious ventricular arrthymias.

Left ventricular function can be assessed by echocardiography or by a gated blood pool scan (MUGA). Accurate assessment of the end-systolic volume is superior to ejection, the measurement of the fraction for predicting survival after acute MI. In patients with lower ejection fractions, the measurement of exercise capacity is useful for further identifying the high-risk patients and also for establishing safe exercise limits before discharge.

In patients with uncomplicated MI, provocable myocardial ischemia can be evaluated by traditional submaximal exercise tests (peak heart rate 70% of maximal predicated rate for the age, and a peak work level of 5 METs) done at 3–5 days after MI or symptom-limited exercise test at

14–21 days after MI. High-risk groups are identified by low exercise capacity and/or development of hypotension, ST-segment depression at low heart rates, and development of angina during exercise testing. Such patients should be referred for cardiac catheterization for revascularization. Patients who cannot exercise because of a physical limitation can be evaluated with a pharmacologic (dipyridamole, adenosine, or dobutamine) myocardial perfusion study with thallium, sestamibi, or dipyridamole stress echocardiography.

Several techniques have been devised to stratify patients who are at increased risk of sudden death after acute MI: signal-averaged ECG, measuring heart rate variability, and baroreflex sensitivity, and invasive electrophysiologic studies. Patients with sustained ventricular tachycardia or ventricular fibrillation that occurs more than 48 hours after acute events are at increased risk for sudden cardiac death and should be considered for diagnostic electrophysiology studies.

22. What interventions are used in secondary prevention of MI?

1. Lifestyle modification: cessation of smoking, treatment of hypertension, treatment of depression after acute MI, supervised rehabilitative exercise program.

2. Modification of lipid profile: Target LDL cholesterol level is less than 100 mg/dl after MI. The most dramatic evidence is the 30% reduction in total mortality and a 42% reduction in coronary artery disease-related death over 5.4 years in patients receiving simvastatin for an elevated cholesterol in the Scandinavian Simvastatin Survival Study.

3. Antiplatelet therapy: In 11 randomized trials over 20,000 patients with a prior MI, ASA 80–325 mg per day can lead to a 25% reduction in the risk of recurrent infarction, stroke or vascular deaths. It should be continued indefinitely in the absence of contraindication. Sulfinpyrazone, 400 mg twice daily, or ticlopidine, 250 mg twice daily, can be given to patients with true aspirin allergy.

4. Beta blockers: Beta blockers have been shown to reduce mortality and risk of reinfarction by as much as 33% in postinfarction patients who have a moderate to high risk. It is recommended to start beta blockers as early as possible and continue them for at least 2–3 years.

5. ACE inhibitors: To prevent late remodeling of left ventricle and to decrease recurrent ischemic events, indefinite therapy with an ACE inhibitor is recommended to all patients with clinical congestive heart failure or patients who have a moderate decrease in their global ejection fraction (< 40%), or in patients who have a large regional wall motion abnormality, even when they have normal global ejection fraction.

BIBIOGRAPHY

1. ACC/AHA guidelines for the management of patients with acute myocardial infarction. J Am Coll Cardiol 32, 2000.
2. Antman EM, Milenko J, Thompson B, et al: Cardiac-specific torponin I levels to predict the risk of mortality in patients with acute coronary syndromes. N Engl J Med 335:18:1342–1349, 1996.
3. Braunwald E (ed): Heart Disease: A Textbook of Cardiovascular Medicine, 5th ed. Philadelphia, W.B. Saunders, 1997.
4. Gaspoz JM, Lee TH, Goldman P, et al: Cost effectiveness of the a new short-stay unit to rule-out acute myocardial infarction in low risk patients. J Am Coll Cardiol 24:1249–1259, 1994.
5. Grundy, et al: AHA/ACC Scientific Statement: Assessment of cardiovascular risk by use of multiple-risk-fator assessment equations. J Am Coll Cardiol 34:1348–1359, 1999.
6. Michels KB, Yusuf S: Does PTCA in acute myocardial infarction affect mortality and reinfarction rates? A quantitative overview (meta-analysis) of the randomized clinical trials. Circulation 91:476, 1995.
7. Ohman EM, Armstrong PW,Christenson RH, et al: Cardiac troponin t levels for risk stratification in acute myocardial ischemia. N Engl J Med 335:8, 1333–1341, 1996.
8. Puleo RR, Guadagno PA, Robert R, et al: Early diagnosis of acute myocardial infarction based on assay of subforms of creatine kinase-MB. Circulation 82:759, 1990.
9. Scandinavian Simvastatin Survival Study Group: Randomized trial of cholesterol lowering in 4444 patients with coronary heart disease. Lancet 344:1383, 1994.
10. White HD, Norris RM, Brown MA, et al: Left ventricular end systolic volume as the major determinant of survival after recovery from myocardial infarction. Circulation 76:44, 1987.

28. DYSRHYTHMIAS

Linda Liu, M.D.

1. What is the normal sequence of cardiac depolarization?

Pacemaker cells in the sinoatrial (SA) node spontaneously depolarize and a wave of depolarization spreads over the atria and into the atrioventricular (AV) node. After a brief delay in the node, the impulse enters the bundle of His and right and left bundle branches. The interventricular septum is the first to depolarize, followed by the apical ventricular myocardium, then the bulk of the left and right ventricular free walls, with the last area activated being the superior portion of the left ventricular free wall or the right ventricular outflow tract.

2. Discuss causes and treatment options for sinus tachycardia.

Sinus tachycardia is probably the most frequently seen rhythm disturbance in the intensive care unit (ICU). It may be a sign of hemorrhage, hypoxia, hypercapnea, thyrotoxicosis, alcohol withdrawal, cardiac tamponade, pulmonary embolism, pneumothorax, infection, pain, or anxiety. Appropriate treatment involves removing or treating the underlying cause. Pharmacologic measures such as beta blockade are rarely indicated.

3. Describe the evaluation of narrow complex tachycardia.

In conscious patients, further diagnostic information, such as a 12-lead ECG, should be collected. If the mechanism of tachycardia is still unclear, carotid massage in patients without significant cerebrovascular disease, Valsalva maneuver, or immersion of the face in ice water may enhance vagal tone to the sinus and AV nodes. Vagal maneuvers have different effects, dependig on the rhythm. Sinus tachycardia may be slowed and transiently reveal P waves before each QRS. AV reentrant tachycardia and AV nodal reentrant tachycardia may be terminated. In atrial flutter or atrial fibrillation, the ventricular response may be transiently slowed enough so that diagnosis is possible. If vagal maneuvers fail to slow the rhythm for diagnosis, adenosine is the preferred agent because of its short half-life and decreased likelihood of causing problematic hypotension. Indications for emergent or urgent treatment of tachyarrhythmias with direct-current cardioversion include impairment of consciousness, hypotension, hypoxia, and cardiac ischemia.

4. How does adenosine work? What are its side effects?

Adenosine is a naturally occurring nucleoside used for the treatment of supraventricular tachycardia (SVT). It inhibits adenylate cyclase, decreases intracellular cyclic adenosine monophosphate (cAMP), and slows AV nodal conduction. Adenosine can terminate reentry SVT and aid in the diagnosis of other arrhythmias by causing a brief high-degree AV block. Because of its rapid metabolism, adenosine has a half-life of 10 seconds. Side effects include flushing, headache, bronchoconstriction, and chest discomfort. Phosphodiesterase inhibitors such as theophylline and caffeine, which elevate cAMP, oppose the effects of adenosine.

5. Describe preexcitation.

Preexcitation occurs when ventricular activation occurs earlier than would be expected using the normal AV conduction system. Wolff-Parkinson-White (WPW) syndrome involves an accessory atrioventricular pathway that connects the atrium and the ventricle and bypasses the AV node. The PR interval is usually shortened (< 0.12 sec) and the QRS duration is usually increased (> 0.12 sec). The initial slurring of the QRS complex with the remainder of the ventricular depolarization is called the delta wave. Digoxin has been reported to shorten refractoriness in the accessory pathway and accelerate the ventricular response. Thus, it is advised not to use digoxin as a single drug in patients with WPW. Surgical ablation is a therapeutic option for young patients or those who do not wish to take chronic beta-blocking therapy.

6. What are the three most common accessory pathways associated with preexcitation syndromes?

1. Kent fibers bridge the atrium and ventricle without passing through the AV node.
2. James fibers bypass the AV node and attach to the bundle of His.
3. Mahaim fibers bypass from the bundle of His or either bundle branch into the intraventricular septal myocardium.

7. What are the most common causes of atrial fibrillation?

1. Mitral valve disease	6. Thyrotoxicosis
2. Ischemic heart disease	7. Cardiomyopathies
3. Congenital heart disease	8. Accessory pathways
4. Alcohol consumption	9. Chronic obstructive pulmonary disease (COPD)
5. Hypertension	10. Perioperative cardiac surgery

8. What are the manifestations of digoxin toxicity? What are the therapeutic options?

Digoxin toxicity commonly manifests as visual changes or GI distrubances. In general, therapy requires simply withholding the drug and monitoring the patient. For occasional premature ventricular contractions or brief runs of bigeminy, additional potassium supplementations, if indicated, may also suffice. Symptomatic bradyarrhythmias should be treated with atropine or transvenous pacing. Tachyarrhythmias can be treated with antiarrhythmic agents such as lidocaine, phenytoin, and propranolol. Digoxin-induced arrhythmias are frequently made worse by cardioversion; therefore, this therapy should be reserved for ventricular fibrillation or any other hemodynamically unstable rhythm.

9. Describe ibutilide.

Ibutilide fumarate, a new antiarrhythmic drug for intravenous use, has been approved for the acute termination of recent-onset atrial fibrillation or flutter. Recent trials completed by the manufacturer included 200 patients with new-onset fibrillation or flutter. Fourteen (45%) of 38 patients who received 0.015 mg/kg over 10 minutes and 19 (48%) of 40 patients who received 0.025 mg/kg converted to sinus rhythm. The success rate for conversion was better for atrial flutter (48–70%) than for atrial fibrillation (22–43%). Comparison of ibutilide with electrical cardioversion is pending. Side effects of ibutilide include torsade de pointes (up to 8% of treated patients) and, in rare instances, AV block or heart failure. Concurrent use with other antiarrhythmics or nonsedating antihistamines may increase the incidence of torsade de pointes and should be avoided.

10. What are the risks of stroke in patients with atrial fibrillation?

The annual incidence of stroke in nonanticoagulated patients with atrial fibrillation is about 5%. Most strokes are embolic and occur within 2 years after the onset of atrial fibrillation. Factors associated with an increased risk of stroke include left atrial enlargement, hypertension, left ventricular dysfunction, and increased age. Several randomized trials have shown that oral anticoagulation with warfarin reduces the risk of stroke secondary to emboli in this population.

11. What is the appropriate level of anticoagulation for patients in atrial fibrillation?

The recommended target international normalized ratio (INR) is 2.0–3.0. A recent study demonstrated a lower stroke rate in warfarin-treated patients (1.9%) than in aspirin-treated patients (2.7%), but the difference was not statistically significant. The risk of major hemorrhagic complications was significantly increased in elderly patients taking warfarin. Further studies are needed, but evidence suggests that aspirin may be a reasonable alternative to warfarin in selected patients with chronic atrial fibrillation, particularly elderly patients and patients at low risk for thromboembolism or high risk for bleeding.

12. How long should a patient be anticoagulated before elective cardioversion?
The Second American College of Chest Physicians (AACP) Conference on Antithrombotic Therapy strongly recommends anticoagulation to an INR of 2–3 if atrial fibrillation has been present for longer than 2 days. Anticoagulation should be at therapeutic levels for at least 3 weeks before elective cardioversion and should be continued until sinus rhythm has been maintained for 2–4 weeks.

13. How is the diagnosis of ventricular tachycardia (VT) established during wide QRS complex tachycardia?
The overwhelming majority of wide QRS complex tachycardias are due to ventricular tachycardia (81%) as opposed to SVT with aberrant conduction (14%) or antegrade conduction over an accessory pathway (5%). The presence of AV dissociation proves the diagnosis of VT. Other morphologic criteria favoring VT include:
- QRS duration >140 ms with right bundle-branch block (RBBB) morphology
- QRS duration >160 ms with left bundle-branch block (LBBB) morphology
- Positive QRS concordance in all precordial leads
- Extreme left axis deviation (–90° to 180°)
- Different QRS morphology during the tachycardia than at baseline in patients with preexisting bundle-branch block

14. According to advanced cardiac life support (ACLS) protocols, what drug is recommended for treatment of VT/ventricular fibrillation unresponsive to defibrillation?
As one of the changes in the International Guidelines 2000, vasopressin, 40 U intravenously, or epinephrine, 1 mg intravenously, is recommended as the primary vasoconstrictor before another attempt at defibrillation. Antiarrhythmics that should be tried next include amiodarone, lidocaine, magnesium sulfate, and procainamide. Bretylium has been removed from the guidelines because of a high occurrence of side effects, availability of more efficacious agents, and limited supply.

15. What is vasopressin?
Vasopressin is a naturally occurring antidiuretic hormone that acts as a nonadrenergic peripheral vasoconstrictor by direct stimulation of smooth muscle V_1 receptors. Vasopressin has a longer half-life than epinephrine (10–20 minutes vs. 2–3 minutes). During cardiopulmonary resuscitation (CPR), vasopressin causes peripheral vasoconstriction of skin, skeletal muscle, intestine, fat, and coronary and renal vascular beds. It also leads to vasodilation of the cerebral vasculature. Preliminary evidence indicates that vasopressin can enhance the return of spontaneous circulation in humans with out-of-hospital ventricular fibrillation.

16. List the causes of torsade de pointes.
Torsade de pointes translates to "twisting of the points" and describes a type of ventricular tachycardia in which the QRS complexes appear to rotate along an axis. It occurs in the setting of a prolonged QT interval, which is associated with:
1. Congenital or idiopathic causes
2. Drugs: type 1A and 1C antiarrhythmics and psychoactive drugs (i.e., phenothiazines, butyrophenones, tricyclic antidepressants)
3. Severe bradycardia
4. Metabolic abnormalities: hypokalemia, hypomagnesemia, hypocalcemia
5. Liquid protein diets
6. Neurologic disease: subarachnoid hemorrhages, strokes, encephalitis
7. Arsenic poisoning
8. Myocardial infarction or ischemia

Arrhythmia is treated with administration of magnesium sulfate, removal of the offending agent, correction of electrolyte imbalances, and atrial or ventricular pacing. Lidocaine is ineffective, and treatment with class 1A antiarrhythmics should be avoided.

17. Summarize the Vaughan-Williams classes of antiarrhythmics, their site of action, and their extracardiac side effects.

Site of Action	Class	Name	Extracardiac Side Effects
Block fast sodium channels	1A	Quinidine	GI upset, thrombocytopenia, hepatic toxicity
		Procainamide	Lupus-like syndrome, agranulocytosis, prolonged QT interval
	1B	Lidocaine	Confusion, seizures
		Tocainide	Confusion, seizures, pulmonary fibrosis, agranulocytosis
		Mexiletine	GI upset, confusion, seizures
	1C	Encainide,	Dizziness, headache, visual disturbances
		Flecainide	Same as encainide
		Propafenone	Same as encainide
Beta blockers	II	Propranolol	Lethargy, attenuated hypoglycemia response, bronchospasm
		Esmolol	Same as propranolol
Delayed repolarization (possible potassium channel blockers)	III	Amiodarone	Vasodilation, hypotension, tremor, ataxia, pulmonary fibrosis, liver and thyroid dysfunction
Calcium channel blockers	IV	Verapamil	Constipation, hypotension
		Diltiazem	Same as verapamil

18. Discuss the electrophysiology, pharmacology, and toxicity of amiodarone.

Amiodarone prolongs the action potential duration and repolarization time by inhibition of potassium ion fluxes and by acting as a weak sodium channel antagonist, giving it class I and class III antiarrhythmic activity. The drug is only 50% bioavailable after oral dosing and is highly protein and lipid bound with an estimated volume of distribution of 50 liters. The elimination half-life is long ($\approx$ 52 days), secondary to avid binding to poorly perfused adipose tissue. Amiodarone is effective in patients with recent MIs, cardiomyopathy, nonsustained VT, atrial fibrillation, and survivors of sudden death. Side effects include conduction abnormalities in the AV node, congestive heart failure secondary to its negative inotropic actions, pulmonary fibrosis or interstitial pneumonitis, liver and thyroid dysfunction, peripheral neuropathy and tremors, corneal microdeposits, allergic rashes, and a blue-gray skin discoloration.

19. When should impaired clearance of lidocaine be suspected?

Impaired clearance should be suspected in conditions where hepatic blood flow is decreased (i.e., congestive heart failure) and when liver function is decreased (i.e., liver disease, hypotension). Lidocaine clearance is also decreased in the elderly, during infusions lasting greater than 24 hours, and with concomitant administration of beta blockers and cimetidine. Signs and symptoms of lidocaine toxicity should also be monitored in patients receiving infusions greater than 2 mg/min.

20. What arrhythmias are not amenable to electrical cardioversion?

Electrical cardioversion is ineffective against tachycardias that arise from enhanced automaticity. Arrhythmias in this category include sinus tachycardia, multifocal atrial tachycardia, accelerated junctional rhythms, any rhythm that occurs in the setting of digoxin intoxication, and ventricular tachycardia caused by class 1C antiarrhythmics.

BIBLIOGRAPHY

1. Chauhan VS, Krahn AD, Klein GJ, et al: Supraventricular tachycardia. Med Clin North Am 85:193–224, 2001.
2. Faber TS, Zehender M, Just H: Drug-induced torsade de pointes—incidence, management and prevention. Drug Safety 11(6):463–476, 1994.

3. Foster RH, Wilde MI, Markham A: Ibutilide: A review of its pharmacological properties and clinical potential in the acute management of atrial flutter and fibrillation. Drugs 54:312–330, 1997
4. Guide to the international ACLS algorithms: Guidelines 2000 for cardiopulmonary resuscitation and emergency cardiovascular care. Circulation 102(Suppl I):I-142–I-157, 2000.
5. Passman R, Kadish A: Polymorphic tachycardia, long Q-T syndrome, and torsades de pointes. Med Clin North Am 85:321–342, 2001.
6. Pelosi F, Morady F: Evaluation and management of atrial fibrillation. Med Clin North Am 85:225–244, 2001.

29. AORTIC DISSECTION

Timothy R. White, M.D., Ph.D., and David E. Schwartz, M.D., F.C.C.P.

1. What is aortic dissection?

Dissection of the aorta occurs with a tear in the intima of the artery. Blood is propelled under pressure through the tear and dissects into the media of the aorta. The hematoma can progress along the course of the aorta and occlude any of the arterial branches of the aorta, including branches of the arch of the aorta or the mesenteric arteries. Retrograde dissection can involve the coronary arteries. The right coronary artery is more frequently involved than the left. Retrograde dissection can also result in loss of commissural support for one or more of the aortic valve cusps and result in acute aortic insufficiency.

The false channel that is created is located in the outer half of the aortic media. The outer wall of this channel is only one-fourth as thick as the original media. This explains the high frequency of rupture of the aorta in patients with aortic dissection. Rupture of the aortic arch occurs most frequently into the mediastinum, the descending thoracic aorta into the left pleural space, and the abdominal aorta into the retroperitoneum. Because the parietal pericardium is attached to the ascending aorta just proximal to the origin of the innominate artery, rupture of any portion of the ascending aorta can lead to cardiac tamponade from hemopericardium.

2. Where is the intimal tear located?

In approximately 70% of patients, the intimal tear, which is the beginning of the dissection, is located in the ascending aorta. In 10% of patients, the laceration is located in the aortic arch, and in approximately 20% of patients the tear is in the descending thoracic aorta. Only rarely is an intimal tear identified in the abdominal aorta.

3. What are the frequency and mortality of aortic dissection?

There are at least 2,000 new cases of aortic dissection per year in the United States. The incidence of aortic dissection has been reported as between 5 and 20 cases per million population per year. In autopsy series of patients with sudden nontraumatic death, aortic dissection is found as the cause in 1.5%. If left untreated after diagnosis, the mortality of aortic dissection is 90% at 3 months.

4. What factors predispose to aortic dissection?

Hypertension is the most important etiologic factor; it is present in 70–90% of patients who develop dissection. **Congenital disorders** associated with aortic dissection include Marfan syndrome, Ehlers-Danlos syndrome, a congenitally bicuspid aortic valve, aortic coarctation, Turner syndrome, giant-cell aortitis, and relapsing polychondritis. There is also an association with **pregnancy**. Half of all dissections in women under the age of 40 have been reported to occur during pregnancy, most frequently in the third trimester. Like acute myocardial infarction, sudden cardiac death, and cardiac arrest, aortic dissection is associated with **circadian and seasonal variations** in incidence. Aortic dissections occur with higher frequency in the morning hours compared with other times of day and in winter months compared with other times of year. This variation seems to be correlated with physiologic variations in blood pressure.

In addition, aortic dissection has been described **after medical or surgical procedures**, including procedures in which the aorta is entered, aortic counterpulsation devices are inserted, and the aorta or its main branches have been cannulated. Iatrogenic aortic dissection is thought to be a rare complication. For example, aortic dissection after cardiac surgery has been reported in 0.12–0.16% of cases in retrospective reviews. Compared with spontaneous dissection, iatrogenic dissections tend to occur in patients who are older (71.4 ± 4.8 years vs. 62.4 ± 13.8 years, p < 0.001) and have a higher incidence of atherosclerotic disease. Trauma is an infrequent cause of aortic dissection. Pathologically aortic dissection is associated with cystic medial necrosis. Dissections are more frequent in males (male-to-female ratio = 3:1).

5. How has aortic dissection been classified?

The first classification system for aortic dissection was that of DeBakey, who described three types of aortic dissection. In type I the dissection begins in the aortic root and extends beyond the ascending aorta. Type II is confined to the ascending aorta. Type III dissections begin distal to the takeoff of the left subclavian artery. In type IIIA the dissection is limited to the thoracic aorta, whereas type IIIB dissection descends below the diaphragm. Rarely type III dissections progress retrograde toward the aortic arch and ascending aorta. The simpler, more recent Stanford classification includes two types: type A dissections, which involve the ascending aorta, and type B dissections, which are distal to the left subclavian artery.

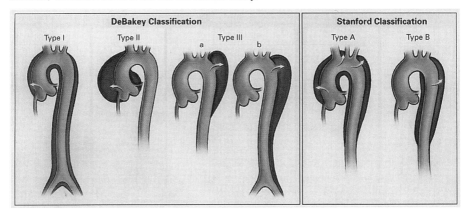

Classification systems for aortic dissection. (From Kouchoukos NT, Dougenis D: Surgery of the thoracic aorta. N Engl J Med 336:1876–1888, 1997, with permission.)

The DeBakey system includes three types of aortic dissection. In type I and II dissections, the intimal tear is proximal to the origin of the left subclavian artery. DeBakey type I dissections involve the ascending aorta, the arch, and variable lengths of the descending thoracic and abdominal aorta. In type II, the dissection is confined to the ascending aorta. Type III dissections are divided into types IIIa and IIIb. In type IIIa the dissection is confined to the descending thoracic aorta, whereas with type IIIb it may extend into the abdominal aorta and iliac arteries. This type of dissection may extend proximally to involve the arch or ascending aorta.

The Stanford classification has only two types. Type A includes all cases of dissection in which the intimal tear is in the ascending aorta, with or without involvement of the arch or descending aorta. Type B includes cases in which the intimal tear is in the descending thoracic aorta. Type B also includes proximal and distal extension of the dissection.

6. What pathophysiologic mechanisms are thought to initiate an aortic dissection?

Current evidence supports two mechanisms for the generation of an aortic dissection: rupture and tearing of the intima of the aorta, and the development of an intramural hematoma. An intimal tear occurs in the wall of the aorta, usually related to hypertension and/or dilatation of the vessel. The pulsatile force of the blood separates the layers of the aorta. The origin of the intimal tear is most frequently in the ascending aorta just above the aortic sinuses: in 60% of patients the tear will be found on the convex portion of the ascending aorta. In 30% of patients, the intimal disruption is located distal to the left subclavian artery, while in the remaining 10% the location of the dissection is the aortic arch.

Recently, a second mechanism for the initiation of aortic dissection has been identified. Spontaneous rupture of the vaso vasorum occurs in less than 10% of patients with aortic dissection. Rupture of these vessels leads to an intramural hematoma of the aorta which spreads within the layers of the media, eventually disrupting the intima. This process has been documented by serial echocardiography.

7. What are the clinical features of aortic dissection?

The most striking clinical manifestation of acute aortic dissection is the abrupt onset of symptoms. Some features of the pain of aortic dissection may be helpful in differentiating it from other causes of acute pain, including myocardial infarction. The onset of sudden severe chest pain usually heralds aortic dissection. Pain may be present in up to 90% of patients. Patients with aortic dissection often localize the pain in the anterior chest with extension to the back. They frequently describe the pain as ripping or tearing in quality. The pain is usually of maximal intensity from its inception and is frequently unremitting. The pain may migrate along the path of the dissection. In contrast, the pain of myocardial infarction has more of a crescendo nature and is frequently described as pressure or a crushing sensation.

In cases of iatrogenic dissection, the above clinical picture may not apply. Patients are less likely to have abrupt pain, and the pain is less likely to migrate. Absence of pain is more prevalent in iatrogenic dissection, as is the presence of ischemia and hypotension.

8. What physical findings and clinical manifestations are suggestive of aortic dissection?

On physical examination patients with aortic dissection may appear to be in shock. However, more than half of patients with distal dissection are hypertensive. Hypotension suggests cardiac tamponade (rupture into the pericardium), rupture of the dissection into the intrapleural or intraperitoneal spaces, or occlusion of the brachial arteries resulting in "pseudohypotension." The loss of peripheral pulses is an important clue to presence of an aortic dissection. This occurs in approximately one-half of patients with proximal dissection and signifies involvement of the brachiocephalic vessels. Only one-sixth of patients with a distal dissection have diminution of a peripheral pulse.

Acute aortic regurgitation may be present in 50% of patients with proximal dissection and can be due to simple widening of the aortic annulus or actual disruption of the aortic valve leaflets. Cardiac tamponade and pleural effusions may indicate rupture of the aortic dissection. These findings portend a poor prognosis and should be searched for carefully. Pleural effusions, which occur most frequently in the left chest, can be caused by rupture of the dissection into the pleural space or from weeping of fluid from the aorta as the result of an inflammatory reaction to the dissection.

Additional physical findings include Horner's syndrome, caused by compression of the cervical sympathetic ganglion, mottling of the flanks, which suggests rupturing of the aneurysm into the retroperitoneal space, and myocardial infarction due to dissection of the coronary arteries. The right coronary artery is most frequently involved, and myocardial infarction is seen in 1–2% of patients with dissection. Mesenteric ischemia or infarction occurs in less than 1% of patients. Severe hypertension with diastolic pressure as high as 160 mmHg has been encountered in patients with distal dissections. This severe hypertension may be secondary to renal ischemia. Hypotension is an ominous finding and is detected in approximately one-fifth of patients with an ascending aortic dissection. It is suggestive of external rupture or cardiac tamponade.

Other less frequent manifestations of aortic dissection include vocal cord paralysis from compression of the left recurrent laryngeal nerve, compression of the pulmonary arteries by the expanding aorta, and complete heart block from extension of the aortic hematoma into the area of the atrioventricular node. Hemoptysis from rupture into the tracheal bronchial tree and hematemesis from perforation into the esophagus have been reported.

9. What laboratory and radiologic data are helpful in confirming the diagnosis of aortic dissection?

Laboratory data are usually unrevealing. Patients may be anemic due to loss of blood into the false lumen of the dissection. Patients may have moderate leukocytosis with white blood cell counts of 10,000–14,000 white cells/ml. Lactic acid dehydrogenase and bilirubin levels are sometimes elevated because of hemolysis within the false lumen. Disseminated intravascular coagulation has been reported. The electrocardiogram (ECG) may be helpful because it shows no signs of ischemia in a patient with severe chest pain. This scenario should suggest the diagnosis of aortic dissection. As noted above, however, in cases of iatrogenic dissection, ischemia may be a prominent feature. Therefore, the presence of ischemic ECG signs does not rule out dissection.

Radiographic examination of the chest often provides valuable information. In 90% of patients there is an abnormality in the aorta seen on chest x-ray. The most frequent finding is simply widening of the aorta and the mediastinum. The most specific sign on chest x-ray may be separation of calcium that is present in the intima of the aorta from the outer border of the false channel. Normally this distance is no more than 0.5 cm. A distance greater than 1 cm is highly suggestive of aortic dissection—the so-called calcium sign. In cases of iatrogenic dissection, radiographic signs are much less reliable. Visualization of mediastinal widening, abnormal aortic contour, intimal flap, or patent false lumen is roughly half as common in iatrogenic dissection as in spontaneous dissection.

10. What procedures or imaging modalities are useful in confirming the diagnosis of aortic dissection?

The following table reviews the assets and limitations of the major diagnostic tests used in evaluating patients with suspected aortic dissection.

Major Characteristics of Common Tests Used in the Diagnosis of Aortic Dissection

	SENSITIVITY	SPECIFICITY	MAJOR ASSETS	MAJOR LIMITATIONS

Angiography	80–90%	90–95%	Shows entry site
			Shows aortic branches
			Shows dependency of
			  aortic branches
				Time and personnel
				Nephrotoxic agents
				Misses intramural
				  hematoma

Conventional CT	65–85%		Easiness and rapidity	Misses entry site
Ultrafast CT scan	80–100%	95–100%		Partial analysis of aortic branches
MRI	95–100%	95–100%	Precise flow analysis Shows aortic branches No contrast material	Transfer of patient Acquisition time and surveillance High cost

Echocardiography
  (transthoracic and
  transesophageal)
	95–100%	85–90%	Rapidity
			Bedside examination
			Assesses aortic
			  regurgitation
			Assesses pericardial
			  effusion
			Assesses myocardial
			  function
				Misses the distal
				  ascending aorta
				Misses branch
				  involvement
				Misses entry site
				Requires expertise
				Uncomfortable on the
				  awake patient

MRI = magnetic resonance imaging.

Echocardiography (transthoracic and transesophageal) has become an important technique in the diagnosis of aortic dissection. It allows rapid assessment of patients and can be carried out in any location. The diagnosis of aortic dissection is based on the finding of an intimal flap separating a true and false aortic lumen. In 75% of patients with type A dissection, transthoracic echocardiography is diagnostic, whereas this technique identifies 40% of type B dissections.

Echocardiography also allows assessment of valvular function (aortic regurgitation, the presence of pericardial effusion and ventricular function). In most cases an additional diagnostic technique is used to confirm the diagnosis and to localize, if possible, the origins of the dissection.

Transesophageal echocardiography (TEE) is being used with increasing frequency for evaluation of the thoracic aorta and has a sensitivity of 80% and a specificity of up to 96% in demonstrating an intimal flap in dissections of the ascending aorta. However, only 70% of distal dissections are demonstrated by transesophageal echo. Unstable patients can be rapidly evaluated using TEE in the emergency room, critical care unit, or operating room. Additional information can be gained from this technique during the surgical procedure. The competency of the aortic valve can be evaluated during the procedure, and if repair is deemed necessary, the adequacy of that repair can be assessed. In addition, the presence and extent of atherosclerotic disease of the aorta can be evaluated using TEE. For these reasons and because of its portability, TEE is emerging as the most useful diagnostic tool in the evaluation of patients with aortic dissection.

Other imaging techniques include conventional computed tomography (CT), ultrafast CT, magnetic resonance imaging (MRI), and angiography. These techniques all require that the patient be in stable condition and tolerate transfer to the radiology department. CT is frequently used for the diagnosis of thoracic aortic disease. It is noninvasive and is particularly valuable in demonstrating intramural hematoma and penetrating atherosclerotic ulcers of the thoracic aorta. In addition, CT scanning will demonstrate aortic dissection as two channels within the aortic silhouette. The diagnostic accuracy of CT is at best 85%. This technique requires the use of intravenous contrast medium, which is associated with worsening of renal function in some patients. CT scanning is most useful for following patients in whom the diagnosis of aortic dissection has already been made and who are being treated medically. Ultrafast CT scanning is more sensitive and specific in the diagnosis of aortic dissection than is conventional CT.

MRI is highly accurate and specific in evaluating possible aortic dissection. It provides excellent imaging in both type A and B dissections, and can accurately identify the intimal entry point (see figure on following page). MRI also allows examination of the major branches of the aorta without the use of intravenous contrast agents. Additional information that can be obtained using MRI includes evaluation of the aortic valve, pericardium, and the function of the left ventricle. Its utility is limited by the inability of critically ill patients to tolerate the long duration of the procedure.

Angiography is the definitive modality for diagnosing aortic dissection and is usually required for patients undergoing elective operations on the thoracic aorta. Angiography allows determination of the site of dissection, the extent of the dissection, and the integrity of the principal arterial trunks that arise from the aorta. Most of the time, both the true and false arterial channels can be identified. Other clues to the presence of aortic dissection on angiography include a linear lucency, which represents the intima and media of the aorta separating the two channels, distortion of the contrast column, and flow reversal or stasis in the aorta. Insufficiency of the aortic valve can also be demonstrated by angiography.

11. What should be considered in the differential diagnosis of aortic dissection?

The differential diagnosis of acute aortic dissection includes acute myocardial infarction, pulmonary embolism, cerebrovascular accidents, acute aortic regurgitation, thoracic nondissecting aneurysm, mediastinal cysts or tumors, pericarditis, cholecystitis, pleuritis, musculoskeletal pain, and atherosclerotic emboli.

12. How should patients in whom acute aortic dissection is suspected be managed?

The initial management is directed at halting the progression of the dissection. The patient's condition should be stabilized prior to additional studies to confirm the diagnosis. A cardiothoracic surgeon should be consulted immediately. Patients should be admitted to an intensive care unit for monitoring and therapy. The patient's clinical condition and symptoms, as well as blood pressure, cardiac rhythm, and urine output, should be monitored carefully. It may be necessary to

Types B and A aortic dissection. *A,* Type B aortic dissection using a sagittal, spin-echo magnetic resonance image. The dissection begins at the origin of the left subclavian artery. The proximal entry is clearly defined 3 cm distal to the origin and appears as a disruption of the flap (arrow). The distal part of the false lumen appears partially thrombosed (arrowhead). (From Nienaber CA, von Kodolitsch Y, Brockhoff CJ, et al: Comparison of conventional and transesophageal echocardiography with magnetic resonance imaging for anatomical mapping of thoracic aortic dissection: A dual noninvasive imaging study with anatomical and/or angiographic validation. Int J Card Imaging 10:1–14, 1994, with permission.)

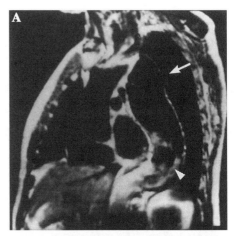

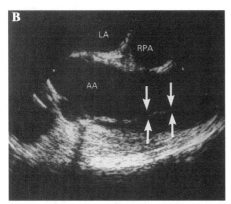

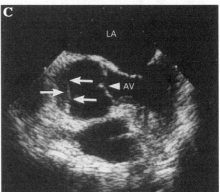

B and *C,* Transesophageal echocardiograms of a type A aortic dissection. This longitudinal-plane image of the ascending aorta (AA) shows the intimal flap (arrows) extending from the aortic root to the distal ascending aorta. In *C,* a transverse-plane image shows the intimal flap (arrows) in the aortic root. LA is left atrium, RPA is the right pulmonary artery, and AV is the aortic valve. (From Kouchoukos NT, Dougenis D: Surgery of the thoracic aorta. N Engl J Med 336:1876–1888, 1997, with permission.)

monitor central venous pressure and/or pulmonary artery pressures and cardiac output. An intraarterial catheter should be placed to monitor blood pressure.

The initial goals of medical therapy are to treat hypertension, decrease the velocity of left ventricular ejection, and treat the patient's pain. Most authorities believe that systolic blood pressure should be lowered to 100–120 mmHg, a mean pressure of 60–65 mmHg, or to the lowest level that is compatible with perfusion of the vital organs. Wheat and associates were the first to describe the successful reduction in the frequency of aortic rupture by aggressively lowering arterial blood pressure. These investigators pointed out the importance of the rate of rise of aortic pressure as the component of stress on the aortic wall that may cause and propagate a dissection.

In addition to management of blood pressure, supportive care should include determining if the patient has myocardial ischemia or infarction, and making sure that sufficient blood is availble in the blood bank in case of rupture of the dissection.

13. What is the role of sodium nitroprusside in management of acute aortic dissection?

Sodium nitroprusside is a potent vasodilator and is recommended as the initial therapy to lower systemic blood pressure in patients with aortic dissection. Nitroprusside alone, however, causes an increase in the velocity of left ventricular ejection and contributes to worsening of the dissection. Therefore, therapy with nitroprusside should be combined with a beta-adrenergic blocking agent. Esmolol, a short-acting intravenous beta blocker that is administered by continuous infusion, is appropriate for control of heart rate and rate of rise of the aortic pressure wave that is a contributing factor in propagation of aortic dissection. Esmolol is administered as a bolus of 500 µg/kg and then started as a continuous infusion of 50–100 µg/kg/min. Repeat bolus doses can be administered as needed to control heart rate, as well as increasing the maintenance dose in 50 µg/kg increments. Propranolol has also been used for aortic dissection. Beta-adrenergic blocking agents may be contraindicated in presence of bradycardia, asthma, and congestive heart failure.

Sodium nitroprusside acts directly on smooth muscles, causing both arterial and venous dilatation. It lowers blood pressure within 1–2 minutes of initiating the infusion, and the effect is terminated within 2 minutes of stopping the drug. The initial dose is 0.25–0.5 µg/kg/min, titrated slowly to control blood pressure. The side effects of this drug include nausea, restlessness, somnolence, and hypotension. The potential for cyanide and/or thiocyanate toxicity exists.

14. Are there alternatives to sodium nitroprusside?

Yes. If nitroprusside is ineffective or poorly tolerated by a patient, then most authorities believe that trimethaphan, a ganglionic blocking agent, should be used. The initial infusion rate is 1 mg/min, and the dose should be titrated to blood pressure. This drug has the advantage of decreasing left ventricular ejection, and beta blockade is not necessary. Complications of this drug include profound hypotension, tachyphylaxis to its effect, somnolence, and sympathoplegia with constipation, urinary retention, ileus, and pupillary dilatation. This drug is usually not effective for more than 48 hours. Other agents that have been used to treat acute aortic dissection include reserpine and calcium channel antagonists.

15. What are the toxic complications of sodium nitroprusside therapy? How are they recognized and treated?

Cyanide and the thiocyanate toxicity. It is recommended that doses no larger than 10 µg/kg/min be administered to patients and that the total dose given not exceed 3–3.5 mg/kg. Cyanide toxicity can be recognized by increasing tolerance to the drug, elevated mixed venous oxygen content, and the development of lactic acidosis. Thiocyanate toxicity is characterized by muscle weakness, hyperreflexia, confusion, delirium, and coma. When the drug is being infused at rates higher than 3 µg/kg for periods exceeding 72 hours, thiocyanate levels should be measured. Thiocyanate levels below 10 mg/100 ml are generally well tolerated. Cyanide poisoning can be treated with amyl nitrite, sodium nitrite, and sodium thiosulfate. For patients with severe thiocyanate toxicity, hemodialysis has been performed.

16. Once the patient has been stabilized medically, what are the options for therapy?

There is now general agreement that patients with a proximal (type A) dissection should be treated surgically, whereas patients with acute distal (type B) dissections may be managed medically. The goals of surgical therapy are to resect the aortic segment containing the proximal intimal tear, to obliterate the false channel, and to restore aortic continuity by using a graft or reapproximating the transected ends of the aorta. In most cases of proximal aortic dissection, cardiopumonary bypass is used. For patients with aortic insufficiency, it may be possible to resuspend the aortic valve, but in some cases, replacement of the aortic valve is necessary. In some cases of proximal dissection, reimplantation of the coronary arteries may be required. The surgical mortality rate for patients with type A dissection is approximately 15–20% in the medical centers with the most experience. Recent studies have reported that the risk of reoperation after type A repair is increased when the initial presentation involves severe aortic insufficiency and that such patients therefore merit an aggressive proximal repair to reduce the rate of this complication. Other recent discussion has raised the issue that elderly patients have higher morbidity and mortality rates and poorer quality of life after type A repair than younger patients. Whether aggressive therapy is justified in elderly patients remains controversial.

Recently an endovascular technique was developed for treating the subset of type A dissections with intimal tear in the descending thoracic aorta and extension of the dissection back into the ascending aorta. Traditional surgical repair of such lesions is especially difficult and carries a poor prognosis. The new technique involves endovascular placement of a stent-graft via the femoral artery, which then closes the intimal tear and allows the false lumen to thrombose. A recent trial reported a 100% success rate in achieving this result with no procedure-related complications.

Definitive therapy for type B dissection is usually medical. Wheat and colleagues in 1965 described a series of patients with distal dissections who were successfully treated medically. Surgery is indicated if medical therapy is failing. This includes evidence of continued dissection, rupture, ischemia of an organ or extremity due to the dissection, and pain that is not relieved with medical therapy. It is believed that patients with distal dissection do better with medical therapy than with surgical therapy because they tend to be older, have extensive atherosclerotic vascular disease, and have complicating medical conditions including cardiac and pulmonary disease. Most patients with distal dissection can be managed medically; however, one-third of patients will eventually require surgery for an enlarging aneurysm and/or dissection. Patients with distal dissection are treated chronically with beta blockers and other standard antihypertensive medications. They should be followed closely for progression of their dissection, with frequent visits to their physician and noninvasive assessment of the extent of the dissection.

BIBLIOGRAPHY

1. Bavaria JE, et al: New paradigms and improved results for the surgical treatment of acute type A dissection. Ann Surg 234:336–343, 2001.
2. Chaudhry A, Romereo L, Pugatch RD, et al: Diagnosis of aortic dissection by computed tomography. Ann Thorac Surg 35:322–325, 1983.
3. DeSanctis RW, Doroghazi RM, Austen WG, Buckley MJ: Aortic dissection. N Engl J Med 317: 1060–1067, 1987.
4. Doroghazi RM, Slater EE, DeSanctis RW, et al: Long-term survival of patients with treated aortic dissection. J Am Coll Cardiol 3:1026–1034, 1984.
5. Eagle KA, Quetermous T, Kritzer GA, et al: Spectrum of conditions initially suggesting acute aortic dissection but with negative aortograms. Am J Cardiol 57:322–326, 1986.
6. Erbel R, Zamorano J: The aorta: Aortic aneurysm, trauma and dissection. Crit Care Clin 12:733–766, 1996.
7. Granato JE, Dee P, Gibson R: Utility of two-dimensional echocardiography in suspected ascending aortic dissection. Am J Cardiol 56:123–129, 1985.
8. Januzzi J, et al: Iatrogenic aotic dissection. Am J Cardiol 89:623–626, 2002.
9. Kato N, et al: Transluminal placement of endovascular stent-grafts for the treatment of type A aortic dissection with entry tear in the descending thoracic aorta. J Vasc Surg 34:1023–1028, 2001.
10. Kirsch M, Soustelle C, Houël R, et al: Risk factor analysis for proximal and distal reoperations after surgery for acute type A aortic dissection. J Thorac Cardiovasc Surg 123:318–325, 2002.
11. Kouchoukos NT, Dougenis D: Surgery of the thoracic aorta. N Engl J Med 336:1876–1888, 1997.
12. Larson EW, Edwards WD: Risk factors for aortic dissection: A necropsy study of 161 cases. Am J Cardiol 53:849–855, 1984.
13. Neri E, et al: Operation for acute type A aortic dissection in octogenarians: Is it justified? J Thorac Cardiovasc Surg 121:259–267, 2001.
14. Pretre R, Von Segresser LK: Aortic dissection. Lancet 349:1461–1464, 1997.
15. Pumphrey CW, Fay T, Weir I: Aortic dissection during pregnancy. Br Heart J 55:106–108, 1986.
16. Roberts WC: Aortic dissection: Anatomy, consequences, and causes. Am Heart J 101:195–214, 1981.
17. Slater EE, DeSanctis RW: The clinical recognition of dissecting aortic aneurysm. Am J Med 60:625–633, 1976.
18. Sumiyoshi M, et al: Circadian, weekly, and seasonal variation at the onset of acute aortic dissection. Am J Cardiol 89:619–623, 2002.
19. Tinker JH, Michenfelder JD: Sodium nitroprusside: Pharmacology, toxicology and therapeutics. Anesthesiology 45:340–354, 1976.
20. Wheat MW, Palmer RF, Bartley TD, Seelman RC: Treatment of dissecting aneurysms of the aorta without surgery. J Thorac Cardiovasc Surg 50:364–373, 1965.

30. VALVULAR HEART DISEASE

Timothy R. White, Ph.D., M.D., and David E. Schwartz, M.D., F.C.C.P.

MITRAL REGURGITATION

1. Describe the mitral valve apparatus.

The mitral valve apparatus consists of an annulus, an anterior and posterior leaflet, multiple chordae tendineae, and two papillary muscles as well as portions of the left ventricular wall. The anterior leaflet is more mobile than the posterior leaflet and accounts for roughly two-thirds of the valve area but attaches along only one-third of the annular circumference. The relatively immobile posterior leaflet fills the the remaining third of the area and attaches along the remaining two-thirds of the annulus.

2. What are the causes of mitral regurgitation?

Abnormalities in any of the above structures may result in an incompetent mitral valve, and the presentation may be acute or chronic. Acute cases are typically traumatic (e.g, rupture of chordae or papillary muscle, fenestration of a valve leaflet due to to acute endocarditis or blunt trauma to the heart). Papillary muscles may rupture after severe myocardial infarction. More chronic dysfunction arises from conditions such as rheumatic heart fever, myxomatous degeneration, chronic ischemia of papillary muscles, or left ventricular enlargement with dilatation of the annulus.

3. Describe the pathophysiology of mitral regurgitation.

The incompetent mitral valve provides a low-pressure path for emptying of the left ventricle during systole. There are three immediate physiologic consequences: (1) less emptying of left ventricular flows through the aortic valve as cardiac output to the systemic circulation; (2) backward flow into the left atrium, which results in pressure and volume load on the atrium and pulmonary circulation; and (3) return of the regurgitated volume to the left ventricle during the next diastole, which leads to volume overload of the ventricle. The volume overload of the atrium and ventricle leads to ventricular dilatation, which can worsen mitral regurgitation.

4. How does acute mitral regurgitation present?

With mitral regurgitation of acute onset, the pathophysiology described in question 3 is poorly tolerated. The normal left atrium is ill prepared for the large volume load and high pressures, remaining small and noncompliant. The regurgitant volume, therefore, is imposed on the pulmonary circulation, resulting in pulmonary venous congestion and hypertension. The large volume load on the left ventricle results in stretching of the myocardium to near maximum. Contractility is increased by the Frank-Starling mechanism, whereas end-systolic pressure is decreased because of the low-pressure path through the incompetent mitral valve. Left ventricular volume, therefore, increases, but since a large fraction is sent back into the atrium, forward stroke volume is diminished. While the myocardium is functioning normally, the presentation consists of left-sided congestive failure with decreased cardiac output and pulmonary congestion.

5. Describe the natural history of chronic mitral regurgitation.

Mitral regurgitation of chronic onset is typically well tolerated for variable lengths of time; patients with mild cases may remain symptom-free for their entire lives. The heart is able to compensate for a gradually evolving volume load on the atrium and ventricle. The left atrium enlarges to accommodate a large volume at low filling pressures, thereby protecting the pulmonary circulation from congestion. Meanwhile, the cardiomyocytes of the left ventricle lengthen by adding sarcomeres in series, allowing the ventricle to increase stroke volume as compensation for

153

the regurgitated fraction. The forward stroke volume is preserved while the ventricular volume has enlarged at relatively normal filling pressure.

With severe disease, the left ventricle ultimately begins to fail with loss of intrinsic muscular function. The ventricle dilates further, forward stroke volume decreases, and regurgitant volume increases with increasing atrial and pulmonary pressures. The symptoms of left-sided congestive failure then ensue.

6. What causes the decompensation in chronic mitral regurgitation?

The ventricle hypertrophies eccentrically in chronic volume overload, whereas in chronic pressure overload the hypertrophy is concentric. Unlike concentric hypertrophy, eccentric hypertrophy is not associated with an increase in protein synthesis. Some research suggests a decrease in the myosin content of the myocardium, and other research suggests a decrease in the production of cyclic adenosine monophosphate. The mass-to-volume ratio of the volume-overloaded heart decreases, resulting in a relatively thinner ventricular wall and subsequent increase in wall stress. With the increase in stroke work demanded by the greatly increased stroke volume, the work performed per gram of myocardium also increases, despite the low-pressure unloading through the regurgitant valve. In dogs with decompensated regurgitation, beta blockers have been shown to return ventricular and cellular function to near-normal levels, suggesting that adrenergic overstimulation may be a mechanism for left ventricular failure in chronic mitral regurgitation.

7. Which studies are helpful in the diagnosis of mitral regurgitation?

The **electrocardiogram** (ECG) shows left atrial enlargement. One-third of patients also have evidence of left ventricular enlargement. Atrial fibrillation is occasionally present. Chest x-ray findings include enlargement of left atrium and ventricle along with pulmonary congestion.

Echocardiography can help to diagnose both presence and cause of mitral regurgitation and to quantify the degree of regurgitaiton. Typical findings include a dilated left atrium and a dilated, hyperdynamic left ventricle. Evidence of disrupted valve leaflets, chordae, or papillary muscles; valvular prolapse; or valvular vegetation leads to immediate diagnosis of the underlying cause. Doppler echocardiography can quantitate the amount of regurgitation by several methods, including visual examination, jet mapping, proximal isovelocity surface area, vena contracta, and quantitative echocardiographic Doppler. Transesophageal echocardiography should be performed before surgery to assess the feasibility of valve repair.

Cardiac catheterization is rarely necessary for diagnosis or quantification. However, if other modalities are discordant, it may provide useful information. Left ventriculography allows visualization of regurgitant flow rather than simply flow velocity and may help to define the problem. Likewise, once surgery is planned, arteriography is indicated to establish the degree of concomitant coronary artery disease.

Severe mitral regurgitation is suggested by findings of mitral regurgitant orifice area greater than 0.3 cm², regurgitant fraction greater than 50%, or V wave on pulmonary artery catheter that is 2–3 times the mean wedge pressure. No method of quantification, however, has been shown to predict outcome.

8. How should patients with mitral regurgitation be managed in the intensive care unit?

Most patients who present to the intensive care unit have acute mitral regurgitation and pulmonary edema. The goals of care are hemodynamic stabilization and identification of the cause of mitral regurgitation. The mainstays of treatment are diuretics to reduce right-sided filling pressures and pulmonary congestion and vasodilators to reduce afterload and promote forward emptying of the left ventricle, thereby reducing the regurgitant fraction. The resultant decrease in left ventricular size may further reduce regurgitation by relieving strain on the mitral valve annulus. Nitroprusside is the vasodilator of choice, starting at a dose of 3–6 μg/kg/min and increasing the dose until symptoms are relieved or systolic pressure drops below 100 mmHg. Toxicity from nitroprusside is unusual during the first 24 hours of therapy. If patients are hypotensive with acute mitral regurgitation, they may benefit from inotropic agents such as dopamine or dobutamine. However, because of its alpha agonist activity, dopamine may elevate systemic vascular resistance and worsen the regurgitant fraction. In patients with refractory hypotension, early use of aortic balloon counterpulsation reduces afterload and increases the forward ejection fraction. The increase in coronary perfusion with the balloon pump may help to reduce regurgitation due to papillary muscle ischemia. If patients remain in cardiogenic shock, emergency catheterization and valve replacement must be performed.

9. What are the surgical options for patients with mitral insufficiency?

Mitral regurgitation is ultimately a mechanical problem and requires a surgical solution. Surgical options include valve repair and valve replacement with or without preservation of the chordae. Preservation of as much of the native apparatus as possible is critical to left ventricular function; ablation results in a immediate and irreversible decrease of roughly 25% in left ventricular function. Although the cause is unclear, presumably the mitral valve apparatus helps to optimize ventricular shape and/or coordination. Clearly valve repair is the preferred option whenever feasible because it preserves the native apparatus and avoids the issue of anticoagulation. Repair also carries a lower operative mortality rate than replacement (2–4% vs. 5–10%).

MITRAL STENOSIS

10. What are the causes of mitral stenosis?

Rheumatic heart disease is by far the most common cause in adults. Congenital forms of mitral stenosis occur in infants and children. Infrequently mitral stenosis is a complication of systemic lupus erythematosus, rheumatoid arthritis, and malignant carcinoid.

11. Describe the natural history of mitral stenosis.

Mitral stenosis is the sole valvular lesion in approximately 25% of patients with rheumatic heart disease, whereas an additional 40% have combined mitral stenosis and mitral regurgitation. Mitral stenosis and aortic regurgitation may also occur together. Women are affected twice as frequently as men. The latency period between the initial episode of rheumatic fever and the development of symptomatic valvular heart disease ranges from three to four decades.

12. How is mitral stenosis graded?

The normal mitral valve area is approximately 4–6 cm^2. When the valve area decreases to approximately 2 cm^2, mild mitral stenosis exists and an abnormal pressure gradient is generated between the left atrium and left ventricle. Mitral stenosis is considered critical when the valve area is less than 1 cm^2. Critical mitral stenosis usually is associated with a gradient of approximately 20 mmHg between left atrial pressure and left ventricular diastolic pressure. Such high hydraulic pressures in the pulmonary vasculature overcome the negative oncotic pressure that normally prevents pulmonary edema.

13. Describe the pathophysiologic abnormalities associated with mitral stenosis.

As valve area decreases, a larger pressure gradient between the left atrium and the left ventricle is needed to generate flow, resulting in substantial elevations in left atrial pressure. This elevated pressure in turn raises pulmonary venous and capillary pressures. As pulmonary capillary pressure exceeds plasma oncotic pressure, fluid is filtered into the interstitium. As the pressure continues to rise, the pulmonary lymphatic system can no longer pump out the fluid, which begins to fill the lung interstitium and alveoli. Pulmonary arteriolar resistance increases and impedes right ventricular ejection. The right ventricle hypertrophies to accommodate the increased load. Eventually the ventricle dilates and fails. As left atrial pressure rises, the left atrium also dilates and becomes substantially enlarged, predisposing to the development of atrial fibrillation and the loss of effective atrial contraction. In most patients left ventricular diastolic pressure and volume are normal.

14. Why do patients with mitral stenosis tolerate tachycardia poorly?

As heart rate increases, diastole shortens more than systole. This decreases the time available for flow across a stenotic mitral valve and results in underfilling of the left ventricle. In addition, patients with mitral stenosis do not tolerate atrial fibrillation. When atrial contraction is lost, cardiac output may be decreased by 20%. Thus, it is desirable to maintain both sinus rhythm and a slow heart rate.

15. What are the signs and symptoms of mitral stenosis?

Most patients report dyspnea and progressive limitations of physical exertion. Orthopnea, paroxysmal nocturnal dyspnea, fatigue, weakness, and hemoptysis are also common. As mitral stenosis advances, symptoms of right heart failure occur, including nausea, anorexia, right upper quadrant pain, ascites, and peripheral edema. Hoarseness has also been described (Ortner's syndrome), and is thought to be due to compression of the left recurrent laryngeal nerve by a dilated left atrium or an enlarged pulmonary artery. Chest pain may occur in 10–20% of patients with mitral stenosis and may be difficult to distinguish from classic angina pectoris. Thromboembolism is a serious complication of mitral stenosis and, before the development of surgical therapy, occurred in 20% of patients. Risk factors for embolization include age over 40 years, low cardiac output, and atrial fibrillation. Anticoagulation should be considered in these patients.

16. Describe the typical physical examination of a patient with mitral stenosis.

Patients characteristically have ruddy cheeks, a normal or reduced left ventricular impulse, and often a right ventricular heave. A prominent S_1 is heard, as is a loud P_2, signifying pulmonary hypertension. An opening snap after S_2 is a classic finding. The murmur of mitral stenosis, typically a low-pitched diastolic rumble that begins with the opening snap of the mitral valve, is best heard at the apex with the bell of the stethoscope and the patient in the left lateral decubitus position.

17. How is the diagnosis of mitral stenosis established?

Electrocardiographic evidence includes left atrial enlargement (P mitrale), right-axis deviation, and right ventricular hypertrophy. Atrial fibrillation also may be seen. A chest x-ray may show signs of left atrial enlargement, such as an elevated left mainstem bronchus, double cardiac density, and prominent left heart border. Evidence of increased lung water also may be seen on chest x-ray (e.g., pulmonary vascular redistribution, interstitial edema, Kerley B lines). Signs of pulmonary hypertension may be present.

Echocardiography is the diagnostic method of choice. Two-dimensional (2-D) echocardiography is more useful than M-mode because the assessment of the anatomic orifice is not influenced by the presence of mitral regurgitation, cardiac output, and other factors that affect catheterization-determined valve areas. Physical findings on 2-D echocardiography include doming of the mitral valve leaflets and restriction of their motion. Thickening of the mitral valve is also frequently seen. An enlarged left atrium is expected. The valve orifice can often be imaged and measured directly. The extent of calcification and pliability can also be assessed by 2-D echocardiography, which may allow selection of appropriate patients for mitral valvulotomy. Echocardiography allows assessent of the other cardiac valves for abnormalities. Doppler echocardiography is also useful in assessing the severity of mitral stenosis. Cardiac catheterization is not required for the diagnosis of mitral stenosis but may be performed to evaluate the extent of coronary artery disease either in patients who have symptoms suggestive of angina or in elderly patients.

18. How should patients with mitral stenosis be managed?

Patients who are asymptomatic or minimally symptomatic can be managed medically. Medical management should be directed at prophylaxis against endocarditis, management of atrial fibrillation, prophylaxis against systemic embolization, and treatment of right heart failure, if present. In patients with an abnormal mitral valve, prophylaxis with antibiotics prior to dental or surgical procedures is mandatory. Atrial fibrillation with rapid ventricular response is poorly tolerated by patients with mitral stenosis and should be treated aggressively with agents to decrease ventricular response. Digoxin is the drug of choice, but it is much less effective when patients exercise. The combination of digoxin and a beta-adrenergic blocking agent is effective in controlling ventricular rate when digoxin alone fails. Beta blockers should not be used alone, however, as they may reduce exercise capacity. Calcium channel blockers such as verapamil and diltiazem have also been used to control ventricular response in atrial fibrillation. Problems exist with verapamil, both because of its negative inotropic effect and because it can decrease renal clearance of digoxin, which may lead to elevated serum digoxin concentrations and digoxin toxicity. Diltiazem may be a better choice when combined with digoxin to control ventricular response in atrial fibrillation because diltizem does not alter digoxin clearance. Combination therapy with diltiazem and digoxin has been shown to adequately control ventricular response at rest and with exercise in patients with atrial fibrillation.

Pharmacologic or electrical cardioversion to restore sinus rhythm is desirable if at all possible. Frequently cardioversion involves the administration of quinidine or a similar antiarrhythmic agent. Patients should be anticoagulated for 2–3 weeks before the attempt at cardioversion. Patients who remain in atrial fibrillation, have heart failure, or have previously experienced embolic phenomena should be maintained on oral anticoagulation with warfarin unless it is contraindicated.

Diuretic therapy and digoxin may help to relieve the symptoms of right heart failure. However, when patients become more symptomatic, surgical therapy should be considered. Once symptoms are severe, patients have a rapid downhill course. Options include catheter balloon valvuloplasty, mitral commissurotomy (either open or closed), and mitral valve replacement.

19. How is a balloon mitral valvuloplasty performed?

This technique presents an alternative to the surgical treatment of mitral stenosis. The procedure is performed by advancing a small balloon flotation catheter across the intraatrial septum and then through the stenotic mitral valve. The balloon is then inflated for short periods to enlarge the mitral valve area. The mechanisms responsible for improvement in valvular function are thought to include fracture of calcium deposits and commissural separation. This procedure can be done with a single- or double-balloon technique.

20. What are the surgical options for patients with mitral stenosis?

Surgical therapy consists of open commissurotomy or mitral valve replacement. Closed commissurotomy is rarely performed in the United States. Indications for mitral valve replacement or commissurotomy include symptomatic heart failure that is New York Heart Association Class II or higher, pulmonary hypertension, or a mitral valve area less than 1 cm². In addition, patients who have had systemic embolization from the stenotic mitral valve should undergo valve replacement even though they are without other significant symptoms.

AORTIC INSUFFICIENCY

21. What causes aortic insufficiency?

Processes that involve either the aortic valve leaflets or the aortic root may cause aortic insufficiency. A common condition affecting the leaflets is rheumatic fever, in which fusion of the commissures restricts valve motion, resulting in both insufficiency and stenosis. Other conditions that may affect the leaflets include infective endocarditis, connective tissue diseases such as Marfan's syndrome and Ehlers-Danlos syndrome, and myxomatous degeneration. The most common condition affecting the aortic root is annulocysticectasia, which is dilation due to systemic hypertension and aging. Other causes include cystic medionecrosis, syphilis, ankylosing spondylitis, and connective tissue orders. Trauma or aortic dissection also may disrupt the aortic root. Aortic insufficiency may present acutely or chronically.

22. Describe the pathophysiology of aortic insufficiency.

As in mitral regurgitation, the fundamental abnormality of aortic insufficiency is volume overload of the left ventricle. During diastole some fraction of the ejected volume in the aortic root flows back into the relaxing ventricle through the incompetent aortic valve. Desite this superficial similarity, the loading conditions of the ventricle and the physiologic responses are quite different in the two lesions. Unlike mitral regurgitation, in which the ventricle unloads its enlarged stroke volume into the low-pressure atrium, in aortic insufficiency the entire stroke volume is ejected against the high systemic pressure. Thus, the left ventricle faces both volume and pressure overload, resulting in a combination of concentric and eccentric hypertrophy. The mass-to-volume ratio remains normal, whereas it is is decreased in mitral regurgitation. The average systolic pressure and wall thickness are also greater in aortic insufficiency. Modest decreases in ejection in aortic insufficiency may be due to increased afterload rather than ventricular decompensation.

23. What are the signs and symptoms of chronic aortic insufficiency?

Patients with chronic aortic insufficiency may be asymptomatic for many years and may not have many physical findings consistent with aortic insufficiency. Pulse pressure is widened because of elevated systolic pressures and a relatively low diastolic pressure. This discrepancy is created by the rapid runoff of blood from the aorta back into the left ventricle. Diastolic pressures may be recorded close to 0 mmHg. Carotid pulses are bounding and may have a bisferious quality with a double systolic impulse. Other physical findings include:

- Corrigan's pulse, which is described as rapid upstroke and collapse of the pulse in peripheral arteries.
- De Musset's sign, which is head bobbing with each heartbeat.
- Duroziez's sign, which is the diastolic murmur auscultated when the stethoscope compresses the femoral artery.
- Quincke's pulse, which refers to the visible pulsation in the capillaries of the nail bed.

Chronic aortic regurgitation is associated with inferior and lateral displacement of the left ventricular impulse. S_1 and A_2 may be diminished. S_3 and S_4 gallops are frequently heard. The hallmark of aortic insufficiency is a high-pitched, blowing, diastolic murmur heard at the right upper sternal border, the left sternal border, and the cardiac apex. This murmur is best heard with the patient sitting up and leaning forward. A mid-diastolic rumble is frequently heard at the cardiac apex, simulating mitral stenosis. This Austin Flint murmur is due to turbulent flow across the mitral valve, which is partially closed by the regurgitant jet from the incompetent aortic valve.

24. What are the signs and symptoms of acute aortic insufficiency?

The presentation differs markedly in acute and chronic aortic insufficiency. In the acute condition, the left ventricle does not have time to accommodate the large regurgitant volume. Systemic cardiac output decreases, because the ventricle is unable to increase stroke volume sufficiently to overcome the regurgitant fraction. A sudden increase in left ventricular end-diastolic volume is accompanied by an increase in end-diastolic pressure in the noncompliant ventricle, which in turn leads to elevated left atrial presssures. The results are symptoms of decompensated left-sided heart failure, such as exertional dyspnea, orthopnea, paroxysmal nocturnal dyspnea, and fatigue. Tachycardia and intense peripheral vasoconstriction are present. Angina is an occasional complaint due to reduced diastolic pressures.

25. Which diagnostic studies are useful in aortic insufficiency?

In chronic aortic insufficiency, ECG shows left ventricular hypertrophy and atrial enlargement. Chest x-ray shows a massively enlarged heart (cor bovinum) and possibly a widened aortic root. Signs of pulmonary congestion may be present. The echocardiogram provides the greatest amount of information. Degree of insufficiency can be quantified by various methods, including size of the regurgitant jet, regurgitant orifice size, quantitative Doppler echocardiography, and Doppler pressure half-time estimation.

26. How should patients with acute, severe aortic insufficiency be managed in the intensive care unit?

Acute, severe aortic insufficiency is a surgical disease. Medically managed patients may have a mortality rate as high as 75%, whereas mortality is reduced to 25% with surgery. In preparation for surgery, the patient must be stabilized medically, although this goal may be difficult to achieve. Vasodilators may help to reduce afterload and promote forward flow, but they also may worsen hypotension, resulting in increased cardiac ischemia and dysfunction. Pressors to treat hypotension result in increased afterload and worsened regurgitation. Aortic balloon counterpulsation is contraindicated because it, too, worsens regurgitation. General supportive measures include supplemental oxygen as well as diuretics, nitrates, and morphine sulfate to reduce pulmonary congestion. Mechanical ventilation may be required to maintain adequate oxygenation. Invasive monitoring of systemic and pulmonary artery pressures may be indicated. Judicious use of nitroprusside may be attempted to reduce afterload and promote forward flow. Ventricular performance may need to be supported. Dobutamine, which is devoid of intrinsic alpha-adrenergic agonist activity, may be useful. An infusion can be started at 3–5 μg/kg/minute and titrated to improve cardiac output. The side effect of tachycardia may be helpful in patients with aortic insufficiency because the decrease in diastole may further reduce the regurgitant volume per beat. In patients with severe pulmonary edema and hypoxemia, vasodilators such as nitroprusside can worsen hypoxemia by overcoming hypoxic pulmonary vasoconstriction. This scenario may require the administration of higher oxygen concentrations and/or the use of higher levels of end-expiratory pressures.

In the intensive care unit, the cause of aortic insufficiency should be diagnosed. For patients with infective endocarditis, appropriate antibiotic therapy should be instituted as soon as possible. For patients with aortic insufficiency due to dissection, surgical therapy is indicated as quickly as possible. Patients with aortic dissection should have blood pressure controlled and should receive therapy to decrease the shear force in the ascending aorta (left ventricular dp/dt). Management is aimed at preparing patients for surgical valve replacement, which is the mainstay of therapy for acute aortic insufficiency.

AORTIC STENOSIS

27. What causes aortic stenosis?

Aortic stenosis may be the result of a congenitally abnormal aortic valve. Unicuspid valves usually produce severe obstruction in infancy. More common is the congenitally bicuspid valve. Premature calcification of a bicuspid valve is the single most common cause of isolated aortic stenosis in the Western world, accounting for approximately 50% of cases. The abnormal architecture of the valve induces turbulent flow, which causes trauma to the leaflets and ultimately leads to fibrosis and calcification of the leaflets. Patients usually become symptomatic in the fourth or fifth decade of life. Congenitally malformed valves can also be tricuspid, with the cusps of unequal size. There may be commissural fusion. Abnormal flow characteristics through these valves may predispose to premature calcification. Rheumatic heart disease accounts for 30% of cases of aortic stenosis. Most patients with rheumatic aortic stenosis have associated mitral valve disease. Rheumatic disease is an unlikely cause of isolated aortic stenosis.

Degenerative disease of the relatively normal aortic valve also may lead to stenosis. Aortic sclerosis, defined as calcific changes and thickening without aortic obstruction, occurs in about 25% of adults over 65 years of age. Lipocalcific changes increasing valve leaflet stiffness are seen in 2–9% of elderly adults. With senile-calcific aortic stenosis, calcium accumulates in the pockets of the aortic cusps, which leads to eventual fibrosis and commissural fusion. Symptoms usually do not occur until the ages of 60–70 years. Obstruction to outflow of the left ventricle also can be caused by hypertrophic obstructive cardiomyopathy and supravalvular or subvalvular stenosis. Discussion of these subjects is beyond the scope of this chapter. Risk factors associated with aortic stenosis include male gender, increasing age, shorter stature, increased serum levels of low-density lipoprotein and lipoprotein (a), hypertension, and current smoking. It is unclear whether modifying any of the last three factors affects disease progression. There is also an association between gastrointestinal bleeding and aortic stenosis.

28. When is aortic stenosis considered critical?

Normal aortic valve area is 2.6–3.5 cm^2. Obstruction to outflow of the left ventricle is considered critical when the aortic valve area is either less than 0.75 cm^2 in the average-sized adult or approximately 0.4 cm^2/m^2 body surface area. This value corresponds to a peak systolic pressure gradient between the aorta and left ventricle of 50 mmHg in the presence of normal cardiac output.

29. How is valve area calculated?

In evaluating a patient with a stenotic valve in either the aortic or mitral position, calculation of valve area is based on a measurement of the pressure gradient and the flow across the valve. These formulas are called the Gorlin equations.

$$\text{Aortic valve area (cm}^2) = \frac{F}{44.3\sqrt{\Delta P}}$$

$$\text{Mitral valve area (cm}^2) = \frac{F}{37.7\sqrt{\Delta P}}$$

In these formulas, flow (F) is equal to flow across the valve in milliliters/second, and change in pressure (ΔP) is equal to the mean pressure gradient in mmHg across the orifice. The constants 44.3 and 37.7 relate to turbulence of flow across the valves and differ between the aortic and mitral valves. Flow is derived by the equation:

$$\text{Flow (F) (ml/sec)} = \frac{\text{Cardiac output (ml/min)}}{\text{DFP (sec/min) or SEP (sec/min)}}$$

For the mitral valve, diastolic filling period (DFP) is derived by measuring the time from mitral valve opening to closure per beat and multiplying by the heart rate. For the aortic valve, systolic ejection period (SEP) is equal to the systolic ejection time (aortic valve opening to closure) multiplied by the heart rate.

It is apparent from these formulas that calculation of valve area depends on flow rates and that with low flows, these estimates may be in error. If regurgitation coexists with stenosis of a valve, valve area calculations will be falsely lowered because the actual flow across a valve per beat is greater than that calculated using the systemic cardiac output.

30. Describe the pathophysiology of aortic stenosis.

Obstruction to aortic outflow at the aortic valve results in a pressure gradient developing from the left ventricle to the aorta. The left ventricle compensates by developing concentric hypertrophy. The consequences of left ventricular hypertrophy include reduced diastolic compliance, a rise in left ventricular end-diastolic pressure, and an increase in myocardial oxygen consumption. This increase in oxygen consumption is related mainly to increased left ventricular wall tension. Potential imbalances in myocardial oxygen demand-supply relationships can result because of compromised subendocardial coronary blood flow related to high subendocardial intramural pressure. This explains why patients may develop signs of coronary ischemia without having concomitant coronary artery disease.

As left ventricular hypertrophy increases and ventricular compliance falls, there is an increase in left ventricular pressure. With time this increase leads to elevations of left atrial pressure and pulmonary venous and capillary pressures, which in turn may lead to transudation of fluid into the lungs with resulting dyspnea and other signs of congestive heart failure. In addition, because of the decrease in left ventricular compliance, patients with aortic stenosis are dependent on organized atrial contraction for ventricular filling. Patients with aortic stenosis poorly tolerate atrial fibrillation with the loss of "atrial kick." Also, because cardiac outflow through a stenotic valve is limited, patients with aortic stenosis do not tolerate reductions in afterload.

31. What are the signs and symptoms of aortic stenosis?

The most common sign of aortic stenosis is a systolic murmur, characteristically a crescendo-descrescendo murmur maximal at the second right intercostal space. This murmur is often well transmitted along the cardiac vessels to the neck and to the apex of the heart. In mild disease, the peak occurs early in systole, but as the stenosis worsens, the murmur peaks later and may soften with decreasing cardiac output. On physical examination, a patient with significant aortic stenosis has a delayed carotid upstroke with a prominent anacrotic notch. With left ventricular failure the cardiac impulse is displaced inferiorly and laterally and is sustained. Auscultation usually reveals a normal S_1 and a single S_2 because of calcification of the aortic valve. An S_4 gallop is also frequently heard.

The traditional triad of symptoms in patients with aortic stenosis includes angina, syncope, and heart failure. Congestive heart failure may occur in 60% of patients, angina in 50%, and syncope in 40%. Cardiac catheterization reveals coexisting coronary artery disease in 60% of patients with aortic stenosis. However, patients with angina may or may not have significant coronary stenosis. Once angina develops, life expectancy is approximately 5 years. Syncope is frequently exertional and may result from peripheral vasodilatation with exertion. Because of the relatively fixed cardiac output in patients with aortic stenosis, compensation for this vasodilation is ineffective. Once syncope develops, survival is approximately 3 years. With the onset of left ventricular failure, survival averages 2 years. In view of the ominous natural history of severe aortic stenosis, symptomatic patients with valve area < 0.7 cm^2 are generally referred for immediate aortic valve replacement.

32. Which studies aid in the diagnosis of aortic stenosis?

With significant aortic stenosis, the cardiac silhouette on **chest x-ray** is enlarged because of a prominent left ventricle. A dilated ascending aorta, due to poststenotic dilatation, also may be seen. With left ventricular failure, pulmonary venous congestion and pulmonary edema can be seen.

ECG evidence of aortic stenosis includes left ventricular hypertrophy, left atrial enlargement, left-axis deviation, and conduction defects. With severe aortic stenosis atrial fibrillation can occur.

Echocardiography using both the two-dimensional mode and Doppler techniques is helpful in diagnosis and management. With two-dimensional echocardiography, doming of the leaflets occurs with valvular aortic stenosis. The valve also may be heavily calcified and immobile. Doppler echocardiography can be used to measure the peak and mean transvalvular gradients, the latter of which corresponds well to the information obtained at cardiac catheterization.

Transesophageal echocardiography (TEE) may be useful in some circumstances in the assessment of aortic stenosis. The improved visualization of the aortic valve afforded by the esophageal window allows improved assessment of the stenotic orifice. In measurement of the aortic valve area, it is important to obtain true short-axis views of the aortic leaflets.

Cardiac catheterization allows calculation of valve area and visualization of coronary arteries.

33. How should patients with aortic stenosis be managed medically?

Patients should have prophylaxis for endocarditis with dental and surgical procedures. They should be counseled to report the symptoms of syncope, heart failure, and angina quickly to their physician. Although atrial arrhythmias occur in less than 10% of patients with isolated aortic stenosis, patients with frequent atrial premature contraction should receive agents to maintain a normal sinus rhythm. If atrial fibrillation does occur, patients may experience significant symptoms, including congestive heart failure, angina, and significant hypotension. These symptoms may necessitate emergency electrical cardioversion. Medications should then be administered to preserve normal sinus rhythm.

The timing of surgery for patients with aortic stenosis is currently based on presence of symptoms. Patients may be asymptomatic for many years. However, once symptoms develop, life expectancy is shortened unless surgical intervention is performed. If the operative procedure is carried out in patients with left ventricular failure or a depressed ejection fraction, the operative mortality rate is 10–25%, which is nearly 5 times higher than in patients with normal ventricular function. Therefore, close monitoring for the onset of ventricular decompensation is essential.

Currently, aortic replacement is not recommended in asymptomatic patients because of the known risks of surgery and the lack of data supporting improved outcome. However, it is reasonable to replace a moderately or severely stenotic valve in an otherwise asymptomatic patient at the time of coronary artery bypass surgery.

34. Is percutaneous balloon valvuloplasty an alternative to surgical therapy in patients with critical aortic stenosis?

Aortic balloon valvuloplasty has had less success in patients with aortic stenosis than in patients with mitral stenosis. In patients with critical aortic stenosis, percutaneous balloon valvuloplasty results in an increase in valve area and a reduction in the gradient across the aortic valve. Patients show an improvement in functional classification. However, restenosis is common, and valve area increases on the average by only 50%. The final valve area after balloon valvuloplasty averages from 0.9 to 1.0 cm^2 in most series. Most authorities recommend balloon valvuloplasty of the aortic valve only in specific patients, including those who are inoperable because of extremely high surgical risk and those who decline valve replacement. In most other patients, aortic valve replacement remains the standard of therapy. The operative mortality rate for aortic valve replacement in most centers ranges from 2% to 8%. Risk factors include impairment of left ventricular function, advanced age, and presence of other valvular lesions. After successful valve replacement, symptoms and hemodynamics are improved. Ventricular performance may return to normal in most patients after successful aortic replacement for aortic stenosis. There also may be regression of left ventricular mass. In patients with aortic stenosis and coronary artery disease, valve replacement and myocardial revascularization should be performed at the same time.

During the surgical procedure, the calcified aortic valve must be removed carefully because of the risk of embolization. Some evidence indicates that the consequences of systemic embolization can be lessened by anesthetic techniques that include high doses of sodium thiopental.

35. What types of valves are available for replacement?

Two types of prosthetic valves are available for replacement in both the mitral and the aortic position: mechanical prostheses and bioprostheses. Mechanical valves can be categorized into the ball-and-cage valves, such as the Starr-Edwards valve, and valves that use a tilting disk design. The Starr-Edwards valve remains the standard because it has the longest record of durability. Its disadvantages include bulky design and a higher incidences of hemolysis. The valve ring has been covered with cloth to reduce the incidence of thromboembolism. Because of its bulky design, it may be inappropriate for patients with a small aortic annulus or small left ventricular cavity. Tilting disk valves are now made of pyrolite, which is almost diamond-hard. Differences in the mode of retention of the disk allow varying degrees of valve opening. Tilting disk valves are less bulky and have a lower profile than the Starr-Edwards valve. Two serious problems with these valves have been reported: thrombosis and strut fracture. Changes in the design of the valve have been and are being made in an attempt to overcome these problems. The St. Jude Medical valve is constructed of pyrolite and consists of two semicircular disks that pivot between open and closed positions without the need for supporting struts. Some surgeons believe that this valve has more favorable flow characteristics and produces lower gradients across the prosthetic valve. Other disk valves include Medtronics, Duromedics, and Carbomedics. All of these mechanical prosthetic valves appear to be quite durable. However, no study has prospectively compared the advantages and disadvantages of the various tilting disk valves.

Patients should be anticoagulated for life when a mechanical valve is used in either the mitral or aortic position. Anticoagulation decreases the risk of thromboembolism by one-third. Prosthetic-valve thromboses have a reported incidence of 0.1–5.7% per patient year. The major contributing factors are inadequate anticoagulation therapy and mitral location of the prosthesis. Valve thrombosis occurs with similar frequency in patients with bioprosthetic valves and those with mechanical valves who receive adequate anticoagulant therapy.

Tissue valves were developed to overcome the risk of thromboembolism. The most common tissue valves are porcine heterografts. They include porcine valves that are fixed and sterilized using glutaraldehyde, which greatly decreases the antigenicity of the valves. The valves are then mounted on manufactured frames. Biologic valves have also been manufactured from porcine pericardium. Examples of tissue valves include the Carpenter-Edwards porcine valve, Carpentier-Edwards pericardial valve, Ionescu-Shiley valve, and Hancock valve. All of these biologic valves are minimally thrombogenic. Patients should be anticoagulated for the first 3 months after surgery while the valve sewing ring becomes endothelialized, because this period is associated with a high likelihood of thromboembolism. Patients can then safely discontinue anticoagulation. The major problem with tissue valves is their limited durability; degeneration and calcification can become sufficiently severe that the patient requires repeat valve replacement. Failures usually begin to appear within the fourth or fifth postoperative year. By 10 years, the rate of valve failure requiring replacement may be 20–30%.

BIBLIOGRAPHY

1. Aikawa K, Otto C: Timing of surgery in aortic stenosis. Progr Cardiovasc Dis 43:477–493, 2001.
2. Braunwald E: Valvular heart disease. In Braunwald E (ed): Heart Disease: A Textbook of Cardiovascular Medicine, 6th ed. Philadelphia, W.B. Saunders, 2001.
3. Carabello BA: Progress in mitral and aortic regurgitation. Progr Cardiovasc Dis 43:457–475, 2001.
4. Carabello BA, Crawford BA: Medical progress: Valvular heart disease. N Engl J Med 337:32–41, 1997.
5. Nishimura RA, Holmes DR, Reeder GS: Percutaneous balloon valvuloplasty. Mayo Clin Proc 65:198–220, 1990.
6. Otto C: Evaluation and management of chronic mitral regurgitation. N Engl J Med 345:740–746, 2001.
7. Safian RD, Berman AD, Diver DJ, et al: Balloon aortic valvuloplasty in 170 consecutive patients. N Engl J Med 319:125–130, 1988.
8. Sutherland GR, Roelandt JR, et al: Transesophageal Echocardiography in Clinical Practice. London, Gower Medical Publishing, 6.1–9.1, 1991.

31. PERICARDIAL DISEASE (PERICARDITIS AND PERICARDIAL TAMPONADE)

Maria A. deCastro, M.D., and David E. Schwartz, M.D., F.C.C.P.

1. What is the pericardium?

The pericardium is an invaginated sac that extends from the great vessels to enclose the heart. The sac is composed of a fibrous outer layer and an inner serous membrane formed from a single layer of mesothelial cells. The visceral pericardium adheres to the epicardial surface of the heart and reflects back upon itself to form the parietal pericardium. The space between the serous layers of the visceral and parietal pericardium normally holds up to 50 ml of an ultrafiltrate of plasma. The protein concentration of this fluid is one-third that of plasma, and this fluid also contains phospholipids that serve as a lubricant. Normally, as well as in disease, the visceral pericardium is the source of pericardial fluid.

2. What is the function of the pericardium?

The pericardium functions to reduce friction between the heart and the other structures of the mediastinum. It also serves as a barrier to protect the heart from inflammatory processes that involve the lungs or pleura. The pericardium limits acute cardiac dilatation and may prevent kinking of the great vessels. Pericardial pressure is a determinant of the transmural distending pressure of the cardiac chambers. This pressure is the difference between intracardiac and intrapericardial pressure. The pressure in the pericardial space is similar to intrapleural pressure and varies from –5 to +5 cm H_2O during respiration. The relationship between pressure and volume in the pericardial space is exponential. Once the pericardium is filled, any further increase in volume is accompanied by a sharp rise in intrapericardial pressure. Normally the pericardial space can acutely accomodate only 100–200 ml of fluid before there is a significant increase in pressure. However, if fluid accumulates slowly, the pericardium can stretch to accommodate 1–2 liters of fluid without reaching the steep portion of the pressure-volume curve. Although the pericardium serves many functions, congenital absence of the pericardium is usually asymptomatic. Very rarely, complete and partial deficiency of the pericardium may lead to incarceration of cardiac tissue or cardiac valvular insufficiency precipitated by severe displacement of the tricuspid valve.

3. What is acute pericarditis?

Acute pericarditis is inflammation of the pericardial sac. Pathologically, pericarditis involves influx of leukocytes, deposition of fibrin, and an increase in vascularity of the pericardium with increased permeability. This inflammatory process may also involve the myocardium and can lead to adhesions between the epicardium and the pericardium. The visceral pericardium may produce excess fluid in reaction to the injury. This leads to effusive pericarditis.

4. What causes acute pericarditis?

The most common causes of pericarditis are viral and bacterial infections, tuberculosis, uremia, myocardial infarctions, trauma, and malignancies. Even after appropriate evaluation, many cases are of unknown etiology. Pericarditis is more common in men than in women. The incidence ranges from 2–6% in autopsy series, although it is diagnosed in only 1 of 1000 hospital admissions.

5. What are the clinical manifestations of acute pericarditis?

Clinically the syndrome of acute pericarditis is characterized by chest pain, a pericardial friction rub, and frequently fever. Often there is no clinical evidence of pericardial fluid, but small effusions may be detected by echocardiogram. These usually do not progress to produce hemodynamic embarrassment.

The pain of pericarditis is sharp and pleuritic and is located retrosternally or in the left precordial region. Pain with swallowing is frequently described. The pain is exacerbated by the supine position and lessened by sitting up and leaning forward. Radiation of the pain to the trapezius ridge may be helpful in differentiating pericarditis from acute myocardial infarction (MI).

A pericardial friction rub is pathognomonic for acute pericarditis. These rubs are evanescent and best detected with the diaphragm of the stethoscope placed firmly at the lower left sternal border while the patient is sitting up and leaning forward. The classic rub is described as having three components that are related to the motion of the heart during a cardiac cycle. The components of the rub are produced by atrial contraction, ventricular systole, and rapid ventricular filling during diastole. The loudest sound is that of ventricular contraction, while the least commonly detected is the early diastolic sound of rapid ventricular filling. With atrial fibrillation the presystolic component due to atrial contraction is absent, and only a two-component rub is heard. Pericardial friction rubs can be detected in the presence of pericardial effusions.

6. What are the typical electrocardiographic (EKG) changes of acute pericarditis?

EKG abnormalities appear in approximately 90% of cases of acute pericarditis. There are four recognized stages of ST and T wave abnormalities in paricarditis: Stage I changes are diagnostic of pericarditis and usually occur with the onset of pain. These consist of ST segment elevation, in which the ST segment is concave upward and is present in all leads except aVr and V_1. The T waves are usually upright. These features distinguish the stage I changes of pericarditis from the EKG changes seen in acute MI. Stage II follows in several days when the ST segments return to baseline. Stage III is inversion of the T waves. In stage IV the T waves revert to normal. Almost 50% of patients with acute pericarditis will have all four EKG stages. PR-segment depression can occur during stage I or II, and may be seen in over 70% of patients. However, in patients with acute MI and pericarditis detected by the development of a pericardial friction rub, only 1 of 31 patients had EKG changes diagnostic of pericarditis.

In patients with pericarditis and a pericardial effusion, low voltage of the ventricular complex may be seen in association with a normal amplitude of the P wave in the limb leads. This is explained by the absence of an effusion over the posterior surface of the atria, which is partially without a pericardial covering. Electrical alternans, which is variation in the amplitude of the ventricular complexes due to changes in cardiac position with rotation of the heart, is also seen in patients with pericarditis and a pericardial effusion.

Sinus tachycardia is often seen in patients with pericarditis who are not febrile or hemodynamically unstable. Atrial arrhythmias are infrequent in uncomplicated cases of pericarditis.

7. What other laboratory findings are helpful in diagnosing pericarditis?

Pericarditis is associated with signs of inflammation, including an elevation of the erythrocyte sedimentation rate and an elevated white blood cell count. Slight increases of the MB fraction of creatine phosphokinase have been described when epicardial inflammation occurs in acute pericarditis. In uncomplicated cases of pericarditis, the chest x-ray is nonspecific. If there is a large pericardial effusion in association with pericarditis, the chest x-ray will show enlargement and changes in shape of the cardiac silhouette. In one-fourth of patients with pericarditis, pleural effusions are found. These are usually left-sided, or, if bilateral, are larger on the left. In contrast, right-sided pleural effusions are the rule in patients with congestive heart failure. The chest x-ray may also reveal an etiology for the development of pericarditis such as a malignancy or an infection.

Echocardiography is the most sensitive method of detecting the presence of a pericardial effusion in patients with pericarditis. With small effusions, fluid is first detected during both systole and diastole and may be present anteriorly. In massive effusions, the heart may "swing" within the pericardium. This may be responsible for the phenomenon of electrical alternans.

8. Is pericardial biopsy or pericardiocentesis helpful in the diagnosis of the etiology of acute pericarditis?

If, after a routine history and physical examination and laboratory studies, the common etiologies of pericarditis have been ruled out and the illness has lasted over 1 week, it may be appropriate to obtain pericardial tissue or fluid. In 231 consecutive patients with acute pericardial disease, this approach yielded a diagnosis in only 14% of patients. In patients with large pericardial effusions, the diagnostic yield of pericardial biopsy and drainage is higher. In 57 patients with large pericardial effusions, 53 of 57 patients had a diagnosis made. Large pericardial effusions were defined as having anterior and posterior fluid collections and 0.5 cm of fluid either anteriorly or posteriorly during diastole on 2-dimensional echocardiography. Diagnoses included malignancy, infection (which included viral, mycobacterial, and mycoplasma), radiation-induced inflammation, collagen-vascular disease, and uremia. These results suggest that if tissue and fluid are carefully evaluated in patients with large pericardial effusions, a diagnosis may be made that will affect therapy. However, for uncomplicated cases of acute pericarditis, invasive techniques are neither helpful nor necessary.

9. How should the patient with acute pericarditis be managed?

The first determination to be made is whether the patient has hemodynamic compromise from the presence of a pericardial effusion. Next, the etiology of the pericarditis should be determined if possible, and appropriate treatment instituted. If, on echocardiogram, the patient has no evidence of an effusion or has an effusion that is not of hemodynamic significance, then the patient is best managed conservatively. (The management of patients with tamponade is discussed later.) The patient should be hospitalized to exclude MI or an infectious etiology. Careful observation is warranted because of subsequent development of a pericardial effusion that could cause hemodynamic embarrassment. Patients should be kept on bed rest. Oral anticoagulants should be discontinued. If anticoagulation is absolutely necessary, it is safest to administer intravenous heparin, which can be quickly reversed by discontinuing the infusion or by administering protamine. The treatment of viral or idiopathic pericarditis includes pain relief with nonsteroidal anti-inflammatory agents (NSAIDs) or, in severe cases, a short course of corticosteroids.

10. What is the natural history of acute pericarditis?

Most patients with viral or idiopathic pericarditis recover with only symptomatic therapy. In others, recurrent or relapsing pericarditis may follow acute pericarditis. Often these patients require therapy with corticosteroids. Management of this syndrome includes slowly tapering the steroid dose. In extreme cases that require steroids for prolonged periods, pericardiectomy has been performed to relieve pain. The prognosis for patients with other forms of pericarditis varies with the prognosis of the underlying disease.

There are life-threatening complications of pericarditis, including the development of a pericardial effusion under pressure, which can result in cardiac tamponade. Pericarditis can also become chronic and lead to the development of fibrosis and calcification of the pericardium. This may result in constriction of the heart.

11. What is cardiac tamponade?

Cardiac tamponade is the accumulation of pericardial contents to the point that there is hemodynamically significant compression of the cardiac chambers.

12. What are the characteristics of cardiac tamponade?

It is characterized by elevated intracardiac pressures, a decrease in filling of the ventricles, and a reduction in stroke volume. In patients with acute cardiac tamponade from penetrating cardiac wounds, Beck described, in 1935, the triad of (1) falling arterial blood pressure, (2) elevated systemic venous pressure, and (3) a small quiet heart. Patients in whom the cardiac compression developed more slowly usually presented with ascites, a small quiet heart, and high central venous pressure.

13. What causes cardiac tamponade?

Cardiac tamponade can result from any cause of either acute or chronic pericarditis. It may result when the pericardial space is filled with transudative or exudative fluid, blood, frankly infected maerial, or gas. In the Mayo Clinic database of 1002 consecutive echo-guided pericardiocentesis procedures, the four most frequent causes were malignancy, surgical complication, cardiac perforation from catheter-based procedures, and infectious agents. Together they accounted for over 70% of the effusions causing tamponade. Other rarer causes included connective tissue disease, radiatdion therapy, ischemia, renal failiure, and idiopathic causes.

Pneumopericardium under tension, which has been well described in children and adults, is a life-threatening complication of mechanical ventilation. The mortality rate for patients with tension pneumopericardium has been reported to be as high as 56%.

Cardiac tamponade also results from trauma to the heart, most commonly from stab wounds. It is thought that after a stab wound to the heart, the pericardium is able to seal itself, allowing the accumulation of blood in the pericardial space. Pacemaker insertion, cardiac catheterization, and placement of central venous lines have all been associated with cardiac tamponade. Tamponade associated with central venous line placement is usually due to perforation of the right atrium, usually occurs 24 hours following placement of the line, and has a mortality approaching 80%. It is recommended that the tips of central venous catheters be positioned in the superior vena cava to avoid this potentially lethal complication.

14. Describe the pathophysiology of cardiac tamponade.

The addition of fluid to the pericardium at a rate exceeding the ability of the pericardium to stretch will increase intrapericardial pressure. As pericardial pressure rises, it approaches atrial and ventricular diastolic pressures. When these pressures are equal, the transmural pressure distending the cardiac chambers approaches zero. Atrial collapse in tamponade can be recognized echocardiographically. Increases in pericardial pressure are reflected by a rise in central venous pressure. In contrast to other conditions in which atrial pressure is increased, plasma atrial natriuretic factor levels are decreased in patients with tamponade. In hypovolemic patients the rise in central venous pressure and pericardial pressures is less prominent, and the diagnosis of cardiac tamponade may be difficult to make.

As intrapericardial pressure rises further, the heart is compressed and ventricular diastolic volumes fall. Stroke volume also falls, and cardiac output is maintained by activation of the sympathetic nervous system. With cardiac tamponade, mean arterial pressure is reduced, as is the pulse pressure, because of this fall in stroke

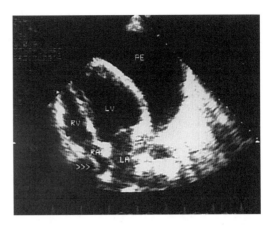

Acute cardiac tamponade. There is marked right atrial wall collapse *(arrows)*. (From Susini G, Pepi M, Sisillo E, et al: Percutaneous pericardiocentesis versus subxiphoid pericardiotomy in cardiac tamponade due to postoperative pericardial effusion. J Cardiothorac Vasc Anesth 7:178–183, 1993, with permission.)

volume. Increased adrenergic tone results in an increase in heart rate and contractility. With severe tamponade, blood pressure is maintained by an increase in systemic vascular resistance, which allows blood pressure to be maintained at the expense of a fall in cardiac output. As tamponade progresses, systemic arterial pressure cannot be maintained and organ perfusion declines. Reduction in coronary perfusion leads to ischemia of the endocardium. Sinus bradycardia, which has been described in cases of severe pericardial tamponade, may be due to sinoatrial node ischemia and heralds cardiovascular collapse and death.

15. What changes are seen in the arterial and venous pulses with cardiac tamponade?

With cardiac tamponade, characteristic phasic changes occur in arterial and venous pressure wave forms. Normally with inspiration there is an increase in venous return that results in an increase in preload of the right ventricle and a small decrease in left ventricular volume. This leads to a decrease in systolic blood pressure of no more than 10 mmHg. Pulsus paradoxus is a hallmark of cardiac tamponade in which there is a fall in arterial systolic pressure with inspiration of greater than the normal value of 10 mmHg. In patients with pericardial tamponade, pulsus paradoxus is seen because of an exaggerated increase in venous return to the right heart during inspiration. This increase in right ventricular volume shifts the intraventricular septum leftward, decreasing left ventricular end-diastolic volume, which results in a fall in output of the left ventricle and of systolic arterial pressure. On physical examination pulsus paradoxus can be detected by a decrease in strength or, in severe cases, loss of a patient's pulse with inspiration. Pulsus paradoxus is not specific to cardiac tamponade and is seen in patients with severe heart failure, asthma and obstructive lung disease, and massive pulmonary embolism.

There are also characteristic changes in the venous waveforms with cardiac tamponade. Normally the venous system has three positive waveforms. The **a wave** is related to atrial contraction, and the **c wave** to closure of the tricuspid valve. The **v wave** results from filling of the atrium during ventricular contraction with the tricuspid valve closed. The **X descent** represents atrial relaxation. The **Y descent** occurs when the tricuspid valve opens and the atrium empties into the ventricle during diastole. In patients with cardiac tamponade, the X descent is preserved, whereas the Y descent is abolished (see figure on following page). These changes occur because the decreased cardiac volume during systole allows atrial pressure to fall and preserves the X descent. However, in diastole the increase in intrapericardial pressure prevents diastolic filling of the ventricle and the Y descent is truncated.

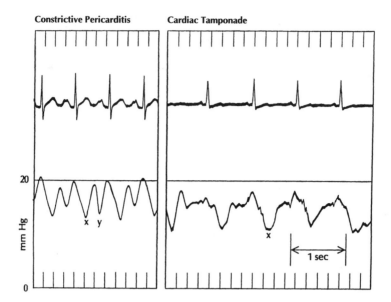

Pressure tracings from the right atrium illustrate the different waveforms in constrictive pericarditis and cardiac tamponade. In chronic constrictive pericarditis, an "M" or "W" contour is formed by prominent dips in both systolic (X descent) and diastolic (Y descent) pressure. In cardiac tamponade, only the systolic dip (X descent) is prominent.

16. What is helpful in making the diagnosis of cardiac tamponade?

The presence of jugular venous distention was the most common physical finding in 56 medical patients with cardiac tamponade. Pulsus paradoxus was present in over 70% of these patients. Kussmaul's sign, an increase in central venous pressure with inspiration, is not seen in patients with pericardial tamponade unless there is an element of pericardial constriction. In patients with tension pneumopericardium, shifting tympany can be demonstrated over the precordium, and a characteristic murmur (bruit de moulin) due to the presence of air and fluid in the pericardium is heard.

Findings on chest x-ray and EKG are nonspecific. Two-dimensional and Doppler echocardiography are most helpful in diagnosing the presence of a hemodynamically significant pericardial effusion. Characteristic echocardiographic features of tamponade are listed in the following table.

Echocardiographic Doppler Features of Cardiac Tamponade

1. Abnormal respiratory changes in ventricular dimensions	5. Dilated inferior vena cava with lack of inspiratory collapse
2. Right atrial compression	6. Left atrial compression
3. Right ventricular diastolic collapse	7. Left ventricular diastolic compression
4. Abnormal respiratory variation in tricuspid and mitral flow velocities	8. Swinging heart

From Fowler NO. Cardiac tamponade: A clinical or an echocardiographic diagnosis? Circulation 87:1738–1741, 1993, with permission.

Transesophageal echocardiography (TEE) may aid in the diagnosis of pericardial tamponade when transthoracic echocardiography is inadequate or when loculated pericardial effusion or clot is suspected. For both of these reasons, TEE has proved particularly useful in the postoperative setting.

Hemodynamic monitoring and cardiac catheterization are invaluable in making the diagnosis of tamponade. The typical finding of loss of the Y descent in the right atrial pressure tracing with preservation of the X is suggestive of tamponade. Intraarterial pressure measurement can help to document the presence of pulsus paradoxus. If pericardial pressure is measured at the time of cardiac catheterization, it should equal atrial and ventricular diastolic pressures. Placement of a pulmonary artery catheter will show elevation and equilibration of diastolic pressures within 3–4 mmHg of each other, termed a "pressure plateau."

Despite the characteristic findings on physical exam and the availability of accurate diagnostic tools, tamponade must be considered early in the course of the disease to allow timely treatment. A review of 50 patients who presented with tamponde to the Montreal Heart Institute revealed an average delay from onset of symptoms to consultation with a cardiologist of 6.6 ± 5.8 days. The diagnosis of tamponade was not initially considered in 80% of these patients. Most were incorrectly diagnosed with heart failure. Clinical deterioration resulted before pericardial drainage was noted in approximately one-third of the patients in this series.

17. What should be considered in the differential diagnosis of tamponade?

Clinical conditions that can be confused with cardiac tamponade include massive pulmonary embolism, tension pneumothorax, severe exacerbation of obstructive lung disease, constrictive pericarditis, restrictive cardiomyopathy, and cardiogenic shock from right ventricular infarction.

18. How should the patient with tamponade be treated?

In the acute setting, medical stabilization of the patient involves maintaining filling pressures with volume expansion to try to prevent diastolic collapse of the heart. Hemodynamic support of the patient with tamponade may also be required. Because the compensatory activation of the sympathetic nervous system results in an increase in systemic vascular resistance, some authorities have recommended inotropic support with isoproterenol to maintain heart rate and contractility as well as to lower afterload. This may be dangerous in patients with marginal blood pressure or inadequate preload. Agents such as dopamine or norepinephrine, which increase the inotropic state of the heart and maintain blood pressure, may be useful in the medical stabilization of the patient. In a dog model of pericardial tamponade, dobutamine infusion delayed the onset of lactic acidosis by maintaining cardiac output and tissue oxygen delivery. Positive-pressure ventilation in patients with cardiac tamponade is associated with a fall in cardiac output, because the decrease in venous return is associated with increased intrathoracic pressure. If at all possible, spontaneous ventilation should be maintained for all patients with tamponade. If supportive measures do not result in improvement, drainage of pericardial fluid needs to be performed emergently.

Definitive therapy for patients with cardiac tamponade involves drainage of the pericardium so that cardiac compression is relieved. This can be done percutaneously or surgically. Percutaneous pericardiocentesis can be performed blindly or guided by two-dimensional echocardiography. The use of echocardiography to guide pericardiocentesis has improved the safety of the procedure. In a series of 117 patients undergoing 132 percardiocenteses, there were no deaths related to the procedure. Patients who have tamponade from a traumatic cause are unlikely to benefit from pericardiocentesis for a prolonged period of time because of the rapid reaccumulation of pericardial fluid. These patients require surgical management. Patients with malignant pericardial effusions who develop tamponade have a high recurrence rate after pericardiocentesis and may require permanent drainage.

Therapy for effusive pericardial disease can involve complete pericardiectomy or pericardiotomy, usually using a subxiphoid approach, with creation of a pericardial window for drainage. In unstable patients, pericardial window can be performed using only local anesthesia. This allows maintenance of spontaneous ventilation. If an unstable patient requires a more extensive procedure, then pericardiocentesis may need to be performed prior to the induction of anesthesia. Limited pericardiectomy allows drainage of the pericardial fluid into the left hemithorax. Recently, percutaneous balloon pericardiotomy (which is performed in the cardiac catheterization laboratory) has been described as an alternative to surgical pericardiotomy. Complete pericardiectomy is performed using either a left anterior thoracotomy or a median sternotomy. Cardiopulmonary bypass is frequently used for complete pericardiectomy. Choice of technique depends on the etiology of the effusion (benign vs. malignant) and the medical condition of the patient.

19. Following cardiac surgery, can a patient in whom the pericardium is open suffer cardiac tamponade?

Yes. Although the pericardium may be left open after cardiac surgery, patients are still at risk for the development of cardiac tamponade. The accumulation of blood in the mediastinum can compress the heart, which can occur because of occlusion of thoracostomy tubes placed during the surgical procedure in 2% of patients following cardiac surgery. Patients with hypotension, low cardiac output, elevated intravascular pressures, and a fall in the output of mediastinal drainage tubes should be suspected of having cardiac tamponade. Marked widening of the mediastinum on chest x-ray may be seen. Obtaining a chest x-ray should not delay therapy. Emergency thoracotomy in the intensive care unit for patients with cardiac tamponade after cardiac surgery is the treatment of choice. The incidence of wound infection is 5% and is not increased by closing the patient's chest in the ICU.

20. What is constrictive pericarditis?

Constrictive pericarditis is the restriction of diastolic filling of the heart produced by the adhesion of a thickened, often calcified, pericardium to the heart. This usually affects all chambers of the heart equally. In most cases the visceral and parietal pericardium are fused. Patients frequently present with dyspnea and the symptoms and signs of elevated venous pressures. Those with longstanding constriction will have peripheral edema, ascites, and a wasted appearance. Elevation of jugular venous pressure is nearly always present, and Kussmaul's sign (a paradoxical increase in venous pressure with inspiration) may be found in patients with constriction. If the patient's neck is examined carefully, the rapid Y descent in the jugular venous waveform can often be seen. On auscultation, an early systolic sound called the pericardial knock may be heard and is fairly specific for constrictive pericarditis.

21. What are the causes of constrictive pericarditis?

Anything that can cause acute pericarditis can result in constrictive pericarditis. The major causes include infections, connective tissue disorders, neoplastic diseases, trauma, metabolic abnormalities, radiation therapy, and myocardial infarction. Worldwide, tuberculosis is the most common etiologic agent, but it accounts for less than 20% of cases in the developed world.

22. How does the cardiac compression due to constrictive pericarditis differ from that of cardiac tamponade?

With thickening of the pericardium, there is restriction of the diastolic enlarging of the ventricles that limits ventricular filling. Filling is normal during the first third of diastole. However, in the last two-thirds of diastole, continued ventricular filling is abruptly halted by the thickened pericardium. This pattern of filling is exemplified by the classic dip and plateau pressure waveform seen in constrictive pericarditis. There is an early diastolic fall in pressure that is immediately followed by a steep rise in pressure to a plateau level.

The presence of Kussmaul's sign and the absence of pulsus paradoxus helps to distinguish constrictive pericarditis from pericardial tamponade. In addition, a prominent Y descent in the right atrial pressure waveform (see figure on p. 178) is seen in constrictive pericarditis and is absent in tamponade. Thickening or calcification of the pericardium seen on echocardiogram or computed tomography may help in making the diagnosis of constrictive pericarditis. Oh et al. have reviewed the Doppler echocardiographic features of constrictive pericarditis.

BIBLIOGRAPHY

1. Callaham M: Pericardiocentesis in traumatic and nontraumatic cardiac tamponade. Ann Emerg Med 13:924–945, 1984.
2. Callahan JA, Seward JB, Nishimura RA, et al: Two-dimensional echocardiographically guided pericardiocentesis: Experience in 117 consecutive patients. Am J Cardiol 55:475–479, 1985.
3. Corey GR, Campbell PT, Van Tright PV, et al: Etiology of large pericardial effusions. Am J Med 95:209–213, 1993.

4. Cummings RG, Wesly RL, Adams DH, Lowe JE: Pneumopericardium resulting in cardiac tamponade. Ann Thorac Surg 37:511–518, 1984.
5. Edwards H, King TC: Cardiac tamponade from central venous catheters. Arch Surg 117:965–967, 1982.
6. Fairman RM, Edmunds LH: Emergency thoracotomy in the surgical intensive care unit after open cardiac operation. Ann Thorac Surg 32:386, 391, 1981.
7. Fowler NO: Cardiac tamponade: A clinical or an echocardiographic diagnosis? Circulation 87:1738–1741, 1993.
8. Fowler NO: Constrictive pericarditis: New aspects. Am J Cardiol 50:1014–1017, 1982.
9. Fowler NO, Gabel M: The hemodynamic effects of cardiac tamponade: Mainly the result of atrial, not ventricular, compression. Circulation 71:154–157, 1985.
10. Griffin S, Fountain W: Pericardio-peritoneal shunt for malignant pericardial effusion. J Thorac Cardiovasc Surg 98:1153–1154, 1989.
11. Guberman BA, Fowler NO, Engel PJ, et al: Cardiac tamponade in medical patients. Circulation 64:633–640, 1981.
12. Hancock EW: On the elastic and rigid forms of constrictive pericarditis. Am Heart J 100:917–923, 1980.
13. Krainin FM, Flessas AP, Spodick DH: Infarction-associated pericarditis: Rarity of diagnostic electrocardiogram. N Engl J Med 311:1211–1214, 1984.
14. Krikorian JG, Hancock EW: Pericardiocentesis. Am J Med 65:808–814, 1978.
15. Laham RJ, Cohen DJ, Kuntz RE, et al: Pericardial effusion in patients with cancer: Outcome with contemporary management strategies. Heart 75:67–71, 1996.
16. Larose E, Ducharme A, Mercier LA, et al: Prolonged distress and clinical deterioration before pericardial drainage in patients with cardiac tamponade. Can J Cardiol 16:331–336, 2000.
17. McCaughan BC, Schaff HV, Piehler JM, et al: Early and late results of pericardiectomy for constrictive pericarditis. J Thorac Cardiovascular Surg 89:340–350, 1985.
18. McGregor M: Pulsus paradoxus. N Engl J Med 301:480–482, 1979.
19. Oh JK, Hatle LK, Seward JB, et al: Diagnostic role of doppler echocardiography in constrictive pericarditis. J Am Coll Cardiol 23:154–162, 1994.
20. Panayiotou H, Haitas B, Hollister AS: Atrial wall tension changes and the release of atrial natriuretic factor on relief of cardiac tamponade. Am Heart J 129:960–967, 1995.
21. Permanyer-Miralda G, Sagrista-Sauleda J, Soler-Soler J: Primary acute pericardial disease: A prospective series of 231 consecutive patients. Am J Cardiol 56:623–630, 1985.
22. Surawicz B, Lasseter KC: Electrocardiogram in pericarditis. Am J Cardiol 26:471–474, 1970.
23. Susini G, Pepi M, Sisillo E, et al: Percutaneous pericardiocentesis versus subxiphoid pericardiotomy in cardiac tamponade due to postoperative pericardial effusion. J Cardiothorac Vasc Anesth 7:178–183, 1993.
24. Tsang SM, Oh JK, Seward JB: Diagnosis and management of cardiac tamponade in the era of echocardiography. Clin Cardiol 22:446–452, 1999.
25. Vanson JA, Danielson GK, Schaff HV, et al: Congenital partial and complete absence of the pericardium. Mayo Clin Proc 68:743–747, 1993.
26. Weiss JM, Spodick DH: Association of left pleural effusions with pericardial disease. N Engl J Med 308:696–697, 1984.
27. Zhang H, Spapen H, Vincent JL: Effects of dobutamine and norepinephrine on oxygen availability in tamponade-induced stagnant hypoxia: A prospective, randomized, controlled study. Crit Care Med 22:299–305, 1994.
286. Ziskind AA, Pearce C, Lemmon CC, et al: Percutaneous balloon pericardiotomy for the treatment of cardiac tamponade and large pericardial effusions: Description of technique and report of the first 50 cases. J Am Coll Cardiol 21:1–5, 1993.

32. ECHOCARDIOGRAPHY IN INTENSIVE CARE

Olivia Vynn Adair, M.D., and Colleen Hubbard, R.T., R.D.M.S., R.D.C.S.

1. Why has echocardiography emerged as an important imaging technique in the management of the intensive care patient?

Success in the management of patients in the intensive care unit (ICU) often depends on prompt and precise diagnosis. Echocardiography is, therefore, particularly advantageous, as it provides both anatomic and physiologic assessment of the heart noninvasively or minimally so with transesophageal echocardiography (TEE). The results are immediately available and serial examinations can easily be performed on unstable patients at the bedside with reliability.

2. Name the various echocardiographic imaging techniques.

The imaging techniques of echocardiography are M-mode, two-dimensional (2-D), TEE, color-flow mapping, and Doppler ultrasound. M-mode contributes information on wall motion, valve excursion, and chamber size, and aids in timing of events during the cardiac cycle. 2-D Echocardiography provides an image of all chambers, outflow tracts, valves, aortic root, descending aorta, and the great vessels. Color-flow and Doppler imaging provide information on blood velocity, direction, and turbulence across the valves, within the chambers, across any shunts, and in the thoracic aorta. TEE permits close evaluation of the heart and aorta from the esophagus and stomach.

3. What are some indications for echocardiographic imaging of the ICU patient?

Hemodynamic instability with suspected cardiac etiology (e.g., tamponade, cardiac dysfunction, low perfusion rate)

Chest pain

Chest trauma

Valve disease

Regurgitation or stenosis, especially with pulmonary edema or syncope

Cerebrovascular or systemic thromboembolic event

Aortic disease

Sepsis, possibly due to endocarditis

4. Why is echocardiography an important diagnostic imaging technique in cardiac tamponade?

Cardiac tamponade has a high mortality rate if not accurately and promptly diagnosed and treated. Echocardiography is the most sensitive technique for the detection and localization of a pericardial effusion, and is highly valuable in evaluating the hemodynamic significance of the effusion. Echocardiography should be considered routinely when tamponade is suspected, as it is quickly performed at bedside, is very sensitive, and can identify effusions as small as 15 ml. Tamponade often may be detected echocardiographically in the absence of physical signs.

5. What are the findings on echocardiography in cardiac tamponade? How sensitive and specific is this imaging technique for tamponade?

The typical findings on echocardiography in tamponade are late diastolic collapse of the right atrial wall (the earliest change) and early diastolic right ventricular free wall collapse or indentation. These findings are highly sensitive, 80–92%, and specific, approximately 100%. The changes on echocardiography occur when the cardiac output has decreased as little as 20% and before a drop in sytemic arterial blood pressure occurs. These echocardiographic findings may be absent in hypertrophy, in elevated right-sided pressures, and after cardiac surgery because of adhesions to the free walls of the heart chambers. If the echocardiogram is not diagnostic of tamponade, but clinical suspicion is high, especially with hemodynamic compromise, a Swan-Ganz catheter should be placed to evaluate for equalization of pressures, an indication of cardiac tamponade.

6. How is echocardiography useful in pericardiocentesis?

All patients undergoing pericardiocentesis should have a 2-D echocardiogram to determine whether the routine approach for the aspiration needle and catheter is appropriate. With an apical four-chamber view providing continuous imaging during the procedure, the needle is visualized as it enters the pericardial sac (agitated saline may be incorporated as an aid if needed). Catheter placement is then verified, and the decrease in pericardial fluid monitored with 2-D echocardiography.

7. Describe the technique of TEE and its risks.

TEE uses a modified flexible gastroscope with an ultrasound transducer mounted on the tip and has the capacities of M-mode and 2-D echocardiography as well as Doppler and color-flow imaging. After the patient has been premedicated with an oral topical anesthetic and a short-acting intravenous relaxant, the probe, 9 mm in diameter and 100 cm long, is introduced as an upper endoscope to approximately 50 cm (to the stomach). Although anesthesiologists quickly adopted TEE for intraoperative monitoring of left ventricular function and ischemia, it is now routinely used in ambulatory, critical care, and emergency room settings. The study can be completed in approximately 20 minutes at the bedside and with minimal risk to the patient. There have been only three reported associated fatalities—two secondary to perforation of the esophagus and one to bradycardia. Minor throat irritation is the most common complaint. Because the probe is introduced blindly, a relative contraindication is esophageal disease, i.e., varices, strictures, diverticuli, or scleroderma. Severe oral injury or neck instability may also make passing the scope difficult or impossible. In these cases, laryngeal scope-assisted probe introduction without neck flexure is sometimes successful. Nasal-gastric and feeding tubes should be removed prior to TEE, as tangling of the tubes as been reported.

8. What are the indications and benefits of transesophageal compared with transthoracic echocardiography in the critical care patient?

The retrocardiac vantage of TEE circumvents interference from interposing structures (skin, bone, lungs) and poor imaging windows that may be due to chest wall abnormalities, bandages, or injuries, thus negating the 10% of studies that are technically difficult with transthoracic echocardiography (TTE) to increase the success rate of TEE to > 98%. In studies of prosthetic valves, TEE eliminates the shadows and artifacts seen on TTE. Also, because of the angle of approach, color-flow Doppler evaluation of intraseptal shunts and valvular regurgitant flow are markedly improved with TEE. Evaluation of both native and prosthetic valve vegetations in endocarditis is much more sensitive with TEE; especially in smaller (< 5 mm) vegetations, TEE is four times more sensitive than TTE. Patients presenting with cerebrovascular events benefit from TEE imaging, as the entire left atrium is easily visualized, including the left atrial appendage, which is rarely viewed with TTE and is the major location of a cardiac emboli source. Another important use of TEE is imaging of the thoracic aorta for aneurysm, dissection, and an intimal flap. All areas of the aorta are accessible, and the accuracy of diagnosing an aortic dissection with TEE is 93–100%.

9. Is echocardiography an acceptable technique in the diagnosis and management of thoracic aorta dissection compared with other imaging techniques?

Aortic dissection is rapidly fatal if not promptly diagnosed and treated, and requires confirmation by a diagnostic imaging technique such as aortography, echocardiography, computed tomography (CT), or magnetic resonance imaging (MRI). Aortography used to be considered the gold standard, but its sensitivity and specificity in recent studies are only 88% and 94%, respectively, and aortography has the disadvantages of time delay, the invasiveness of aortic catheterization and contrast material, and radiation exposure, making the initial study and serial studies less desirable.

In comparison, combined transesophageal and transthoracic echocardiography is rapid (study time 15–20 minutes), mobile, easily done at bedside, and accurate (sensitivity 99%, specificity 98%), and allows on-line, immediate interpretation. In addition, no contrast material is required, and the entry tear of the dissection is identified in > 87% of patients. Echocardiography also provides additional data (e.g., aortic insufficiency, other valve disease, cardiac function, pericardial effusion). CT, although relatively noninvasive, requires contrast material, involves a moderate time delay, often does not permit identification of entry tear, and has a low sensitivity, 83% (specificity 100%). MRI has the advantages of high sensitivity and specificity (95% and 98%, respectively), noninvasiveness, and provision of additional cardiac data. Disadvantages are that the patient must be relatively stable to be transported, support equipment may not be able to be brought into the imaging suite, a relative time delay, unavailability of equipment and emergency staff, and identification of entry tear identified in only 39% of patients. Therefore, echocardiography (combined transthoracic and transesophageal) should be performed when dissection of the thoracic aorta is suspected as the first study for diagnosis, for location of entry tear, and for identification of aortic insufficiency and other cardiac abnormalities.

10. Should all patients with blunt chest trauma undergo echocardiography?

Cardiac contusion from blunt chest trauma remains a challenge in ICU management because the picture is often complicated by major injuries and fractures. Cardiac complications associated with such trauma include myocardial contusion, laceration or rupture, valve damage or rupture, and marked myocardial depression. Although echocardiography offers immediate noninvasive imaging, the incidence of functional cardiac abnormalities due to blunt trauma is low (< 20%), even with a high incidence of major injuries and fractures (50%). Also, because the course is usually benign, even in patients sustaining contusion, the additional cost of echocardiography is not warranted routinely in patient management. The deaths in this group of patients in a large study were not related to cardiac abnormalities but rather to other injuries. Therefore, echocardiography should be based on clinical findings that suggest cardiac complications (murmur, rub, congestive heart failure, and unusual chest pain with associated symptoms) or unexpected deterioration in the clinical course of the patient.

11. Do patients with penetrating chest wall injury require echocardiography routinely?

A higher proportion of patients presenting with penetrating chest injury have cardiac complications than do those sustaining blunt chest trauma. For example, up to 33% of patients with penetrating chest wall injury have silent hemopericardium. Other findings include regional wall abnormalities, pneumopericardium, and foreign bodies. Therefore, a low threshold for echocardiography should be entertained in patients presenting with penetrating chest wall trauma.

12. What is the sensitivity of transesophageal versus transthoracic echocardiography in the diagnosis of endocarditis?

TEE improves detection of vegetation on both native and prosthetic valves. The sensitivities of TEE and TTE are 100% and 63%, respectively, whereas the specificities are the same (98%). Larger vegetations (> 10 mm) are visualized by both techniques, but only 25% of smaller vegetations (< 5 mm) are detected by TTE compared with 100% by TEE. Also, 20–30% of TTE studies are technically inadequate and the overall success rate in diagnostic studies of patients presenting with possible endocarditis.

13. Is a baseline echocardiogram recommended for all patients with endocarditis?

Bacterial endocarditis results in high morbidity and a mortality rate of 33%. Specific high-risk patients are more likely to develop complications and require surgery, and therefore should have an echocardiogram. For example, patients with native aortic valve involvement in endocarditis and patients with a history of intravenous drug abuse have a 2.5 times increased risk of periannular infection and local extension of infection (occurring in 50%). Because of the seriousness of such sequelae, these patients should have serial echocardiography for follow-up. Other complications to be evaluated are the development of annular abscesses, aneurysms, and fistulous communications. Patients with echocardiographically evident vegetations vs. silent endocarditis (no vegetation visualized) require surgery 93% vs. 15%, have major embolic events 47% vs. 15%, and mortality is 35% vs. 23%. Therefore, it is reasonable to perform echocardiography early in the absence of an immediate response to appropriate therapy to evaluate for the presence of a vegetation. Also, because the initial study may be negative and clinical signs of complications (congestive heart failure, arrhythmias, heart block, pericarditis, and valve destruction) are late findings, serial echocardiograms may be required to plan early surgery, as emergent surgery is associated with high mortality.

14. What complications of endocarditis can be diagnosed by echocardiography?

Two complications that are identifiable echocardiographically are regurgitant flow and obstructive flow (with large vegetations) across the valves. These abnormal flow profiles may be associated with leaflet destruction or rupture. Perivalvular abscess and local extension of infection may be visualized, as may fistula formation, rupture or abscess of the sinus of Valsalva, myocardial or root abscess, mycotic aneurysm, pericardial effusions, and unexpected multiple valve involvement. Because increased morbidity and mortality are associated with the complications of endocarditis, their recognition is extremely important. Often TEE will be required to obtain the highest resolution, especially in prosthetic valve endocarditis.

15. What diagnostic role does echocardiography play in the evaluation of an AIDS patient admitted with respiratory distress and hemodynamic instability?

Recent studies have identified cardiac abnormalities in as many as 70% of patients with AIDS, and they are more common in hospitalized patients. These abnormalities include pericardial effusions, tamponade, pericardial and myocardial tumors, valve disease, myocarditis, and cardiomyopathy. Because the presenting symptoms may not be specifically pulmonary or cardiac in origin and because their management may be drastically altered, it is recommended that these patients undergo early echocardiography. Cardiac implications of AIDS (e.g., tamponade, endocarditis, and myocarditis) may be fatal if not treated promptly, and many are treatable or at least manageable.

16. What is the appropriate imaging modality for a patient admitted with acute pulmonary edema and a prosthetic valve?

Any patient with a prosthetic valve who presents with evidence of acute pulmonary edema or cardiac dysfunction should have prompt investigation of the valve for dysfunction or endocarditis with an echocardiogram. Failure rates of approximately 7% and 9% per year are expected for aortic and mitral prosthetic valves, respectively. The most sensitive imaging techniques for this purpose are TEE and color-flow Doppler imaging. Information desired includes regurgitant or stenotic flow, movement of leaflets or mechanical processes, paravalvular regurgitation, vegetations, dehiscence of valve ring, and atrial and ventricular thrombi.

17. What diagnostic benefits are gained from echocardiography for the patient admitted with a new cerebral embolic event?

Echocardiography plays an important role in the search for a potential cardiac source of the emboli in the evaluation of patients with transient ischemic attacks or strokes. Approximately one-sixth of all cerebral infarcts are due to cerebral embolism of cardiac origin. Thrombi may be located in the chambers, aorta, and great vessels. Also, possible myxoma, other cardiac tumors, valvular vegetations, intracardiac shunts, and patent foramen ovale may be the source of embolization and are identifiable with an echocardiogram. Echocardiography is particularly beneficial in identifying the source of embolism and are identifiable with an echocardiogram. Echocardiography is particularly beneficial in identifying the source of embolism in younger patients (< 45 year sof age), with one study demonstrating a positive echocardiogram in 37% of these patients presenting with a stroke. Likewise, patients with a history of cardiac disease are much more likely to have a cardiac source of cerebral emboli. In addition, other individuals without a known source of embolus should undergo echocardiography, and TEE may be required.

18. When should stroke patients undergo TEE?

TEE permits, with better resolution than TTE, detailed imaging of important areas that have a high potential for being a cardiac source of the emboli. These areas include the left atrium, especially the appendage (rarely visualized on TTE), and intraseptal defects, including patent foramen ovale. TEE has been shown to be four times more sensitive in imaging small valvular vegetations (< 5 mm), which serve as a source of emboli. A recent study demonstrated that in patients presenting with an unexplained stroke, a cardiac source was identified in 57% of cases by TEE compared with 15% by TTE. TEE also provided a diagnosis in 40% of patients without a cardiac history. Therefore, it is recommended that patients with a stroke of unknown etiology, even with a normal TTE, undergo TEE.

19. A 58-year-old woman presented with recurrent transient ischemic attacks (TIAs) and a history of poorly treated hypertension due to poor compliance. Work-up, including echocardiogram, was negative. The patient was discharged with a prescription for Plavix. While being escorted to the hospital lobby, she experienced a TIA and was rushed to the ICU. An immediate TEE was ordered. Since the echocardiogram was normal, was this procedure necessary?

Because TEE is more specific, it is warranted in patients with cerebrovascular accident or TIA, especially in a recurrent pattern. The findings clearly explain the symptoms of transient and recurrent episodes of emboli (see figure below). A thrombus was located through a patent foramen ovale (PFO). The thrombus in both atria was unstable, and bits were actually floating off. A bubble study confirmed the PFO. The patient was taken to surgery that night for repair of PFO and thrombus.

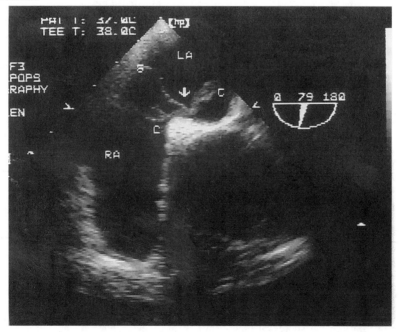

TEE of patient with recurrent TIAs. A thrombus (C) is located in the left atrium (LA) and right atrium (RA), passing through the patent foramen ovale (PFO). The thrombus is very mobile, and tiny fragments can be seen floating off the unstable thrombus.

20. A 36-year-old man with a history of Marfan's syndrome and proximal aorta repair 3 years ago was admitted to the ICU for cardiac evaluation one day after eye surgery with complaints of chest and back pain. He also had severe headaches, nausea, and vomiting. TEE was performed. What were the findings?

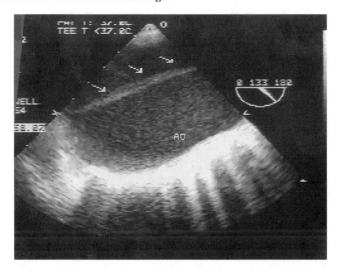

The aorta (Ao) displays a large dissection occupying one-third of the aorta (noted by arrows).

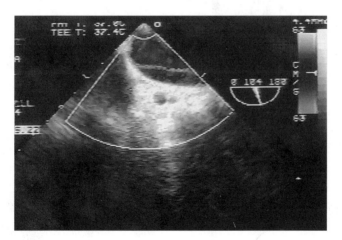

Color flow Doppler displays flow in the dissection with evidence of thrombus. The dissection extended from the arch distal to the renal arteries.

Although the previous repair had been performed because of the inherent medial degenerative disease of the aorta, further aneurysmal development and a high risk of sudden death are chronic concerns.

BIBLIOGRAPHY

1. Adair OV, Randive N, Krasnow N: Isolated toxoplasma myocarditis in acquired immune deficiency syndrome. Am Heart J 118:856–857, 1989.

2. Ballal RS, Nanda NL, et al: Usefulness of transesophageal echocardiogram in assessment of aortic dissection. Circulation 84:1903–1914, 1991.
3. Bolger A: Beyond the annulus [editorial]. J Am Coll Cardiol 39:1210–1212, 2002.
4. Dressler FA, Roberts WC: Infective endocarditis in opiate addicts: Analysis of 80 cases studied at necropsy. Am J Cardiol 63:1240–1257, 1989.
5. Fisher EA, Goldman ME: Transesophageal echocardiography: A new view of the heart. Ann Intern Med 113:91–93, 1990.
6. Graupner C, Vilacosta J, Roman J, et al: Periannular extension of infective carditis. J Am Coll Med.
7. Hossack KF, Moreno CA, Vanway CW, Burdick DC: Frequency of cardiac contusion in nonpenetrating chest injury. Am J Cardiol 61:391–394, 1988.
8. Hunaiker PR, Keller D, et al: Bedside quantification of atherosclerosis severity for cardiovascular risk stratification: A prospective cohort study. J Am Coll Cardiol 7:702–709, 2002.
9. Khandheria BK: Suspected bacerial endocarditis. To TEE or not to TEE. J Am Coll Cardiol 21:222–224, 1993.
10. Klodas E, Edwards WD, Khandheria B: Use of transesophageal echocardiography for improving detection of valvular vegetations in subacute bacterial endocarditis. J Am Soc Echo 2:386–389, 1989.
11. Krozon I, Tunick P: Transesophageal echocardiogram as a tool in the evaluation of patients with embolic disease. Drug Cardiovasc Dis 36:39–60, 1993.
12. Moten M, Pandian NG: Echocardiography in cardiac tamponade. Cardiovasc Reviews & Reports 9(9):46–49, 1988.
13. Pavlides GS, Hauser AM, O'Neill WJ, Timmis GC: Transesophageal echocardiography: Current indications. J Intervent Cardiol 1:123–132, 1989.
14. Pearson AC, Labovitz AJ, Tatineni S, Gomez CVR: Superiority of transesophageal echocardiography in detecting cardiac source of embolism in patients with cerebral ischemia of uncertain etiology. J Am Coll Cardiol 17:66–72, 1991.
15. Raymond R, Hinderliter A, Willis P, et al: Echocardiographic predictors of adverse outcomes in primary pulmonary hypertension. J Am Coll Cardiol 39:1127–1132, 2002.
16. Schwammenthal E, Schwammenthal Y, Tanne D, et al: Transcutaneous detection of aortic arch. J Am Coll Cardiol 39:1127–1132, 2002.
17. Scott PJ, Ettles DF, Wharton GA, Williams GJ: The value of transesophageal echocardiography in the investigation of acute prosthetic valve dysfunction. Clin Cardiol 13:541–544, 1990.
18. Singh S, Wann S, Schuchard G, et al: Right ventricular and right atrial collapse in patients with cardiac tamponade: A combined echocardiographic and hemodynamic study. Circulation 70:966–971, 1984.
19. Wilbers C, Carrol CL, Hnilica MA: Optimal diagnostic imaging of aortic dissection. Texas Heart Inst J 17:271–278, 1990.
20. Zenker G, Erbel R, Kramer G, et al: Transesophageal two-dimensional echocardiography in young patients with cerebral ischemic events. Stroke 19:345–348, 1988.

V. Infectious Disease

33. SEPSIS SYNDROME

Jason Widrich, M.D., and Michael A. Gropper, M.D., Ph.D.

1. What is the incidence of sepsis?

Severe sepsis and septic shock are common and associated with substantial mortality and consumption of health care resources. There are an estimated 751,000 cases (3.0 cases per 1000 population) of sepsis or septic shock in the United States each year. Sepsis and septic shock are responsible for as many death each year as acute myocardial infarction (215,000, or 9.3% of all deaths).The incidence and mortality rate of sepsis are substantially higher in elderly than in younger people. The projected growth of the elderly population in the United States will contribute to an increase in incidence of 1.5% per year, yielding an estimated 934,000 and 1,110,000 cases by the years 2010 and 2020, respectively. The present annual cost of sepsis and septic shock is estimated at $16.7 billion.

2. Explain the nomenclature for disorders related to sepsis.

The nomenclature for disorders related to sepsis was defined in the 1990s by the American College of Chest Physicians and the Society of Critical Care Medicine. The following terms describe the progression of signs and symptoms of sepsis syndrome.

Systemic inflammatory response syndrome (SIRS): characterized by (1) temperature > 38°C or < 36°C; (2) heart rate > 90 beats/minute; (3) respiratory rate > 20 breaths/minute or the need for mechanical ventilation; and (4) white blood cell count > 12,000 cells/mm^3 or < 4,000 cells/mm^3.

Sepsis: SIRS plus a documented source of infection.

Severe sepsis: sepsis with dysfunction of one or more organs.

Septic shock: sepsis-induced hypotension (< 80 mmHg) that persists despite adequate fluid resuscitation plus hypoperfusion, abnormal organ function or organ dysfunction (oliguria < 0.5 ml/kg/hr, lactic acidosis, and alteration in mental status evaluated without sedative drugs).

Multiple organ dysfunction syndrome (MODS): failure in more than one organ system that requires acute intervention.

3. How does the nomenclature relate to outcome?

Previous studies have shown that as the disorder progresses from SIRS to septic shock, the mortality rate increases. Additional studies have shown that the mortality rate in patients who meet three or four criteria for SIRS but have no documented infection is the same or slightly higher than the mortality rate in patients with sepsis. Whether this finding is due to a shortfall in the ability to diagnose infection or other occult processes remains to be elucidated.

Sepsis progresses to MODS with tragic consequences. The mortality rate for patients with acute renal failure in the setting of sepsis ranges from 50% to 80%. For most patients with sepsis syndrome, the failure of three or more organ systems results results in a mortality rate > 90% The organ systems most often affected early in the process are pulmonary, hematologic, renal, and cardiovascular.

4. Discuss current understanding of the pathogenesis of sepsis and septic shock.

Sepsis syndrome begins with the invasion and growth of microorganisms (gram-positive, gram-negative, fungal, or viral) in a normally sterile tissue space. The endothelium is damaged by infection, trauma, or other insult, and activation of the host immune response begins. Tumor necrosis factor alpha, interleukin (IL)-6, and IL-8 are associated with the activation of an inflammatory cascade and chemotaxis of leukocytes, monocytes, and macrophages. Anti-inflammatory substances such as IL-4, IL-10, prostaglandins, and other components of the immune system work to maintain homeostasis in the face of an infectious insult. Sepsis syndrome develops when the balance between the pro- and anti-inflammatory substances is lost.

The coagulation pathway plays a critical role in sepsis. The complement system, vasoregulatory system (nitric oxide, bradykinin, prostaglandins), the coagulation cascade (tissue factor, protein C, thrombin, antithrombin III), and fibrinolysis (fibrin, plasmin, and plasminogen-activating factor) play a role as well. The result is the development of a vicious cycle that promotes, both locally and systemically, further inflammation, release of oxygen free radicals, and deposition of microvascular thrombi, resulting in ischemia, reperfusion injury, and tissue hypoxia. Global tissue hypoxia independently contributes to endothelial activation and further disruption of the homeostatic balance among coagulation, vascular permeability, and vascular tone. These are key mechanisms leading to microcirculatory failure, refractory tissue hypoxia, and organ dysfunction.

It is becoming clear that the processes of coagulation and inflammation are tightly linked. Recent studies have shown that patients with severe sepsis have depleted levels of protein C, protein S, and antithrombin III. Administration of protein C to patients with severe sepsis appears to decrease mortality by both regulating the coagulation pathway and decreasing inflammation.

5. Which microorganisms are most commonly associated with sepsis?

A recent study of patients admitted for severe sepsis and septic shock found the following infecting organisms:

Gram-positive: *Staphylococcus aureus* (20%), coagulase-negative staphylococci (about 10%), enterococci (3–5%). *Streptococcus pneumoniae* and beta-hemolytic streptococci were the most common.

Gram-negative: *Serratia* sp., *Salmonella* sp., *Proteus* sp., *Pseudomonas* sp. (3–5%), *Cirobacter* sp., *Escherichia coli* (23–28%), and *Klebsiella* sp. (3–5%).

Anaerobes (3–4%): *Candida* sp. and fungi (1–3%), viral (< 1%).

Although such data are useful for understanding general trends, each hospital or intensive care unit may vary based on the community patient population, on-site strains of resistance, lapses in infection control, nosocomial vs. community-acquired infection, and level of immunocompromise. Much of this information can be found for specific areas in the hospital's infection control department or department of public health.

6. What are the most common sources of infection?

Lung (36%), blood (20%), abdomen (19%), urinary tract (13%), skin (7%), other (5%).

7. What can be done to control the source of infection and prevent nosocomial infection?

Numerous measures can be taken to limit the spread and severity of infections and to prevent new infection in septic or critically ill patients. Source control consists of surgical debridement of wounds, drainage of an abscess or empyema, care for pressure points and ulcers, and proper contact precautions (even stethoscopes and personal pagers have been implicated as sources of pathogenic bacteria). In addition, antibiotic therapy that is begun empirically and promptly and then focused on appropriate sensitivities is life-saving and prevents antibiotic resistance. Other measures include appropriate ventilator management, enteral nutrition, gastrointestinal prophylaxis, and indwelling catheter management.

8. How often should the central lines in septic patients be changed?

The Infectious Disease Society of America recommendations for percutaneous central venous catheters (CVCs) emphasize (1) the clinical picture of the patient with regard to the infectious process and (2) the results of cultures drawn from peripheral sites and/or the central line.

- If the patient with a CVC has a fever or symptoms/signs of an infection and no other obvious site of infection, change the line over a guidewire and order peripheral percutaneous and central catheter blood cultures.
- If another source of infection can explain the clinical picture, then the catheter should remain in place.
- If the blood cultures are negative, but the patient has no other site of infection to explain the clinical picture or is deteriorating rapidly or immunocompromised, insert a new line at a new site and remove the suspected line. The search for other sources of infection should be continued. The decision to administer empirical antibiotic coverage should be based on the clinical picture, and different centers and countries have different thresholds for their use. Empirical antibiotics may be used in patients with a worsening clinical picture, but a more extensive work-up for septic emboli, endocarditis, and/or osteomyelitis also should be considered.
- If the blood cultures are positive, a new central line site is necessary. Infection should be treated empirically (for 10–14 days) and then tailored when sensitivity results are available.
- If an infection is complicated (e.g., *S. aureus*, *Candida* sp., or multiple organisms), further work-up or long-term antibiotic coverage (6–8 weeks) may be needed to prevent the sequelae of bacteremia (endocarditis, septic phlebitis or thrombosis, and osteomyelitis).

9. Discuss the role of antibiotic-coated catheters.

CVCs impregnated with a combination of chlorhexidine and silver sulfadiazine or minocycline and rifampin appear to be effective in reducing the incidence of both catheter colonization and catheter-related bloodstream infection in high-risk patients. A recent head-to-head trial of the two combinations reported that catheters with minocycline and rifampin were superior in reduction of infections.

10. How does management differ in immunocompromised patients with neutropenic sepsis?

1. A more diffuse or quicker progression of infection and symptoms is possible. A high index of suspicion is required in neutropenic patients, who may be unable to mount the usual febrile response or leukocytosis.

2. Suspicion for fungal and viral infection should be higher. Empirical treatment should include broad-spectrum antibacterial, antiviral, and antifungal medications.

11. What clinical signs and symptoms should raise suspicion of SIRS, sepsis, and underlying organ dysfunction?

Respiratory: cyanosis, tachypnea, orthopnea, increased sputum (yellow or green, frothy), hypoxemia ($PaO_2/FiO_2 < 300$), oxygen saturation < 90%.

Cardiovascular: chest pain, pulmonary edema, arrhythmias, need for pressors, cardiac index < 2.5, heart rate > 100 beats/minute, decreased systemic vascular resistance, increased cardiac output.

Renal: urine output < 0.5 ml/kg/hr, increased blood urea nitrogen, increased creatinine, acute renal failure, acidosis, increasing base deficit, metabolic acidosis (usually lactate).

Hepatic: elevated aspartate aminotransferase, alanine aminotransferase, or gamma-gluytamyl transferase; prolonged bleeding time; asterixis; encephalopathy; elevated bilirubin.

Immunologic: fever > 38°C or hypothermia, chills, increased white blood cell count or left shift, neutropenia.

Hematologic: weakness, pallor, poor capillary refill, easy bruising, spontaneous bleeding, anemia, increased prothrombin or partial thromboplastin time, decreased fibrinogen, disseminated intravascular coagulation (elevated D-dimers).

Gastrointestinal: anorexia, ileus, inability to tolerate tube feeds, nausea, vomiting, hypoalbuminemia.

Endocrine: hyperglycemia, hypoglycemia, adrenal insufficiency, weight loss.

Neurologic: weakness, confusion, delirium, psychoses, seizures.

12. What should be the hemodynamic goals for resuscitation of patients in severe sepsis or septic shock?

The hemodynamic goals most commonly used include the following:
- Perfusion pressure (mean arterial pressure [MAP] > 65 mmHg)
- Central venous pressure: 8–13 mmHg
- Cardiac index > 2.5 L/min/m²
- Pulmonary artery occlusion pressure (PAop): 12–19 mmHg
- Urinary output > 0.5 ml/kg/hr

13. How should fluids, pressors, and blood products be used to meet these goals?

1. The most important initial therapy is early, adequate fluid resuscitation. No data show an improvement in mortality rates with the use of colloids vs. crystalloids.

2. If the fluid-resuscitated patient is still hypotensive, pressor therapy should be initiated to achieve a MAP of 60–65 mmHg. A recent small cohort study reported significant improvement in mortality rates when norepinephrine is used instead of high-dose dopamine in patients with septic shock; thus, norepinephrine is probably the pressor of choice. No data indicate that dopamine (in low or high doses) confers renal protection or improves mortality rates. Vasopressin is approved by the FDA only for use in the advanced cardiac life support algorithm and and currently has no role in the management of septic shock. Some patients may require addition of dobutamine if cardiac output is very low, but few data support a specific oxygen delivery target.

3. Multicenter trials have shown that outcome is no worse in patients with hemoglobin concentrations of 7.0–9.0 gm/dl compared with patients transfused to keep the hemoglobin concentration between 10 and 12 gm/dl. The exception to these recommendations is patients with coronary heart disease, in whom an optimal hemoglobin concentration is probably closer to 10 gm/dl.

14. Discuss the goals of oxygenation in patients with sepsis.

The bulk of evidence from numerous studies suggests that inducing supranormal oxygen delivery with inotropes either does not improve or worsens outcome. One recent prospective, randomized trial reported significant improvement with attempts to achieve a balance between supply and demand as determined by central venous oxygen saturation. The goals for oxygenation included central venous oxygen saturation > 70% and arterial oxygen saturation > 90%. The investigators transfused blood to a hematocrit no higher than 30% and provided pressor support to a cardiac index of 2.5 L/min/m² with dobutamine and low-dose dopamine. Therapy was initiated on the patient's arrival at the emergency department, whereas most centers start aggressive hemodynamic management after arrival in the intensive care unit. This study and others like it may pose new questions for the choice of pressor and the optimal hematocrit for septic patients.

15. Should a pulmonary artery (PA) catheter be used in patients with sepsis?

Controversial. Recent meta-analyses found no increase or decrease in mortality rates associated with the use of PA catheters. In patients with septic shock, cardiac output is expected to be high and systemic vascular resistance is expected to be low. Most clinicians and centers use PA catheters to follow a specific trend (mixed venous oxygen saturation or correlation of wedge pressure to cardiac index or urine output) or to answer a specific question:
- Does the patient have left-sided myocardial dysfunction?
- Does the patient have renal failure or an abnormal response to a fluid challenge?
- Does the patient have right-sided heart failure or pulmonary hypertension?

It should be kept in mind that the PA catheter is merely a monitor—not a therapy. If significant benefit cannot be provided by the information obtained from the catheter, the patient is exposed to the risks of catheterization for no sound reason.

16. What guidelines for respiratory management can improve outcome in septic patients?

The lungs are the most common organ system to fail in septic patients, many of whom eventually require mechanical ventilation. The lungs are the most likely source of initial infection, and patients are at great risk for nosocomial and ventilator-associated pneumonias. Pulmonary hygiene and strict attention to the management of pneumonia, effusions, empyemas, and other pulmonary diseases is essential to improving outcome.

The recent definitions and guidelines for management of acute lung injury (ALI) and acute respiratory distress syndrome (ARDS) have made a significant impact on identification of patients with these disorders. Diagnosis of ALI and ARDS are based on the following criteria: bilateral infiltrates, $PaO_2/FiO_2 < 300$ (ALI) or < 200 (ARDS), and no evidence of a cardiac source (e.g., left atrial hypertension) for respiratory distress. Volutrauma caused by large tidal volumes not only leads to release of inflamatory mediators (e.g., IL-6) that can provoke a septic response but also allows translocation of bacteria across damaged alveolar membranes. The ARDS Network (a multicenter organization aimed at treating ARDS) has identified a protective ventilation strategy, based on lower tidal volumes and use of positive end-expiratory pressure (PEEP), that significantly decreases the mortality rate of patients with ARDS. According to their study, patients with ALI or ARDS should be ventilated with a tidal volume of 6 ml/kg ideal body weight.

Another technique to decrease the number of days on the ventilator and the incidence of pneumonia and sepsis is the use of daily trials of spontaneous breathing (as opposed to pressure support or intermittent ventilation) to wean patients from ventilator dependence. Nearly all patients with respiratory failure should have such trials; if the trials are successful, patients should be extubated (see Chapters 10 and 23).

17. What guidelines for nutrition and gastrointestinal management should be kept in mind?

Many of the recommendations for nutrition and GI prophylaxis in critically ill patients also apply to septic patients. Septic patients are in a hypercatabolic state and often have difficulty in using glucose stores. In addition, some cases of sepsis cause an ileus, which is exacerbated by the use of sedatives and narcotics. Enteral feedings improve nutritional and immunologic status compared with starvation or total parenteral nutrition. A feeding tube should be considered early in the course of admission to intensive care. Recent studies have shown a lower risk for aspiration and a lower incidence of associated pneumonia and sinusitis with jejunal feedings (vs. gastric feeding tube placement) and reduction in nasogastric instrumentation. To decrease the incidence of stress ulceration, GI bleeding, and bacterial translocation, H_2 blockers, proton pump inhibitors, and sucralfate (alone or in combination) are now commonplace treatments in most critically ill patients, although the optimal agent is not known.

18. Discuss the prevention and management of venous thromboemoblism.

The interaction of the inflammatory, coagulative, and fibrinolytic pathways in sepsis leads to thrombosis (deep venous thrombosis, pulmonary embolism, disseminated intravascular coagulation). When possible, prophylaxis should include subcutaneous heparinization, compression stocking, or use of an inferior vena cava filter. A high level of suspicion for thrombogenic process is essential to improve patient care.

19. What new therapies have emerged? Have any therapies aimed at coagulation been useful?

Activated protein C (APC) is a vitamin K-dependent anticoagulant activated by the complex of thrombin and thrombomodulin. It inactivates coagulation factors Va and VIIIa (with the help of protein S) in the coagulation cascade, reduces plasmin-activating inhibitor 1 to promote fibrinolysis, and decreases tumor necrosis factor alpha and the endothelial adhesion of leukocytes in the inflammatory pathways. Proteins C and S levels have been found to be reduced in sepsis, and depletion of APC has been found to correlate with the severity of sepsis syndrome. A recent large, randomized, prospective study of the use of APC in patients with severe sepsis and septic shock demonstrated a significant decrease in inflammatory cytokines, D-dimer, and mortality rates. APC recently was approved for clinical use by the FDA. Significant side effects include a 3–5% incidence of bleeding secondary to its anticoagulant-like effects.

Tissue factor pathway inhibitor (TFPI) and **antithrombin III** showed promise in phase II clinical trials as strategies for modulating the coagulation pathway but have been unsuccessful in large phase III trials.

Continuous venovenous hemofiltration (CVVH) has been considered as a strategy for removing harmful plasma factors from patients with sepsis. To date, the recommendations for use of hemodialysis and CVVH have not expanded to include sepsis, and both have inherent risks and side effects. CVVH, however, is useful for management of renal failure in hypotensive patients with septic shock (see Chapter 45).

20. Why have no therapies directed at binding inflammatory mediators been successful?

Numerous products have been tried to block or promote many of the pro- and anti-inflammatory cytokines involved in sepsis. To date, none have successfully reduced mortality rates if given after the infectious insult, although some have shown positive results if given before a known infectious insult in the laboratory. Currently there are two perceptions of the basic problem: (1) the inflammatory process may be too intricate to be controlled by a single anti-inflammatory agent, and (2) it may be vital to the immune system for all circulating cytokines to be present and functioning to some extent.

21. Do steroids have a role in the treatment of sepsis?

Various studies have evaluated the role of steroids and other immunosuppressive therapies in the treatment of sepsis. To date, few data indicate a significant benefit from use of steroids. Most study groups have been of insufficient size to lend confirm reports of beneficial effects. A significant minority of septic patients, who are refractory to pressor use because of underlying adrenal insufficiency, may obtain benefit from steroids—if they can be identified for treatment. The classic description is a hemodynamically compromised patient, refractory to all pressors, who exhibits a dramatic stabilizing response to steroid administration.

BIBLIOGRAPHY

1. Acute Respiratory Distress Network: Ventilation with lower tidal volumes as compared with traditional volumes for acute lung injury and the acute respiratory distress syndrome. N Engl J Med 342:1301–1308, 2000.
2. American Heart Association: Emergency Cardiovascular Care. Dallas, American Heart Association, 2000.
3. Angus DC, et al: Epidemiology of severe sepsis in the United States: Analysis of incidence, outcome, and associated costs of care. Crit Care Med 29:1303–1309, 2001.
4. Balk RC, et al: Pathogenesis and management of multiple organ dysfunction or failure in severe sepsis and septic shock. Crit Care Clin 16:337–352, 2000.
5. Bernand G, et al: Efficacy and safety of human activated protein C for severe sepsis. N Engl J Med 344, 2001.
6. Bernand GR: The National Heart, Lung, and Blood Institute and Food and Drug Administration Workshop Report: Pulmonary artery catheterization and clinical outcomes. JAMA 283:2568–2572, 2000.
7. Bochud PY, Glauser MP, Calandra T: Antibiotics in sepsis. Intens Care Med 27(Suppl 1):S33–S48, 2001.
8. Bone RC, et al: American College of Chest Physicians/Society of Critical Care Medicine Consensus Conference: Definitions for sepsis and organ failure and guidelines for the use of innovative therapies in sepsis. Chest 101:1644–1655, 1992.
9. Brun-Buisson C: Microbiology of sepsis. Intens Care Med 26:564–574, 2000.
10. Choi PT, Yip G, Quinonez LG, Cook DJ: Crystalloids vs. colloids in fluid resuscitation: A systematic review. Crit Care Med 27:200–210, 1999.
11. DeWitt, et al: The gut's role in metabolism, mucosal barrier function, and gut immunology. Infect Dis Clin North Am 13:465–481, 1999.
12. Emanuele R, et al: Early goal directed therapy in the treatment of sepsis and septic shock. N Engl J Med 345:1368–1378, 2002.
13. Gropper M: A momentary pause [editorial]. Br J Anesth 86(6):746–748, 2001.
14. Herbert PC, et al: A multicenter, randomized, controlled trial of transfusion requirements in critical care. N Engl J Med 340:409–417, 1999.
15. Jimenez MF: Source control in the management of sepsis. Intens Care 27(Suppl): S49–S62, 2001.
16. Krieger BP, Isber J, Brietenbucher A, et al: Serial measurements of the rapid-shallow-breathing index as a predictor of weaning outcome in elderly medical patients. Chest 112:1029–1034, 1997.
17. Martin C, Viviand X, Leone M, Thirion X: Effect of norepinephrine on the outcome of septic shock. Crit Care Med 28:2758–2765, 2000.
18. Mermel LA, et al: Management guidelines for catheter infections. CID 32:1249, 2001.

19. National Center for Health Statistics, 2001.
20. Opal SM, et al: Clinical trials for severe sepsis: Past failures and future hopes. Infect Dis Clin North Am 13:285–297, 1999.
21. Rangel-Faustino MS, et al: The natural history of SIRS. JAMA 273:117–123, 1995.
22. Surgenor SD, et al: Hemofiltration in sepsis: Is removal of bad humors the answer? [editorial]. Crit Care Med 28:3751–3752, 2000.
23. Tobin M: Advances in mechanical ventilation. N Engl J Med 344:1986–1996, 2001.
24. Veenstra DL: Efficacy of antiseptic-impregnated central venous catheters in preventing catheter-related bloodstream infection: A meta-analysis. JAMA 281:261–267, 1999.
25. Warren BL, et al: High-dose ATIII (KyberSept Trial). JAMA 286:15, 2001.
26. Wheeler AP, Bernard GRL Treating patients with severe sepsis. N Engl J Med 340:207–214, 1999.

34. ENDOCARDITIS

Ira M. Dauber, M.D.

1. How do you know whether a patient has endocarditis?

Endocarditis is usually a bacteremic febrile illness. Positive blood cultures are the sine qua non of endocarditis. Clinically both cardiac and extracardiac manifestations occur. A new regurgitant heart murmur is the most common characteristic cardiac finding. Congestive heart failure due to valvular dysfunction (usually regurgitation), myocardial invasion with abscess formation (often signaled by bundle branch), and heart block can occur. Extracardiac manifestations are due to embolization (both septic and nonseptic emboli) and immune-complex manifestations (e.g., glomerulonephritis).

Two or more sets of blood cultures should be collected. In the absence of other sources of bacteremia, positive blood cultures are diagnostic. The presence of valvular vegetations on an echocardiogram is strongly suggestive of endocarditis but not diagnostic for active disease (they may be old). An echocardiogram without vegetations or valvular abnormalities makes the diagnosis of endocarditis unlikely. Endovascular infections such as endocarditis should be strongly considered in patients with the combination of fever and new-onset heart failure or a new regurgitant heart murmur and in patients with continuous bacteremia.

2. Do negative blood cultures rule out endocarditis?

No. Approximately 10% of patients with endocarditis may have "culture-negative" endocarditis. Prior antibiotic therapy is the most common cause of negative blood cultures. Slow growing or fastidious organisms (nutritionally deficient bacteria, fungi, *Chlamydia* sp.) and right-sided endocarditis (up to 22% of cases) are also associated with culture-negative endocarditis. Some patients with culture-negative endocarditis are not infected and have nonbacterial thrombotic (marantic) endocarditis.

3. What type of heart murmur is usually associated with endocarditis?

Regurgitant murmurs (aortic, mitral, or tricuspid regurgitation) secondary to valvular injury are the most common murmurs. Valvular stenosis is rarely due to endocarditis, but it is more likely in prosthetic than native valve endocarditis. In many patients, a murmur may not audible. Acute and severe mitral and aortic insufficiency may have short murmurs, which are further obscured by tachycardia. Tricuspid or pulmonic insufficiency murmurs can be difficult to appreciate on exam. Echocardiography with Doppler is a valuable method for evaluating and detecting cardiac murmurs due to endocarditis.

4. Are acute and subacute endocarditis different diseases?

No. Time course and clinical features can vary in relation to the aggressiveness of the underlying bacteriologic agent. Acute endocarditis has a rapid onset (days to weeks) and progresses as an acute toxic febrile illness with major cardiac symptoms, including congestive heart failure, valvular insufficienc,y and conduction abnormalities. In contrast, subacute endocarditis is an indolent, chronic (weeks to months) illness associated with weight loss, malaise, persistent fever, heart murmur, and anemia, which may or may not present with cardiac manifestations. Peripheral manifestations such as splenomegaly, hematuria, Osler nodes, Janeway lesions, and Roth spots are more common with subacute endocarditis.

5. How do right-sided and left-sided endocarditis differ? Does the difference matter?
They differ in the location of the infected valve (tricuspid or pulmonic vs. aortic or mitral), which leads to important clinical differences. Left-sided endocarditis is more common overall. Left-sided valvular dysfunction has greater hemodynamic consequences and is more likely to be associated with congestive heart failure. Left-sided lesions are associated with systemic embolization (brain, kidney, spleen). Right-sided endocarditis is more common with IV drug abuse. Right-sided lesions embolize to the lung, presenting as lung abscess, pneumonia or pulmonary emboli. Right-sided endocarditis may not be associated with an audible murmur (one-third of cases), usually has few peripheral manifestations, and is more likely to be culture-negative.

6. Which valves are most commonly affected?
The answer depends on the etiology of the endocarditis:
• Native valve (acute or subacute): mitral > aortic > tricuspid.
• Prosthetic valve: aortic > mitral
• Fungal: right > left-sided valves
• IV drug abuse: right > left-sided valves

7. What is nonbacterial thrombotic endocarditis (NTBE)?
NTBE (marantic) endocarditis is a condition in which platelet-fibrin deposits form on cardiac valves in patients with endothelial injury of the valve and a hypercoagulable state but without infection. Valvular dysfunction can develop as with infectious endocarditis. Predisposing conditions include malignancy, systemic lupus erythematosus, disseminated intravascular coagulation, uremia, burns, and intracardiac catheters.

8. Describe the initial approach to the treatment of endocarditis.
The importance of obtaining a specific microbiologic diagnosis cannot be overemphasized; antibiotic therapy should be delayed until adequate numbers of blood cultures have been obtained. The hemodynamic consequences of endocarditis can be severe. Specific therapy tailored to the observed hemodynamic alterations should be initiated as soon as possible. Empirical antibiotic therapy can be started for acute endocarditis before isolation of a causative organism. Initial intravenous therapy with penicillin, a beta-lactamase resistant penicillin (e.g., nafcillin), and an aminoglycoside provides effective empirical therapy for the majority of patients. Because of the increased frequency of methicillin-resistant staphylococci in IV drug abusers and prosthetic valve infections, vancomycin should be substituted for the penicillins.

9. What organisms most commonly cause endocarditis?
This answer also depends on the etiology of the endocarditis:
• Native valve (acute): *Streptococcus* sp.   30–45%
                          Staphylococcus aureus   15–35%
                          Enterococci   10-20%
• Native valve (subacute): usually *Streptococcus viridans*
• Prosthetic valve infections: *S. aureus* and *Staphylococcus epidermidis*
• IV drug abusers: *S. aureus* and gram-negative organisms
• Fungal : *Candida* sp.

10. Discuss the antimicrobial approach to treating endocarditis.
Native valve bacterial endocarditis: Usually responds to antibiotic treatment alone. Treatment with bactericidal antibiotics is required usually for 4–6 weeks. Choice of specific antibiotics is based on the isolated organism(s). Commonly used choices include the following:

- Streptococci (nonenterococcal): penicillin G
- Enterococci: penicillin G + gentamicin
- Staphylococci (methicillin-sensitive): nafcillin or oxacillin + gentamicin
- Staphylococci (methicillin-resistant): vancomycin
- Gram-negative: penicillin/cephalosporin + aminoglycoside (depends on organism)

Fungal endocarditis: Because of their poor outcome with medical therapy alone, patients with fungal endocarditis usually require surgical intervention. Intravenous antifungal therapy (amphotericin B + 5-fluorocytosine) should be initiated and continued postoperatively.

Prosthetic valve endocarditis: Early (< 2 months after insertion) and late prosthetic valve endocarditis are treated differently. Early infections are more commonly due to *S. epidermidis*, gram-negative organisms, and diptheroids. Initial therapy with vancomycin and gentamicin is indicated. Late infections have a similar spectrum to native valve endocarditis.

Culture-negative endocarditis: For acute endocarditis, initial therapy with vancomycin and gentamicin aimed at the bacterial causes of culture-negative endocarditis can be initiated. Further therapy is aimed at likely causes based on the clinical situation. In patients at risk for fungal endocarditis (immunosuppression, prior use of broad-spectrum antibiotics, fungal infection elsewhere) or in whom empirical antibiotics result in no clinical improvement, amphotericin B + 5-fluorocytosine should be added. For subacute endocarditis, therapy should be withheld until there is a specific diagnosis.

Note: Therapy should be modified for patients with penicillin allergy or renal dysfunction.

11. Are there any new "bugs" to worry about?

New bugs are here. HACEK group members (*Haemophilus, Actinobacillus, Cardiobacterium, Eikenella, and Kingella* spp.) are isolated in up to 10% of new cases of endocarditis. Previous therapy for these uncommon organisms consisted of ampicillin and gentamicin for 4 weeks. The American Heart Association now recommends treatment with ceftriaxone, 2 gm/day intramuscularly or intravenously for 4 weeks, because many of these organisms have become resistant to ampicillin. Ampicillin plus gentamicin is appropriate if the organism is sensitive to ampicillin.

12. Have any old bugs developed new tricks? What should I do?

Enterococci have become increasingly resistant to penicillin, aminoglycosides, and vancomycin. Management strategies include the following:

- Early in vitro testing is crucial for selecting antimicrobial therapy.
- Unusual antibiotic combinations may be needed (e.g., flouroquinolones and rifampin).
- Effective combinations are unlikely to be found for organisms resistant to penicillin G and vancomycin; consider suppression with chloramphenicol or tetracycline and early surgery.

13. What are the indicators of poor outcome or high mortality rate in endocarditis?

Native valve infections usually respond to adequate antibiotic treatment. Prosthetic valve and fungal infections have a lower response and higher mortality rates. The presence of congestive heart failure, involvement of the aortic or a prosthetic valve, systemic embolization, large (> 10 mm) vegetations, or an infecting organism other than streptococci are associated with a worse outcome. Neurologic events or immunosuppression due to HIV increase the risks. The mortality rate for *S. viridans and bovis* is 4–16%; for enterococci, 15–25%; for *S. aureus,* 25–47%; and for gram-negative or fungal organisms, > 50%.

14. How do I recognize treatment failure?

Treatment failure is evident as persistent infection, progressive cardiac dysfunction, or persistent hemodynamic instability. Failure to eradicate the infection may be due to emergence of resistant organisms, unsuspected multiple organisms (especially in IV drug abusers), inadequate drug levels, and/or the presence of a perivalvular or myocardial abscess. Fever usually resolves within 1 week of treatment. Persistent fever may be due to other causes besides treatment failure (drugs, immune-complex nephritis, thrombophlebitis). Despite successful treatment of the infection, hemodynamic instability may continue because of severe valve injury and the limited ability of the heart to compensate for acute volume overload (e.g., with aortic or mitral regurgitation).

15. What are the late consequences of endocarditis despite successful treatment?
Embolization risk can persist for up to 6 months (until endothelialization of vegetations and injured endocardial surfaces is complete). Mycotic aneurysms can present months or years after an episode of endocarditis. Congestive heart failure may develop due to persistent valve dysfunction.

16. Which cardiac conditions are associated with endocarditis? Is antibiotic prophylaxis recommended by the American Heart Association (AHA) for all of these conditions?
High risk for endocarditis (prophylaxis recommended)
• Prosthetic heart valves (including bioprostheses and homografts)
• Complex cyanotic congenital heart disease (e.g., tetralogy of Fallot, transposition)
• Previous infectious endocarditis
• Surgically constructed systemic or pulmonary shunt
Moderate risk for endocarditis (prophylaxis recommended)
• Other congenital heart disease (except low-risk type listed below)
• Acquired valvular heart disease (e.g., rheumatic or calcific disease)
• Hypertrophic cardiomyopathy
• Mitral valve prolapse with regurgitation and/or thickened valve leaflets
Negligible risk for endocarditis (prophylaxis *not* recommended)
• Mitral valve prolapse without regurgitation
• Atrial septal defect (isolated secundum type)
• Surgically repaired atrial or ventricular septal defect and patent ductus arteriosus
• Cardiac pacemakers/implanted defibrillators
• Prior coronary artery bypass surgery
• Trivial valvular regurgitation on echocardiography without structural abnormality
• Previous rheumatic or Kawasaki disease without residual valvular dysfunction
• Physiologic, functional, or innocent heart murmurs

17. List the common procedures for which the AHA recommends antibiotic prophylaxis for patients at risk for endocarditis. Which procedures do not require prophylaxis?

Prophylaxis recommended	Prophylaxis not recommended
• Esophageal dilation/sclerotherapy of varices	• Gastrointestinal endoscopy with or without biopsy*
• Cystoscopy/urethral dilation	• Laparoscopy
• Rigid bronchoscopy	• Flexible bronchoscopy with or without biopsy
• Vaginal delivery if infection present	• Vaginal delivery in absence of infection
• Urethral catheterization if urinary infection present	• Urethral catheterization in absence of urinary infection
• Complex dental procedures (bleeding likely)	• Simple dental procedures (bleeding unlikely)
• Incision and drainage of infected tissue	• Endotracheal intubation
• Urinary tract surgery including prostate	• Cardiac catheterization
• Gallbladder surgery	• Transesophageal echocardiography
• GI surgery involving intestinal mucosa	• Cesarean section
• Tonsils, adenoids, upper respiratory mucosa surgery	• Tympanostomy tube insertion

* Prophylaxis optional for high-risk procedures.

18. Which antibiotics does the AHA recommend for effective prophylaxis?
For dental, oral, respiratory tract, or esophageal procedures

Standard prophylaxis	Amoxicillin, 2 gm orally 1 hour before procedure
Inability to take oral medications	Ampicillin, 2 gm intramuscularly or intravenously within 30 min before

Penicillin allergy	Clindamycin, 600 mg orally 1 hour before, *or*
	Cephalexin, 2 gm orally 1 hour before, *or*
	Cephadroxil, 2 gm orally 1 hour before, *or*
	Azithromycin, 500 mg orally 1 hour before, *or*
	Clarithromycin, 500 mg orally 1 hour before
Penicillin allergy and inability to take oral medications	Clindamycin, 600 mg intravenously within 30 min before, *or* Cefazolin, 1 gm intramuscularly or intravenously within 30 min before

For genitourinary or gastrointestinal (excluding esophageal) procedures

High risk	Ampicillin, 2 gm intramuscularly or intravenously, *and*
	Gentamicin, 1.5 mg/kg within 30 min before *and*
	6 hr later, ampicillin, 1 gm intramuscularly or intravenously *or* amoxicillin, 1 gm orally
High risk and penicillin allergy	Vancomycin, 1 gm intravenously, *and* Gentamicin, 1.5 mg/kg intravenously, completed within 30 min before
Moderate risk	Amoxicillin, 2 gm orally 1 hour before, *or* Ampicillin, 1 gm intramuscularly or intravenously within 30 min before
Moderate risk and penicillin allergy	Vanocomycin, 1 gm IV completed within 30 min before

19. Discuss the role of echocardiography in the diagnosis and treatment of endocarditis.

Echocardiography (transthoracic [TTE] or transesophageal [TEE]) has evolved from a previously controversial to a currently important role in the evaluation of patients with suspected endocarditis. It is also helpful in assessing the ongoing treatment of established endocarditis. Although echocardiography alone should not be used to rule out endocarditis, it can be used to determine the presence of vegetations and/or regurgitant valvular lesions TTE has a 60–70% sensitivity for vegetations, but imaging may be inadequate in up to 20% of patients. TEE is more sensitive (75–95%) than TTE for detecting abnormalities associated with endocarditis; TEE also has excellent specificity (75–95%), especially for evaluation of prosthetic valve endocarditis (85–98%).

A negative TTE effectively rules out endocarditis if the clinical pretest probability of endocarditis is low. In patients with intermediate pretest probability, the initial use of TEE is more efficient, because a negative TTE does not exclude endocarditis and a follow-up TEE is necessary. A negative TEE has a 92% negative predictive value and is clinically satisfactory to rule out endocarditis. TEE should be used for the initial assessment of all cases of suspected prosthetic valve endocarditis because of the poor imaging usually obtained with TTE.

In established endocarditis, echocardiography can be used to assess ongoing treatment, look for evidence of treatment failure, and measure the effects of valvular dysfunction on myocardial function. Serial echocardiograms can measure the presence, size, and number of vegetations. Evidence of treatment failure, such as myocardial abscess, perivalvular extension of infection, or enlarging vegetation size, also can be imaged. Myocardial dysfunction, which may require valve replacement regardless of the success of treatment of the infection, can be diagnosed early. TEE is generally more useful than TTE for this purpose.

20. Discuss the role and optimal timing of surgery in the management of endocarditis.

Indications for surgery are based on clinical criteria, type of valve (native or prosthetic), and infecting organism. The role of surgery continues to expand in the treatment of endocarditis as operative mortality improves and antibiotic-resistant organisms are more often involved.

Clinical indications for surgery, regardless of organism or valve type, are hemodynamic instability (moderate-to-severe heart failure due to valvular insufficiency or obstruction), uncontrolled infection (persistent bacteremia, lack of an effective antimicrobial regimen), intramyocardial or perivalvular extension of infection, and recurrent emboli after appropriate antibiotic therapy.

The infecting organism also plays a role in the need for surgery. Organisms likely to require surgery are fungi (regardless of valve type), gram-negative organisms (with native valve dysfunction or on any prosthetic valve), enterococci without available bactericidal therapy, staphylococcal infection of a prosthetic valve, and relapse after optimal therapy.

Prosthetic valve infections are more likely to require surgery than native valve infections. In addition to the above indications, surgery is indicated for prosthetic valve endocarditis with an unstable prosthesis, large (>10 mm) or hypermobile vegetations, and culture-negative endocarditis with persistent (> 10 days) fever. Large native valve vegetations are a borderline indication for surgery; most patients do not embolize.

Timing of surgery is determined by the indication(s). **Emergent surgery** (within hours) is indicated for unstable prosthetic valves or refractory congestive heart failure. **Early surgery** (2–7 days) is indicated for hemodynamically unstable patients, uncontrolled infection, and vegetations with recurrent systemic emboli. Early surgery has been suggested for patients with large vegetations (because of the increased risk for subsequent emboli) and with infections unlikely to respond to medical therapy alone (fungal or nonstreptococcal infections, prosthetic valve infections). Prolonged courses of ineffective antibiotic therapy are associated with poor survival if surgery is necessary (10% survival rate after 4–6 weeks of therapy vs. 83% if surgery is performed within 10 days of starting therapy). Hemodynamic status at the time of surgery is the most important predictor of outcome. Thus, early surgery can reduce the risks of progressive hemodynamic deterioration in patients who need (or will need) surgery.

The placement of a foreign body into an infected surgical field is not without problems. Postoperative endocarditis occurs in up to 10% of patients with active infections at the time of surgery, and the incidence of valve dehiscence is higher without prior antibiotic therapy. In hemodynamically stable patients, a 7- to 10-day course of antibiotics before surgery seems reasonable. In patients with neurologic injury, a 10-day delay may reduce the risk of intracranial hemorrhage. A 21-day delay in surgery is recommended for patients with intracranial hemorrhage.

CONTROVERSY

21. Is antibiotic prophylaxis recommended for mitral valve prolapse?

Prophylaxis has been recommended because mitral valve prolapse is the most common predisposing factor for native valve endocarditis. It accounts for 10–30% of new cases. However, it is present in 2–4% of the overall population(more often in young women). Thus, antibiotic prophylaxis presents a considerable public health problem. The relative risk of endocarditis with mitral valve prolapse is low: an estimated 0.5 per 10,000 patient years, which is comparable to the risk of endocarditis in the general population. Increased risk of endocarditis is associated with presence of an audible mitral regurgitation murmur, age > 45 years, systemic hypertension, and male sex. The presence of mitral regurgitation is associated with a 10-fold increase in the risk of endocarditis. That risk is comparable to the risk of isolated bicuspid aortic valve but still 100-fold less than the risk of underlying rheumatic valvular disease.

Conclusion: Prophylaxis is recommended for high-risk mitral valve prolapse: prolapse with mitral regurgitation or with echocardiographically definite myxomatous valve abnormalities. It is not recommended for mild abnormalities without valvular dysfunction.

BIBLIOGRAPHY

1. Bayer AS, Bolger AF, Taubert KA, et al. Diagnosis and management of infective endocarditis and its complications. Circulation 98:2936–2948, 1998.
2. Bonow RO, Carabello B, de Leon AC, et al: Guidelines for the management of patients with valvular heart disease: ACC/AHA Task force on Practice Guidelines. J Am Coll Cardiol 32:1486–1503, 1998.
3. Cheitlin MD, Alpert JS, Armstrong WF, et al: ACC/AHA guidelines for the clinical application of echocardiography: Executive summary. J Am Coll Cardiol 29:862–879, 1997.
4. Dajani AS, Taubert KA, Wilson W, et al: Prevention of bacterial endocarditis. Recommendations by the American Heart Association. Circulation 96:358–366, 1997.

5. Delay D, Pellerin M, Carrier M, et al: Immediate and long-term results of valve replacement for native and prosthetic valve endocarditis. Ann Thorac Surg 70:1219–1226, 2000.
6. Karchmer AW: Infective endocarditis. In Braunwald E (ed): Heart Disease: A Textbook of Cardiovascular Medicine, 5th ed. Philadelphia, W.B. Saunders, 1997, pp 1077–1104.
7. Kaye D: Treatment of infective endocarditis. Ann Intern Med 124:606–608, 1996.
8. Lick SD, Zwischenberger JB: Endocarditis: When to operate? ACC Curr J Rev 12:21–23, 1995.
9. Li JS, Sexton DJ, Mick N, et al: Proposed modifications to the Duke criteria for the diagnosis of infective endocarditis. Clin Infect Dis 30:633–638, 2000.
10. Mylonakis E, Calderwood SB: Infective endocarditis in adults. N Engl J Med 345:1318–1330, 2001.
11. Wilson WR, Karchmer AW, Dajani AS, et al: Antibiotic treatment of adults with infective endocarditis due to streptococci, enterococci, staphylococci, and HACEK microorganisms. JAMA 274:1706–1713, 1995.

35. MENINGITIS

David Lehman, M.D., Ph.D., and Randall Reves, M.D.

1. What clinical and pathophysiologic features distinguish meningitis from other central nervous system infections?

Meningitis is an infection localized to the subarachnoid space, resulting in varying degrees of meningismus. The inflammatory process may involve the entire leptomeningeal surface of the brain and spinal cord and spread through the foramina of Luscha and Magendie to produce ventriculitis. With meningitis, neurologic dysfunction is usually limited to depressed sensorium and seizures. Focal cerebral signs or cranial nerve defects are seen in 14–20% of cases and result from the inflammation surrounding cranial nerves that traverse the subarachnoid space or increased intracranial pressure. Subdural empyema or epidural abscess within the cranium or spinal canal, brain abscess, encephalitis, myelitis, and neuritis tend to produce more localized signs or symptoms than those seen with meningitis.

2. What signs and symptoms should place meningitis in the differential diagnosis?

Symptoms of a recent upper respiratory infection followed by the development of headache, nuchal rigidity, vomiting, confusion, or lethargy should always prompt consideration of acute meningitis. The classic triad of fever, neck stiffness, and altered mental status is present in about half of cases. Symptoms are often more subtle in infants, the elderly, or patients who develop meningitis associated with neurosurgical procedures.

3. What are the differences in acute, subacute and chronic presentations of meningitis?

Individuals presenting with a rapidly progressive illness of less than 24 hours' duration usually have bacterial meningitis. The acute presentation is seen in about 25% of cases of bacterial meningitis. A subacute presentation of up to 7 days' duration is seen in nearly all cases of meningitis due to viruses and in three-quarters of cases due to bacteria. The distinction between the acute and subacute presentation has important diagnostic, therapeutic, and prognostic implications. Chronic meningitis is usually due to tuberculosis or fungi and has a more gradual onset of meningeal symptoms or even presents as dementia.

4. When should one make an exception to the adage "If you think of doing a spinal tap, do one"?

Lumbar punctures generally should be avoided in the presence of brain abscess or other localized brain lesions in which the risk for herniation is deemed significant. Precautions should also be taken to avoid passing the spinal needle through an infected area such as infected skin or through an epidural abscess. In some situations, neurosurgical consultation may be required to sample cerebrospinal fluid (CSF) via cervical or cisternal approaches. Correction of severe coagulopathies or thrombocytopenia may be required before performing a spinal tap.

5. **When should a CT scan be done before a spinal tap in a patient presenting with meningitis?**
CT scanning is **not** needed before a spinal tap in most patients with suspected meningitis—only those at risk for mass lesions. The risk factors for mass lesions are age over 65 years; history of central nervous system (CNS) disease, immunosuppression, or seizure (in the past seven days); and physical findings of papilledema, focal neurologic deficits, or unconsciousness. To avoid critical delays in therapy, empirical therapy can be initiated immediately after obtaining blood cultures. The spinal tap can be done if the CT scan has resolved the issue of a mass lesion.

6. **What is the goal of initiation of antibiotic treatment in patients with bacterial meningitis?**
The goal is to begin appropriate therapy within 1 hour of patient contact. Delays in treatment can be expected to increase the frequency of death and neurologic complications in survivors. Achieving this 1-hour goal is difficult, requiring rapid recognition, triage, and initation of treatment.

7. **In addition to prompt, effective treatment, what determines prognosis for community-acquired bacterial meningitis?**
The etiologic agent is important. Fatality rates are 11% for cases due to *Neisseria meningitidis*, 24% for cases due to *Streptococcus pneumoniae*, and up to 40% for cases due to *Listeria monocytogenes*. Hypotension at presentation, seizures, and altered mental status are independent predictors. Poor outcomes are noted in 9%, 33%, and 56% of patients with none, one, or more than two of these factors, respectively.

8. **What CSF findings in meningitis should prompt initiation of antimicrobial therapy?**
Patients with an acute, rapidly progressive course should receive empirical therapy, pending analysis of CSF results. In subacute presentations, indications for and choice of antimicrobial therapy should be based on prompt assessment of CSF studies as well as clinical and epidemiologic features. Gram stains of spun sediment of CSF are positive in 80–90% of culture-documented cases of meningitis and usually provide rapid information about likely etiologic agents. In the presence of negative Gram stain, analysis of other CSF parameters can be used to assist in the decision concerning empirical therapy. CSF cell count > 1000/mm^3, protein > 150 mg/dl, or glucose < 30 mg/dl indicates a high probability of bacterial meningitis rather than a viral etiology and warrants appropriate antimicrobial therapy, pending the results of cultures and other studies. None of these guidelines alone or in combination can be used to rule out bacterial etiologies or preclude antimicrobial therapy; clinical judgment, frequent reassessment, and repeat spinal taps may be indicated. Bacterial antigen tests appear to have no useful diagnostic value.

9. **How are CSF findings interpreted in the setting of prior antimicrobial therapy?**
Up to 50% of patients with meningitis present after having received up to several days of antimicrobial therapy, usually by the oral route. Prior antimicrobial therapy reduces the frequency of positive cultures. Several days of therapy are generally required to alter the high CSF cell count and the low glucose levels in patients with bacterial meningitis.

10. **What recent changes have occurred in the likely bacterial pathogens causing meningitis?**
Bacterial meningitis has become primarily an adult disease. In 1995 the median age was 25 years for patients with meningitis due to the five major pathogens (*S. pneumoniae, N. meningitidis*, group B streptococci, *L. monocytogenes,* and *Haemophilus influenzae*). In 1986 children between 1 month and 5 years of age accounted for two-thirds of the cases of bacterial meningitis. Between 1986 and 1995, the rate of meningitis declined in this age group as a result of *H. influenzae* type b vaccine. *S. pneumoniae* causes the majority of adult cases. The prevalence of penicillin resistance among pneumococci has increaesd in recent years, and penicillin can no longer be considered the first choice for empirical therapy of bacterial meningitis in adults.

11. What is the role of empirical therapy in meningitis?

An etiologic diagnosis should be obtained in the great majority of cases of bacterial meningitis, and initial empirical therapy should be continued, altered, or discontinued after results of CSF studies and other clinical data are available.

12. What are the likely bacterial pathogens causing meningitis and recommended antimicrobial agents for empirical therapy when the CSF Gram stain is nondiagnostic?

To treat immunocompetent patients for the most common bacteria, *S. pneumoniae*, *H. influenzae* or *N. meningitidis*, a broad-spectrum cephalosporin (cefotaxime or ceftriaxone) is the preferred antibiotic. In patients at increased risk for *S. agalactiae* or *L. monocytogenes*, specifically infants under 3 months or adults over 50 years of age, ampicillin should be added to the cephalosporin. Patients who are immunocompromised have increased risk for *L. monocytogenes* and gram-negative bacilli and should receive ampicillin plus ceftazidime. Staphylococci and gram-negative bacilli are more common in cases developing after head trauma or neurosurgical procedures; empirical therapy should include vancomycin and ceftazidime.

13. What are the recommended antimicrobial agents for meningitis when Gram stain or culture identifies common bacterial pathogens?

In recent years recommendations have changed for patients whose CSF contains gram-positive cocci. Treatment should be initiated with vancomycin plus ceftriaxone (cefotaxime for neonates), pending susceptibility testing of the *S. pneumoniae*. Penicillin G is the treatment for gram-negative cocci, *N. meningitidis*. For gram-positive bacilli (*L. monocytogenes*), ampicillin plus gentamicin is recommended. Gram-negative bacilli are initially treated with a broad-spectrum cephalosporin (cefotaxime or ceftriaxone) plus an aminoglycoside. For head trauma or neurosurgery patients, ceftazidime is the preferred broad-spectrum cephalosporin. Cefotaxime or ceftriaxone is recommended for *H. influenzae* because of decreased rates of subsequent hearing loss.

14. How long should therapy for bacterial meningitis be continued?

Meningitis due to *N. meningitidis* and *H. influenzae* should be treated for 7 days in most cases, and follow-up spinal taps are not routinely done. The recommended duration of therapy for *S. pneumoniae* is 10 days. The suggested duration for *L. monocytogenes* and *S. agalactiae* is 14–21 days. For gram-negative bacilli other than *H. influenzae*, 21 days of therapy are recommended.

15. What is the role for repeat spinal taps in the management of meningitis?

Routine follow-up spinal taps are not necessary for the typical cases of pneumococcal or meningococcal meningitis. Patients who fail to respond clinically should be reassessed, especially those with gram-negative bacilli, and consideration should be given to intrathecal aminoglycosides, in particular for *P. aeruginosa*.

16. What are the causes of recurrent meningitis?

Recurrent bacterial meningitis can result from persistent unrecognized or undrained parameningeal foci. Recurrence can also result either from abnormal communications with the upper respiratory tract or skin or from immunologic defects. CSF leaks into the nasopharynx, middle ear, or paranasal sinuses can result from congenital defects or be acquired following trauma; pneumococci are the usual etiologic organism, except in patients receiving antibiotics, who are more likely to acquire gram-negative bacilli. Recurrent meningitis from a variety of organisms, including gram-negative bacilli, can result from infected dermal sinuses that communicate with the subarachnoid space, usually in the lumbosacral region. Immunologic defects associated with recurrent meningitis include splenectomy, hypogammaglobulinemia, and inherited deficiencies of complement components.

17. Which studies are mandatory and which should also be considered in evaluation of the aseptic meningitis syndrome?

Aseptic meningitis is a syndrome of meningitis with negative Gram stains and cultures and typically a normal CSF glucose. It is not synonymous with viral meningitis. Secondary syphilis and "parameningeal foci" may produce CSF pleocytosis; parameningeal foci include localized suppurative processes in or adjacent to the meninges. Bacterial endocarditis may also present as aseptic meningitis. The evaluation of aseptic meningitis should always include blood cultures and serum rapid plasma reagin (RPR) or Venereal Disease Research Laboratory (VDRL) test. Testing of CSF alone is inadeqate, because CSF is usually negative in secondary syphilis. Sinus radiographs should be considered in all cases, and CT or MRI scans of the head or spine may be indicated in some instances to rule out brain abscess, epidural abscess, and subdural empyema as parameningeal foci.

Tuberculosis, fungi, and some fastidious organisms, such as *Leptospira, Borrelia,* and *Brucella* species, may present with the aseptic meningitis syndrome and require specific additional testing for diagnosis. Patients with aseptic meningitis and hypoglycorrhachia following fresh-water exposure may be at risk for parasitic meningitis due to *Naegleria* sp. Rocky Mountain spotted fever should be considered in potentially exposed patients presenting with symptoms of meningitis and CSF studies that are normal or suggestive of aseptic meningitis.

18. What are the noninfectious causes of meningitis?

The clinical presentation of meningitis can result from inflammatory reactions to intrathecal medications or from systemically administered drugs such as trimethoprim/sulfamethoxazole or nonsteroidal anti-inflammatory agents. A murine monoclonal antibody, OKT3, and azathioprine have been associated with meningitis in transplant recipients. Other noninfectious causes include carcinomatosis (usually with hypoglycorrhachia), inflammatory reactions to necrotic tumors, Mollaret's syndrome, sarcoidosis, and connective tissue diseases. A slowly leaking cerebral aneurysm may be responsible for aseptic meningitis with xanthochromic CSF.

19. What form of empirical therapy should always be considered in chronic meningitis?

Acid-fast smears and cultures of CSF are negative in up to 90% and 60% of patients, respectively, in case series of tuberculous meningitis. To avoid sequelae associated with delays in diagnosis and treatment of tuberculous meningitis, and pending 6-week culture results and evaluation of clinical response, empirical therapy should be considered in any chronic, undiagnosed cases of meningitis, especially in patients at risk for tuberculosis (e.g., birth in a developing country, chest x-rays compatible with tuberculosis). The "typical" cell and chemical parameters are notoriously nonspecific in tuberculous meningitis, and normal levels of CSF glucose do not exclude the diagnosis.

20. In the patient infected with HIV, what meningitides should be considered in the differential diagnosis?

Cryptococcal meningitis and aseptic meningitis (possibly caused by HIV) are the most common HIV-related meningitides. Other etiologies include tuberculosis, syphilis, herpes simplex, histoplasmosis, coccidioidomycosis, metastatic lymphoma, and *L. monocytogenes*. The relative risk of purulent meningitis is 150 times greater in HIV-infected patients than in the general population.

21. How sensitive are India ink examination and cryptococcal antigen testing for cryptococcal meningitis?

The sensitivity of India ink examination of CSF for the diagnosis of cryptococcal meningitis is 50%. Cryptococcal antigen testing of CSF is positive in 85%, and the sensitivity is increased to 94% by testing both CSF and serum. Cryptococci are the most common cause of meningitis in patients with AIDS, occurring in about 3%. In the setting of AIDS, it is common to find little or no indication of inflammation in the CSF.

22. How contagious is meningitis?

Among adults, meningococcal meningitis is the only bacterial agent in which risk of disease transmission has been documented. Among household members, the risk of secondary cases within a month of onset of the index case has been determined to be < 1% (about 6 per 1000). Although cases have been reported among medical personnel caring for patients with meningococcal disease, the risk is probably considerably lower than that among household members. Two days' treatment with rifampin or a single dose of oral ciprofloxacin is recommended for household or other intimate contacts to interrupt nasopharyngeal carriage. Prophylactic therapy may be offered to those with intense exposure, such as occurs in performing intubation, but is not indicated for medical personnel in general. Cases should be reported promptly to the local/state public health department, which can be very helpful in locating individuals who should receive prophylaxis. The enteroviruses that cause the majority of cases of viral meningitis are contagious, but most infected contacts are either asymptomatic or manifest febrile illnesses other than meningitis.

CONTROVERSIES

23. What is the role of steroids in bacterial meningitis?

For meningitis caused by *H. influenzae*, type b among children, dexamethasone has been shown to reduce adverse neurologic outcomes, particularly hearing loss. Dexamethasone has not been shown to be beneficial for pneumococcal or meningococcal meningitis, but only a small number of patients have been studied. The long-term adverse effects of dexamethasone on children have not been studied. Studies of dexamethasone use in experimental penicillin-resistant pneumococcal meningitis show reduced CSF levels of ceftriaxone and vancomycin and decreased clearance of pneumococci from CSF cultures. Some experts recommend adding rifampin to ceftriaxone for therapy of penicillin-resistant pneumococci if steroids are used. The changing spectrum of bacterial meningitis (decreased incidence of *H. influenzae* and increased drug-resistant pneumococcus) adds to the uncertainty concerning any recommendation of routine dexamethasone use. Among adults, bacterial meningitis is usually due to *S. pneumoniae* or *N. meningitidis*, and steroid use is controversial. Some experts recommend steroids in adults with papilledema or increased intracranial pressure. If steroids are used, a 2-day course of dexamethasone at 0.15 mg/kg every 6 hours may be optimal; treatment should be started before or shortly after the first dose of antibiotics.

24. When should *N. meningitidis* vaccine be used?

Vaccination is recommended for epidemic conditions, defined by a threshold of 15 cases/100,000 population per week for two consecutive weeks. In a meningitis outbreak, close contacts should be given chemoprophylaxis and also vaccinated if the serogroup of the incident case is included in the vaccine. Close contacts include boy- or girlfriend(s), daycare center members, and anyone who frequently sleeps and eats in the same housing unit with the index patient.

BIBLIOGRAPHY

1. Attia J, Hatala B,Cook DJ, Wong JG: Does this adult patient have meningitis? JAMA 282:175–181, 1999.
2. Carpenter RR, Petersdorf RG: The clinical spectrum of bacterial meningitis. Am J Med 33:262–275, 1962.
3. Hasbun R, Abrahams J, Jekel J, Quagliarello VJ: Computed tomography of the head before lumbar puncture in adults with suspected meningitis. N Engl J Med 345:1727–1733, 2001.
4. Hirschmann JV: Bacterial infections of the central nervous system. In Dale DC, Federman DD (eds): Scientific American Medicine. New York, Scientific American, 2001, section xxxvi, pp 1–16.
5. Hussein AS, Shafran SD: Acute bacterial meningitis in adults: A 12-year review. Medicine (Baltimore) 79:360–368, 2000.
6. McIntyre PB, Berkey CS, King SM, et al: Dexamethasone as adjunctive therapy in bacterial meningitis: A meta-analysis of randomized clinical trials since 1988. JAMA 278:925–931, 1997.
7. Morris A, Low DE: Nosocomial bacterial meningitis, including central nervous system shunt infections. Infect Dis Clin North Am 13:735–750, 1999.
8. Quagliarello VJ, Scheld WM: Treatment of bacterial meningitis. N Engl J Med 336:708–716, 1997.
9. Schuchat A, Robinson K, Wenger JD: Bacterial meningitis in the United States in 1995. N Engl J Med 337:970–976, 1997.
10. Tunkel AR, Scheld WM: Acute meningitis. In Mandell GL, Bennett JE, Dolin R (eds): Principles and Practice of Infectious Diseases, 5th ed. New York, Churchill Livingstone, 2000, pp 959–997.

36. URINARY TRACT INFECTIONS

Raymond N. Blum, M.D., and Kathleen D. Liu, M.D., Ph.D.

1. What are the risk factors associated with urinary tract infection (UTI) in the ICU?

Approximately 80% of nosocomial UTIs are associated with catheterization. The rate of acquisition of bacteriuria with a catheter in place is about 5–10% per day, with about 50% of patients bacteriuric by day 8. Other known risk factors include female sex, diabetes, and absence of systemic antibiotic use.

2. What is the pathogenesis of a catheter-related UTI?

Most catheter-related UTIs begin with colonization of the meatus and urethra, followed by an ascending infection. Some are related to colonization of the collection system and an intraluminal, ascending infection. Occasionally, bacteremic seeding of the kidneys can occur.

3. When should presence of a UTI be considered in a critically ill patient?

Signs and symptoms in a critically ill patient are often subtle but can include fever, leukocytosis, bacteremia, and lower abdominal and low-back pain. Of all nosocomial infections, 30% are infections of the urinary tract. Thus, in evaluating a hospitalized patient for infection, the clinician must pay attention to the urinary tract. The urinary tract is the source of nosocomial sepsis and bacteremia in up to 15% of cases.

4. How is the diagnosis of UTI established?

The gold standard of bacteriuria has been $\geq 10^5$ cfu/mm^3 in a urine culture. However, the presence of this level of bacteriuria may represent only colonization. Also, in ambulatory women, as few as 10^2 cfu/mm^3 have been associated with a true infection. In catheterized patients, most with low concentrations of bacteria will progress over a few days to $\geq 10^5$ cfu/ml. Supporting evidence of a true infection (in a non-neutropenic patient) is the presence of pyuria or hematuria as well as signs and symptoms.

5. What organisms are likely to be involved in UTI in catheterized patients?

The likely pathogens depend on the length of catheterization and the use of antimicrobial agents. Immediately after catheterization, gram-positive organisms such as *Staphylococcus epidermidis* and *Staphylococcus aureus* can be seen. Otherwise, *Escherichia coli*, *Klebsiella*, and enterococci are more common. Resistant gram-negative organisms, such as those from the *Serratia*, *Proteus*, and *Pseudomonas* species, are more common in patients receiving broad-spectrum antimicrobials.

6. What are the complications of UTI?

Complications of nosocomial UTI include fever, pyelonephritis, perinephric abscess, bacteremia, sepsis, metastatic infections, and death. A three-fold increase in mortality is associated with UTI from an indwelling catheter in hospitalized patients. About 1% of hospitalized patients with nosocomial UTI experience bacteremia. Catheter-associated UTI has been shown to increase hospital stays by 2–3 days. Metastatic infections can include endocarditis, especially in patients with valvular heart disease, osteomyelitis, and epidural abscess. In males, infections of the epididymis and testes can occur.

7. When is therapy indicated?

Therapy is indicated for all episodes of symptomatic bacteriuria. Treatment of episodes of asymptomatic bacteriuria without the removal of the catheter may lead to the emergence of resistant organisms. Therapy may be indicated for asymptomatic bacteriuria under special circumstances, including patients undergoing urologic or other significant surgical procedures in which prostheses may be left in place as well as patients at high risk for serious complications (e.g., pregnant women, neutropenic patients, organ transplant recipients).

8. What antimicrobial agents should be used?

Initial empirical therapy in patients with evidence of sepsis should include agents that are active against both gram-positive and gram-negative organisms, such as vancomycin or ampicillin, and a third-generation cephalosporin or an aminoglycoside. Alternatively, a fluroquinolone with good urinary concentration, such as ciprofloxacin, may be considered. Therapy can be guided additionally by a Gram stain of the urine. Coverage should be narrowed as quickly as possible based on susceptibility testing. Therapy for mild symptoms may include oral agents such as trimethoprim/sulfamethoxazole.

9. What should be done with the catheter during infections?

If no longer required, the catheter should be removed. If there are leaks or evidence of obstruction in the catheter system, it should be replaced. Use of a condom catheter or intermittent catheterization should be considered.

10. What are the risk factors associated with candiduria?

Candiduria is associated with broad-spectrum antimicrobials, catheterization, diabetes, corticosteroids, female sex, and stasis of urine. A systemic fungal infection must always be considered when candiduria is found. Candiduria has been reported in up to 5–10% of catheterized patients.

11. How should candiduria be managed?

Removal of the catheter is paramount to the elimination of candiduria. If this is not possible, bladder irrigation can be used. The role of systemic antifungal therapy, including amphotericin and fluconazole, should be reserved for serious infections or when there is evidence of systemic fungal infection. If candiduria does not resolve after catheter removal, the urinary tract is evaluated for obstruction. Treatment of asymptomatic candiduria in a catheterized patient may be replaced by bacteriuria.

12. What is the role of bladder irrigation in managing candiduria?

Irrigation of the bladder with amphotericin using a triple-lumen catheter can help to decrease candiduria. This is usually done with a solution of 50 mg of amphotericin/L of D5W instilled either as a continuous infusion over 24 hours for 5–7 days or instilling 200–300 ml and clamping the catheter for 60–90 minutes at regular intervals for 5–7 days. It is especially useful when short-term catheterization is anticipated.

13. What are key features in preventing nosocimial UTI?

Elimination of unnecessary use of catheterization in the intensive care unit is the most important measure in decreasing the incidence of nosocomial UTIs. Aseptic insertion, meticulous care to avoid breaching the closed system, use of sterile technique in obtaining all urine specimens, and not changing the catheter unless obstruction or malfunction occurs can help to decrease the risk of UTI. Follow-up urinalysis and culture should be done in all catheterized patients.

CONTROVERSIES

14. Is there a role for amphotericin bladder irrigation in treating candiduria?

For: Bladder irrigation with amphotericin is a safe and effective method for control of candiduria. Cure rates of up to 90% have been reported. The urine may be a source of both upper tract infections and dissemination of candidal organisms.

Against: Candiduria may represent colonization in a catheterized patient on broad-spectrum antibiotics. Treatment of this colonization without catheter removal leads to replacement with bacteria (often more resistant organisms). In addition, candiduria may represent dissemination and should be treated with a systemic agent such as fluconazole.

15. Should asymptomatic bacteriuria in short-term catheterized patients be treated?

For: There is a significant risk of bacteremia and sepsis in catheter-related bacteriuria. Hospital mortality is increased in patients with catheter-associated bacteriuria, and there is a 10–20% risk of UTI associated with an indwelling catheter even if it is removed. Absence of antimicrobial therapy is associated with bacteriuria sooner in catheterized patients.

Against: It is virtually impossible to maintain sterile urine in patients who require catheterization. Treating episodes of asymptomatic bacteriuria will lead to colonization with more resistant and perhaps more virulent organisms such as Pseudomonas and Serratia. If followed with daily urine cultures, most patients who develop symptomatic bacteriuria do so on the first day that bacteriuria is detected.

BIBLIOGRAPHY

1. Fisher JF, Chew WH, Shadomy S, et al: Urinary tract infections due to *Candida albicans*. Rev Infect Dis 4:1107–1118, 1982.
2. Fisher JF, Newman CL, Sobel JD: Yeast in the urine. Solutions for a budding problem. Clin Infect Dis 20:183–189, 1995.
3. Garibaldi RA, Burke JP, Britt MR, et al: Meatal colonization and catheter-associated bacteriuria. N Engl J Med 303:316–319, 1980.
4. Garibaldi RA, Burke JP, Dickman ML, Smith CB: Factors predisposing to bacteriuria during indwelling urethral catheterization. N Engl J Med 291:215–219, 1974.
5. Givens CD, Wenzel RP: Catheter-associated urinary tract infections in surgical patients: A controlled study on the excess morbidity and costs. J Urol 124:646–648, 1980.
6. Jacobs LG, Skidmore EA, Cardoso LA, et al: Bladder irrigation with amphotericin B for treatment of fungal urinary tract infections. Clin Infect Dis 18:313–318, 1994.
7. Krieger JN, Kaiser DL, Wenzel RP: Urinary tract etiology of bloodstream infections in hospitalized patients. J Infect Dis 148:57–62, 1983.
8. Kunin CM: Care of the urinary catheter. In Detection, Prevention and Management of Urinary Tract Infections, 4th ed. Philadelphia, Lea & Febiger, 1988.
9. Platt R, Polk BF, Murdock B, Rosner B: Risk factors for nosocomial urinary tract infections. Am J Epidemiol 124:977–985, 1986.
10. Platt R, Polk BF, Murdock B, Rosner B: Mortality associated with nosocomial urinary-tract infection. N Engl J Med 307:637–642, 1982.
11. Saint S, Lipsky BA: Preventing catheter-related bacteriuria. Arch Intern Med 159:800–808, 1999.
12. Schaeffer AJ: Catheter-associated bacteriuria. Urol Clin North Am 13:737–747, 1986.
13. Turck M, Stamm W: Nosocomial infection of the urinary tract. Am J Med 70:651–655, 1981.
14. Wagenheimer FME, Naber KG: Hospital-acquired urinary tract infections. J Hosp Infect 46;171–181, 2000.
15. Warren JW: Catheter-associated urinary tract infections. Infect Dis Clin North Am 1:823–854, 1987.

37. DISSEMINATED FUNGAL INFECTIONS

Mark W. Bowyer, M.D.

1. How common are fungal infections in hospitalized patients?

The total number of fungal infections in hospitalized patients increased from 6% in 1980 to 10.4% in 1990 and may be as high as 20% in some hospitals in 2002.

2. Why has the incidence of fungal infections increased so dramatically?

Fungi generally do not cause invasive infection in healthy people. Increases in the number of patients with immunosuppression due to cancer, chemotherapy, transplantation, or HIV infection; use of vascular and urinary catheters; and use of broad-spectrum antibiotics have led to an explosion of deep-seated funal infections in clinical practice.

3. Which fungi are responsible for invasive infections in humans?

Over 250 fungal species have been reported to produce human infections. Nearly 80% of these infections are caused by *Candida* species. *C. albicans* is the most common (60–90% of all candidal infections). *C. tropicalis, C. glabrata*, and *C. krusei* account for the most of the remainder. The other major cause of human infection are the *Aspergillus* species, which account for 15–20% of fungal infections. Rarer causes of infection in humans include *Histoplasma, Blastomyces, Torulopsis, Fusarium, Scedosporium, Cryptococcus, Tricosporon, Rhizopus*, and *Rhizomucor* species.

4. List the risk factors for disseminated fungal infection.

1. Prolonged, multiple (≥ 3), or broad-spectrum antibiotics
2. *Candida* sp. isolated from multiple sites other than blood
3. Hemodialysis
4. Foreign bodies (central venous, arterial, or urinary catheters)
5. Age > 40 years
6. Immunocompromise
   - Diabetes mellitus
   - Serum glucose > 200 mg/dl
   - HIV
   - Hematologic malignancy
   - Immunosuppressive therapy (for cancer or organ transplant)
   - Acute renal failure
   - Steroid therapy
   - Parenteral nutrition (especially with high lipid content)
7. Deep abdominal surgery
8. Severe trauma
   - Second- and third-degree burns
   - Severe head injury
   - Multiple organ system trauma
9. Serious infection
   - Gram-negative sepsis
   - Acute peritonitis
   - Intra-abdominal abscess
10. Care in the ICU (especially with mechanically ventilation)

Low risk = < 3 risk factors, high risk = ≥ 3 risk factors.

5. List the diagnostic criteria for disseminated fungal infection.

Definitive: (1) fungus cultured from tissue, (2) burn wound invasion, (3) endophthalmitis, or (4) fungus cultured from peritoneal fluid.

Suggestive: (1) two positive blood cultures ≥ 24 hours apart (without a central line) or two positive blood cultures with the second obtained 24 hours after the removal of a central line, or (2) three confirmed colonized sites.

6. How reliable are these criteria?

The above criteria are positive in only 30–50% of patients with disseminated fungal infection.

7. If disseminated candidiasis is suspected, where should you look for it?

In blood cultures, on the retina (endophthalmitis), on heart valves (endocarditis), in bones (osteomyelitis), in wounds, and in the liver, spleen, or kidneys (renal abscesses and candiduria).

8. What is the overall mortality rate associated with candidemia?

The overall mortality rate associated with candidemia is 40–60%, with an attributable mortality rate of 38%.

9. Should antifungal therapy be delayed until blood cultures are positive for fungus?

No. Blood cultures have been found to be only 40–68% sensitive. Systemic antifungal therapy should be strongly considered, especially in a patient that is at high risk for disseminated fungal infection, under the following conditions:

1. A fever persists despite antibiotics and negative blood cultures.
2. High-grade funguria occurs in the absence of a bladder catheter.
3. Funguria persists after the removal of a bladder catheter.
4. Fungus is cultured from at least two body sites.
5. Visceral fungal lesions are confirmed.

10. How do the antifungals work?

Fluconazole and itraconazole, which are triazoles, are fungistatic. They inhibit C-14 α-demethylase, a cytochrome p450-dependent fungal enzyme required for the synthesis of ergosterol, the major sterol in the fungal cell membrane. This alters cell membrane fluidity, thereby decreasing nutrient transport, increasing membrane permeability, and inhibiting cell growth and proliferation. Amphotericin B, a polyene, is fungicidal. It binds irreversibly to ergosterol (but not to cholesterol, the major sterol in mammalian cell membranes), creating a membrane channel that allows leakage of cytosol, which leads to cell death. Flucytosine is used in conjunction with amphotericin B and has synergistic action against *Candida* and *Cryptococcus* species. Flucytosine acts directly on fungal organisms by competitive inhibition of purine and pyrimidine uptake.

11. Compare the efficacy of fluconazole and amphotericin B for treatment of candidemia.

Randomized multicenter trials in non-neutropenic patients have found no statistically significant difference in the efficacy of fluconazole and amphotericin B in terms of clearing fungemia or survival at the end of therapy. Meta-analysis has shown that fluconazole treats candidemia more successfully than amphotericin B in neutropenic patients.

12. What advantages does fluconazole offer over amphotericin B in the treatment or prevention of disseminated fungal infections?

1. Fluconazole is available in both intravenous (IV) and oral (PO) forms. Patients have been successfully treated with 7 days of IV fluconazole, followed by the oral form, if the patient is capable of oral ingestion. able. PO administration is easier and less costly than IV administration.
2. Fluconazole is not nephrotoxic and has fewer overall adverse effects than amphotericin B, which can cause hypokalemia, fever, and chills.
3. Systemic fluconazole is equally effective against fungal urinary tract infections (UTIs) as amphotericin B bladder irrigation but has fewer of the above adverse effects.

13. Are there any limitations to the use of fluconazole?

Yes. Fluconazole is not active against *Aspergillus* sp. or *Candida krusei*, whereas itraconazole and amphotericin B are. Also, fluconazole may cause hepatotoxicity, increase phenytoin and cyclosporine levels, and potentiate the anticoagulant effects of warfarin. Nonetheless, fluconazole has fewer overall adverse effects than amphotericin B.

14. What should be done when a candidal infection fails to respond to fluconazole?

If the diagnosis is confirmed, the underlying risk factors have been minimized, the drug regimen is being administered correctly, the dosage has been maximized (up to 800 mg/day), and drug-drug interactions are ruled out (rifampin decreases fluconazole levels), the next step is to try another azole such as itraconazole. Amphotericin B is a less desirable alternative, but no one should hesitate to use it for life-threatening infections that do not respond to other treatments.

15. Are less toxic forms of amphotericin B available?

Yes. To reduce the toxicity associated with amphotericin B, lipid formulations have been produced. The earliest and most widely studied is Ambisome, which in randomized trials was shown to be safer than amphotericin B with many fewer side effects. Other lipid-associated, nonliposomal products include amphotericin B lipid complex (Abelcet) and amphotericin B colloidal dispersion (Amphocil), both of which appear to be similar to Ambisome in efficacy and toxicity. The disadvantage of these alternative forms is their currently high cost.

16. What new antifungal drugs are currently under investigation?

Two classes of antifungal compounds are currently in late-stage clinical trials: new, improved triazoles and inhibitors of glucan synthesis. The new triazoles include voriconazole and ravuconazole, which have improved potency against a much broader spectrum of clinically relevant fungal species. Both are active orally; voriconazole also can be administered intravenously.

A group of compounds known as candins are derivatives of naturally occurring antibiotics that cause osmotic fragility and lysis of fungal cells. Candins are potently fungicidal, and several semisynthetic derivatives are under development for clinical use. Caspofungin (Cancidas) has received FDA approval for patients with aspergillosis who are refractory to or intolerant of standard therapies. Anidulafungin and micafungin are in phase II trials for the treatment of candidiasis and aspergillosis.

17. How can health care providers help prevent the spread of fungal colonization in the ICU?

Easily. Wash hands and wear gloves when working directly with patients. *Candida* species were found on the hands of 33–75% of ICU staff in one study.

BIBLIOGRAPHY

1. Anaissie EJ, Darouiche RO, Abi-Said D, et al: Management of invasive candidal infections: Results of a prospective, randomized, multicenter study of fluconazole versus amphotericin B and review of the literature. Clin Infect Dis 23:964–972, 1996.
2. Ascioglu S, dePauw BE, Meis JFGM: Prophylaxis and treatment of fungal infections associated with haematological malignancies. Int J Antimicrob Agents 15:159–168, 2000.
3. Boogaerts M, Maertens J: Clinical experience with itraconazole in systemic fungal infections. Drugs 61(Suppl 1):39–47, 2001.
4. Hann IM, Prentice HG: Lipid-based amphotericin B: A review of the last 10 years of use. Int J Antimicrob Agents 17:161–169, 2001.
5. Jarvis WR: Epidemiology of nosocomial fungal infections, with emphasis on *Candida* species. Clin Infect Dis 20:1526–1530, 1995.
6. Lewis RE, Kelpser ME: The changing face of nosocomial candidemia: Epidemiology, resistance, and drug therapy. Am J Health Syst Pharm 56:525–536, 1999.
7. Rabkin JM, Orloff SL, Corless CL, et al: Association of fungal infection and increased mortality in liver transplant recipients. J Surg 179:426–430, 2000.
8. Rex JH, Bennett JE, Sugar AM, et al: A randomized trial comparing fluconazole with amphotericin B for the treatment of candidemia in patients without neutropenia. N Engl J Med 331:1325–1330, 1994.
9. Tkacz JS, DiDomencio B: Antifungals: What's in the pipeline. Curr Opin Microbiol 4:540–545, 2001.
10. Verdun-Lunel FM, Meis JFGM, Voss A: Nosocomial fungal infections: Candidemia. Diagn Microbiol Infect Dis 34:213–220, 1999.

38. TOXIC SHOCK SYNDROMES

Mary Bessesen, M.D.

1. What are the toxic shock syndromes (TSSs)?

Two TSSs are commonly recognized, one caused by *Staphylococcus aureus*, the other by *Streptococcus pyogenes* (commonly called group A streptococci).

2. What are the cardinal clinical features of the TSSs?

Fever, hypotension, and multiorgan failure. A diffuse erythroderma that progresses to desquamation is commonly seen in staphylococcal TSS.

3. Describe the basic pathophysiology of the TSSs.

Bacterial endotoxins function as superantigens. Conventional antigens presented in the context of major histocompatibility molecules on antigen-presenting cells must be recognized by multiple elements of the T-cell receptor and stimulate 1/10,000 T cells. Superantigens are recongized by the **V chain** and may stimulate up to 20% of all T cells. The result is massive release of cytokines, leading to capillary leak syndrome.

4. What are the clinical differences between staphylococcal and streptococcal TSS?

Staphylococcal TSS is rarely associated with bacteremia, whereas streptococcal TSS is associated with bacteremia in 60–100% of cases. Soft tissue infections causing staphylococcal TSS may be clinically subtle; streptococcal TSS often is associated with myositis or necrotizing fasciitis. The mortality rate of staphylococcal TSS is less than 3%; the mortality rate of streptococcal TSS is 30–70%.

5. What risk factors predispose to staphylococcal TSS?

The classic case profile is a young (15–25 years old), menstruating female. However, any staphylococcal infection can predispose to TSS, including surgical wound infections, furuncles, and abscesses. Postpartum cases can occur after vaginal or cesarean delivery. Nasal reconstructive surgery carries an especially high risk of TSS. Cases also may occur after nasal packing for epistaxis.

6. What are the signs and symptoms of staphylococcal TSS?

The typical presentation includes high fever, rash, and confusion. There may be a prodrome of myalgias, vomiting, and diarrhea. Patients are listless, but focal neurologic findings are not seen. Examination of patients with menstruation-associated TSS reveals vaginal hyperemia and exudate that yields *S. aureus* on culture. In nonmenstrual cases, a careful examination usually reveals a focus of staphylococcal infection. It is important to note that this focus is frequently subtle. The drainage from a wound infection causing TSS may be only serous-appearing, rather than grossly purulent. This is a toxin-mediated disease, and the local appearance is not one of intensive purulence. Drainage of local infections is a key point in management.

7. How does nonmenstrual TSS differ from menstrual TSS?

Nonmenstrual TSS is much more often nosocomial, and renal and CNS involvement is much more common. Toxic shock syndrome toxin 1 (TSST-1) is produced by the isolates that cause most cases of menstruation-associated TSS. TSST-1 can be absorbed across intact mucous membranes. In cases not associated with menstruation, the majority of staphylococcal isolates also produce TSST-1; a substantial minority, however, produce staphylococcal enterotoxin B (SEB) or C (SEC). SEB and SEC are not absorbed across mucous membranes but can cause TSS in cases of staphylococcal infection of wounds.

8. What are the common laboratory findings in staphylococcal TSS?

Leukocytosis with marked left shift, thrombocytopenia, azotemia, sterile pyuria, and elevated transaminases are common but not invariable findings. Blood cultures are usually sterile, as are cerebrospinal fluid (CSF) cultures. Cultures of the local site of infection are usually positive for *S. aureus*.

9. Describe the treatment of staphylococcal TSS.

The primary intervention consists of fluid resuscitation and supportive care. Any focus of staphylococcal infection must be drained. In women, a vaginal examination must be performed as soon as the patient is stabilized and any foreign bodies (such as tampon or diaphragm) removed. After cultures of the local site and the blood are obtained, antistaphylococcal therapy should be administered intravenously. For nosocomial TSS or menstrual TSS in patients at high risk for carriage of oxacillin-resistant *S. aureus* (i.e., health care workers, nursing home residents, intravenous drug users), vancomycin should be used until culture and sensitivity results return. If an oxacillin-sensitive strain is recovered, therapy with oxacillin or nafcillin may then be substituted.

In community-acquired menstrual TSS with no risk factors for oxacillin-resistant *S. aureus*, initiation of therapy with oxacillin or nafcillin is appropriate. Based on in vitro evidence that clindamycin inhibits toxin production and animal data showing improved survival, many clinicians treat with clindamycin in addition to oxacillin, nafcillin, or vancomycin.

10. Can staphylococcal TSS recur?

Yes. After an episode of staphylococcal TSS, 50% of patients fail to mount a serum antibody response to TSST-1. As a result, recurrent episodes are seen.

11. What is the differential diagnosis of TSS?

Streptococcal scarlet fever, measles, leptospirosis, Rocky Mountain spotted fever, Stevens-Johnson syndrome, and Kawasaki's disease can mimic TSS. Multiorgan involvement is usually absent in streptococcal scarlet fever, and the primary focus yields *S. pyogenes*. Exclusion of measles, leoptospirosis, and Rocky Mountain spotted fever requires both a careful history for potential exposures and serologic testing. Stevens-Johnson syndrome is characterized by target lesions and is commonly associated with antecedent drug use. Kawasaki's disease is characterized by fever and rash without multisystem involvement. It is most commonly seen in children under the age of 6 years and is associated with thrombocytosis rather than thrombocytopenia.

12. Why do some people develop TSS when exposed to a toxin-producing strain whereas others do not?

The absence of preexisting antibody to the pertinent bacterial toxin appears to be a critical host factor in TSS. Among patients with menstruation-associated TSS, 90% have no preexisting antibody to TSST-1. In contrast, more than 90% of healthy people over the age of 25 years are seropositive. Lack of preexisting antibody to streptococcal pyrogenic exotoxins has been shown to be important in the pathophysiology of streptococcal TSS.

13. Discuss the role of intravenous immunoglobulin (IVIG) in streptococcal TSS.

In vitro evidence indicates that immunoglobulins neutralize superantigen activation of cytokine release by *S. pyogenes*. In addition, a case control study demonstrated a significantly improved outcome among patients treated with IVIG.

CONTROVERSY

14. What antibacterial agents should be used to treat streptococcal TSS?

Penicillin has maintained efficacy against S. pyogenes for decades. There is no evidence of emergence of resistance. Penicillin has been shown to reduce the incidence of rheumatic fever after streptococcal pharyngitis. Its narrow spectrum of activity reduces antimicrobial selective pressure in the intensive care unit. Penicillin is very well tolerated.

Clindamycin is also highly active *S. pyogenes*. In animal models of streptococcal myositis, clindamycin was more effective than penicillin. This finding may be due to greater activity against high burdens of organisms (inoculum effect). An alternative explanation is that inhibition of protein synthesis blocks toxin production by the pathogen and reduces production of tumor necrosis factor by the host. A case control study demonstrated improved outcomes among children with invasive *S. pyogenes* infections whose therapy included a protein synthesis inhibitor in the first 24 hours. The risk of *Clostridium difficile*-associated diarrhea is high among patients treated with clindamycin.

BIBLIOGRAPHY

1. Bartlett P, Reingold AL, Graham DR, et al: Toxic shock syndrome associated with surgical wound infections. JAMA 247:1448–1450, 1982.
2. Hoge CW, Schwartz B, Talkington DF, et al: The changing epidemiology of invasive group A streptococcal infections and the emergence of streptococcal toxic shock-like syndrome: A retrospective population-baesd study. JAMA 269:384–389, 1993.

3. Jacobson JA, Kasworm EM, Crass BA, Bergdoll MS: Nasal carriage of toxigenic *Staphylococcus aureus* and prevalence of serum antibody to toxic-shock syndrome toxin 1 in Utah. J Infect Dis 153:356–358, 1986.
4. Kaul R, McGeer A, Norby-Teglund A, et al: Intravenous immunoglobulin therapy for streptococcal toxic shock syndrome: A comparative observational study. The Canadian Streptococcal Study Group. Clin Infect Dis 28:800–807, 1999.
5. McCormick JK, Yarwood JM, Schlievert PM: Toxic shock syndrome and bacterial superantigens: An update. Annu Rev Microbiol 55:77–104, 2001.
6. Todd J, Fishaut M, Kapral F, Welch T: Toxic shock syndrome associated with phage-group-1 staphylococci. Lancet 2:1116–1118, 1978.
7. Zimbelman J, Palmer A, Todd J: Improved outcome of clindamycin compared with beta-lactam antibiotic treatment for invasive *Streptococcus pyogenes* infection. Pediatr Infect Dis J18:1096–1100, 1999.

39. HIV/AIDS IN THE INTENSIVE CARE UNIT

Kristina Crothers, M.D., Laurence Huang, M.D., and Leslie H. Zimmerman, M.D.

1. What is the most common indication for ICU admission in patients with human immunodeficiency virus infection/acquired immunodeficiency syndrome (HIV/AIDS)?

Acute respiratory failure accounts for 40–50% of ICU admissions. Other causes include central nervous system (CNS) dysfunction, sepsis, and gastrointestinal (GI) bleeding. Patients with HIV/AIDS also may be admitted to the ICU for reasons unrelated to immunodeficiency, such as asthma, chronic obstructive pulmonary disease (COPD), cardiac disease, metabolic alterations (diabetic ketoacidosis [DKA]), drug overdose, trauma, or postoperative care.

2. How has the spectrum of disease in patients with HIV/AIDS changed in the era of highly active antiretroviral therapy (HAART)?

HAART, a combination of potent antiretroviral therapies, including new protease inhibitors, was introduced in 1996. Subsequently, mortality rates have declined, and the incidence of opportunistic infections has decreased. Therefore, future studies may show that the spectrum of diseases requiring ICU admission has shifted toward diseases unrelated to immunodeficiency. Even in the era of HAART, however, some patients may be unaware of their HIV status and thus may not be on antiretroviral therapy. The initial diagnosis of HIV/AIDS may be made during an ICU admission.

3. What is the overall mortality rate of patients with HIV/AIDS in the ICU?

Before the introduction of HAART, the mortality rate in the ICU was 30–40%. The effect of HAART on mortality rates is as yet unclear.

4. What factors predict mortality in patients with HIV/AIDS in the ICU?

Mortality is related to several factors, including severity of acute illness and preadmission health status. Predictors of increased mortality rates include the need for mechanical ventilation and more severe disease at baseline (as assessed by different scoring systems, such as the simplified acute physiology score [SAPS I]). Patients with lower albumin values and a history of weight loss also may have a higher mortality rate. Although predictive of long-term mortality, CD4+ T-cell count has not been predictive of short-term mortality during ICU stays in studies done before the introduction of HAART.

5. What factors are relevant in patients on HAART therapy?

Antiretroviral medications have numerous drug interactions, resulting in toxic side effects and changes in drug levels. Common medications that can interact with antiretroviral therapies include antibiotics (fluoroquinolones, macrolides, and certain antifungal agents), antacids (H_2 blockers and proton pump inhibitors), and seizure medications (phenytoin, carbamazepine, and phenobarbital).

HIV-protease inhibitors in particular can have numerous interactions with drugs such as antiarrhythmics, sedatives, hypnotics, and statins. Each patient's medications should be reviewed carefully to prevent or minimize adverse effects when new therapies are initiated in the ICU.

In addition, some patients may experience a paradoxical worsening of an underlying opportunistic infection after starting HAART therapy. Diseases such as mycobacterial and cryptococcal infections, cytomegalovirus retinitis, and *Pneumocystis carinii* pneumonia (PCP) have been reported to worsen transiently after the initiation of HAART, presumably because of increased inflammatory responses related to immune reconstitution.

6. Which CD4+ T-cell count reflects a patient's risk for opportunistic infections: the current count or the nadir (lowest) count?

The current count reflects the current risk for opportunistic infections. It was initially unclear whether the rise in CD4+ T-cell count in response to antiretroviral therapy reflected a restoration of immune function. It is now clear, however, that immune function can be restored with HAART. Thus, primary and secondary prophylaxis for opportunistic infections can be safely stopped in most patients who have had a significant and sustained response to HAART. For example, primary and secondary prophylaxis against PCP can be stopped in patients who have responded to HAART with an increase in CD4+ T cells above 200 for at least 3 months. Primary prophylaxis against *Mycobacterium avium* complex (MAC) can be stopped in patients with an increase in CD4+ T cells above 100 for at least 3 months.

RESPIRATORY DISEASE

7. What is the most common cause of acute respiratory failure in patients with HIV/AIDS?

PCP is responsible in approximately 50% of cases. Other causes include the following:
   a. Infections
       i. Bacterial infections (most common pathogens: *Streptococcus pneumoniae*, *Haemophilus influenzae*, *Staphylococcus aureus*, *Pseudomonas aeruginosa*)
       ii. Mycobacterial infections (most common pathogen: *M. tuberculosis*)
       iii. Fungal infections (including *Cryptococcus neoformans* and *Aspergillus fumigatus*, and, in endemic areas, *Histoplasma capsulatum* and *Coccidioides immitis*)
       iv. Viral infections (including influenza, cytomegalovirus [CMV], herpes simplex virus [HSV], measles)
   b. Neoplasms
       i. Kaposi's sarcoma
       ii. Non-Hodgkin's lymphoma
       iii. Bronchogenic lung carcinoma
   c. Miscellaneous
       i. Pulmonary edema (noncardiogenic, cardiogenic)
       ii. Asthma/COPD
       iii. Pulmonary embolism
       iv. Lymphocytic interstitial pneumonitis (LIP) (rare in adults)
       v. Nonspecific interstitial pneumonitis (NIP)
       vi. Primary pulmonary hypertension

8. Name the most likely diagnosis in a patient with HIV/AIDS who presents with respiratory failure and the following signs, symptoms, and chest radiographic findings.
   a. Progressive dyspnea, dry cough, and fevers over several weeks; CD4+ T-cell count of 150; and diffuse pulmonary infiltrates without intrathoracic adenopathy or pleural effusions (Fig. 1).
   These findings are suggestive of PCP with a CD4+ T-cell count < 200. Other diseases to consider include bacterial (especially *Haemophilus influenzae*), fungal (especially *C.*

neoformans), mycobacterial, parasitic (especially *Toxoplasma gondii*), or viral (especially CMV) pneumonia, LIP/NIP, pulmonary edema, and pulmonary hemorrhage.

b. **Acute onset of fever, chills, and cough with purulent sputum; CD4$^+$ T-cell count of 350; and multilobar consolidation in the right lung** (Fig. 2).

These findings are suggestive of a bacterial, community-acquired pneumonia (CAP), especially since the CD4$^+$ T-cell count is > 200. Another major diagnosis to consider is tuberculosis. CAP is often complicated by parapneumonic pleural effusion in patients with HIV/AIDS.

c. **Progressive dyspnea, cough, fevers, and weight loss; CD4+ T-cell count of 50; and diffuse miliary pulmonary infiltrates with slightly enlarged hilar regions, suggestive of intrathoracic adenopathy** (Fig. 3).

These findings are suggestive of disseminated mycobacterial or fungal disease in a severely immunocompromised patient. Other diagnoses to consider include malignancy and, less commonly, PCP.

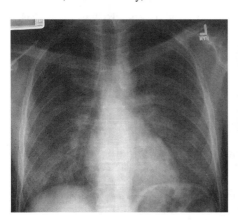

FIGURE 1

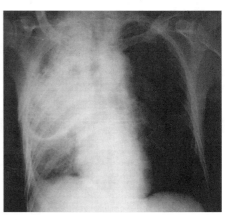

FIGURE 2

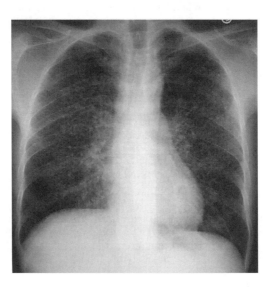

FIGURE 3

9. Describe the diagnostic work-up of respiratory failure in patients with HIV/AIDS.

Sputum and blood cultures should be obtained when a pulmonary infection is suspected. Sputum or tracheal aspirate specimens can be sent for Gram stain, acid-fast and fungal smears, and cultures. A routine expectorated sputum specimen is not as useful for diagnosing PCP. Blood cultures for bacterial, mycobacterial, and fungal pathogens should be ordered. A significant proportion of patients with AIDS have disseminated disease and positive blood cultures.

Thoracentesis should be considered for patients with pleural effusions. Pleural fluid should be sent for routine analysis and cultures. In patients with suspected non-Hodgkin's lymphoma, pleural fluid cytology is often diagnostic.

Sputum induction is a useful method to diagnose PCP. Because *P. carinii* cannot be cultured, the diagnosis of PCP relies on microscopic visualization of the characteristic cysts and trophozoites (trophic forms) on stained respiratory specimens. Unfortunately, in patients on high flow oxygen therapy, sputum induction is difficult, and in patients on mechanical ventilation, it is not technically feasible. In these critically ill patients, a more invasive diagnostic approach is necessary.

Bronchoscopy with bronchoalveolar lavage (BAL) is a sensitive method to diagnose pulmonary infections. Many institutions report a diagnostic sensitivity > 95–98% for PCP. In addition, bronchoscopy can diagnose mycobacterial, fungal, and some viral pathogens. Furthermore, approximately 15% of patients with pulmonary Kaposi's sarcoma do not have mucocutaneous involvement, and visual inspection of the tracheobronchial tree may be the first indication of the disease.

Nonbronchoscopic lavage using a control tipped catheter has successfully diagnosed PCP in mechanically ventilated patients and should be considered when bronchoscopy is unavailable.

Transbronchial biopsy allows microbiologic as well as pathologic examination of a small piece of lung tissue. It can lead to diagnosis of a number of diseases, including mycobacterial, fungal, and viral infections and neoplastic diseases. Some of these diseases require tissue confirmation for diagnosis. However, transbronchial biopsy also carries a risk of pneumothorax and therefore should not be performed unless other diagnostic modalities have been exhausted. Mechanical ventilation increases the risk for pneumothorax.

Open lung biopsy may be necessary for patients in whom the diagnosis remains elusive despite sputum and blood cultures and bronchoscopy. An open lung biopsy is rarely necessary to establish a diagnosis of PCP. Biopsy of an abnormal lymph node often yields a diagnosis of malignancy or mycobacterial or fungal infection; therefore, a thorough physical examination should be performed.

10. What are the treatment options for patients with PCP and respiratory failure?

Trimethoprim-sulfamethoxazole (TMP-SMX) administered intravenously is the treatment of choice (see below). TMP-SMX is a fixed combination drug and should be dosed at 15–20 mg/kg/day of the TMP component divided in 6- to 8-hour intervals. For patients unable to tolerate TMP-SMX, treatment options include intravenous pentamidine, intravenous clindamycin plus oral primaquine, or intravenous trimetrexate plus oral dapsone (combined with leucovorin). Unfortunately, no study has compared these three regimens. The choice of which regimen to use in the setting of either intolerance to TMP-SMX or perceived TMP-SMX treatment failure is unclear and often depends on clinician preferences.

Patients with moderate-to-severe PCP, defined as a room air arterial oxygen pressure ≤ 70 mmHg or an alveolar-arterial oxygen difference ≥ 35 mmHg, should receive adjunctive corticosteroids. Corticosteroid therapy instituted within 24–72 hours of PCP therapy can prevent the initial deterioration often seen in patients with PCP and reduces the rate of respiratory failure and death.

Establishing a definitive diagnosis is preferable to instituting empirical therapy for PCP. Empirical therapy has been associated with higher morbidity and mortality rates (presumably because of incorrect diagnoses). In critically ill patients with respiratory failure, the potential consequences of a missed or delayed diagnosis are considerable. Definitive diagnosis is always preferable.

Treatment Options for Moderate-to-Severe Pneumocystis carinii *Pneumonia*

TREATMENT OPTION	DOSE(S), ROUTE, FREQUENCY
Trimethoprim-sulfamethoxazole[1]	15–20 mg/kg (TMP) IV, divided every 6–8 hr
OR	
Pentamidine[2]	3–4 mg/kg IV once daily
OR	
Trimetrexate[3] +	45 mg/m^2 IV once daily +
Leucovorin ±	20 mg/m^2 PO every 6 hr ±
Dapsone[4]	100 mg PO once daily
OR	
Clindamycin[5] +	1800 mg IV, divided every 6–8 hr +
Primaquine (base)[6]	30 mg PO once daily
PLUS	
Prednisone	40 mg PO twice daily for 5 days, then
	40 mg PO once daily for 5 days, then
	20 mg PO once daily for 11 days

[1] Side effects include rash, pruritus, fever, nausea, vomiting, elevated liver enzymes, and neutropenia.
[2] Side effects include nephrotoxicity manifested by hyperkalemia, hypocalcemia, and hypomagnesemia, cytopenias (especially neutropenia and thrombocytopenia), and pancreatic toxicity manifested by hyper-amylasemia, hypoglycemia, and hyperglycemia.
[3] Side effects include neutropenia, rash, fever, and elevated liver enzymes.
[4] Side effects include rash, nausea, vomiting, hemolytic anemia (check glucose-6-phosphate dehydrogenase level), and methemoglobinemia.
[5] Side effects include rash, fever, nausea, vomiting, and diarrhea.
[6] Side effects include hemolytic anemia (check glucose-6-phosphate dehydrogenase level) and methemo-globinemia.

11. Does the development of pneumothorax in a mechanically ventilated patient with PCP portend a worse prognosis?

Yes. Data collected through the early 1990s suggest that the mortality of PCP-related acute respiratory failure requiring mechanical ventilation is around 75%. Of the subgroup of patients who develop pneumothorax while on mechanical ventilation, the mortality rate appears to be close to 100%.

12. How has the mortality from PCP-associated acute respiratory failure changed over the course of the AIDS epidemic?

The first data about the outcome of mechanical ventilation in patients with PCP and acute respiratory failure from the early to mid 1980s revealed dismal survival rates (0–13%). Beginning in 1987, several reports described an improved survival rate of 30-45%. The reasons for the improved outcome are unclear. Possible explanations include a change in the selection of patients admitted to the ICU, improved management in the ICU, increased use of adjunctive corticosteroids for moderate-to-severe PCP, and use of antiretroviral medication. Studies of data collected through the 1990s suggest that approximately 60–70% of patients with PCP-related acute respiratory failure survive to ICU discharge, but only about 30–40% survive to hospital discharge.

CENTRAL NERVOUS SYSTEM DYSFUNCTION

13. What are the most common causes of CNS dysfunction that require ICU admission?

CNS dysfunction requiring ICU admission is usually due to either mass lesions or meningitis, often resulting in coma or seizures. The most common causes of mass lesions are *T. gondii* infection and primary CNS lymphoma; the most common cause of meningitis is *C. neoformans* infection.

14. How does the development of CNS dysfunction affect the critical care of an HIV-infected person?

CNS dysfunction can affect a patient's ability to participate in making clinical decisions about care. Neurologic dysfunction also influences a patient's perceived quality of life.

15. Name the most likely diagnosis in a patient with HIV/AIDS who presents with neurologic changes and a focal lesion on CT scan of the head.

The most likely diagnosis is CNS lymphoma, followed by toxoplasmosis. Although toxoplasmosis usually causes multiple CNS lesions, it may present with a single lesion on CT scan (see question 16). Other possible causes include fungal, bacterial, and mycobacterial abscesses.

16. Describe the diagnostic work-up for this patient.

1. **Toxoplasma IgG.** CNS toxoplasmosis is believed to result from reactivation of latent infection, and the serum toxoplasma IgG is positive in ≥ 97% of cases. Therefore, it is an excellent screening test. Patients with a negative toxoplasma IgG (especially if only a single lesion is visible on CT scan) are unlikely to have CNS toxoplasmosis. In these cases, a diagnostic brain biopsy to evaluate for neoplastic and other infectious etiologies should be strongly considered. Patients with a positive toxoplasma IgG and a focal lesion on CT scan should probably undergo further neuroimaging (see below).

2. **Magnetic resonance imaging (MRI).** MRI is a more sensitive neuroimaging study than CT scan. An MRI often reveals multiple lesions when a CT scan revealed either no lesions or only a single lesion. The finding of multiple lesions (especially bilateral, ring-enhancing lesions that involve the basal ganglia and/or hemispheric corticomedullary junction) is more suggestive of CNS toxoplasmosis than CNS lymphoma. For patients with a positive toxoplasma IgG and multiple lesions on neuroimaging (MRI or CT scan), empiric therapy for toxoplasmosis is reasonable. However, such patients must be followed closely, and a repeat study should be performed in 7–14 days to assess for radiographic response. Patients who fail to respond clinically and radiographically should undergo a diagnostic brain biopsy. For patients with a positive toxoplasma IgG and a single lesion on MRI, a diagnostic brain biopsy to evaluate for neoplastic and other infectious etiologies should be strongly considered.

3. **Lumbar puncture (LP).** An LP is usually not necessary in patients with a mass lesion on CT scan and is contraindicated in patients with evidence of mass effect on CT scan of the head.

17. What are the treatment options for patients with cryptococcal meningitis?

Patients with cryptococcal meningitis that is severe enough to require critical care should be treated with amphotericin B and flucytosine (5-FC). The dose of amphotericin B is 0.7–1.0 mg/kg/day IV for a minimum of 2 weeks, followed by fluconazole at 400 mg/day for a minimum of 8 weeks; the dose of 5-FC is 100 mg/kg/day for 2 weeks. Fluconazole is an effective drug to treat cryptococcal meningitis. In critically ill patients, however, it probably should be viewed as a second-line option.

Amphotericin B is associated with significant side effects, including nausea, vomiting, fevers, rigors, hypokalemia, and hypomagnesemia. Renal toxicities can result in a rise in serum creatinine and renal tubular acidosis, and bone marrow toxicities can result in anemia and thrombocytopenia.

A frequent complication of cryptococcal meningitis is increased intracranial pressure (ICP). Therefore, opening pressure should be measured. For patients with an opening pressure ≥ 250 mm H_2O, many authorities recommend a daily lumbar puncture to maintain a pressure < 250 mm H_2O. Approximately 20–25 ml of cerebrospinal fluid can be safely removed daily. Occasionally, a lumbar drain or ventriculostomy should be placed in patients with persistently elevated opening pressures.

GASTROINTESTINAL DISORDERS

18. What GI conditions may require ICU admission?

The most common GI disorder requiring ICU admission in patients with HIV/AIDS is GI bleeding. In 40–60% of cases, the specific cause was reported to be a consequence of HIV infection.

Examples include Kaposi's sarcoma, AIDS-associated lymphoma, CMV enterocolitis, and MAC. Peritonitis and bowel perforation also may require ICU admission. The most common cause of life-threatening abdominal pain is CMV-related peritonitis from small bowel or colon enteritis with or without demonstrable perforation. Bowel perforations also have been reported as a result of Kaposi's sarcoma, lymphoma, and mycobacterial infection. Patients also may present with pancreatitis (consider alcohol and HIV-related medications, including pentamidine and many of the antiretrovirals) and AIDS cholangiopathy. The presentation of AIDS cholangiopathy, which may be caused by a variety of infectious and neoplastic processes, ranges from asymptomatic elevation in liver function tests to fulminant biliary sepsis.

19. Describe the diagnostic and therapeutic alternatives that should be considered in critically ill patients with HIV/AIDS and GI disorders.

In patients with GI bleeding, procedures that can be diagnostic as well as therapeutic include endoscopy, colonoscopy, and surgery. In patients with acute abdominal pain, diagnostic procedures include radiographic studies such as abdominal CT or ultrasound; if an acute abdomen is suspected, emergency surgery may be necessary. For critically ill patients with a GI source of sepsis, fluids and broad-spectrum antibiotics directed against gram-negative bacteria should be instituted. In septic patients with a suspected biliary source of sepsis (based on ultrasonographic evidence of common bile duct dilation), endoscopic retrograde cholangiopancreatography (ERCP) with sphincterotomy may be palliative.

BIBLIOGRAPHY

1. Afessa B, Green B: Clinical course, prognostic factors, and outcome prediction for HIV patients in the ICU. The PIP (Pulmonary complications, ICU support, and Prognostic factors in hospitalized patients with HIV) study. Chest 118:138–145, 2000.
2. Bedos JP, Chastang C, Lucet JC, et al: Early predictors of outcome for HIV patients with neurological failure. JAMA 273(1):35–40, 1995.
3. Casalino E, Mendoza-Sassi G, Wolff M, et al: Predictors of short- and long-term survival in HIV-infected patients admitted to the ICU. Chest 113:421–429, 1998.
4. Curtis JR, Yarnold PR, Schwartz DN, et al: Improvements in outcomes of acute respiratory failure for patients with human immunodeficiency virus-related *Pneumocystis carinii* pneumonia. Am J Respir Crit Care Med 162:393–398, 2000.
5. Gill JK, Greene L, Miller R, et al: ICU admission in patients infected with the human immunodeficiency virus: A multicentre study. Anaesthesia 54:727–732, 1999.
6. Huang L, Stansell JD: *Pneumocystis carinii* pneumonia. In Sande MA, Volberding PA (eds): The Medical Management of AIDS, 6th ed. Philadelphia, W.B. Saunders, 1999, pp 305–330.
7. Lazard T, Retel O, Guidet B, et al: AIDS in a medical intensive care unit: Immediate prognosis and long-term survival. JAMA 276:1240–1245, 1996.
8. Levy RM, Berger JR: Neurologic critical care in patients with human immunodeficiency virus 1 infection. Crit Care Clin 9:49–72, 1993.
9. Lew E, Dieterich D, Poles M, Scholes J: Gastrointestinal emergencies in the patient with AIDS. Crit Care Clin 11:531–560, 1995.
10. Nickas G, Wachter RM: Outcomes of intensive care for patients with human immunodeficiency virus infection. Arch Intern Med 160:541–547, 2000.
11. Palella FJ Jr, Delaney KM, Moorman AC, et al: Declining morbidity and mortality among patients with advanced human immunodeficiency virus infection. HIV Outpatient Study Investigators. N Engl J Med 338:853–860, 1998.
12. Piscitelli SC, Gallicano KD: Interactions among drugs for HIV and opportunistic infections. N Engl J Med 344:984–986, 2001.
13. Rosen MJ, Clayton K, Schneider RF, et al: Intensive care of patients with HIV infection: Utilization, critical illnesses, and outcomes. Pulmonary Complications of HIV Infection Study Group. Am J Respir Crit Care Med 155:67–71, 1997.
14. Saag MS, Graybill RJ, Larsen RA, et al: Practice guidelines for the management of cryptococcal disease. Infectious Disease Society of America. Clin Infect Dis 30:710–718, 2000.
15. Zimmerman LH, Huang L: Critical Care of HIV Infected Patients. In Cohen PT, Sande MA, Volberding PA (eds): The AIDS Knowledge Base, 3rd ed. New York, Little, Brown, 1997.

40. MULTIDRUG-RESISTANT BACTERIA

John W. Crommett, M.D., and Mark W. Bowyer, M.D.

1. What multidrug-resistant bacteria are of concern to critical care practitioners?

With the increasing use of broad spectrum antibiotics, several bacteria have developed resistance to these drugs. Of particular concern to critical care practitioners are gram-positive organisms such as vancomycin-resistant enterococci (VRE), methicillin-resistant (MRSA) and vancomycin-resistant *Staphylococcus aureus* (VRSA), multidrug-resistant *Streptococcus pneumoniae*, and multidrug-resistant gram-negative rods, particulary imipenem- and ceftazidime-resistant *Pseudomonas aeruginosa, Acinetobacter baumanii, Serratia* spp., *Stenotrophomonas* spp., *Enterobacter cloacae*, and *Klebsiella* spp.

2. What conditions put a patient at increased risk for VRE colonization and infection?
- Previous vancomycin, cephalosporin, or metronidazole therapy
- Severe underlying disease
- Immunosuppression associated with organ transplantation and hematologic malignancies
- Intra-abdominal or cardiothoracic surgery, particularly repeated intra-abdominal surgeries
- Indwelling central venous or urinary catheter
- Previous or prolonged hospitalization
- High score on the Acute Physiology, Age, and Chronic Health Evaluation (APACHE) II

3. What are the sources of VRE infection?

Enterococci are part of the normal flora of the mouth, gastrointestinal tract, female reproductive tract, urethra, and perineum. In the above predisposing conditions, resistant strains of enterococci can develop, and these colonized areas can be the source of an infection. A colonized person can also be the source of patient-to-patient transmission via contamination of patient-care equipment, environmental surfaces, and hospital personnel.

4. How long does VRE last on inanimate objects and hands? Does cleaning remove VRE?

A significant factor contributing to VRE transmission is the presence and persistence of these orgtanisms on inanimate objects, particularly linen and objects exposed to body fluids, such as bedpans. VRE has been seen to persist on countertops for up to 7 days, on a dry surface for up to 45 days when suspended with organic material, on bed rails for 24 hours, on telephone handpieces for 60 minutes, and on the diaphragms of stethoscopes for 30 minutes. Chlorine compounds are probably a better option than phenols or quaternary ammonium compounds for removal of VRE from environmental surfaces. Both gloved and ungloved hands may carry VRE for over 60 minutes. While hand-washing with soap for 5 seconds decreases the VRE bacterial count, a 30-second soap scrub is required to eradicate it completely from the hands.

5. What factors are responsible for the high risk of VRE colonization and serious infections in patients with orthotopic liver transplant?
1. Extensive abdominal surgery
2. Selective pressures of broad-spectrum antibiotics
3. High-dose immunosuppressive therapy
4. Prolonged postoperative stay in the intensive care unit

6. MRSA is resistant to which drugs?

All penicillins and cephalosporins; some isolates are also resistant to aminoglycosides.

7. What are the risk factors for MRSA?
- Previous antimicrobial therapy
- Previous or prolonged hospitalization
- Serious underlying disease
- Intravenous drug use

8. One of your patients has been found to be colonized or infected with VRE or MRSA. What isolation precautions should be taken to prevent patient-to-patient transmission?

1. Place VRE/MRSA patients in single rooms or in the same room with other patients colonized or infected with the same organism.

2. All persons entering the room should wear disposable gloves. In addition, people who will have substantial contact with the patient or environmental surfaces in the room should wear a disposable gown. These items should be removed before leaving the room, taking care that clothing does not contact any surfaces or the patient.

3. Wash hands vigorously with antiseptic soap for 30 seconds immediately on leaving the room. VRE can persist on hands for 1 hour and MRSA for more than 3 hours.

4. Dedicate items such as stethoscopes and sphygmomanometers to be used with this particular patient or room during this particular admission. Dispose of them or adequately clean them after the patient leaves.

5. Obtain stool cultures or rectal swabs of roommates of patients found to be newly colonized or infected with VRE.

6. Make sure that, whenever possible, unit or floor staff caring for VRE patients have as little contact as possible with other patients.

9. In the search for the source or spread of a MRSA outbreak in the ICU, what areas and surfaces should be checked for colonization?

The most common mechanism of MRSA introduction is a colonized or infected patient. Useful sites for culture are wounds, intravascular catheter sites, tracheostomy sites, sputum from intubated patients, or rectal/perineal swabs. Patients with dermatitis are at especially high risk for acquisition and dissemination of MRSA, probably due to epidermal exfoliation. Rare cases of airborne MRSA have been seen in burn units. The principal mode of patient-to-patient transmission within an institution, however, is via temporarily colonized hands of hospital personnel. To track this colonization, swab the anterior nares, a major reservoir. Rates of hospital personnel colonization during MRSA outbreaks have been seen to range from 0.8% in an institution with an isolated outbreak, to 56% in an institution with chronic, endemic MRSA.

10. How should MRSA and VRE infections be treated?

MRSA: Intravenous vancomycin is the drug of choice. Alternatives include teicoplanin, which has the advantage of less frequent dosing and less nephrotoxicity and ototoxicity and can even be given intramuscularly; the streptogramin antibiotic combination quinupristin-dalfopristin; and the oxazolidinone compounds, linezolid and eperezolid.

VRE: Teicoplanin may be effective, but cross-resistance may occur in Van A or Van B types of enterococcal resistance. Quinupristin/dalfopristin or linezolid should be strongly considered for patients with VRE infections. If an anatomic focus of infection can be found, surgical removal or drainage should be performed. Consultation with infectious disease specialists is prudent when a patient is first diagnosed with VRE colonization or infection.

11. Describe the mechanisms of action, toxicities, and usual dose ranges of quinupristin-dalfopristin and linezolid.

The combination of **quinupristin-dalfopristin** inhibits bacterial protein synthesis by binding irreversibly to different sites on the 50S ribosomal subunit. Quinupristin actually inhibits peptide chain elongation, whereas dalfopristin inhibits peptidyl transferase. The combination is synergestic with other antimicrobials against a wide variety of gram-positive bacteria and has limited bactericidal activity against the enterococci. The most common toxicity in clinical trials was inflammation at the injection site. Also noted were some increases in conjugated bilirubin and gamma-glutamyl transferase. The usual dose for treatment of serious nosocomial infections is 7.5 mg/kg of actual body weight in a 5% dextrose solution, delivered over 1 hour 2 or 3 times/day for 7–10 days.

Linezolid. The oxazolidinones also bind to the 50S ribosomal subunit, preventing the binding of the 30S subunit and formation of the 70S initiation complex. Binding is competitively inhibited by chloramphenicol and lincomycin. Toxicities were mild, including diarrhea, tongue discoloration, folliculitis, and headache. Also of note is weak monoamine oxidase inhibition. The intravenous dosing is 500 or 625 mg twice daily. Further trials are under way to evaluate this class of drugs in skin and soft tissue infections as well as pneumonia.

12. What is the role of tetracycline, chloramphenicol, and other antimicrobials in the treatment of VRE?

These drugs may exhibit in vitro activity against VRE, but their only effect is bacteriostasis and clinical failures have been documented. Most enterococci (80–90%) are resistant to macrolides such as erythromycin. The fluoroquinolones also have in vitro activity against the enterococci and may be useful for treating VRE infections of the urinary tract; however, their effectiveness in treating other enterococcal infections has not been convincingly demonstrated. Increasing resistance to fluoroquinolones is likely to affect their potential utility.

13. Give examples of appropriate and inappropriate use of vancomycin.

Appropriate use includes:
- Infections due to MRSA
- Empirical coverage in a setting where MRSA is very likely
- Serious infections due to gram-positive organisms in a patient with a serious allergy to beta-lactam antimicrobials
- *Clostridium difficile* colitis failing to respond to metronidazole (orally)
- Prophylaxis for major surgery involving implantation of prosthetic materials at institutions with a high rate of MRSA infections

Inappropriate use includes:
- Routine prophylaxis for surgery, indwelling catheters, endocarditis, very low-birth-weight infants, peritoneal or hemodialysis patients
- Routine empirical therapy in febrile patients
- Methicillin-susceptible staphylococcal infections
- Neonates with persistent MRSA bacteremia (try combination therapy with rifampin plus an aminoglycoside)
- Eradication of MRSA colonization
- Primary treatment of *C. difficile* colitis
- Topical application or irrigation

14. What effect does vancomycin have on MRSA-colonized/infected surgical wounds?

Bacterial count decreases by about 50%.

15. When is it permissible to take VRE and MRSA patients out of isolation?

In consultation with the infectious disease service, establish requirements that must be met for the patient to be moved out of isolation or discharged. For example, three consecutive VRE/MRSA-negative cultures taken at least 1 week apart from all sites previously found to be VRE/MRSA-positive may be required before a patient may be moved out of isolation.

16. Do MRSA patients have to test negative before being discharged?

No. MRSA patients should be discharged as soon as other medical or surgical conditions allow. Outside the hospital, there is little risk that MRSA will spread to ambulatory, healthy persons in the same household. If patients are on a decolonization regimen, they can complete it at home. If the patient is being transferred to a chronic care facility, the institution should be notified of the patient's MRSA status so that the appropriate isolation steps can be instituted.

17. What are the features of multidrug-resistant *Streptococcus pneumoniae*?

Once thought to be universally susceptible to penicillin, some strains of *S. pneumoniae* are now resistant to numerous antibiotics. In the United States up to 35% of isolates are no longer susceptible to penicillin, and some strains are now susceptible only to vancomycin. Although not currently a major problem in ICUs, there are concerns that if vancomycin resistance should jump from enterococci to pneumococci, *S. pneumoniae* infection may become untreatable.

18. What can be done to limit the spread of drug-resistant pneumococci?

Public health authorities recommend widespread use of the pneumococcal vaccine for all persons 2 years or older who have underlying medical conditions associated with increased risk for pneumococcal disease.

19. Which gram-negative bacteria have developed multidrug resistance?

Sporadic outbreaks of *Enterobacteriaceae* resistant to third-generation cephalosporins are being reported with increasing frequency. Reservoirs for multidrug-resistant bacteria have been identified in ICUs, and stool colonization is a risk factor in long-term ICU patients. To date, *Klebsiella pneumoniae*, *Escherichia coli*, *P. aeruginosa*, *Serratia* spp., and *Acinetobacter* spp. have demonstrated multidrug resistance. Imipenem is the only agent that is consistently bactericidal against these isolates, and some isolates, particularly of *Pseudomonas* spp., are imipenem-resistant.

20. What is all the fuss about *Acinetobacter* infections in the ICU?

Overall, the number of infections caused by *Acinetobacter* species, particularly *A. baumanii*, has increased in recent years. The organisms have few nutritional requirements and are highly resistant to antimicrobials. Infections of the respiratory tract and bloodstream seem to predominate, although all organs are susceptible. A host does not need to be compromised to develop *A. baumanii* bacteremia. Administration of systemic antibiotics favors infection and colonization and does not seem to prevent the development of bacteremia, even if the antibiotics have activity against the organisms. Imipenem is currently the most effective agent, but resistant strains exist. The treatment of choice has not yet been established, and many recommend double coverage when *A. baumanii* is believed to be the cause of a serious infection. Surgical treatment of the source, as always, is indicated and may be curative. Measures are certainly needed to prevent and control infections caused by *Acinetobacter* species and to improve the use of antimicrobial agents to delay the appearance of resistant strains.

21. What other problems with multidrug resistance are lurking on the horizon?

Recent problems include vancomycin-resistant *Staphylococcus aureus* and emerging imipenem resistance in some of the gram-negative rods such as *Pseudomonas* and *Acinetobacter* species. Most worrisome, however, is the development of resistance to the newer streptogramin antibiotics (already reported) and the oxazolidinones. As always, development of new antibiotics is essential, but unless we continue to address inappropriate uses and infection control practices, the utility of new agents will be short-lived.

CONTROVERSY

22. What is the significance of clearance in long-term care patients colonized with VRE?

Overall, little is known about the persistence of colonization with VRE in the nononcologic, non-ICU patient. A recent study by Baden et al. revealed the following:

1. Patients who receive long-term medical care, even without oncologic disease, may shed VRE for at least 5 years.

2. Despite multiple negative VRE cultures, approximately 25% of patients remain colonized with VRE.

3. Current culture techniques often fail to detect VRE.

4. Recent antibiotic use leads to increased detection of VRE excretion.

5. Criteria for determining genetic relationships in the long-term care setting must be developed, because the criteria for outbreaks may be misleading.

Based on these findings, it is unclear what impact attempted clearance of organisms such as VRE will have on individual patients or patients in general. Certainly, if our detection techniques fail a significant portion of the time, we cannot reliably determine if clearance indeed has been achieved. In addition, the cost of attempted clearance in terms of future antibiotic resistance has not been fully comprehended.

BIBLIOGRAPHY

1. Archibald L, Phillips L, Monnet D, et al: Antimicrobial resistance in isolates from inpatients and outpatients in the United States: Increasing importance in the intensive care unit. Clin Infect Dis 24:211–215, 1997.
2. Baden LR, Thiemke W, Skolnik A, et al: Prolonged colonization with vancomycin-resistant *Enterococcus faecium* in long-term care patients and the significance of clearance. Clin Infect Dis 33:1654–1660, 2001.
3. Cetron MS, Farley MM, McCraken GH: Multidrug-resistant *S. pneumoniae*: What can be done? Patient Care Jan 15, 1997, pp 20–33.
4. Chien JW, Kucia ML, Salata RA: Use of linezolid, an oxazolidinone, in the treatment of multidrug-resistant gram-positive bacterial infections. Clin Infect Dis 30:146–151, 2000.
5. Cisneros JM, Reyes MJ, Pachon J, et al: Bacteremia due to Acinetobacter baumanii: Epidemiology, clinical findings, and prognostic features. Clin Infect Dis 22:1026–1032, 1996.
6. Fridkin SL, Edwards JR, Courval JM, et al: The effect of vancomycin and third-generation cephalosporins on prevalence of vancomycin-resistant enterococci in 126 U.S. adult intensive care units. Ann Intern Med 135:175–183, 2001.
7. Hierholzer WJ, et al (Hospital Infection Control Practices Advisory Committee): Recommendations for preventing the spread of vancomycin resistance: Recommendations of the Hospital Infection Control Practices Advisory Committee (HICPAC). Am J Infect Control 23:87–94, 1995.
8. Monteclavo MA, Jarvis WR, Ulman J, et al: Infection control measures reduce transmission of vancomycin-resistant enterococci in an endemic setting. Arch Intern Med 131:269–272, 1999.
9. Mulligan ME, Murray-Leisure KA, Ribner BS, et al: Methicillin-resistant *Staphylococcus aureus*: A consensus review of the microbiology, pathogenesis, and epidemiology with implications for prevention and management. Am J Med 94:313–328, 1993.
10. Murray BE: Vancomycin-resistant enterococci. Am J Med 102:284–293, 1997.
11. Wenzel RP, Edmond MB: Vancomycin-resistant *Staphylococcus aureus*: Infection control considerations. Clin Infect Dis 27:245–251, 1998.
12. Winston DJ, Emmanouilides C, Kroeber A, et al: Quinupristin/dalfopristin therapy for infections due to vancomycin-resistant *Enterococcus faecium*. Clin Infect Dis 30:790–797, 2000.

41. CATHETER-RELATED INFECTIONS AND ASSOCIATED BACTEREMIA

Carlos E. Girod, M.D.

1. Define the different types of catheter-related infections.

The Centers for Disease Control and Prevention have proposed the following definitions:

- **Catheter colonization:** presence of ≥ 15 colony-forming units (CFUs) in a semiquantitative culture or $> 10^3$ CFUs in a quantitative culture from a proximal or distal catheter segment in the absence of clinical symptoms.
- **Exit-site infection:** erythema, tenderness, induration, or purulence within 2 cm of the exit site of the catheter.
- **Tunnel infection:** erythema, tenderness, and induration in the tissues overlying the catheter and > 2 cm from the exit site.

- **Catheter-related bloodstream infection (CR-BSI):** isolation of the same organism from a semiquantitative culture of catheter segment and from the blood (preferably a peripheral blood culture) in a patient with clinical symptoms of bloodstream infection.

2. Is catheter-related infection a rare syndrome associated only with inexperience?

No. Catheter-related infections remain among the top three causes of hospital-acquired infections, with an estimated incidence of 4–17%. Mortality rates attributable to nosocomial bloodstream infections have been reported to be as high as 10–20%. The infection rate varies within a wide range, depending on the type of ICU. In the burn unit there are 30.2 infections per 1000 central catheter days, whereas in the respiratory ICU there are 2.1 infections per 1000 central catheter days.

3. What are the portals of entry in catheter-related infections?

(1) Most studies have clearly shown that the skin around the insertion site is the most common portal of entry of infection. Analysis of catheter segments by Gram stain and semiquantitative cultures shows predominance of bacteria along the outer surface from tip to skin entry. Bacterial adherence followed by migration along catheter is the major mechanism. (2) The second most common portal of entry of bacteria is through contamination of the catheter hub during its manipulation. (3) Hematogenous dissemination from a distal infectious focus with catheter colonization is less common and is associated with yeasts, enterococci, and *Klebsiella* sp. Case reports of catheter colonization from the infused solution have been described with pathogens such as *Pseudomonas* and *Enterobacter* spp. (4) Other sources, such as contaminated transducer kits, disinfectants, and infusion lines, are rare causes of catheter-related infections.

4. What are important risk factors for catheter-related infections?

AIDS	Granulocytopenia
Diabetes mellitus	Loss of skin integrity
Altered host defense	Malnutrition
Multiple medical problems	Distal infection
Age < 1 year, > 60 years	Total parenteral nutrition (TPN)
Immunosuppressive therapy	Sepsis

Review of the literature suggests that the presence of sepsis is the most important patient-related risk factor.

5. What are non–patient-related risk factors for catheter infections?

Alteration of skin flora	Inadequate maintenance
Lack of sterile procedure	Hypertonicity of infusate
Catheter adherence properties	Location and duration
Catheter size	Type of catheter
Lumen number	Skill of inserting physician

Duration of catheterization is the most important non–patient-related risk factor for catheter-related infection.

6. Is any specific type of catheter linked to increased infection?

Clinical trials have shown that tips of peripheral intravenous catheters have a significant risk for contamination 72 hours after insertion. Nevertheless, when changed every 72 hours, these catheters are less often associated with infection than central, pulmonary, and arterial catheters. The insertion site should be the upper extremity or external jugular vein. Use of a lower-extremity site carries a greater risk of infection.

Arterial catheters are associated with infection less often than pulmonary artery and central venous catheters. They are a rare source of bacteremia in ICU patients, probably because high arterial flow around the catheter decreases adherence of bacteria. Infections associated with arterial catheters most commonly are related to contamination of the transducer chamber fluid.

Central venous catheters carry a definite increased risk of related infection and bacteremia compared with peripheral and arterial catheters. Numerous studies have shown an incidence of bacteremia in triple-lumen catheters of 7–19% vs. 3.7% in single-lumen catheters.

Pulmonary artery (PA) catheters have an estimated incidence of bloodstream infection of 3–5% when left in place for more than 72 hours. A recent review by Maki recommends that PA catheters be left in place for no more than 5 days. If further hemodynamic monitoring is needed, a new PA catheter should be placed at a new puncture site. The increased risk of infection is attributed to the number of manipulations performed with PA catheters.

7. Are physician experience and timing at insertion important?

The skill and experience of the physician inserting the catheter are important factors. Experience with fewer than 25 prior insertions carries an 18–20% incidence of catheter-related infection vs. 8–12% for experience with more than 25 prior insertions. A recent report by Sherertz et al. demonstrated that physicians in training who attended a 1-day infection control course were able to reduce the rate of catheter-related infections by 35%. Elective catheterization carries less risk of infection than emergency insertion. An increased incidence of catheter-related infection has been described when the catheter is placed after a 6-day ICU course and is probably a marker of severity of patient's illness.

8. How long can an intravascular catheter be used without risk of catheter-related infection?

Prolonged catheterization is the most important risk factor for related infection. No catheter should be left in place any longer than absolutely necessary. Recommended duration of catheter use prior to removal should be determined on a patient-to-patient basis, taking into account the host and nonhost factors listed in questions 4 and 5. Of note, a study by Cobb et al. demonstrated no difference in rate of infection between scheduled routine line changes (every 3 days) vs. replacement when a clinical indication was present. Nevertheless, catheters should **not** be left in place indefinitely.

9. Do routine guidewire or new site changes every 48–72 hours decrease the incidence of catheter-related infection?

In the past, anecdotal reports suggested that routine guidewire catheter exchanges reduced the risk of infection. A randomized controlled study of 160 patients demonstrated that routine replacement of central venous catheters every 3 days did not prevent the development of infection. This finding applied to both techniques of replacement: new site or guidewire exchanges. This study clearly demonstrated an increased risk for bleeding or pneumothorax in patients receiving insertion of catheters at new sites. Currently routine replacement of catheters is not recommended; the catheter should be replaced when clinically indicated.

10. Is changing an intravascular catheter over a guidewire associated with less risk of related infection than a new site replacement?

Guidewire changes are usually preferred over new site insertion because of less risk of pneumothorax or bleeding complications. It is an effective method for changing central venous catheters, ruling out catheter-related infection in a febrile, nonseptic patient. Every attempt must be made to sterilize the entire external portion of the catheter, guidewire, and surrounding skin. The removed catheter should be cultured; if it is infected, the guidewire-placed catheter must be removed. This technique should not be performed in the setting of confirmed or clinically suspected sepsis. A recent review by Cook et al. concluded that guidewire exchanges are associated with increased catheter colonization, exit site infection, and bacteremia.

11. Which site is more at risk for catheter-associated infection: internal jugular or subclavian?

The internal jugular site has a higher incidence of catheter-related infection than the subclavian site (12% vs. 7%). This finding is supported by retrospective chart reviews and prospective studies with statistical significance. The increased risk is believed to be due to (1) increased oral and nasal secretions that pool in the neck site of a supine patient, (2) the inability to apply an occlusive dressing to the neck site, and (3) higher skin temperature. Nevertheless, the internal jugular site is preferred by many physicians because of its lower risk of pneumothorax.

12. What is the most sensitive and specific means of diagnosing catheter-related infections?

Physical exam is unreliable. Local inflammation or purulence at the entry site is seen in less than half of cases. Fever, leukocytosis, and positive peripheral blood cultures are also not reliable indicators of catheter-related infection.

The most widely used and reliable test is removal of the catheter and culture of its tip by rolling it over a blood-agar plate, as described by Maki et al. in 1977. Growth of > 15 colonies per plate is associated with a specificity of 76–96% and a positive predictive value of 16–31% for catheter-related bloodstream infection or sepsis. Another laboratory method is quantitative broth culture of the intravascular and subcutaneous catheter segments. Cleri et al. reported that > 10^3 CFUs was predictive of catheter-related bloodstream infection. This technique is highly sensitive but has low specificity and poor positive predictive value.

13. What organisms cause catheter-related infections?

Microbiology of Device-Associated Bacteremia

Staphylococcus aureus	*Candida* species[b]
Staphylococcus epidermidis	*Pseudomonas aeruginosa*[c]
Klebsiella species[a]	*Pseudomonas cepacia*[c]
Enterobacter species[a]	*Citrobacter freundii*[a]
Serratia marcescens[a]	*Corynebacterium* species (especially
Candida albicans[b]	JK strains)[d]

[a] Frequently associated with contaminated infusate.
[b] Most often associated with TPN; usually along the catheter path, but occasionally as a result of contaminated infusate.
[c] May arise from a water source (e.g., infusate) or may reflect cutaneous colonization.
[d] JK bacteremia occurs almost exclusively in severely immunosuppressed patients who are or have been receiving broad-spectrum antibiotics and who have indwelling intravascular devices.
From Mandell GL, et al (eds): Principles and Practice of Infectious Diseases. New York, Churchill Livingstone, 1990, p 2191, with permission.

14. Where should blood cultures be obtained to document catheter-related bacteremia?

Blood cultures should be drawn from both catheter and peripheral sites. Blood cultures drawn through the catheter are associated with a high false-positive rate for the diagnosis of catheter-related bacteremia. The diagnosis is best made by removal of the catheter with semi-quantitative tip culture.

15. Describe the treatment of catheter-related infection.

Treatment depends on the stage of infection and the pathogen. As a general rule, if catheter-related bloodstream infection or septicemia is strongly suspected, the catheter must be removed and replaced if access is needed. Most of the infectious complications are self-limited and resolve after removal of the catheter. If empirical antibiotic therapy is needed, vancomycin is the drug of choice while awaiting cultures because of an increased incidence of oxacillin-resistant staphylococci.

Coagulase-negative staphylococci can be treated in nonimmunosuppressed patients by removal of catheter alone and/or intravenous antibiotics for 3 days.

Staphylococcus aureus-associated bacteremia should be treated with removal of catheter and IV antibiotics for 2–3 weeks because of a higher association with endocarditis.

Yeast colonization or infection of catheter can be treated with removal of catheter. The presence of positive blood cultures, persistent fever despite catheter removal, retinal lesions, or immunosuppression mandates a prolonged course of amphotericin B.

16. What are other ways to prevent catheter infection?

Recently reported new techniques that seem to prevent infection:

• **Chlorhexidine gluconate:** skin decontamination before insertion of the catheter leads to greater reduction of infection than use of iodine solutions.

• **PNB ointment** (polymyxin-neomycin-bacitracin): at skin entry site.

• **Specialized teams:** Eggimann et al. demonstrated a 3-fold reduction in catheter-related infection with a specialized team devoted to placement and maintenance of central and peripheral venous catheters.

• **Vitacuff** (a subcutaneous collagen cuff at the catheter entry site impregnated with silver): its use has been associated with a 3-fold reduction in colonization and a 4-fold reduction in bacteremia. Its drawbacks are cost and the need for specialized training.

• **Antibiotic-impregnated catheters** (either minocycline and rifampin or chlorhexidene and silver sulfadiazene): reduced rates of catheter colonization and bloodstream infection have been reported. In a recent article by Darouiche et al., central venous catheters impregnated with minocycline and rifampin were significantly less likely to be colonized or to cause a bloostream infection than those impregnated with chlorhexidene and silver sulfadiazene.

17. Is it necessary to wear a mask and sterile gown during central line placement?

Two prospective studies have recently demonstrated a reduction in catheter-associated infections when physicians used long-sleeved surgical gowns and masks and full-length sterile drapes to cover patients.

CONTROVERSIES

18. Should femoral lines be used routinely?

For: Easier technique with no risk of pneumothorax. No randomized, controlled trial has demonstrated that this location is associated with an increased risk of catheter-related infection.

Against: Close location to urogenital and rectal areas with their associated gram-negative bacteria flora. Higher rate of colonization with a reported incidence of 34% (5 times the rate seen with subclavian catheter location). The femoral location also has a greater risk for arterial cannulation with complication of distal embolization. Recent reports suggest an increased risk for local and deep venous thrombosis.

19. What is the role of new methods for the diagnosis of catheter-related bloodstream infections that do not require catheter removal?

For: In a recent study by Blot et al., catheter-related infection was ruled out by studying the differential time to positivity (DTP) between a blood culture obtained from the hub of the catheter and a peripheral blood culture site. A positive hub blood culture at least 2 hours before a positive peripheral blood culture had a high sensitivity (94%) and specificity (95%) for catheter-related bloodstream infection. Another recent advance in catheter-sparing culture techniques was reported by Kite et al. Their technique uses 100 µl of blood drawn from the catheter hub. This blood is processed for Gram stain and an acridine-orange leukocyte cytospin (a technique that detects bacterial DNA). The presence of bacteria or bacterial DNA had a high sensitivity (96%) and specificity (92%) for catheter-related bloodstream infection.

Against: Both studies focused on long-term vascular access for hemodialysis or chronic TPN and chemotherapy administration. Therefore, the populations tested had a high prevalence of catheter-related infection. Further studies validating these techniques in patients with short-term arterial and central venous catheters are needed.

BIBLIOGRAPHY

1. Bach A: Central venous catheter infections [letter]. Intens Care Med 22(6):613, 1996.
2. Badley AD, Steckelberg JM, Wollan PC, et al: Infectious rates of central venous pressure catheters: Comparison between newly placed catheters and those that have been changed. Mayo Clin Proc 71:838–846, 1996.

3. Benezra D, Kiehn TE, Gold JW, et al: Prospective study of infections in indwelling central venous catheters using quantitative blood cultures. Am J Med 85:495–498, 1988.
4. Blot F, Nitenberg G Chachaty E, et al: Diagnosis of catheter-related bacteraemia: A prospective comparison of the time of positivity of hub-blood versus peripheral-blood cultures. Lancet 354:1071–1077, 1999.
5. Bozzetti F, Terno G, Bonfanti G, et al: Prevention and treatment of central venous catheter sepsis by exchange via guidewire. Ann Surg 198:48–52, 1983.
6. Cercenado E, Rodriguez M, Romero T, et al: A conservative procedure for the diagnosis of catheter-related infections. Arch Intern Med 150:1417–1420, 1990.
7. Cobb DK, High KP, Sawyer RG, et al: A controlled trial of scheduled replacement of central venous and pulmonary-artery catheters. N Engl J Med 327:1062–1068, 1992.
8. Collignon PJ, Soni N, Pearson IY, et al: Is semiquantitative culture of central vein catheter tips useful in the diagnosis of catheter-associated bacteremia? J Clin Microbiol 24:532–535, 1986.
9. Cook D, Randolph A, Kernerman P, et al: Central venous catheter replacement strategies: A systematic review of the literature. Crit Care Med 25:1417–1424. 1997.
10. Cooper GL, Hopkins CC: Rapid diagnosis of intravascular catheter-associated infection by direct Gram staining of catheter segments. N Engl J Med 312:1142–1147, 1985.
11. Corona ML, Peters SG, Narr BJ, et al: Infections related to central venous catheters. Mayo Clin Proc 65:979–986, 1990.
12. Darouiche RO, Raad II, Heard SO, et al: A comparison of two antimicrobial-impregnated central venous catheters. N Engl J Med 340:1–8, 1999.
13. Eggimann P, Harbath S, Constantin MN, et al: Impact of a prevention strategy targeted vascular-access care on incidence of infections acquired in intensive care. Lancet 355:1864–1868, 2000.
14. Flowers RH, Schwenzer KJ, Kopel RF, et al: Efficacy of an attachable subcutaneous cuff for the prevention of intravascular catheter-related infection. JAMA 261(6):878–883, 1989.
15. Fraenkel DJ, Rickard C, Lipman J: Can we achieve consensus on central venous catheter-related infections? Anaesth Intens Care 28:475–490, 2000.
16. Graeve AH, Carpenter CM, Schiller WR: Management of central venous catheters using a wire introducer. Am J Surg 142:752–755, 1981.
17. Gregory JA, Schiller WR: Subclavian catheter changes every third day in high-risk patients. Am Surg 51;534, 1985.
18. Hampton AA, Sheretz RJ: Vascular-access infections in hospitalized patients. Surg Clin North Am 68:57–71, 1988.
19. Henderson DK: Infections due to percutaneous intravascular devices. In Mandell GL, Douglas RG, Bennett JE (eds): Principles and Practice of Infectious Diseases. New York, Churchill Livingstone, 2000, pp 3005–3020.
20. Hilton E, Haslett TM, Borenstein MT, et al: Central catheter infections: Single- versus triple-lumen catheters. Am J Med 84:667–671, 1988.
21. Kite P, Dobbins BM, Wilcox MH, McMahon MJ: Rapid diagnosis of central-venous-catheter-related bloodstream infection without catheter removal. Lancet 354:1504–1507, 1999.
22. Maki DG: Risk factors for nosocomial infection in the intensive care unit. Arch Intern Med 149:30–35, 1989.
23. Mantese VA, German DS, Kaminski DL, et al: Colonization and sepsis from triple-lumen catheters in critically ill patients. Am J Surg 154:597–600, 1987.
24. Myers ML, Austin TW, Sibbald WJ: Pulmonary artery catheter infections. Ann Surg 201:237–241, 1985.
25. Norwood S, Ruby A, Civetta J: Catheter-related infections and associated septicemia. Chest 99:968–975, 1991.
26. Raad II, Baba M, Bodey GP: Diagnosis of catheter-related infections: The role of surveillance and targeted quantitative skin cultures. Clin Infect Dis 20:593–597, 1995.
27. Reed CR, Sessler CN, Glauser FL, et al: Central venous catheter infections: Concepts and controversies. Intensive Care Med 21:177–183, 1995.
28. Senagore A, Waller JD, Bonnell BW, et al: Pulmonary artery catheterization: A prospective study of internal jugular and subclavian approaches. Crit Car Med 15:35–37, 1987.
29. Sherertz RJ, Ely EW, Westbrook DM, et al: Education of physicians-in-training can decrease the risk of vascular catheter infection. Ann Intern Med 132:641–648, 2000.

42. BIOTERRORISM

Leoncio L. Kaw, M.D., and Mark W. Bowyer, M.D.

1. What biologic agents have the potential to be used as weapons of mass destruction?

Bacterial Agents	Viral Agents	Biologic Toxins
Anthrax	Smallpox	Botulinum
Tularemia	Viral hemorrhagic fevers	Ricin
Plague	Venezuelan equine encephalitis	Staphylococcal enterotoxin B
Brucellosis		T-2 mycotoxins
Q fever		
Glanders and melioidosis		

2. What epidemiologic clues should raise suspicion that a disease outbreak is due to bioterrorism?
- Large epidemic with a similar disease or syndrome, especially in a discrete population
- Unusually numerous cases of unexplained diseases or deaths
- Disease that is unusual to the geographic area or transmission season
- Multiple simultaneous or serial epidemics of different diseases in the same population
- Disease outbreaks of the same illness in noncontiguous areas
- Disease known to be transmitted by a vector that is not present in the local area
- Single case of a disease due to an uncommon agent (e.g., smallpox)
- Unusual age distribution for common diseases
- Unusual strains or variants of organisms or antimicrobial resistance patterns different from those circulating in the local area
- More severe disease than expected for known pathogen or failure to respond to standard therapy
- Similar genetic type of agents isolated from distinct sources at different times or locations
- Unusual routes of exposure for a pathogen (e.g., inhalational route for a disease that normally develops through other exposure)

3. What is smallpox?
Smallpox is a viral, exanthematous disease caused by the orthopox virus, variola. There are two principal forms of the disease, variola major. and a much milder form, variola minor. The disease spreads from person to person primarily by droplet nuclei or aerosols expelled from the naso- or oropharynx of infected persons and by direct contact. Contaminated clothing or bed linens can also spread the virus. There are no known animal or insect reservoirs or vectors.

4. Describe the typical clinical presentation of smallpox.
The disease usually begins after a 12- to 14-day incubation period (range: 7–17 days) and consists of high fever, malaise, and prostration with headache and backache. These symptoms are followed by the appearance of a maculopapular rash that progresses to papules (1–2 days after appearance of rash), vesicles (4th–5th day), pustules (by 7th day), and finally scab lesions (14th day). Other organs are seldom involved. Death, which commonly occurs during the second week of illness, most likely results from the toxemia associated with circulating immune complexes and soluble variola antigens.

5. What clinical features distinguish smallpox from other viral diseases such as measles and chickenpox?
1. Smallpox presents with a characteristic rash in a centrifugal in distribution (i.e., more abundant in the face and extremities).

2. Lesions on any given part of the body are generally synchronous in stage of development.

3. Lesions are also seen on the palms of the hands and soles of the feet.

4. The skin lesions are deeply embedded in the dermis and generally leave depressed depigmented scars on healing.

6. How is the diagnosis of smallpox confirmed?

The diagnosis can be rapidly confirmed in the laboratory by demonstration of characteristic virions on electron microscopy of vesicular or pustular fluid or scabs. Findings of aggregations of variola virus particles called Guarnieri bodies under light microscopy are also diagnostic. The Gispen's modified silver stain is another rapid but relatively insensitive test for Guarnieri bodies in vesicular fluid, in which cytoplasmic inclusions appear black.

The above tests, although extremely useful, cannot discriminate variola from the other members of the genus orthopoxvirus (i.e., vaccinia, monkeypox, cowpox). Definitive identification and characterization of the virus require growth of the virus in cell culture or on chorioallantoic egg membrane and characterization of strains by polymerase chain reaction (PCR) techniques or restriction fragment-length polymorphisms.

7. What are the treatment options for infected or exposed patients?

At present, no drug or substance has been proved effective for the treatment of smallpox. Supportive therapy and antibiotics as indicated for treatment of secondary bacterial infections are the best that can be offered. Vaccination administered within 4 days of first exposure has been shown to offer some protection against acquiring infection and significant protection against a fatal outcome. Cidofovir, a nucleoside analog DNA polymerase inhibitor, also has been shown to have significant in vitro and in vivo activity in experimental animals, although at present no evidence indicates that it is more effective than immediate postexposure vaccination in humans.

8. What factors make smallpox an extremely potent bioterrorism agent?

1. Virtually nonexistent immunity to smallpox among the population at risk because of the absence of naturally occurring disease and the discontinuation of routine vaccination in the early 1970s.

2. Potentially delayed recognition of the disease by health personnel because of its rarity and presumed eradication of the disease.

3. Increased mobility and crowding of the population.

These factors give smallpox the potential for rapid spread and the ability to cause illness that can certainly overwhelm existing medical and public health systems. A single suspected case of smallpox should be treated as a national health emergency, and the proper authorities should be promptly notified.

9. What is botulism?

Botulism is a clinical syndrome brought about by ingestion or inhalation of the toxins produced by the spore-forming bacillus *Clostridium botulinum*. These toxins, which exist in seven distinct antigenic types, exert their cytotoxic effect by preventing acetylcholine release at the neuromuscular junction, resulting in blockade of neuromuscular transmission and flaccid muscle paralysis.

The syndrome generally presents with the classic triad of (1) symmetric, descending, and progressive flaccid paralysis that always begins in bulbar musculature in (2) an afebrile patient with (3) a clear sensorium. The bulbar palsies are prominent and can be summarized in part as the 4 D': diplopia, dysarthria, dysphonia, and dysphagia. Anticholinergic signs and symptoms, such as dry mouth, ileus, constipation, and urinary retention, are often present. Sensory changes however, are not observed. Because the toxins do not cross the blood-brain barrier, central nervous system symptoms are absent.

10. How do you differentiate botulism clinically from other neuromuscular disorders?

A cluster of cases of acute flaccid paralysis is more suggestive of botulinum intoxication than Guillain-Barré syndrome, myasthenia gravis, or tick paralysis. Patients should be asked whether they know of other persons with similar symptoms, along with a careful travel and dietary history. Botulism differs from other neuromuscular disorders in its prominent cranial nerve palsies, which are disproportionate to milder weakness and hypotonia below the neck; its symmetry; its absence of sensory changes; its normal cerebrospinal fluid findings; and its distinctive finding of reduced amplitude of evoked muscle potentials with incremental response to repetitive stimulation at 50 Hz on electromyography (EMG). Distinguishing features of commonly misdiagnosed conditions are outlined below.

Condition	Features that Distinguish Condition from Botulism
Guillain-Barré syndrome	History of antecedent infection; paresthesia; often ascending paralysis; elevated protein levels in cerebrospinal fluid without pleocytosis; reduced conduction velocity and abnormal F response on EMG
Myasthenia gravis	Recurrent paralysis; sustained response to anticholinesterase therapy; decremental response of muscle action potential with repetitive nerve stimulation on EMG
Tick paralysis	Paresthesias; ascending paralysis; presence of tick in scalp or skin
Stroke	Asymmetric paralysis; abnormal cerebrospinal fluid and/or cranial computed tomography studies
Poliomyelitis	Antecedent febrile illness; asymmetric paralysis; cerbrospinal fluid pleocytosis
Atropine overdose	Symptoms of central nervous system excitation (hallucinations and delirium)

11. How is the diagnosis of botulism established?

Laboratory testing is generally not critical to the diagnosis of botulism. The standard test is the mouse bioassay, in which type-specific antitoxin protects mice against any botulinum toxin in the sample. Sample specimens include serum, gastric aspirates, stool, and respiratory secretions. Polymerase chain reaction may be used to detect *C. botulinum* genes in an environmental sample.

12. How is botulinum intoxication treated?

Supportive care and passive immunization with equine antitoxin are the cornerstones of therapy for botulism. Antibiotics have no known direct effect. A licensed trivalent antitoxin, which contains neutralizing antibodies against botulinum toxin types A, B, and E, is available from the Centers for Disease Control and Prevention (CDC) and is given as a 10-ml dose of a 1:10 dilution in 0.9% saline solution. A skin test is required before administration. An investigational heptavalent (ABCDEFG) antitoxin developed by the U.S. Army Medical Research Institute of Infectious Diseases is available for cases involving other toxin types. Early administration of antitoxin is critical because it can neutralize only the circulating toxins in patients with progressive symptoms. When symptom progression ceases, the circulating toxins are consumed; thus, the antitoxin no longer exerts any effect. Supportive management, such as enteral tube or parenteral feeding, mechanical ventilation, bowel and bladder care, and prevention of decubitus ulcers, deep venous thromboses, and nosocomial infections, is extremely important, especially in patients with generalized muscle paralysis and prolonged illness.

13. What is anthrax?

Anthrax is primarily a zoonotic disease of herbivores caused by the gram-positive, spore-forming soil organism *Bacillus anthracis*. Humans generally acquire the disease from contact with infected animals or contaminated animal products, ingestion of poorly cooked infected meat, or inhalation of aerosolized spores. The disease thus manifests clinically as three distinct syndromes: cutaneous, inhalational, and gastrointestinal anthrax. Involvement of the meninges may occur rarely.

14. Describe the classic appearance of the cutaneous form of anthrax.

Cutaneous anthrax is initiated when spores of *B. anthracis* are introduced into the skin through cuts or abrasions or by biting flies. The primary lesion—a painless, pruritic papule—

appears 1–7 days after the introduction of the endospore and is usually seen in the exposed areas of the arms and face. After 1–2 days, the lesion forms a vesicle that is surrounded by a nonpitting, gelatinous edema (often out of proportion to the vesicular size) and by a number of satellite vesicles. The lesion then enlarges and undergoes central necrosis and drying, forming an ulcer covered by a characteristic black eschar.

15. Describe the clinical presentation of inhalational anthrax.

The typical presentation of inhalational anthrax is biphasic. The initial phase follows an incubation period of 1–10 days and begins with the insidious onset of mild fever, myalgia, malaise, nonproductive cough, some chest or abdominal pain, and, in some cases, nausea and vomiting. The second phase develops within 1–3 days and begins abruptly with acute dyspnea, diaphoresis, further fever, and cyanosis. Stridor may result from tracheal compression by enlarged mediastinal lymph nodes. In up to 50% of cases, obtundation, seizures, and nuchal rigidity may develop as a result of complicating anthrax meningitis. This stage is rapidly progressive; shock, associated hypothermia, and death occur within 24–36 hours. A chest radiograph typically shows widening of the mediastinum and pleural effusions.

Recent events, however, have revealed cases wherein the clinical course was in some ways different from the classic bimodal pattern described above. One patient presented with progressively worsening headache of 3 days' duration, accompanied by nausea, chills, and night sweats but no respiratory complaints. Physical examination was notable only for pulse rate elevated out of proportion to either symptoms or fever, diffuse rhonchi, and decreased breath sounds in both lung bases.

16. What laboratory tests are used in the diagnosis of anthrax?

Presumptive identification of infection is made by direct Gram's stain of a smear of the skin lesion (vesicular fluid or eschar), cerebrospinal fluid, or blood. A positive test shows encapsulated, broad, gram-positive bacilli. Diagnosis also can be based on growth of nonhemolytic colonies and large, nonmotile, nonencapsulated, gram-positive, spore-forming rods on sheep's blood agar. Confirmatory laboratory tests include growth of heavily encapsulated bacilli on nutrient agar in the presence of 5% carbon dioxide, susceptibility to lysis by gamma phage, and direct fluorescence-antibody staining of cell-wall polysaccharide antigen. Supportive laboratory tests include evidence of *B. anthracis* DNA by PCR, demonstration of *B. anthracis* in a clinical specimen by immunohistochemical staining for the cell wall antigen, and serologic tests that may be validated by laboratory confirmation.

The CDC defines a confirmed case of anthrax as (1) a clinically compatible case of cutaneous, inhalational, or gastrointestinal disease that is laboratory confirmed by isolation of *B. anthracis* from an affected tissue, or (2) other laboratory evidence of *B. anthracis* infection based on at least two supportive laboratory tests.

17. How is anthrax treated?

The recommended initial therapy for adults with clinically evident inhalational anthrax, severe cutaneous anthrax, and gastrointestinal anthrax is 400 mg of ciprofloxacin given intravenously every 12 hours. Doxycycline, 100 mg IV every 12 hours, is a suitable alternative. A triple-therapy regimen of parenteral ciprofloxacin, 400 mg every 8 hours; rifampicin, 300 mg every 12 hours; and clindamycin, 900 mg every 8 hours was recently reported with 100% survival rate at one institution.

For benign cases of cutaneous anthrax, oral treatment with ciprofloxacin, 500 mg every 12 hours, is recommended. Oral doxycycline, 100 mg every 12 hours, and amoxicillin, 500 mg every 8 hours, are suitable alternatives in susceptible strains.

Total duration of treatment should be 60 days.

18. Should exposed but asymptomatic persons be treated?

Postexposure prophylaxis is indicated to prevent inhalational anthrax after a confirmed or suspected aerosol exposure. The drug regimen is similar to that used to treat cutaneous anthrax.

BIBLIOGRAPHY

1. Arnon SS, Schechter R, Inglesby TV, et al: Botulinum toxin as a biological weapon: Medical and public health management. JAMA 285:1059–1070, 2001.
2. Borio L, Frank D, Mani V, et al: Death due to bioterrorism-related inhalational anthrax: Report of 2 patients. JAMA 286:2554–2559, 2001.
3. Bush LM, Abrams BH, Beall A, Johnson CC: Index case of fatal inhalational anthrax due to bioterrorism in the United States. N Engl J Med 345:1607–1610, 2001.
4. Centers for Disease Control and Prevention: Recognition of illness associated with the intentional release of a biologic agent. MMWR 50(41):893–897, 2001.
5. Centers for Disease Control and Prevention: Update: Investigation of anthrax associated with intentional exposure and interim public health guidelines, October 2001. MMWR 50(41):889–893, 2001.
6. Centers for Disease Control and Prevention: Interim Smallpox Response Plan and Guidelines [draft 2.0]. Atlanta, Centers for Disease Control and Prevention, 2001.
7. Dixon TC, Meselson M, Guillemin J, Hanna PC. Anthrax. N Engl J Med 341:815–826, 1999.
8. Gallagher TC, Strober BE: Cutaneous *Bacillus anthracis* infection. N Engl J Med 345:1646–1467, 2001.
9. Henderson DA, Inglesby TV, Bartlett JG, et al: Smallpox as a biological weapon: Medical and public health management. JAMA 281:2127–2137, 1999.
10. Inglesby TV, Dennis DT, Henderson DA, et al: Plague as a biological weapon: Medical and public health management. JAMA 283:2281–2290, 2000.
11. Kortepeter M, Christopher G, Cieslak T, et al (eds): USAMRIID's Medical Management of Biological Casualties Handbook, 4th ed. Fort Detrick, MD, U.S. Army Medical Research Institute of Infectious Diseases, 1998.
12. Mayer TA, Bersoff-Matcha S, Murphy C, et al: Clinical presentation of inhalational anthrax following bioterrorism exposure: Report of 2 surviving patients. JAMA 286:2549–2553, 2001.
13. Shafazand S, Doyle R, Ruoss S, et al: Inhalational anthrax: Epidemiology, diagnosis, and management. Chest 116:1369–1376, 1999.
14. Swartz MN: Recognition and management of anthrax: An update. N Engl J Med 345:1621–1626, 2001.

VI. Renal Disease

43. HYPERTENSION

Stuart L. Linas, M.D.

1. Define the clinical spectrum of severe hypertension.

Severe hypertension can be classified in many ways, but there are three major categories: hypertensive crisis or emergent hypertension, hypertension with end-organ dysfunction (such as angina), and uncontrolled or urgent hypertension.

Hypertensive crisis is the turning point in the course of hypertension when immediate management of elevated blood pressure plays a decisive role in the eventual outcome. The most common etiologies are malignant and accelerated hypertension. Accelerated hypertension is defined as severe hypertension (diastolic blood pressure usually > 120 mmHg) in the setting of retinal hemorrhage and exudates (cotton wool spots). Malignant hypertension is accelerated hypertension with papilledema.

Hypertension with end-organ dysfunction is a form of severe hypertension in which blood pressure reduction may be associated with relief of clinical signs and symptoms.

Urgent hypertension is elevated blood pressure in the absence of end-organ dysfunction. Because it is only an abnormal "number," urgent hypertension is not associated with the dire consequences of the other types of severe hypertension.

2. Define the two hemodynamic determinants of blood pressure. Which is the predominant problem in malignant hypertension?

Arterial blood pressure is the product of cardiac output and systemic vascular resistance. Malignant hypertension is caused by increased systemic vascular resistance.

3. What are the most common underlying causes of malignant hypertension? Is an evaluation for secondary hypertension necessary?

Even though 95% of all patients with hypertension have essential hypertension, in patients who present with malignant hypertension, essential hypertension accounts for only 50% of the cases. Because secondary hypertension is a precipitant in the remaining 50% of patients with malignant hypertension, an evaluation for secondary causes is usually warranted. The most common secondary causes of malignant hypertension include renal artery stenosis, pheochromocytoma, cocaine, and primary aldosteronism.

4. In what situations should an evaluation for secondary hypertension be warranted?

A work-up for secondary hypertension should be undertaken in the following situations:

1. Initial presentation of malignant hypertension (especially if the patient is white or younger than 30 years of age or older than 60 years).

2. Increase in creatinine after an ACE inhibitor.

3. In compliant patients whose BP is difficult to control after an adequate trial with a combination potent vasodilator, beta-blocker and diuretic.

5. What are the potential complications of untreated and treated malignant hypertension?

Studies from the 1950s and 1960s revealed that the mortality from untreated malignant hypertension was 80–90%. Most of the deaths were due to acute renal failure. With the initiation of prompt antihypertensive therapy and acute dialysis (if necessary), morbidity and mortality have become due primarily to cardiovascular disease (stroke, myocardial infarction, and congestive heart failure).

6. Describe the acute treatment of malignant hypertension.

The acute treatment of choice is intravenous sodium nitroprusside. The initial dose is 0.5 μg/kg/min, and should be increased by 0.5 μg/kg/min every 2–3 minutes until a diastolic blood pressure less than 110 mmHg has been attained. Further acute decreases in blood pressure may result in vital organ hypoperfusion, as blood flow autoregulation may be altered to accommodate chronically elevated blood pressure. Other parenteral drugs that are less ideal (but acceptable) for the acute treatment of malignant hypertension include diazoxide, trimethaphan, and labetalol. Blood pressure should be monitored continuously during therapy. If there is concern about the accuracy of sphygmomanometric readings, monitoring should be done with an indwelling arterial catheter.

7. Outline a chronic antihypertensive regimen to follow successful acute treatment of malignant hypertension.

Because malignant hypertension is mediated by increased systemic vascular resistance, it is recommended that chronic therapy include a vasodilator such as hydralazine, pinacidil, or minoxidil. Vasodilators cause reflex tachycardia and sodium retention; therefore, it is usually necessary also to include a beta blocker and a diuretic. In some cases, chronic blood pressure reduction may be achieved with less potent vasodilators, such as angiotensin-converting enzyme (ACE) inhibitors or calcium channel blockers.

8. Describe the acute antihypertensive treatment in a patient with a pheochromocytoma.

Hypertension from pheochromocytomas is caused by vascular smooth muscle alpha$_1$ receptor activation, which results in vasoconstriction. Thus, the best acute treatment is intravenous administration of the alpha$_1$-blocker phentolamine. Sodium nitroprusside is also a reasonable choice. Beta blockers should initially be avoided because they cause both unopposed peripheral alpha$_1$ receptor stimulation and decreased cardiac output.

9. Describe the acute medical management of a patient with aortic dissection.

The initial therapeutic aim is to decrease both blood pressure and cardiac contractile force (dp/dt). This goal has traditionally been best achieved with sodium nitroprusside plus a beta blocker. Trimethaphan or labetalol is also effective in this setting.

10. What is the treatment for cocaine-induced hypertensive crisis?

Cocaine causes hypertension by inhibiting catecholamine reuptake at nerve terminals. Therefore, alpha$_1$ blockade with phentolamine or labetalol is effective. If hypertension is severe, sodium nitroprusside is the drug of choice.

11. What is the correct treatment for elevated blood pressure in the setting of a cerebrovascular accident (CVA)?

Patients with acute CVA often have high blood pressure for reasons not completely understood. BP < 160/100 mmHg should not be treated, because further blood pressure reduction can result in hypoperfusion of vital organs that have adapted to a chronically elevated BP. BP > 180/110 mmHg should be treated judiciously with parenteral agents such as sodium nitroprusside. Rapid lowering should be avoided; the aim of therapy is to reduce MAP by 25% or to lower DBP to 100 mmHg, whichever is higher, during the first hour. If neurologic status deteriorates, the rate of BP reduction should be slowed. Oral therapy should be instituted before parenteral treatment is discontinued. Avoid using clonidine or methyldopa, which can impair cerebral function.

CONTROVERSIES

12. Why are clonidine, beta blockers, and diuretics undesirable choices for treatment of malignant hypertension?

Each medication works, at least partly, by reducing cardiac output. Although this effect may result in acute blood pressure reduction, it may also further increase systemic vascular resistance. Therefore, vasodilator therapy is a better choice for malignant hypertension treatment.

13. What is the best antihypertensive regimen for a patient with preeclampsia?

Preeclampsia is the combination of hypertension, proteinuria, and edema. It occurs after the 20th week of gestation. The traditional treatments of choice are hydraliazine or alpha-methyl-dopa. If these drugs are ineffective or poorly tolerated, labetalol is a reasonably safe and effective alternative. Medications to be avoided because of potential teratogenesis include sodium nitroprusside, trimethaphan, diazoxide, ACE inhibitors, beta blockers, and calcium channel blockers. Furthermore, the safety of many antihypertensive drugs during pregnancy is unknown. Because preeclampsia and eclampsia may be life-threatening, it may be necessary to prescribe potent antihypertensives (sodium nitroprusside, minoxidil) with uncertain fetal toxicity potential.

14. What should be the approach to treatment of severe hypertension in patients with ischemic heart disease and chest pain?

Hypertension can precipitate ischemic chest pain in patients with severe coronary artery disease. Alternatively, hypertension can be secondary to chest pain, which results in marked increases in catecholamines and secondary reactive hypertension. In either setting, hypertension is associated with an increase in systemic vascular resistance and increases in myocardial oxygen demand. Nitroglycerin and beta blockers are the initial agents of choice. Because nitroprusside increases heart rate and myocardial oxygen demand in this setting, it is a secondary agent.

15. In severe hypertension, lowering of blood pressure can result in increases in serum creatinine and decreases in glomerular filtration rate (GFR). Why?

There are two major causes of loss of GFR after reduction of blood pressure in the setting of severe hypertension:

1. **Renal artery stenosis.** In patients with fixed atherosclerotic lesions of the main renal artery, decreases in blood pressure cause decreases in renal blood flow and GFR. This effect is related to a fixed lesion in a major or secondary renal artery. Decreases in blood pressure lead to decreases in glomerular capillary flow. Usually decreases in pressure are compensated by increases in efferent arteriolar tone. In some circumstances, decreases in flow are so severe that even maximal increases in efferent arteriolar tone cannot compensate. In other circumstances, agents used to reduce blood pressure, such as ACE inhibitors and angiotensin receptor blockers, prevent increases in efferent tone that normally would compensate for decreases in flow.

2. **Long-standing essential hypertension.** In this setting, no macrovascular abnormalities are present; the problem is marked sclerosis of the microvasculature of the kidney, including the afferent artery. Because of afferent arteriolar sclerosis, the afferent artery is unable to vasodilate in response to decreases in systemic blood pressure. Hence, GFR falls when blood pressure is lowered. This effect on GFR is made worse by agents such as ACE inhibitors and angiotensin receptor blockers, which prevent increases in efferent arteriolar tone that normally would offset, at least partially, decreases in blood pressure.

BIBLIOGRAPHY

1. Blumenfeld JD, Laragh JH: Management of hypertensive crises: The scientific basis for treatment decisions. Am J Hypertens 14:1154–1167, 2001.
2. Gifford RW Jr: Management of hypertensive crises. JAMA 266:829–835, 1991.
3. Hanson AS, Linas SL: Accelerated and malignant hypertension. Contemp Issues Nephrol 28:143–180, 1994.
4. Kitiyakara C, Guzman NJ: Malignant hypertension and hypertensive emergencies. J Am Soc Nephrol 133–142, 1998.

5. McRae RP, Liebson PR: Hypertensive crisis. Med Clin North Am 70_749–767, 1986.
6. Nolan CR, Linas SL: Accelerated malignant hypertension. In Schrier RW, Gottschalk CW (eds): Disease of the Kidney, 6th ed. Boston, Little, Brown, 1996, pp 1475–1556.
7. Vaughan CJ, Delanty N: Hypertensive emergencies. Lancet 356:411–417, 2000.

44. ACUTE RENAL FAILURE

Joseph I. Shapiro, M.D.

1. How is acute renal failure (ARF) diagnosed?

ARF is best diagnosed by the observation of a rapid deterioration in renal function, specifically glomerular filtration rate (GFR), over a period of hours to a few days. GFR is clinically best determined by an estimation of the clearance of creatinine. In many cases, if it is simply assumed that creatinine production is constant, a rising serum level of creatinine demonstrates that the clearance of creatinine has fallen. Until the patient achieves a steady state, the level of renal function cannot be assessed by the serum creatinine concentration. If a patient with previously normal renal function suddenly loses all renal function, serum creatinine will rise by only 1–2 mg/dl per day. Blood urea nitrogen (BUN) is another indicator of dereasing glomerular filtration. Of greater importance, a more dramatic rise in BUN compared with creatinine may suggest a prerenal or obstructive (postrenal) etiology. Urine output is another marker of altered renal physiology. Oliguria (urine output < 400 ml/24 hr) and anuria (urine output < 50 ml/24 hr) indicate an excretory capacity below the requirements of daily solute load, assuming normal metabolism.

2. What features distinguish acute from chronic renal failure?

When a patient presents some time after the onset of ARF, this distinction may not be so simple. In other words, when the serum creatinine is already extremely high (10 mg/dl or greater), it may not increase much more. As a rule of thumb, chronic renal failure is more likely to be associated with anemia, hypocalcemia, normal urine output, and small shrunken kidneys on ultrasound examination than is acute renal failure. It has been reported that chronic but not acute renal failure may be associated with an increase in the serum osmolal gap, i.e., the difference between measured and calculated serum osmolality. Most nephrologists agree that if kidneys are of normal size on ultrasound examination, a renal biopsy may be warranted.

3. What is the urine output of patients with ARF?

Although oliguria (urine output < 400 ml/24 hours in adults) implies the presence of ARF, often ARF is associated with normal or even increased urine flow. In the past two decades, non-oliguric ARF has come to be recognized as being as common as oliguric ARF. Generally, however, oliguria denotes a worse prognosis in the setting of acute tubular necrosis. It is important to distinguish between a low GFR and a "normal" urine output, recognizing that decreased plasma clearance of waste products may render the patient uremic.

4. How is ARF classified?

As for many medical disorders, it is generally better to start off with big categories and zoom in to the precise diagnosis. In ARF, the big categories are prerenal, intrarenal or parenchymal, and postrenal or obstructive.

Prerenal azotemia occurs when the renal perfusion pressure falls below the autoregulatory threshold for maintenance of normal GFR. This may occur in states of total body salt and water depletion such as dehydration, in conditions in which total body salt and water are excessive such as heart failure and cirrhosis, or from local lesions that decrease renal perfusion pressure such as renal artery stenosis. Typically such patients have concentrated urine with relatively low sodium concentration and a relatively benign urinalysis and can be treated by optimization of hemodynamic parameters. A special case of prerenal azotemia, called the hepatorenal syndrome, however, usually does not respond to such therapy and generally requires liver transplantation to correct the abnormal renal hemodynamics that result from liver failure. Recent experimental data suggest that the renal hemodynamic alterations associated with liver failure stem from the marked increases in systemic nitric oxide. Many of the precipitating causes of prerenal azotemia may lead to intrinsic renal failure; a therapeutic trial aimed at optimizing hemodynamics may be the only way to distinguish among them.

Intrarenal or parenchymal renal failure may be classified as vascular, glomerular, or tubulointerstitial. Vascular causes include large and small vessel vasculitis, atheroembolic renal disease, and the thrombotic microangiopathies. Acute glomerulonephritis from a variety of causes may cause ARF. Tubulointerstitial causes of ARF are more common and include acute interstitial nephritis, usually resulting from drug allergy; precipitation of myeloma proteins in the tubular fluid seen with myeloma kidney; and acute tubular necrosis, which is the most common tubulointerstitial form. Parenchymal causes of ARF are generally associated with isotonic urine that is high in sodium concentration and an active urinary sediment that contains clues to the etiology of the renal failure.

Postrenal or obstructive renal failure is a common cause of ARF and may result from either intraluminal or extraluminal obstruction at any site from the beginning of the collecting system to the tip of the urethra. Typically the urine (if elaborated) is isotonic or dilute and relatively high in sodium. Although examination of urine sediment may provide clues to the etiology of obstruction, often it does not. In general, bilateral ureteral obstruction is required to manifest renal failure.

5. What pathophysiologic mechanisms are operant in acute tubular necrosis?

Renal ischemia, toxic injury to the kidney, or a combination of these insults can cause prolonged loss of renal function. Physiologically, decreased GFR must result from an alteration in glomerular hemodynamic factors, such as a decrease in the effective surface area or permeability of the glomerulus (Kf), a decrease in glomerular blood flow, or an abnormality in tubular integrity, including obstruction of tubular flow by cellular debris or backleak of ultrafiltrate through a porous tubule. In fact, each of these pathogenetic features can be shown to be operant in some experimental models of ARF. The major mechanism by which renal failure is induced may be different from the primary mechanism by which it is maintained. For example, in ischemic ARF, decreases in renal and glomerular blood flow may cause the initial loss of renal function. However, tubular necrosis, with its attendant obstructing debris and backleak of ultrafiltrate, maintains the low GFR. The tubular mechanisms are usually important in the maintenance of ARF from most causes seen clinically. Therefore, pharmacologic efforts to improve renal blood flow are not, by themselves, generally effective in shortening the duration of ARF.

6. Describe the approach to the differential diagnosis of ARF.

The approach to the patient with ARF requires a good history and physical exam in concert with judiciously ordered laboratory and imaging tests. The history is extremely important in determining whether antecedent renal ischemia may have occurred, settings for which include surgery, other causes of hypotension, or dehydration. In addition, exposure to nephrotoxic drugs, such as aminoglycosides or nonsteroidal anti-inflammatory agents, or endogenous substances can be elicited. The physical examination is most useful in establishing volume status as well as in obtaining clues to any systemic illness (such as vasculitis) that may present as ARF. Evaluation of the neck veins is essential. Although urinary obstruction may be detected by other means, the finding of suprapubic dullness after voiding is a valuable clue to the presence of bladder outlet obstruction.

7. What are the common causes of ARF in the hospital and ICU setting?

ARF that develops in hospitalized patients (not in the ICU) is due to acute tubular nerosis (38%), prerenal azotemia (28%), or other causes (e.g., obstruction, glomerulonephritis, acute interstitial nephritis). In the ICU most cases of ARF are due to acute tubular necrosis (76%) or prerenal azotemia (19%). Patients in the ICU with multiorgan failure have a substantially higher mortali-tyrate (> 70%), even with functional or prerenal failure.

8. **What causes ARF in kidney transplants?**

About one-half of cadaveric kidneys undergo acute tubular necrosis, and about 5–8% have primary nondysfunction in the early postoperative period. Unique causes of ARF in renal transplant recipients are graft rejection, vascular occlusion, and opportunistic infections. Ostruction always should be ruled out. Often a transplant biopsy is required to diagnose the cause.

9. **How does examination of the urine help in the differential diagnosis of ARF?**

Laboratory evaluation begins with careful examination of the urine. A concentrated urine points more to prerenal causes, whereas isotonic urine suggests parenchymal or obstructive causes. Typically, the urine sediment of patients with prerenal azotemia demonstrates occasional hyaline casts or finely granular casts. In contrast, the presence of renal tubular epithelial cells and "muddy" granular casts strongly suggests acute tubular necrosis; microhematuria and red blood cell casts suggest glomerulonephritis; and white cell casts containing eosinophils suggest acute interstitial nephritis. As discussed above, benign urine sediment is quite compatible with urinary obstruction.

10. **What are the implications of urinary electrolytes in the differential diagnosis of ARF?**

The determination of urine electrolyte and creatinine concentrations may be helpful in the differential diagnosis of ARF. When used with serum values, urinary diagnostic indices can be generated. Understanding the concepts behind the interpretation of these indices is easier and better than trying to remember specific numbers. Quite simply, if the tubule is working well in the setting of decreased GFR, tubular reabsorption of sodium and water is avid, and the relative clearance of sodium to creatine is low. Conversely, if the tubule is injured and cannot reabsorb sodium well, the relative clearance of sodium to creatine is not low. Therefore, with prerenal azotemia, the ratio of the clearance of sodium to the clearance of creatine ($\times$ 100), which is also called the fractional excretion of sodium ($FENa = UNa/UCr \times PCr/PNa \times 100$), is typically less than 1.0, whereas with parenchymal or obstructive causes of ARF, the FENa is generally greater than 2.0.

11. **What are important exceptions to the rules about urinary diagnostic indices described above?**

The FENa test is much less useful when patients are nonoliguric. In this setting, the specificity of a low FENa for prerenal azotemia is markedly diminished. In addition to nonoliguria, several causes of ATN, specifically dye-induced acute tubular necrosis or acute tubular necrosis associated with hemolysis or rhabdomyolysis, may typically be associated with a low FENa. Patients who have prerenal azotemia but have either persistent diuretic effect, chronic tubulointerstitial injury, or bicarbonaturia may have a relatively high FENa. In the last case, the fractional excretion of chloride (FECl), which is calculated in an analogous way, will be appropriately low (< 1%). Finally, the early stages of acute renal failure from glomerulonephritis, transplant allograft rejection, or urinary obstruction may be associated with a low FENa.

12. **How is ARF prevented?**

Acute tubular necrosis often results from a combination of insults and is most likely to occur in particular clinical settings as well as in older patients, so that avoidance and prophylaxis are often possible. Acute tubular necrosis usually occurs after surgery or preexisting dehydration. In these settings, nephrotoxic drugs, such as radiocontrast dye, aminoglycosides, amphotericin B, nonsteroidal anti-inflammatory agents, and some cancer chemotherapeutic agents (e.g., cisplatin, methotrexate), are far more potent in causing ARF. Optimizing volume status and establishing a relatively high rate of urine flow minimize the risk of ARF. In specific situations, such as administration of radiocontrast dye or cisplatin and relatively high-risk surgery (e.g., open-heart or biliary tract surgery), mannitol (12.5–25 gm administered as an IV infusion) has been thought to be a useful adjunct in preventing ARF. However, data from Solomon et al. have demonstrated that mannitol actually potentiates ARF following radiocontrast. Contrast nephropathy is best prevented by careful patient and procedure assessment. In high-riskg groups, intravenous hydration remains the only proven safeguard. A recent study supports the use of N-acetyl-cysteine to attenuate radiocontrast ARF during cardiac catheterization. In addition, other reports demonstrate a benefit from the use of low ioinic strength contrast.

13. How is established ARF treated?

The key point in treatment is to make an accurate diagnosis. Different causes of ARF require different therapies. Prerenal azotemia is treated by optimizing hemodynamic factors. The approach obviously differs among patients. In dehydration, simple volume resuscitation is effective. In congestive heart failure, diuresis, by virtue of resultant decreases in afterload, may improve renal perfusion. Urinary obstruction must be relieved.

Parenchymal ARF is also addressed in a diagnosis-directed manner. Acute glomerulonephritis may respond to immunosuppressive medications and/or plasmapheresis. Acute interstitial nephritis usually mandates discontinuation of the offending allergen, usually a drug, and may resolve more quickly with the administration of steroids.

Acute tubular necrosis is best treated, as discussed above, by prevention. Although pharmacologic agents such as calcium channel blockers and atrial natriuretic factor may ameliorate established experimental ARF, these agents are not yet approved for clinical use. Because nonoliguric acute tubular necrosis is associated with lower mortality and morbidity rates than oliguric acute tubular necrosis, there is some excitement about the administration of high-dose loop diuretics (1–3 gm/24 hr given as an IV infusion or as repeated boluses) in concert with renal doses of dopamine (1–3 µg/kg/min). This therapy, which converts some patients with oliguric acute tubular necrosis to a nonoliguric state, certainly facilitates management of volume and nutritional status. Whether this approach actually improves the prognosis is not clear. Optimization of fluid status and avoidance and/or therapy of electrolyte disorders are the mainstays of conservative management of ARF.

14. Which electrolyte disorders accompany ARF?

The most common are hyperkalemia, hypermagnesemia, hyperphosphatemia, hypocalcemia, and acidosis.

15. Describe the approach to hyperkalemia in patients with ARF.

Hyperkalemia most commonly occurs with oliguric acute tubular necrosis or urinary obstruction. It is truly a medical emergency. A serum potassium over 6.0 mandates an EKG, searching for peaked T waves, diminished P-wave amplitude, or prolonged QRS complex. Any of these findings is an indication for parenteral therapy. The quickest-acting parenteral therapy is calcium, administered as chloride, gluceptate, or gluconate salts. This therapy does not affect the serum potassium level but does antagonize the effects of hyperkalemia on the membrane potential of the heart and prevents or reverses the cardiac effects of hyperkalemia. Administration of 1–2 ampules of calcium (4.8–9.6 mEq) has immediate effects, but they persist only as long as the resultant hypercalcemia. Adverse effects include possible precipitation of calcium and phosphate in a hyperphosphatemic patient. Generally, this risk is outweighed by the risk of untreated hyperkalemia. Another rapidly effective approach is the administration of insulin, which drives potassium into cells and lowers the serum potassium level. In patients who have a normal serum glucose, insulin (10 units IV) is generally administered with dextrose (one ampule of D50W or an infusion of D10W). The effects of insulin last somewhat longer than those of calcium and can be prolonged by a constant infusion of insulin, usually administered with glucose to prevent hypoglycemia. Bicarbonate may also be used to raise arterial pH and to shift potassium into cells. Complications include potentially adverse hemodynamic effects of intravenous bicarbonate and volume expansion from sodium load.

Other useful approaches include removal of potassium from the body with potassium-binding resins (Kayexalate), increased urinary excretion with the use of diuretics (if possible), and hemodialysis or peritoneal dialysis. These methods of removing potassium from the body take longer to work than parenteral calcium, insulin, and bicarbonate and therefore must be considered only after the medical emergency is addressed.

16. What abnormalities in calcium, phosphate, and magnesium accompany ARF?

In patients with ARF, phosphate excretion is minimized and hyperphosphatemia generally results. This process is accelerated in conditions in which tissue breakdown with attendant release of phosphate into the extracellular fluid occurs. Increases in serum phosphate concentration cause microprecipitation of calcium and resultant hypocalcemia. Although this is not usually clinically important, occasionally severe hypocalcemia causes tetany, seizures, and cardiac arrhythmias, which are largely preventable by the judicious administration of oral phosphate binders, usually aluminum hydroxide. Rarely, hemodialysis with porous membranes must be undertaken to lower the serum phosphate. If the hyperphosphatemia is extremely severe, a low calcium dialysate bath should be used to avoid extensive calcium-phosphate precipitation. Hypermagnesemia generally results in patients with ARF who are receiving magnesium-containing antacids or cathartics. Because the kidney is the usual organ that excretes magnesium, these agents should certainly be avoided in patients with ARF.

17. What abnormalities in acid-base balance accompany ARF?

The kidney is the organ that generally excretes acid generated by metabolism of a typical Western diet; therefore, ARF is often associated with acidosis. Although the degree of metabolic acidosis is generally minor, occasionally other contributing factors, such as ongoing lactic acidosis, cause severe metabolic acidosis.

Oral sodium bicarbonate may be useful in treating metabolic acidosis associated with ARF if the acidosis is relatively mild. It is not clear, however, whether intravenous sodium bicarbonate, especially if administered as a bolus, should be used. In some cases, either intravenous or oral sodium bicarbonate may be contraindicated by coexisting volume expansion. A growing body of literature suggests that the deleterious hemodynamic effects of intravenous bolus of bicarbonate contraindicate its use. The mechanism of these deleterious hemodynamic effects may involve the generation of CO_2 when bicarbonate is mixed with acidotic blood. This CO_2 can diffuse across cell membranes and potentially produce a paradoxical intracellular acidosis in cardiac and vascular tissue. Hemodialysis against a bicarbonate bath may be used to address acidosis in this setting without causing increases in $PaCO_2$; however, most extremely acidotic patients are hemodynamically unstable to start with, making hemodialysis difficult to perform. The therapeutic approach to severe metabolic acidosis with or without ARF failure is controversial.

18. What is the uremic syndrome?

The uremic syndrome is a symptom complex associated with renal failure. It may occur with chronic and acute renal failure and involves virtually all organs of the body. Major manifestations are nausea and vomiting, pruritus, bleeding disorder, encephalopathy, and pericarditis. The syndrome generally mandates initiation of nonconservative therapy for ARF, such as hemodialysis, peritoneal dialysis, or continuous arteriovenous hemofiltration. The pathogenesis of the uremic syndrome is still poorly understood; however, neither urea nor creatinine produces any of the known manifestations of uremia.

19. What are the indications for nonconservative therapy of ARF?

Indications for nonconservative therapy, such as dialysis, include uremic signs or symptoms, fluid overload and/or electrolyte abnormalities that are refractory to conservative management. It has become the standard of care to provide nonconservative therapy when the BUN exceeds 100 mg/dl or the serum creatinine exceeds 10 mg/dl, especially in the setting of oliguric acute tubular necrosis. These latter guidelines are not absolute and must be interpreted in the light of other clinical features.

20. What are the options for nonconservative therapy of ARF?

The three main options for nonconservative therapy of ARF are hemodialysis, peritoneal dialysis, and continuous renal replacement therapy (CRRT). There are, of course, variations of each of these modalities. Hemodialysis involves the pumping of blood through an artificial kidney that removes solutes primarily by dialysis along a concentration gradient; water is removed by ultrafiltration driven by a pressure gradient. Central venous access, anticoagulation, a skilled technician, and expensive equipment are mandatory for this process. Peritoneal dialysis involves the repetitive instillation and removal of fluid into the peritoneal cavity. Solute removal again results primarily by dialysis along a concentration gradient, and fluid removal occurs by ultrafiltration driven by an osmotic pressure gradient. Although this method is less efficient and less rapid than hemodialysis, no central venous access, anticoagulation, skilled technician, or expensive equipment is necessary. Finally, CRRT includes a number of treatments characterized by slow, gradual, continuous removal of fluid and electrolytes. Continuous venovenous hemodialysis (CVVHD) is the most widely used method. It involves solute removal by convection and fluid removal by hydrostatic pressure across high flux membrane.Like conventional dialysis, CVVHD requires central venous access, anticoagulation, skilled staff, and complex equipment. Continuous arteriovenous hemofiltration/dialysis (CAVH/CAVHD) is a technically simple but less efficient form of CRRT. Although each of these techniques has advantages and disadvantages, in general, the expertise of the center is probably the most important factor. Of interest, the biocompatibility of the hemodialysis membrane appears to be an important factor in determining outcome, whereas the intensity of the dialsyis prescription does not appear to be an important factor.

21. What are the advantages of CRRT?

CRRT is theoretically superior to conventional dialysis, but this advantage has not translated into improved survival rates. CRRT provides more hemodynamic stability, which is highly desirable in unstable ICU patients. Large volumes of fluid can be removed over an extended period, and the removal of solutes is more efficient. Hemodynamic stability appears to shorten the time to renal recovery. The high-flux synthetic membranes are more biocompatible, exhibiting less complement and leuckocyte activation. In hypercatabolic critically ill patients, high nutritional requirements mandate a large fluid intake. CRRT can provide an important adjuvant to this therapy, allowing high caloric intake without hypervolemia.

22. What are the disadvantages of CRRT?

As mentioned above, CAVHD requires arterial access and CVVHD requires complex equipment. The need for continuous anticoagulation can pose a significant problem for patients at risk for bleeding. CRRT requires patient immobilization, necessitating disconnection from complex procedures or investigations. CRRT is also more expensive than conventional dialysis.

23. What is SLEDD?

Slow low-efficiency daily dialysis (SLEDD) has many of the advantages of CRRT but does not require the ICU nursing staff to manage the equipment. SLEDD is conventional dialysis using low blood and dialysis flow rates over an extended period, such as 12 hours. Unfortunately, SLEDD also requires central venous access and, like conventional hemodialysis, skilled technicians to operate the hemodialysis hardware.

BIBLIOGRAPHY

1. Anderson RJ, Gabow PA, Gross PA: Urinary chloride concentration in acute renal failure. Min Elect Metab 10:92–97, 1984.
2. Anderson RJ, Linas SL, Berns AS, et al: Nonoliguric acute renal failure. N Engl J Med 296:1134–1138, 1977.
3. Appel BB: Aminoglycoside nephrotoxicity. Am J Med 159:427–443, 1990.
4. Barrett BJ, Parfrey PS, Vavsour HM, et al: Contrast nephropathy in patients with impaired renal function: High versus low osmolar media. Kidney Int 421:1274–1279, 1992.
5. Better OS, Stein JH: Early management of shock and prophylaxis of acute renal failure in traumatic rhabdomyolysis. N Engl J Med 322:825–829, 1990.
6. Cantarovich F, Locatelli A, Fernandez JC, et al: Furosemide in high doses in the treatment of acute renal failure. Postgrad Med J 47:13–17, 1971.
7. Gillum DM, Dixon BS, Yanover MS, et al: The role of intensive dialysis in acute renal failure. Clin Nephrol 25:249–256, 1986..
8. Graziani G, Cantaluppi A, Casati S, et al: Dopamine and furosemide in oliguric acute renal failure. Nephron 37:39–42, 1984.

9. Hakim RM, Wingard RL, Parker RA: Effect of the dialysis membrane in the treatment of patients with acute renal failure. N Engl J Med 331:1338–1342, 1994.
10. Hou SH, Bushinsky DA, Wish JB, et al: Hospital acquired renal insufficiency: A prospective study. Am J Med 74:243–248, 1983.
11. Karsou SA, Jaber BL, Pereira BJ: Impact of intermittent hemodialysis variables on clinical outcomes in acute renal failure. Am J Kidney Dis 35:980–991, 2000.
12. Levinsky NG: Pathophysiology of acute renal failure. N Engl J Med 296:1453–1457, 1977.
13. Maguire WC, Anderson RJ: Continuous arteriovenous hemofiltration in the intensive care unit. J Crit Care 1:54–56, 1986.
14. Malhotra D, Shapiro JI: Pathogenesis and management of lactic acidosis. Concepts Crit Care 2:439–448, 1996.
15. Miller TR, Anderson RJ, Linas SL, et al: Urinary diagnostic indices in acute renal failure. Ann Intern Med 89:47–50, 1978.
16. Paller MS: Drug-induced nephropathies. Med Clin North Am 74:909–917, 1990.
17. Schetz M, Lauwers PM, Ferdinande P: Extracorporeal treatment of acute renal failure in the intensive care unit: A critical review. Intens Care Med 15:349–357, 1989.
18. Schrier RW, Conger JD: Acute renal failure: Pathogenesis, diagnosis, and management. In Schrier RW (ed): Renal and Electrolyte Disorders. Boston, Little, Brown, 1986, pp 423–460.
19. Shapiro JI, Anderson RJ: Urinary diagnostic indices in acute renal failure. AKF Nephrol Let 1:13–16, 1984.
20. Shapiro JI, Anderson RJ: Sodium depletion states. In Brenner BM, Stein J (eds): Topics in Nephrology. New York, Churchill Livingstone, 1985, pp 155–192.
21. Solomon R, Werner C, Mann D, et al: Effects of saline, mannitol, and furosemide to prevent acute decreases in renal function induced by radiocontrast agents. N Engl J Med 331:1416–1420, 1994.
22. Tepel M, van der GM, Scharzfeld C, et al: Prevention of radiographic-contrast-agent-induced reductions in renal function by acetylcysteine. N Engl J Med 343:180–184, 2000.
23. Vanholder R, Van Biesen W, Lameire N: What is the renal replacement method of first choice for intensive care patients? J Am Soc Nephrol 12(Suppl 17):S40–S43, 2001.
24. Venkatsen J, Shapiro JJ, Hemilton R: Dialysis considerations in the patient with acute renal failure. In Henrich WL (ed): Principles and Practice of Hemodialysis, 2nd ed. St. Louis, Mosby, 1998.
25. Venkateswara K, Rao: Posttransplant medical complications. Surg Clin North Am 78, 1998.

45. RENAL REPLACEMENT THERAPY AND RHABDOMYOLYSIS

Ludwig H. Lin, M.D.

RENAL REPLACEMENT THERAPY

1. What are the indications for renal replacement therapy?

Absolute indications for renal replacement include life-threatening situations related to electrolyte imbalances (hyperkalemia and acidosis), fluid overload in the setting of oliguria/anuria (congestive heart failure and hypoxia), potentially lethal drug overdoses (e.g., lithium, theophylline, acetaminophen), and severe complications resulting from uremia (pericardial effusion, pericarditis, or mental status changes).

Relative indications include fluid overload, uremia with a blood urea nitrogen (BUN) concentration higher than 100 mg/dl, and clinical platelet dysfunction due to uremia.

2. What are the indications for continuous renal replacement therapy (CRRT)?

The indications for CRRT include all of the indications for renal replacement in general, along with the additional factor of hemodynamic instability. Critically ill patients often do not tolerate the higher flow rates required in hemodialysis (HD) and develop either hypotension or arrhythmias. CRRT has a slower flow rate and often can be used in patients who otherwise would not tolerate HD. In addition, patients with elevated intracranial pressure (ICP) do not tolerate HD because of the rapid shifts in fluid and blood urea nitrogen (BUN), but they can tolerate CRRT.

Nontraditional (i.e., unproven) indications for CRRT include management of hyperthermia and rhabdomyolysis (see questions at the end of this chapter); inflammatory cytokine removal in systemic inflammatory response syndrome (SIRS); and fluid management in hemodynamically unstable patients. In liver transplant surgeries, for example, anesthesiologists now use intraoperative slow continuous ultrafiltration (SCUF) to remove fluid in patients with anuria/oliguria due to acute renal failure (ARF).

3. **List the different modes for renal replacement therapy.**
   Intermittent renal replacement therapies
   • Peritoneal dialysis (PD)
   • Intermittent hemodialysis (IHD)
   • Plasma ultrafiltration (PUF)
   Continuous renal replacement therapies
   • Slow continuous ultrafiltration (SCUF)
   • Continuous arteriovenous hemofiltration (CAVH)
   • Continuous arteriovenous hemodialysis (CAVHD)
   • Continuous arteriovenous hemodiafiltration (CAVHDF)
   • Continuous venovenous hemofiltration (CVVH)
   • Continuous venovenous hemodialysis (CVVHD)
   • Continuous venovenous hemodiafiltration (CVVHDF)

4. **Define hemofiltration, hemodialysis, and hemodiafiltration.**
   Hemofiltration: Plasma passes through a highly permeable membrane as it flows through the circuit with a pressure gradient driving the "convective" flow.
   Hemodialysis: As blood flows on one side of a semipermeable membrane, the dialysate solution, which contains various electrolytes in different concentrations, flows in the other direction to drive the diffusion of water as well as electrolytes across the membrane as a result of the difference in the concentration gradient.
   Hemodiafiltration: This technique makes simultaneous use of the concepts of hemofiltration and hemodialysis.

5. **What are the components of a CRRT system?**
   The two types of hemofilters used for CRRTs are a flat-plate and a hollow-fiber filter. Flat-plate filters have a semipermeable membrane that lines plates and is housed in a rectangular casing; the hollow-fiber filters are composed of thousands of tiny cylindrical, "straw-like" hollow fibers enclosed in a cylinder-shaped casing. Both systems separate the filter into two compartments: the blood compartment and the ultrafiltrate compartment. The average surface area is 0.6 m^2. The membranes are made of synthetic biocompatible membranes, such as polysulfone or polyacrylonitrile. The other components of a CRRT system include circuit tubing, collection bag, dialysate infusion tubing, anticoagulation tubing, blood pumps, and the machine itself.

6. **What kind of access is ideal for the initiation of renal replacement therapy?**
   The ideal access catheter is short and has a large bore to minimize resistance, yet is not large enough to compromise perfusion or venous return. The arteriovenous (AV) therapies require two large-bore, single-lumen catheters. Adults typically require 7- or 8-French arterial catheters and 7- to 12-French venous catheters. The catheter lengths range from 10 to 20 cm and vary depending on the insertion site. For venovenous (VV) therapies, a dual-lumen venous catheter may be placed, using one lumen for afferent and one for efferent flow. Two single-lumen, large-bore venous catheters can also be placed. Femoral vessels can be safely used but may have problems with decreased flow rates during patient movement, high intra-abdominal pressure, or clots.

7. What are the differences in the equipment used for hemodialysis vs. CRRT?

Hemodialysis uses small-pore membranes and works by diffusion clearance rather than "bulk-flow" convection clearance, which is the operating principle behind CAVH and CVVH. CAVHD and CVVHD add an additional step to dialysis, which provides diffusion clearance in addition to convection clearance. Both acute IHD and CRRT use large-bore, high-flow catheters. Chronic IHD is done with arteriovenous grafts or fistulas, which are accessed by needles during the dialysis sessions.

CRRT uses large-pore membranes that allowr passage of molecules as large as 20–50 KD and now is done on machines with roller pumps to guarantee a steady flow and weight-measuring systems to keep track of the hourly fluid balance. This technique allows precise fluid management.

8. What is the difference between hemofiltration and hemodialysis?

Hemofiltration simply describes the loss of plasma as it flows by convection across a highly permeable membrane. Renal replacement, as defined by clearance of solutes and correction of electrolytes, occurs in hemofiltration through the loss of excessive solutes via bulk flow as well as by replacement of the lost plasma volume with a fluid that has the correct electrolyte concentrations. **Hemodialysis** works as renal replacement by using countercurrent flow to adjust the electrolyte concentrations in plasma as it flows against the flow of a dialysate containing various electrolytes.

9. What kinds of laboratory tests should be ordered regularly for patients on CRRT?

Sodium, potassium, bicarbonate, calcium, and phosphate levels can change quickly in critically ill patients. Hyperphosphatemia occurs in IHD because of inefficient clearance of phosphate, but hypophosphatemia often occurs during CRRT. Hypomagnesemia also can occur, especially when magnesium is complexed with citrate (e.g., for use as an anticoagulant).

10. What other nutritional derangements need to be considered in CRRT?

Glucose loss via filtrated volume can be significant (up to 40–80 gm/day), depending on the volume. This loss must be taken into account in calculating the patient's energy expenditure and nutritional replacement needs. The opposite is true when peritoneal dialysate is used as CRRT fluid, because it contains a high concentration of glucose (between 1240 and 3600 mg/dl) that may lead to hyperglycemia and excessive glucose uptake.

Amino acids are lost in both HD and CRRT. The amino acids present in the highest plasma concentrations have the highest elimination rate; thus, glutamine loss is most pronounced. As a general rule, amino acid supply should be raised by 0.2 gm/kg/day to compensate for renal replacement therapy.

Peptides larger than 20–50 KD are not filtered by CVVH, but the smaller peptides, such as catecholamines and humoral mediators, may be lost. However, because of the sieve ratio for the usual flow rates and membrane pore sizes of conventional CRRT, the amount lost is actually multiples lower than the amount cleared by the body's own metabolism. Studies show that protein catabolism is actually induced by the interaction of blood with the synthetic biocompatible membrane, which can generate additional protein losses.

Water-soluble vitamins are known to be lost in both IHD and CRRT. Vitamin C is lost in appreciable amounts and must be replaced, and in one case report CRRT resulted in vitamin B_1 (thiamine) deficiency, leading to right ventricular dysfunction and persistent acidosis. Fat-soluble vitamins are complexed to plasma proteins and lipoproteins, which are too large to be filtrated through the membrane. Therefore, their levels are not affected by CRRT.

11. What are the criteria for choosing a replacement solution in CRRT?

Renal replacement therapy has three concurrent goals: (1) clearance of toxins, (2) compensation for acidosis, and (3) fluid elimination (if tolerated by the patient's hemodynamic status). In CVVH, the filtrated plasma is set aside as waste and replaced by a solution of the physician's designation. In CVVHD, a dialysate is also run at a constant flow rate to provide additional clearance capability.

The replacement fluids in use include lactate, bicarbonate, and acetate-buffered solutions. The consensus is that acetate buffering systems result in decreased cardiac contractility and hemodynamic instability. Lactate-based solutions have a stable shelf-life and appear to work well in buffering the acidosis of critically ill patients. However, in patients with reduced lactate metabolism (e.g., hepatic failure, liver transplantation, lactic acidosis), the increased systemic levels of lactate resulting from lactate-based buffering solutions may mean increasing acidosis. Therefore, in these patients, a bicarbonate-based replacement fluid should be used. However, bicarbonate-containing solutions are unstable,and need to be mixed fresh at the patient's bedside. This may mean an increased workload for the ICU nursing or pharmacy staff and also introduces the possibility of operator error when each new bag of replacement fluid is mixed.

12. Discuss the role of CRRT in the management of septic shock.

This is one of the most controversial issues related to CRRT. Theoretically, all of the small molecular weight peptides responsible for inflammatory responses (e.g., interleukins 1 and 6, tumor necrosis factor beta, elements of the complement pathway, and other molecules such as leukotrienes and prostaglandins) are cleared by CRRT. Aggressive clearance may ameliorate their effect on the patient. Preliminary studies in both animal models and humans point to a possible role for CRRT in clearing the inflammatory mediators responsible for creating and sustaining the deletrious phenomenon of septic shock or, in a more accurate description of most cases, systemic inflammatory response syndrome (SIRS). In animal models, high-flow CRRT has been demonstrated to decrease systemic levels of inflammatory signals. Although this effect has not been demonstrated in humans, decreased vasopressor requirements have indeed been found in high-flow CRRT.

There are quite a few reasons for the controversy, and clinical studies to date show murky results. Because of the required numbers of subjects and the pathophysiologic diversity of critically ill patients, studies demonstrating favorable outcome are difficult to conduct. Furthermore, in practical terms the clearance of appreciable amounts of inflammatory mediators in humans will be hard to achieve. High-flow CRRT in humans requires an hourly filtration rate of 3–6 liters, which is beyond the capability of current machines. In addition, the sieve ratio of the inflammatory mediators is so nonsignificant that the native clearance rate by the patient's own body still vastly outstrips the clearance rate generated by the convective flow of CRRT. Many experts argue that the decreased levels of inflammatory mediators seen in prior trials probably are due to adsorption onto the filter membranes rather than actual convective clearance and that the frequent changes of filter membranes required to keep up with the adsorptive process will be prohibitively expensive and impractical.

However, because of the strong theoretical possibilities of using CRRT to treat sepsis and/or SIRS and patchy reports of favorable outcomes, this controversy is likely to continue.

13. What is the role of CRRT in liver failure?

Patients with fulminant hepatic failure often have additional complications such as hepatic encephalopathy, possible cerebral edema and increased intracranial pressures, concomitant renal failure, and coagulopathy and thrombocytopenia. These complications make CRRT a likely therapeutic option, although it may technically challenging to initiate. Some clinicians believe that CRRT actually is able to reduce the intracranial pressure (ICP) of patients with cerebral edema and impending herniation; furthermore, IHD can cause perturbations in cerebral perfusion because of the rapid intravascular shifts. In addition, patients with liver failure and concomitant ARF often are hemodynamically unstable and cannot tolerate IHD because of the hemodynamic side effects.

14. What kind of anticoagulation is required for the circuits in CRRT?

CRRT may be done without anticoagulation; however, clotting may occur at a higher frequency. Sites of clotting include the lumen of the access catheter, the hemofilter, and the venous trap of the circuit. Anticoagulation prevents filter and circuit clotting and maximizes the clearance capacity of the hemofilter membrane. The anticoagulant is not administered systemically; it is infused prior to the hemofilter, and the majority is lost then via the convective flow across the filter membrane. Obviously, some anticoagulant remains within the bloodstream.

In patients whose pathophysiology contraindicates heparinization, such as patients with heparin-induced thrombocytopenia, an alternative anticoagulant is trisodium citrate. It is quite efficacious but requires a posthemofilter infusion of calcium to reverse the effects of the anticoagulation,as well as to avoid systemic hypocalcemia. Prostacyclin can also be used, but it is associated with appreciable levels of systemic hypotension.

15. What are the complications of renal replacement therapy?

All of the risks inherent in obtaining central venous access are obviously associated with renal replacement therapy. Air embolization remains an especially constant danger, as does distal limb ischemia due to the use of large-bore arterial catheters in instances of AV renal replacement therapy.

Fluid overload or hypovolemia, electrolyte imbalances, and acid-base disturbances may result if the health care team is not hypervigilant in tracking the patient's physical status frequently.

Normothermic patients may become hypothermic, and febrile patients may become normothermic during CRRT, because both the extracorporeal circuit and the unwarmed replacement fluid bags cause heat loss. This loss may be dangerous if the patient becomes significantly hypothermic or if the lack of a febrile response alters the management algorithm of the critical care physician.

16. Discuss the drug-dosing strategy during renal replacement therapy.

Heparin, vancomycin, metronidazole, amikacin, myoglobin, and hemoglobin are the major compounds that are cleared by the large-pore CRRT membranes compared with the smaller pores of IHD. Otherwise, the clearance of drugs during CRRT is difficult to predict because of additional interactions with hepatic clearance and hepatic perfusion, protein binding by the particular drug involved, and the particular drug's sieve ratio.

The best recommendation is to dose medications initially with the assumption that the patient has a creatine clearance rate of 14 ml/min (which is the clearance rate achieved by a CVVH filtration rate of 20 L/day) and then to check plasma levels frequently to guide dosing.

17. What is the role of peritoneal dialysis in the critical care setting?

Peritoneal dialysis is contraindicated in patients with recent abdominal surgery and intra-abdominal infection or disease (e.g., peritonitis, ileus). These scenarios are common in critically ill patients. In addition, the peritoneal dialysate can decrease diaphragmatic excursion, creating problems with tachypnea and respiratory difficulties.

In patients with coagulopathy, hemodynamic instability, or elevations in ICP that may respond poorly to the rapid fluid shifts of IHD, peritoneal dialysis may be a reasonable alternative, especially if CRRT is not an available option.

RHABDOMYOLYSIS

18. What causes rhabdomyolysis?

The short answer is that muscle ischemia, damage, and eventual necrosis lead to rhabdomyolysis. The various etiologies are grouped into physical and nonphysical causes in the table below. Both groups of causes probably share a common generic pathway in that increased demands on the muscle cells and their mitochondria, whether because of intrinsic deficiencies or extrinsic forces (i.e., decreased oxygen delivery or increased metabolic demands), lead to ischemia and eventual damage.

Causes of Rhabdomyolysis

Physical causes
- Trauma and compression
- Occlusion or hypoperfusion of the muscular vessels
- Strained exercise of muscles
- Electrical current
- Hyperthermia

Table continued on following page

Causes of Rhabdomyolysis (Continued)

Nonphysical causes
- Metabolic myopathies
   McArdle disease
   Mitochondrial respiratory chain enzyme deficiencies
   Carnitine palmitoyl transferase deficiency
   Myoadenylate deasminase deficiency
   Phosphofructokinase deficiency
- Drugs and toxins
   Medications: antimalarials, colchicines, corticosteroids, fibrates, HMG-CoA reductase inhibitors,
      isoniazid, zidovudine
   Drugs of abuse: alcohol, heroin
   Toxins: snake and insect venoms
- Infections
   Local infection with muscular invasion (pyomyositis)
   Systemic infections: toxic shock syndrome, *Legionella* sp., tularemia, *Salmonella* sp., falciparum
      malaria, influenza, HIV, herpes viruses, coxsakievirus
- Electrolyte abnormalities

19. Discuss the symptoms and signs of rhabdomyolysis

The classic presentation of rhabdomyolysis, which consists of myalgia, weakness, and dark urine, is actually quite rare. Rhabdomyolysis does not necessarily lead to visible myoglobinuria, and muscle pain or tenderness do not necessarily occur. However, a history suggestive of muscle compression; a physical exam demonstrating muscle tenderness, especially after fluid resuscitation and muscle reperfusion; and laboratory tests confirming muscle damage lead to a strong presumptive diagnosis.

20. What lab tests should be ordered to diagnose rhabdomyolysis?

Creatine phosphokinase activity is the most sensitive indicator of muscle damage; it may continue to increase several days after admission. Hyperkalemia, hyperuricemia, and hyperphosphatemia also occur. Hypocalcemia dvelops as calcium is chelated and deposited in the damaged muscle tissue. Lactic acidosis and gap acidosis result from release of other organic acids, whereas non-gap acidosis results fromrenal insufficiency and renal failure.

Hyperalbuminemia occurs initially during third-space fluid sequestration and resultant intravascular depletion. Later in the progression of the disease, as malnutrition, catabolism, fluid overload, and capillary leak persist, hypoalbuminemia becomes the predominant feature.

21. What are the complications of rhabdomyolysis?

The most immediate concern is hyperkalemia due to cell necrosis. As cellular death and necrosis occur, the release of myoglobin and its metabolites; DNA and its metabolites (xanthine, hypoxanthine, and uric acid); and other cellular debris form casts in the renal tubules. Together with hypovolemia, they cause renal tubular obstruction. In addition, renal vasoconstriction develops, probably from the degradation of nitric oxide in its interaction with the myoglobin molecule, and direct renal cytotoxicity results from the heme protein molecules. All of these processes result in the development of acute renal failure and oliguria/anuria.

The other immediate concern is hypovolemia. Patients with crush injuries or other causes of compression injury to muscle compartments are severely hypovolemic and have high fluid resuscitation needs.

22. What treatment options are available?

Supportive care, with assurance of intravascular repletion and prevention of continued renal insult, is the main strategy. Continued hydration with sodium bicarbonate-based crystalloids is the main fluid maintenance strategy; mannitol can be used to increase the volume of filtered fluid, to act as an free radical scavenger to counter reperfusion oxidative injury, and to act as an osmotic agent. Allopurinol reduces the production of uric acid and also has free radical scavenge properties. In addition, pentoxyphylline, a purine analog, can be used to enhance capillary flow and to decrease neutrophil adhesion and cytokine release. Control of hyperkalemia and hypocalcemia are also part of the supportive care regimen.

23. What kind of prophylactic management options are possible?

Guidelines for the treatment of catastrophic crush injuries (developed in response to earthquake disasters) recommend resuscitation with 1 L of crystalloid even before extrication and immediate subsequent resuscitation with 2 L of fluid, consisting of 1 L of isotonic saline and 1 L of dextrose 5% with 100 mmol of sodium bicarbonate. The addition of mannitol or other diuretics may be helpful. In the first 24 hours, up to 10 L of intravascular volume may be lost as sequestrated fluid in the affected limb. Administration of up to 10–12 L of fluid is recommended during this period, with careful monitoring of urine output.

24. What drugs need to be avoided in patients with rhabdomyolysis?

Succinylcholine, a drug used for rapid muscle paralysis to achieve airway control, causes generalized depolarization of neuromuscular junctions, and can cause hyperkalemia if the patient has abnormal proliferations of the motor endplates. Patients with rhabdomyolysis can be affected by the same hyperkalemic response, and case reports in the literature support the avoidance of succinylcholine in patients with rhabdomyolysis. The phenomenon is somewhat confounded by the fact that most of the cases described probably resulted from damage to intrinsically vulnerable muscle tissue; most of these patients had undiagnosed myopathies. The severe and lethal nature of these hyperkalemic events, however, warrants caution.

BIBLIOGRAPHY

 1. Bellomo R, Mehta R: Acute renal replacement in the intensive care: Now and tomorrow. New Horiz 3:760–767, 1995.
 2. Bellomo R, Ronco C, Mehta RL: Nomenclature for continuous renal replacement therapies. Am J Kidney Dis 28:S2–S7, 1996.
 3. Bellomo R, Ronco C: Blood purification in the intensive care unit: Evolving concepts. World J Surg 25:677–683, 2001.
 4. Better O, Stein J: Early management of shock and prophylaxis of acute renal failure in traumatic rhabdomyolysis. N Engl J Med 322:825–829, 1990.
 5. Bonnardeaux A, Pichette V, Ouimet D, et al: Solute clearance with high dialysate flow rates and glucose absorption from the dialysate in continuous arteriovenous hemodialysis. Am J Kidney Dis 19:31–38, 1992.
 6. Clark WR, Mueller BA, Kraus MA, et al: Solute control by extracorporeal therapies in acute renal failure. Am J Kidney Dis 28:S21–S27, 1996.
 7. Corwin H, Schreiber M, Fang L: Low fractional excretion of sodium: Occurrence with hemoglobinuric and myoglobinuric-induced acute renal failure. Arch Intern Med 144:981–982, 1984.
 8. Davenport A, Will EJ, Davison AM: Hyperlactatemia and metabolic acidosis during haemofiltration using lactate-buffered fluids. Nephron 59:461–465, 1991.
 9. Druml W: Metabolic aspects of continuous renal replacement therapies. Kidney Int 56:S56–S61, 1999.
10. Eneas J, Schoenfeld P, Humphreys M: The effects of infusion of mannitol-sodium bicarbonate on the clinical course of myoglobinuria. Arch Intern Med 139:801–805, 1979.
11. Forni LG, PJ H: Continuous hemofiltration in the treatment of acute renal failure. N Eng J Med 336:1303–1309, 1997.
12. Frankenfield DC, Reynolds HN, Wiles CE, et al: Urea removal during continuous hemodiafiltration. Crit Care Med 22:407–412, 1994.
13. Gabow P, Kaehny W, Kelleher S: The spectrum of rhabdomyolysis. Medicine 61:141–152, 1982.
14. Glavis C: Continuous arteriovenous hemofiltration. In Parsons PE, Weiner-Kronish JP (eds): Critical Care Secrets. Philadelphia, Hanley & Belfus, 1992, p pp 210–216.
15. Gronert GA: Cardiac arrest after succinylcholine: Mortality greater with rhabdomyolysis with receptor upregulation. Anesthesiology 94:523–529, 2001.
16. Grossman R, Hamilton R, Morse B, et al: Nontraumatic rhabdomyolysis and acute renal failure. N Engl J Med 291:807–817, 1974.

17. Heering P, Ivens K, Thümer O, Braüse M, Grabensec B: Acid-basc balance and substitution fluid during continuous hemofiltration. Kidney Int 56:S37–S40, 1999.
18. Hoffmann JN, Faist E: Removal of mediators by continuous hemofiltration in septic patients. World J Surg 25:651–659, 2001.
19. Kierdorf HP, Leue C, Arns S: Lactate- or bicarbonate-buffered solutions in continuous extracorpeal renal replacement therapies. Kidney Int 56:S32–S36, 1999.
20. Knochel J: Rhabdomyolysis and myoglobinuria. Semin Nephrol 1:75–86, 1981.
21. Koffler A, Fridler R, Massry S: Acute renal failure due to nontraumatic rhabdomyolysis. Ann Intern Med 85:23–28, 1976.
22. Levraut J, Ciebiera J-P, Jambou P, et al: Effect of continuous venovenous hemofiltration with dialysis on lactate clearance in critically ill patients. Crit Care Med 25:58–62, 1997.
23. Llach F, Felsenfeld A, Hawssler M: The pathophysiology of altered calcium metabolism in rhabdomyolysis-induced acute renal failure. N Engl J Med 305:117–123, 1981.
24. Manns M, Sigler MH, Teehan BP: Continuous renal replacement therapies: An update. Am J Kidney Disease 32:185–207, 1998.
25. Morris C, Alexander E, Bruns F, Levinsky N: Restoration and maintenance of glomerular filtration by mannitol during hypoperfusion of the kidney. J Clin Invest 51:155, 1972.
26. Prendergast BD, George CF: Drug-induced rhabdomyolysis-mechanism and management. Postgrad Med 69:333–336, 1993.
27. Ragaller MJR, Theilen H, Koch T: Volume replacement in critically ill patients with acute renal failure. J Am Soc Nephrol 12:S33–S39, 2001.
28. Ron D: Prevention of acute renal failure in traumatic rhabdomyolysis. Arch Intern Med 144:277–280, 1984.
29. Roth D: Acute rhabdomyolysis associated with cocaine intoxication. N Engl J Med 319:637–677, 1988.
30. Sieberth H-G, Kierdorf HP: Is cytokine removal by continuous hemofiltration feasible? Kidney Int 56:S79–S83, 1999.
31. Singh U, Scheld WM: Infectious etiologies of rhabdomyolysis: Three case reports and a review. Clin Infect Dis 22:642–649, 1996.
32. Vanholder R, Sever MS, Erek E, Lameire N: Rhabdomyolysis. J Am Soc Nephrol 11:1553–1561, 2000.
33. Vanholder R, Sever MS, Erek E, Lameire N: Acute renal failure related to the crush syndrome: towards an era of seiso-nephrology? Nephrol Dial Transplant 15:1517–1521, 2000.
34. Ward M: Factors predictive of acute renal failure in rhabdomyolysis. Arch Intern Med 148:1553–1557, 1988.
35. Wynne JW, Goslen JB, Ballinger WE, et al: Rhabdomyolysis with cardiac and respiratory involvement. South Med J 70:1125–1128, 1977.
36. Zager R: Studies of mechanisms and protective maneuvers in myoglobinuric acute renal injury. Lab Invest 60:619–629, 1989.
37. Zager RA: Rhabdomyolysis and myohemoglobinuric acute renal failure. Kidney Int 49:314-326, 1996.

46. HYPOKALEMIA AND HYPERKALEMIA

Stuart L. Linas, M.D.

1. Why is tight regulation of serum potassium (K) critical?

Only about 56 mEq of the body's total 4200 mEq of K is extracellular. Therefore, changes in extracellular fluid (ECF) K, either by compartmental shifts or by net gain or loss, significantly alter the ratio of extracellular to intracellular K. Because this ratio determines the resting membrane potential, small changes in ECF K can profoundly affect neuromuscular excitability.

2. Does a decrease in serum K always reflect a decrease in total body K?

No. Hypokalemia can occur either from transcellular shift of K from extracellular to intracellular compartments (redistribution hypokalemia) or from a decrease in total body K.

3. What controls internal balance of K?

A number of factors move K into cells, including alkalosis, insulin, and catecholamines.

4. What are the causes of hypokalemia secondary to redistribution?

The causes of altered transcellular distribution include alkalosis, insulin excess, beta-adrenergic agonists, hypokalemic periodic paralysis, barium poisoning, cellular proliferation (leukemia or B. lymphoma), and digoxin immune Fab treatment.

5. Does the hypokalemia that occurs with cellular shift need to be treated?

Because this type of hypokalemia does not reflect a true total body deficiency of K, it does not need to be treated except in emergent cases, such as periodic paralysis or myocardial infarction.

6. Total body K is dependent on external balance (i.e., the difference between K intake and excretion). What factors influence urinary excretion of K?

Key factors influencing K secretion include adequate sodium delivery to distal nephron sites (flow rate), aldosterone, and increased distal delivery of anions (such as bicarbonate and ketones).

7. Describe the manifestations of hypokalemia.

By depressing neuromuscular excitability, hypokalemia leads to muscle weakness, with quadriplegia, hypoventilation, adynamic ileus, and orthostatic hypotension. Severe hypokalemia disrupts cell integrity, leading to rhabdomyolysis. Renal effects include the stimulation of renal ammonia production, which can promote encephalopathy in patients with advanced liver disease. Among the most critical are the cardiac consequences, including atrial and ventricular arrhythmias. The EKG shows S-T segment depression and flattened T waves, which result in prominent U waves. Prominent U waves, in turn, give the impression of a prolonged QT interval.

8. What is the diagnostic approach to a patient with hypokalemia?

After eliminating spurious causes (such as leukocytosis), true hypokalemia can be approached on the basis of urinary K, systemic acid-base status and urinary chloride.

A low urinary K (< 20 mEq/day) indicates poor intake or extrarenal losses. Poor intake is seen in elderly, alcoholic, and anorexic patients. Extrarenal losses are usually from gastrointestinal losses, such as diarrhea, which is rich in K.

A high urinary K (> 20 mEq/day) indicates renal losses and can be classified according to the systemic pH. Metabolic acidosis with hypokalemia is seen in renal tubular acidosis (distal and proximal), diabetic ketoacidosis, alcoholic ketoacidosis and ethylene glycol and methanol poisoning. A normal pH with hypokalemia is seen in acute tubular necrosis, postobstructive diuresis, magnesium depletion, and osmolal diuresis such as glucose. Metabolic alkalosis with hypokalemia is further classified according to the urinary chloride. If the urinary chloride is < 10 mEq/L, the cause is either vomiting or recovery from diuretics. If the urinary chloride is > 10 mEq/L in the setting of hypertension, then the renal K loss can be due to hyperaldosteronism, mineralocorticoid excess (congenital adrenal hyperplasia), increased Na channel activity (Liddle's syndrome), or increased glucocorticoids (ectopic or pituitary ACTH). In the absence of hypertension and a urinary chloride > 10, the differential diagnosis includes Bartter's syndrome and its variants (such as Gitelman's syndrome).

9. When does serum K falsely estimate body K?

Intracellular/extracellular K shifting has a profound effect on serum K values. The reciprocal movement of K and H^+ across the cell membrane results in a rise in serum K of approximately 0.6 mEq/L for every drop in pH of 0.1 unit in the case of acidemia, and a fall in serum K of 0.1–0.4 mEq/L for every rise in pH of 0.1 unit in the case of alkalemia. Hormones that drive K into cells include insulin and catecholamines. An example of the importance of acid-base balance and insulin in K homeostasis is in diabetes with ketoacidosis. In this situation, the administration of insulin moves K into cells by both direct and indirect means (correction of acidosis).

10. What drugs cause renal K wasting, hypokalemia, and reductions in total body K?

The most common drugs are diuretics—thiazides, loop diuretics, and acetazolamide. Acetazolamide increases urinary K by blocking sodium bicarbonate reabsorption in the proximal convoluted tubule. Increases in distal delivery of sodium and bicarbonate result in increases in urinary K and hypokalemia. When factored for degree of natriuresis, thiazides may cause more K loss than loop diuretics. The major reason is that thiazides have a substantially longer half-life than most loop diuretics.

Penicillin and penicillin analogs (e.g., carbenicillin, ticarcillin, piperacillin) also cause renal K wasting that is mediated by various mechanisms, including delivery of nonreabsorbable anions to the distal nephron, which results in K trapping in the urine.

Amphotericin, platinum, and aminoglycosides cause renal K wasting even in the absence of decreases in glomerular filtration rate (GFR).

11. How is hypokalemia treated?

In most cases, potassium chloride (KCl) is used. In metabolic acidosis, replacement with K bicarbonate or equivalent (e.g., K citrate, acetate, or gluconate) is recommended to help alleviate the acidosis. Alcoholics and diabetics out of control often have phosphate deficiency and should receive some of the potassium as K phosphate. Oral replacement is the safest route, and administration of doses of up to 40 mEq multiple times daily is allowed. Delayed-release formulations tend to reduce the GI upset seen with the higher doses.

12. When is intravenous replacement necessary? What are the risks?

When oral administration is not possible, as when the GI tract is nonfunctional, or in life-threatening situations such as severe weakness, respiratory distress, cardiac arrhythmias, or rhab-domyolysis, K must be replaced intravenously. Infusion rates must normally be limited to 10 mEq/hr to prevent the potentially catastrophic effect of a K bolus to the heart. In extreme situations, under cardiac monitoring and frequent serum level checks, infusion rates of up to 30 mEq/hr can be used.

13. In what other circumstances is special care in replacement necessary?

• K-depleted patients who are also on digitalis therapy (especially overdose) are prone to serious arrhythmias and must be treated urgently.
• K overload rarely occurs during replacement *except* in the following circumstances: renal failure, use of K-sparing diuretics (spironolactone, amiloride, triamterene), and possibly use of angiotensin-converting enzyme (ACE) inhibitors and angiotensin receptor blockers (ARBs).
• Significant magnesium deficiency causes renal K wasting and often must be corrected before therapy for hypokalemia can be effective.

14. What is the relationship between potassium and magnesium?

Magnesium depletion can cause hypokalemia that is unresponsive to oral or intravenous KCl therapy. Magnesium depletion occurs after diuretic use or sustained alcohol consumption. Severe magnesium depletion causes renal K wasting. The mechanism is unclear, but total body K cannot be repleted with K alone in patients with magnesium depletion. K repletion first requires magnesium repletion. Only then is the kidney able to retain K.

15. Describe the clinical manifestations of hyperkalemia.

Hyperkalemia results in heart block and asystole. Initially the EKG shows peaked T waves, followed by decreasing amplitude of R waves, prolonged P-R interval, and progressive widening of the QRS complex, until QRS and T blend into a sine-wave pattern. Because cardiac arrest can occur at any point in this progression, hyperkalemia with EKG changes constitutes a medical emergency. Other effects of hyperkalemia include weakness and neuromuscular paralysis (without CNS disturbances) and suppression of renal ammoniagenesis, which may result in metabolic acidosis.

16. What degree of chronic renal failure causes hyperkalemia?

Chronic renal failure per se is not associated with hyperkalemia until the GFR is reduced to about 75% of normal (serum creatinine > 4 mg/dl). More than 85% of filtered K is reabsorbed in the proximal tubule. Urinary excretion is determined primarily by K secretion along the cortical collecting tubule and K reabsorption in the medullary and papillary collecting tubules. Hyperkalemia disproportionate to reductions in GFR usually results from decreases in K secretion (secondary either to decreases in aldosterone, as may occur in Addison's disease, or to diabetes with hyporeninemic hypoaldosteronism) or from marked decreases in distal nephron sodium delivery, as may occur in severe prerenal states.

17. What causes hyperkalemia?
   1. **Cellular shifts:** Redistribution of even small amounts out of the large intracellular pool can significantly raise serum K. Causes include acidosis, hyperosmotic state, and insulin deficiency. Certain drugs may contribute, including beta blockers and digitalis.
   2. **Increased endogenous K** release due to tumor lysis, rhabdomyolysis, brisk hemolysis, or heavily catabolic states such as severe sepsis may raise serum K, particularly in the setting of renal failure.
   3. **Increased exogenous K** sources include oral K replacement, K-rich foods, total parenteral nutrition, salt substitutes, and high-dose K penicillin.
   4. **Decreased renal K excretion** is the leading cause, as 90% of K intake is renally excreted under normal circumstances. Only late in the course of chronic renal failure (GFR < 10 ml/min), however, is renal failure the *sole* cause of hyperkalemia. Primary defects in K excretion out of proportion to decrement in GFR are seen in certain diseases: systemic lupus erythematosus, sickle cell disease, obstructive uropathy, and renal transplantation. Drugs that impair K excretion include K-sparing diuretics, ACE inhibitors, nonsteroidal anti-inflammatory drugs, and heparin (by suppression of aldosterone synthesis and secretion). Finally, hypoaldosteronism reduces K excretion. In addition to Addison's disease, hypoaldosteronism is seen in renal diseases associated with impaired renin production, such as diabetes mellitus and chronic interstitial nephritis.

18. What is the transtubular K gradient (TTKG)? In what clinical situation is it useful?
   TTKG is an indirect semiquantitative index of the K secretory process and approximates the effect of aldosterone on tubular K secretion. It is calculated as follows:

$$TTKG = U_K/(U_{OSM}/P_{OSM})/P_K$$

In patients with hyperkalemia, a TTKG < 4 suggests reduced renal mineralocorticoid activity and a TTKG > 6 is consistent with a stimulated renal K secretory process. There are two limitations to using the TTKG: (1) U_{Na} must be > 25 mM (to ensure that sodium delivery is not the limiting factor) and (2) the urine be hypertonic (to ensure that antidiuretic hormone is present for normal K conductance in the distal nephron).

19. Describe the treatment of hyperkalemia.
   The presence of serum K > 6.5, EKG changes, or severe weakness mandates emergent therapy. The general approach is to use therapy from each of the following three categories for definitive treatment.
   1. **Membrane stabilization:** Calcium raises the cell depolarization threshold and reduces myocardial irritability. One or two ampules of IV calcium chloride results in improvement in EKG changes within seconds, but because K levels are not altered, the beneficial effect lasts only about 30 minutes.
   2. **Shift K into cells:** IV insulin (e.g., 10-unit bolus of regular insulin), with glucose administration if necessary to prevent hypoglycemia, begins lowering serum K in about 2–5 minutes and lasts a few hours. Correction of acidosis with IV sodium bicarbonate (e.g., 2 ampules) has a similar duration and time of onset.
   3. **Removal of K:** Loop diuretics can sometimes cause enough renal K loss in patients with intact renal function, but usually a GI K-binding resin must be used (e.g., Kayexalate, 30 gm orally or 50 gm by retention enema). The resin is given with a cathartic to remove the K from the gut and prevent development of a solid mass in the bowel. Note that as K is drawn into the gut lumen, sodium is absorbed, giving the patient a net volume load. Acute hemodialysis is effective at K removal and must be used when the GI tract is nonfunctional or when serious fluid overload is already present.

BIBLIOGRAPHY

1. Linas SL, Berl T: Clinical diagnosis of abnormal potassium balance. In Seldin DW, Giebisch G (eds): The Regulation of Potassium Balance. New York, Raven Press, 1989, pp 177–205.
2. Halperin ML, Kamel SK: Electrolyte quintet: Potassium. Lancet 352:135–140, 1998.
3. Weiner D, Wingo C: Hyperkalemia: A potential silent killer. J Am Soc Nephrol 9:1535–1543, 1998.
4. Weiner D, Wingo C: Hyperkalemia: Consequences, causes, and correction. J Am Soc Nephrol 8:1179–1188, 1997.
5. Gennari FG: Hypokalemia. N Engl J Med 339:451–458, 1998.
6. Osorio FV, Linas SL: Disorders of potassium metabolism. In Schrier RW (ed): Atlas of Diseases of the Kidney, vol. 1. Philadelphia, Current Medicine, 1998, pp 3.2–3.17.
7. Kellerman PS, Linas SL: Disorders of potassium metabolism. In Feehally J, Johnson R (eds): Comprehensive Clinical Nephrology. London, Mosby International, 1999, pp 1–10.

47. HYPONATREMIA AND HYPERNATREMIA

Stuart Senkfor, M.D., Tomas Berl, M.D., and Kathleen D. Liu, M.D., Ph.D.

1. Why is sodium homeostasis critical to volume control?

Sodium and its corresponding anion represent almost all of the osmotically active solutes in the extracellular fluid. As such, its serum concentration reflects the tonicity of body fluids. Under normal circumstances, serum osmolality can be closely calculated by $2 \times [Na^+] + 10$ under normal circumstances (see question 17, formula 1, for pathophysiologic conditions). Slight changes in tonicity are counteracted by thirst regulation, antidiuretic hormone (vasopressin) secretion, and renal concentrating or diluting mechanisms. Preservation of normal serum osmolality (290 mOsm/L) guarantees cellular integrity by regulating net movement of water across cellular membranes.

2. Does hyponatremia simply represent a low sodium state?

No. Hyponatremia is defined as a serum sodium concentration < 135 mEq/L. However, serum sodium concentration tells little about total body sodium or volume status. Hyponatremia can occur in low total body sodium (hypovolemic), normal total body sodium (euvolemic), and excess total body sodium (hypervolemic) states. Physical examination is the major source of volume assessment. Helpful findings include tachycardia, dry mucous membranes, orthostatic hypotension, increased skin turgor (hypovolemia) edema, extra heart sound (S_3), jugular venous distention, and ascites (hypervolemia).

3. How can hyponatremia develop in a hypovolemic patient?

Hypovolemic hyponatremia represents a decrease in total body sodium in excess of a decrease in total body water. Sodium and water loss can be due to renal and extrarenal sources. For example, renal losses can be due to glycosuria, diuretic use, mineralocorticoid deficiency, and intrinsic renal disease. Extrarenal losses include vomiting, diarrhea, excessive sweating, burns, and third spacing. Hypovolemia leads to hyponatremia by limiting the kidney's ability to excrete water. Hypovolemia results in a decrease in renal perfusion, a decrement in glomerular filtration rate (GFR), and an increase in proximal tubule reabsorption, all serving to limit water excretion. More important is the effect of hypovolemia to supersede the expected inhibition of vasopressin release by hypotonicity and thereby maintain the secretion of the hormone. That is, the body protects volume at the expense of tonicity. Continued release of vasopressin limits renal diluting ability, and any water taken in is retained, culminating in hyponatremia. Therefore, hypovolemia results in antidiuretic hormone secretion, decreased renal perfusion, decreased GFR, increased proximal tubular sodium reabsorption, and maximum water reabsorption. The latter occurs despite the presence of hypotonicity due to nonosmotic release of antidiuretic hormone.

4. How does hypervolemic hyponatremia differ from hypovolemic hyponatremia?

Once again, the kidneys are at the center of the problem, due either to intrinsic renal disease or renal compensation secondary to an extrarenal abnormality. Physical examination reveals edema and no evidence of volume depletion. Intrinsic renal disease with markedly decreased GFR (acute or chronic) prevents the adequate excretion of sodium and water. Intake of sodium in excess of what can be excreted leads to hypervolemia (edema); excessive intake of water leads to hyponatremia. Homeostasis is lost and volume overload, hyponatremia, and edema develop. In contrast, in congestive heart failure, hepatic cirrhosis, and nephrotic syndrome the ability of an intrinsically normal kidney to excrete excess sodium and water is limited.

5. Is euvolemic hyponatremia, then, due only to an increase in total body water?

Although there is a decrement in total body sodium, the hyponatremia is primarily due to an increase in total body water as a consequence of nonosmolar release of antidiuretic hormone or production of an antidiuretic-hormone-like substance by tumors. The syndrome of inappropriate antidiuretic hormone secretion (SIADH) is a common cause of euvolemic hyponatremia and is associated with malignancies, pulmonary disease, central nervous system disorders, and drugs. The latter category includes hypoglycemic agents, psychotropics, narcotics, and chemotherapeutic agents. Other causes of euvolemic hyponatremia include psychogenic polydipsia, hypothyroidism, adrenal insufficiency, pain, surgery, and anesthesia.

6. What diagnostic tests are useful in the evaluation of hyponatremia?

The physical examination is critical to the detemination of volume status, as described above. Serum electrolytes and serum and urine osmolality are useful. High urine osmolality despite low serum osmolality suggests SIADH in the euvolemic state or hypovolemic hyponatremia. Very low urine osmolality suggests excessive water intake, as in psychogenic polydipsia. Measurements of TSH and cortisol can be used to assess endocrine causes of hyponatremia.

7. Are hyponatremia and hypo-osmolality synonymous?

No. Hyponatremia can occur without a change in total body sodium or total body water in two settings. The first is pseudohyponatremia, which is only a laboratory abnormality in patients with severe hyperlipidemia or hyperproteinemia; lipids and proteins occupy an increasingly large volume in which the sodium determination is made. Serum sodium is low in these pathologic states when a flame photometry method is used, but normal when an ion-specific electrode is used. Most clinical laboratories now use an ion-specific electrode. The second setting occurs when large quantities of osmotically active substances (such as glucose or mannitol) cause hyponatremia but not hypotonicity. This condition is known as translocational hyponatremia. In such states, water is drawn out of cells to extracellular space, diluting the plasma solute and equilibrating osmolar differences. Serum sodium decreases by approximately 1.6–1.8 mEq/L for every increase of 100 mg/dl over normal glucose levels. In this setting, the serum sodium should not be interpreted without an accompanying serum glucose, and the appropriate correction should be made if the glucose exceeds 200 mg/dl. In addition, use of large quantities of irrigant solutions that do not contain sodium (but instead contain glycine, sorbitol, or mannitol) during gynecologic or urologic surgeries can also cause severe hyponatremia. This hyponatremia has both translocational and dilutional components.

8. What is the difference between acute and chronic hyponatremia?

Acute hyponatremia is a distinct entity in terms of morbidity and mortality as well as treatment strategies. Acute hyponatremia most commonly occurs in the hospital (as in the postoperative setting), in psychogenic polydipsia, and in elderly women taking thiazide diuretics. **Chronic hyponatremia** is defined as a duration > 48 hours. The great majority of patients who present to physicians or to emergency rooms with hyponatremia should be assumed to have chronic hyponatremia.

9. What are the signs and symptoms of hyponatremia?

Hyponatremia is the most common electrolyte disorder, with a prevalence of about 2.5% in hospitalized patients. Although the majority of patients are asymptomatic, symptoms do develop in patients with a serum sodium of less than 125 mEq/L or in whom the sodium has decreased rapidly. Gastrointestinal complaints of nausea, vomiting, and anorexia occur early, but neuropsychiatric complaints such as lethargy, confusion, agitation, psychosis, seizure, and coma are more common. Clinical symptoms roughly correlate with the amount and rate of decrease in serum sodium.

10. Is there a standard therapy for hyponatremia?

Although controversy exists regarding treatment strategies, there is a consensus that not all hyponatremias are alike. Duration (acute versus chronic) and the presence or absence of neurologic symptoms should direct therapy. The dilemma of therapy involves balancing symptoms and cerebral edema versus the risk of a demyelinating syndrome with therapy. In patients with acute symptomatic hyponatremia, the risk of delaying treatment and allowing the consequences of cerebral edema to culminate in a seizure and respiratory arrest clearly outweigh any risk of treatment. Hypertonic saline and furosemide (which promotes free water excretion) should be given until symptoms subside. In contrast, the asymptomatic chronic hyponatremia patient in high-risk categories (alcoholism, malnutrition, and liver disease) is at greatest risk for complications of the correction of hyponatremia, namely central pontine myelinolysis. Such patients are best treated with water restriction.

11. What are some helpful guidelines for treatment of hyponatremia?

Both delay of therapy and overly aggressive therapy, especially in high-risk patients (alcoholism, malnutrition, liver disease), place patients at greater risk for treatment complications.

In chronic asymptomatic patients, simple free water restriction (i.e., 1000 cc/day) allows a slow and relatively safe correction of serum sodium. However, this stretegy requires patient cooperation, which may be difficult to obtain from outpatients. In selected patients, who are resistant to free water restriction, an antidiuretic hormone antagonist (demeclocycline, 600–1,200 mg/day), or a maneuver to increase urinary solute excretion may be necessary.

The most difficult therapeutic dilemma is posed by patients with cerebral symptoms and hyponatremia of unknown duration. Such patients are also at risk of a demyelinating disorder if treated too aggressively, yet the presence of symptoms is reflective of central nervous system dysfunction. These patients should be treated with careful (hourly) monitoring of serum sodium, as hypertonic saline and furosemide are given. The rate of increase should not exceed 1.5 mEq/L/hr, and the total increment should not exceed 8 mEq/24 hr. Acute therapy can be slowed when one of the following endpoints is achieved: (1) symptoms are improved, (2) a "safe" serum sodium level (120–125 mEq/L) is attained, or (3) the total increment goal in serum sodium for that 24-hour period has been achieved.

12. What is central pontine myelinolysis?

Central pontine myelinolysis is a rare neurologic disorder of unclear etiology characterized by symmetric midline demyelination of the central basis pontis. Extrapontine lesions can occur in the basal ganglia, internal capsule, lateral geniculate body, and cortex. Symptoms include motor abnormalities that can progress to flaccid quadriplegia, respiratory paralysis, pseudobulbar palsy, mental status changes, and coma. Central pontine myelinolysis is frequently fatal in 3–5 weeks, but survival with residual deficit is increasingly observed. Magnetic resonance imaging and, to a lesser extent, CT scanning can be used to document the alterations in white matter. Although central pontine myelinolysis can occur in patients without a history of hyponatremia, it is one of the major concerns as a complication of therapy. Risk factors include a change in serum sodium of greater than 20–25 mEq/L in 24 hours, correction of serum sodium to normal or hypernatremic range, symptomatic and coexistent alcoholism, malnutrition, and liver disease.

13. Can hypernatremia also occur in hypovolemic, euvolemic, and hypervolemic states?

Yes, and these categories, based on physical examination, provide a useful framework for understanding and treating patients. However, in contrast to hyponatremia, hypernatremia always reflects an excess of sodium relative to total body water content. Hypovolemic hypernatremia tends to occur in the very young and the very old. It is typically due to extracellular fluid losses and the inability to intake adequate amounts of free water. Febrile illnesses, vomiting, diarrhea, and renal losses are common etiologies.

Euvolemic hypernatremia can also be due to extracellular loss of fluid without adequate access to water or from loss of control of water hemostasis. Diabetes insipidus, either central (inadequate antidiuretic hormone secretion) or nephrogenic (renal insensitivity to antidiuretic hormone), results in the inability to reabsorb filtered water, resulting in systemic hypertonicity but a hypo-osmolar urine.

Hypervolemic hypernatremia, although uncommon, is iatrogenic. For example, sodium bicarbonate injection during cardiac arrest, administration of hypertonic saline, saline abortions, and inappropriately prepared infant formulas are several examples of induced hypernatremia.

14. What are the causes of diabetes insipidus?

Central diabetes insipidus can result from trauma, tumors, strokes, granulomatous disease, and central nervous system infections, but it commonly follows neurosurgical procedures. Nephrogenic diabetes insipidus can occur in acute or chronic renal failure, hypercalcemia, hypokalemia, and sickle cell disease, or it may be drug related (lithium, demeclocycline).

15. What are the signs and symptoms of hypernatremia?

In awake and alert patients, thirst is a prominent symptom. Anorexia, nausea, vomiting, altered mental status, agitation, irritability, lethargy, stupor, coma, and neuromuscular hyperactivity are common.

16. What is the best therapy for hypernatremia?

The first priority is circulatory stabilization with normal saline in patients with significant volume depletion. Once hypotension has been corrected, patients can be rehydrated with oral water, intravenous D5W, or even one half normal saline. Overly rapid correction of long-standing hypernatremia can result in cerebral edema. Water deficit can be calculated with formula in question 17. Some investigators have suggested that in patients with long-standing hypernatremia, the water deficit should be corrected by no more than 10 mEq/day or 0.5 mmol/hr. If the hypernatremia has occured over a short period (hours), it can be corrected more rapidly, with the goal of correcting half of the water deficit in the first 24 hours. In patients with central diabetes insipidus, a synthetic analogue of antidiuretic hormone, namely DDAVP, can be administered, preferably by intranasal route.

17. What are some helpful formulas for assessing sodium abnormalities?

Serum osmolality = 2 $[Na^+]$ + glucose/18 + BUN/2.8 + ethyl alcohol/4.6

Total body water (TBW) = body weight × 0.6

TBW excess in hyponatremia = TBW $(1 - [serum\ Na^+]/140)$

TBW deficit in hypernatremia = TBW $(serum\ [Na^+]/140 - 1)$

BIBLIOGRAPHY

1. Adrogue HJ, Madias, NE: Hypernatremia. N Engl J Med 342:1493–1499, 2000.
2. Adrogue HJ, Madias NE: Hyponatremia. N Engl J Med 342:1581–1589, 2000.
3. Anderson RJ: Hospital-associated hyponatremia. Kidney Int 29:1237–1247, 1986.
4. Arieff AI: Hyponatremia associated with permanent brain damage. Adv Intern Med 32:325–344, 1987.
5. Arieff AI: Osmotic failure: Physiology and strategies for treatment. Hosp Pract May 15:173–194, 1988.
6. Ashraf N, et al: Thiazide-induced hyponatremia associated with death or neurologic damage in outpatients. Am J Med 70:1163–1168, 1981.
7. Ayus CJ, et al: Treatment of symptomatic hyponatremia and its relationship to brain damage. N Engl J Med 317:1190–1195, 1987.
8. Ayus JC, Arieff AI: Glycine-induced hypo-osmolar hyponatremia. Arch Intern Med 157:223–226, 1997.
9. Berl T: Treating hyponatremia: Damned if we do and damned if we don't. Kidney Int 37:1006–1018, 1990.
10. Brass EP, Thompson WL: Drug-induced electrolyte abnormalities. Drugs 24:207–228, 1982.
11. Clifford B: Hyponatremia and the brain. Am Fam Physician 38:119–124, 1988.
12. Gross P: Treatment of severe hyponatremia. Kidney Int 60:2417–2427, 2000.
13. Halterman R, Berl T: Therapy of dysnatremic disorders. In Brady K, Wilcox CS (eds): Therapy in Nephrology and Hypertension. Philadelphia, W.B. Saunders, 1998, pp 257–269.
14. Narins RG, Riley L: Polyuria: Simple and mixed disorders. Am J Kidney Dis 17:237–241, 1991.
15. Zarinetchi F, Berl T: Evaluation and management of hyponatremia. Adv Intern Med 41:25, 1995.

VII. Gastroenterology

48. UPPER AND LOWER GASTROINTESTINAL BLEEDING IN THE CRITICALLY ILL PATIENT

Fernando Velayos, M.D.

1. Do all patients with gastrointestinal (GI) hemorrhage need to be admitted to the ICU?

No. Patients who are actively bleeding, who had significant bleeding, or who are at risk of cardiovascular compromise as a consequence of bleeding should be admitted to an intensive care unit.

2. What is unique about a hospitalized patient who develops GI bleeding?

GI bleeding in an inpatient admitted for an unrelated condition is associated with a high mortality rate. Bleeding that begins during hospitalization has a mortality rate of 25% compared with 3.5–7% for bleeding that begins before admission. The cause of death is usually not the bleeding itself, but rather exacerbation of the primary disease process.

3. Discuss the major causes of GI bleeding.

Ulcers in the duodenum and stomach are the most common cause of bleeding from the **upper GI tract** and account for about 50% of cases. Upper GI bleeding is defined as blood loss originating proximal to the ligament of Treitz. Gastric erosions (23 %), varices (10%), Mallory-Weiss tear (7%), and esophagitis (6%) account for most of the remaining cases. Ulcers and varices are the lesions most likely to produce significant upper tract bleeding that requires ICU admission.

Diverticular bleeding is the most common cause of bleeding from the **lower GI tract** and accounts for 43% of cases. Lower GI bleeding is defined as blood loss originating distal to the ligament of Treitz. Angiodysplasia (20%), undetermined causes (12%), neoplasia (9%) and colitis (9%) account for most of the remaining cases. Diverticula and occasionally angiodysplasia are the lesions most likely to produce significant lower tract bleeding that requires ICU admission.

4. For which causes of GI bleeding are critically ill patients at risk?

Although critically ill patients can have any of the typical causes of bleeding, they are at particular risk for developing stress-induced ulcers in the upper GI tract and hypotension-induced ischemia of the colon.

5. What questions help in assessing the severity of GI bleeding?

1. Does the patient have significant hemodynamic compromise?
2. Is the patient actively bleeding?
3. Is this a high-risk patient (age > 60, variceal bleeding, or comorbid condition)?
4. Is this an upper GI bleed?

6. What factors are associated with a high mortality rate in patients with upper GI hemorrhage?

Multivariable scoring systems have been developed for accurate assessment and management of patients with GI bleeding. These predictors help identify which patients are at highest risk of dying. Such patients benefit from early therapeutic procedures and ICU-level care. Risk factors associated with a high mortality include the following:

1. Age > 60 years
2. Underlying medical conditions (e.g., diabetes, renal failure, coronary artery disease, cancer, liver disease)
3. Persistent hypotension
4. More than 5 units of transfusion
5. Bleeding or rebleeding during hospitalization
6. Bloody nasogastric aspirate
7. Need for emergency surgery
8. High-risk lesions (esophageal varices, high-risk ulcers seen on endoscopy, ulcers > 2 cm, and ulcers located in the lesser curve of the stomach or posterior bulb of the duodenum)

7. What are the steps in early management of a patient with GI bleeding?
1. Place two large-bore (at least 18-gauge) intravenous catheters.
2. Estimate volume loss. A patient in shock has lost at least 40% of total blood volume. A patient with tachycardia and postural hypotension has lost at least 20% of total blood volume. The initial hematocrit poorly reflects the degree of blood loss if the bleeding is acute. There is an equilibration period of 24–72 hours before hematocrit concentrations are reflective of the amount of blood loss.
3. Begin resuscitation with isotonic normal saline and, if appropriate, blood transfusion, at a rate commensurate with the estimated blood volume loss.
4. Consider intubating uncooperative and agitated patients at high risk for aspiration. Vigorous upper GI bleeding poses the greatest risk in patients who are intoxicated or encephalopathic or have altered mental status.
5. Obtain a nasogastric tube aspirate, and perform a rectal exam to localize the bleeding source (upper or lower GI tract) and assess the briskness of bleeding.
6. Correct any underlying coagulopathy with fresh frozen plasma.
7. Give a 50-μg intravenous bolus of octreotide, followed by a continuous infusion of 50 μg/hour if bleeding varices are suspected.

8. Does a nonbloody nasogastric aspirate rule out an upper GI bleed?
No. Up to 15% of patients with an upper GI bleed may have a nonbloody nasogastric (NG) aspirate. This situation can occur when the tip of the NG tube is located in the esophagus or when a competent pyloric sphincter does not allow blood from a duodenal ulcer to reflux into the stomach. Thus, patients with hematochezia, hemodynamic instability, and a negative NG aspirate should still be considered for immediate upper endoscopy.

9. Does passage of an NG tube in a patient with varices precipitate bleeding?
No. No evidence supports the concern that passage of a nasogastric tube precipitates bleeding by traumatizing a varix.

10. What role does endoscopy play in the management of upper and lower GI bleeding?
Endoscopy is important in diagnosing and treating upper and lower GI hemorrhage. Ulcers in the stomach or duodenum are treated either with thermal contact methods (heater probe, electrocoagulation) or injection with a variety of substances (epinephrine, saline, sclerosing agents such as alcohol). Varices are treated with endoscopic band ligation or injection of sclerosing agents such as ethanolamine oleate. Urgent endoscopic therapy of varices and ulcers reduces length of stay, incidence of further rebleeding, and need for surgery and improves survival rates.
Timing of colonoscopy in a patient with an acute lower GI bleed is still being refined. Urgent colonoscopy for acute lower GI bleeding is less established than urgent esophagogastroduodenoscopy (EGD) for acute upper GI bleeding. Diverticula and vascular ectasias may be scattered throughout the colon, and finding the culprit lesion can be difficult with active bleeding or an inadequately prepped colon. More than one potential bleeding source is identified at colonoscopy in 42% of patients with acute lower GI bleeding. Some centers have investigated rapid purge followed by urgent colonoscopy within 12 hours of presentation and have reported success in identifying and

treating the culprit lesion. Colonoscopy within 24 hours may be a more reasonable target whereby the patient can be adequately resuscitated and bowel preparation can be performed. Stratification into low- and high-risk groups for rebleeding has been established for EGD but not for colonoscopy.

11. Discuss the role of tagged red blood cell (RBC) scan and angiography in acute lower GI bleeding.

If blood loss is brisk enough to affect adversely the quality of the colonoscopy, tagged RBC scan followed by angiography can assist in localizing and treating a bleeding lesion in the lower GI tract. Tagged RBC scan is more sensitive than angiography in detecting bleeding but is less accurate in localizing the bleeding. It does not provide therapeutic capabilities but can detect 0.1 ml/min of blood loss. Angiography is superior to tagged RBC scan in localizing the source of bleeding and providing therapy but is less sensitive in detecting blood loss. It can detect 0.5 ml/min of blood loss.

12. What is a stress ulcer?

A stress ulcer is part of a spectrum of mucosal lesions in the stomach and duodenum indicative of injury from severe physiologic stress. This wide spectrum is now known as stress-related erosive syndrome (SRES). Previously SRES has been called stress gastritis, stress-related mucosal disease, erosive gastritis, and hemorrhagic gastritis as well as stress ulcer. These lesions range from diffuse superficial erosions to deeper lesions that can form true ulcers and on occasion perforate. Stress ulcers were initially described by Curling in patients with extensive burns and by Cushing in patients after severe central nervous system trauma. Cushing's ulcers are an interesting subset of SRES because they are always associated with elevated gastrin and gastric acid secretion. In comparison, SRES can occur with high, normal, or low acid output.

13. Which hospitalized patients are at risk for SRES?

As may be expected, increasing severity of underlying illness correlates with increasing risk of clinically significant stress-related bleeding. In a meta-analysis of 2252 patients, Cook et al. identified mechanical ventilation and coagulopathy as the two main risk factors for SRES. Presence of additional risk factors, such as hypotension, sepsis, liver failure, renal failure, extensive burns, or trauma, proportionally increased the risk of significant stress-related hemorrhage.

14. How is SRES diagnosed?

Not all SRES is clinically apparent, although almost all mechanically ventilated patients develop SRES. The lesions may be clinically silent, cause occult bleeding, or cause overt bleeding. About 75–100% of critically ill patients have endoscopic evidence of erosions 12–24 hours after the onset of illness. Only a subset of these erosions is clinically apparent. Occult lesions may only ooze blood and produce a positive fecal occult blood test. Others may cause a slow decrease in serum hemoglobin concentration. Overt lesions may require blood transfusions or may be detected as coffee grounds in a nasogastric tube or as melena. Occult bleeding occurs in over 25% of critically ill patients, whereas overt bleeding occurs in less than 10%.

15. Describe the pathologic mechanism of SRES.

SRES is caused by an imbalance of the classic aggressive and defensive factors. Aggressive factors include acid, pepsin, and bile. The classic stress ulcer causes diffuse ulceration and hemorrhage of the oxynthic gastric mucosa of the proximal stomach and fundus. The high acid output is the aggressive factor that injures the adjacent lining. The classic lesion, however, is not the norm. SRES occurs in the antrum, duodenum, and distal esophagus. It occurs in the setting of high, normal, or low acid output. The recognition that high acid is not the only factor responsible for these lesions highlights how breakdown of defensive factors contributes to SRES. Defensive factors such as mucosal integrity, alkaline mucus buffer, gastric epithelial restitution (migration of gastric epithelial cells to areas of gastric mucosa disruption), and protective mucosal prostaglandin production are affected by hypotension, infection, and systemic acidosis. Defensive factors are significantly impaired in critically ill patients.

16. How can SRES be prevented?

The overall incidence of bleeding from SRES has dramatically decreased since the 1980s because of improvements in ICU care and support (less breakdown of defensive factors) rather than the use of pharmacologic prophylaxis (reduction of aggressive factors such as acid). Even so, prophylaxis has been shown to decrease bleeding from SRES, although it has no impact on mortality.

Maintaining a gastric pH above 4 has been shown to prevent SRES. Antacids, H_2 receptor antagonists, and proton pump inhibitors have been investigated with this strategy in mind. Sucralfate is thought to work primarily as a cytoprotective agent, although stimulation of several growth factors implicated in ulcer healing may be its true mechanism of action.

Antacids were the first medications to demonstrate efficacy in reducing overt and clinically significant bleeding. They are not used more often because they require frequent dosing and nasogastric administration and can cause hypermagnesemia in patients with renal insufficiency. H_2 receptor antagonists effectively increase gastric pH > 4 by blocking histamine stimulation of gastric acid secretion. They are widely used because of availability of an IV formulation and because they have been shown to be effective in SRES prophylaxis. Side effects include thrombocytopenia, CNS effects, and tachyphylaxis. Proton pump inhibitors are effective compared with placebo. In comparison with H_2 receptor antagonists, they more effectively maintain the gastric pH above 4 over a 24-hour period. They do not have the tachyphylaxis of H_2 receptor antagonists. An IV formulation is available in the United States. At this time limited data compare them with H_2 receptor antagonists.

Enteral nutrition is undergoing evaluation, and small trials have demonstrated efficacy in reducing the incidence of SRES.

17. What is ischemic colitis?

Ischemic colitis encompasses a wide spectrum of injury to the colon due to compromised arterial inflow. The spectrum of injury extends from reversible colonopathy (submucosal or intramural hemorrhage, transient colitis) to irreversible disease (chronic ulcerating colitis, fulminant universal colitis, stricture, gangrene).

18. What causes ischemic colitis?

The causes of ischemic colitis can be categorized by the pathophysiologic mechanism of injury. They are either occlusive(e.g., iatrogenic occlusion of the inferior mesenteric artery during aortic surgery) or nonocclusive (e.g., decreased splanchnic blood flow during shock or with cardiac bypass surgery).

In younger patients, ischemia is more likely to be related to (1) systemic conditions such as vasculitides (e.g., systemic lupus erythematosus); (2) infections (cytomegalovirus, *Escherichia coli* 0157:H7); (3) coagulopathies (e.g., protein C and S deficiencies, antithrombin III deficiency, resistance to activated protein C); (4) various medications (e.g., oral contraceptives) or illicit drugs (e.g., cocaine, methamphetamines); or (5) strenuous and prolonged physical exertion (e.g., long-distance running).

19. Which patients are at risk for ischemic colitis?

In the intensive care unit, ischemic colitis tends to occur in middle-aged or elderly patients with atherosclerotic disease (coronary artery disease, peripheral artery disease) in the setting of hypotension, shock in combination with vasoconstrictive drugs, or recent surgical repair of the aorta (particularly aneurysm repair). Ischemic colitis complicates 7% of elective aortic surgical repairs and 60% of surgeries for ruptured abdominal aortic aneurysms. Ischemic colitis is responsible for approximately 10% of deaths after aortic reconstruction.

20. How is ischemic colitis diagnosed?

Many features are variable and nonspecific. Patients often have crampy, left lower quadrant abdominal pain followed by the urge to defecate. Within 24 hours they pass bright red blood or maroon blood mixed with stool. Bleeding is usually not sufficient to require transfusion. The abdomen is usually mildly tender in the affected segment, typically in the left lower quadrant.

Depending on whether the insult continues, superficial ischemia can extend and produce transmural ischemia. In extreme cases, this process can cause abdominal distention, gangrene, and peritonitis. The patient may become febrile and develop leukocytosis. Plain abdominal films may demonstrate "thumbprinting," indicating submucosal edema. A CT scan of the abdomen may reveal a thickened colonic wall in the affected area or may demonstrate pneumatosis (air in the wall of the colon). No serum tests help diagnose early ischemic colitis. Serum lactate, lactate dehydrogenase, creatine phosphokinase, and amylase levels are typically elevated in advanced and severe ischemic damage. Acidosis is also a late finding and occurs in the setting of bowel infarction. A colonoscopy or sigmoidoscopy can make the definitive diagnosis of ischemic colitis. The procedure must be done with caution given the risk of perforation from insufflation of air or lateral wall pressure in the sigmoid colon and at the flexures while the endoscope is advanced. A colonoscopy is contraindicated in patients with peritonitis or significant colonic transmural involvement.

21. What areas of the colon are at greatest risk for occlusive and nonocclusive ischemia?

Much of the blood supply to the GI tract depends on good collateral flow between the celiac artery, superior mesenteric artery (SMA), and inferior mesenteric artery (IMA). Branches of the SMA supply the right, proximal, and mid-transverse colon. Branches of the IMA supply the region from the distal transverse colon to the proximal rectum. The splenic flexure relies on collateral flow between the SMA and IMA, which may be poor in up to 10% of the population. The rectum rarely becomes ischemic because of rich collateral flow between the IMA and internal iliac circulation.

All areas of the colon can be affected by ischemia, but certain causes of ischemic colitis tend to affect certain segments of the colon more often. Nonocclusive ischemia secondary to a low flow state most commonly affects the right colon and is involved in 68% of hypotension-associated ischemic colitis. The arterial anatomy of the right colon contributes to this increased risk because a marginal artery formed from branches of the SMA is incompletely developed or absent in 25–75% of people. Thus, fewer end vessels supply oxygen to the right colon. Low-flow states can also affect the "watershed" areas in the splenic flexure or rectosigmoid junction because of poor collateral flow in 10% of the population. Occlusion of the IMA produces ischemia in the sigmoid colon, the area most remote from collateral flow.

22. Describe the treatment of ischemic colitis.

Most patients with ischemic colitis have mild-to-moderate disease that is reversible and associated with a low mortality rate. If there is no evidence of gangrene or perforation, treatment of suspected nonocclusive ischemic colitis is primarily supportive. Patients with iatrogenic occlusion (e.g., after aortic surgery) may require repeat surgery and revascularization. Patients with evidence of transmural injury or perforation require emergent laparotomy. Mortality is greatly increased by the need for surgery. The mortality rate in patients undergoing surgery is about 60%.

23. List three additional causes of submassive to massive GI bleeding that are cared for in an ICU setting.

Bleeding from aortoenteric fistula, varices, and high-risk ulcers.

24. What are the clinical manifestations of an aortoenteric fistula?

Aortoenteric fistula (AEF) is rare but may be dramatic and catastrophic in presentation. It is defined as a communication between the abdominal aorta and an adjacent loop of bowel. A primary fistula results from erosion of an enlarged abdominal aortic aneurysm into the bowel. A secondary fistula is a complication of abdominal aortic reconstruction. An inflamed or infected prosthetic graft erodes into the adjacent adherent bowel secondary to the constant pulsatile motion of the aorta. It can complicate up to 1.5% of aortic reconstruction surgeries. Although the fistula can occur between the aorta and any portion of the GI tract, 75% of cases affect the duodenum. The third and fourth portions of the duodenum are most often involved because they cross directly anterior to the abdominal aorta.

An AEF presents months to years (average = 3 years) after aortic reconstructive surgery. The patient may present acutely with melena, hematemesis, or. less frequently. hematochezia. Over 20% of cases have the classic history of a "herald bleed," which is a brisk bleeding episode that stops spontaneously before a more massive hemorrhage in the hours to weeks that follow. Alternatively, the patient may have a chronic presentation with intermittent bleeding for weeks to months. The patient may report malaise, weight loss, fever, or pain.

25. How is an AEF diagnosed?
The diagnosis of AEF requires a high rate of clinical suspicion. EGD is useful in ruling out more common causes of GI bleeding. A routine endoscopic evaluation extends from the esophagus through the second portion of the duodenum. Most aortoenteric fistulae occur in the third and fourth portions of the duodenum. Therefore, if AEF is suspected, endoscopy must be performed through the fourth portion of the duodenum. EGD may detect abnormalities in 50% of cases but makes the definitive diagnosis in only about 25% of cases. An abdominal CT scan may be useful in making the diagnosis, although findings can be subtle, and a normal CT scan does not rule out the diagnosis. Angiography is rarely helpful because of the slow and intermittent nature of bleeding. Surgery is mandatory because untreated AEF is uniformly fatal. Surgery entails removal of the infected graft, repair of the aortoenteric fistula, and creation of an extra-anatomic bypass to revascularize the lower extremities.

26. Describe the management of variceal bleeding.
Patients with cirrhosis and portal hypertension are at risk of bleeding from varices. First-time variceal hemorrhage is associated with a 30–50% mortality rate. Varices can cause a large- volume GI bleed because high portal pressures precipitate rupture of varices. Poor hemostasis due to thrombocytopenia and coagulopathy compounds the problem. After carrying out the early management steps described before, patients suspected of having variceal hemorrhage should be started on octreotide while awaiting endoscopy. A loading dose of 50 µg IV is followed by an infusion of 50 µg/hour. Octreotide works by decreasing portal pressures. Patients with acute variceal hemorrhage treated with both octreotide and endoscopy have been found to have significantly lower rebleeding rates than those treated with endoscopic therapy alone. Although the optimal duration of therapy has not been determined, studies have utilized a 5-day infusion.

Prompt endoscopic therapy with either variceal band ligation or sclerotherapy is the cornerstone of treatment. Band ligation and sclerotherapy are two effective options with distinct advantages and vocal proponents. In a meta-analysis, variceal band ligation was found to be more effective in reducing rebleeding rate, mortality rate, and complication rate compared with sclerotherapy. Patients who have persistent bleeding or who rebleed despite endoscopic therapy may require transjugular intrahepatic shunting (TIPS) or, in rare cases, even surgery to decrease portal pressures and control bleeding. Active variceal hemorrhage unresponsive to endoscopic therapy can be temporarily controlled by balloon tamponade. This procedure entails placement of a Sengstaken-Blakemore tube or a Minnesota tube by a gastroenterologist until TIPS or surgery can be performed.

27. Which patients with ulcers require continued ICU care?
EGD stratifies patients with ulcers into groups at high risk and low risk of rebleeding. Endoscopy also can treat high-risk ulcers and decrease the risk of rebleeding. Patients who rebleed have a higher mortality rate than those who do not. A clean-based ulcer carries the lowest risk of rebleeding and does not require endoscopic therapy. These low-risk patients may be discharged within the first 24 hours of hospitalization. High-risk ulcers are defined as those that are actively bleeding, those that are not bleeding but have a visible vessel, and those that are not bleeding but have an adherent clot over them. The highest risk of rebleeding occurs within the first 72 hours after the initial bleeding episode. Surgery is reserved for ulcers that continue to bleed despite endoscopic therapy. Other high-risk lesions include varices, ulcers > 2 cm, and ulcers located in the lesser curve of the stomach or in the posterior bulb of the duodenum.

Ulcer Appearance and Prognosis in Ulcer Disease

	APPEARANCE	PREVALENCE (%)	REBLEED (%)	MORTALITY (%)
Lowest risk	Clean base	42	5	2
↓	Flat spot	20	10	3
	Adherent clot	17	22	7
↓	Visible vessel	17	43	11
Highest risk	Active bleeding	18	55	11

BIBLIOGRAPHY

1. Bastounis E, Papalambros E, Mermingas V, et al: Secondary aortoduodenal fistulae. J Cardiovasc Surg 38:457–464, 1997.
2. Beejay U, Wolfe MM: Acute gastrointestinal bleeding in the intensive care unit: The gastroenterolgist's perspective. Gastroenterol Clin North Am 29:309–336, 2000.
3. Brandt LJ, Boley SJ: AGA technical review on intestinal ischemia. American Gastrointestinal Association practice guidelines. Gastroenterology 118:954–968, 2000.
4. Cook DJ, Fuller HD, Guyatt GH, et al: Risk factors for gastrointestinal bleeding in critically ill patients. N Engl J Med 330:377–381, 1994.
5. Cook DJ, Reeve BK, Guyatt GH, et al: Stress ulcer prophylaxis in critically ill patients: Resolving discordant meta-analyses. JAMA 274:308–314, 1996.
6. Cook D, Heyland D, Griffith L, et al: Risk factors for clinically important upper gastrointestinal bleeding in patients requiring mechanical ventilation. Crit Care Med 27:2812–2817, 1999.
7. Greenwald DA, Brandt LJ. Colonic ischemia. J Clin Gastroenterol 27:122–128, 1998.
8. Hussain H, Lapin S, Cappell MS: Clinical scoring systems for determining the prognosis of gastrointestinal bleeding. Gastroenterol Clin North Am 29:445–464, 2000.
9. Laine L, Peterson WL: Bleeding peptic ulcer. N Engl J Med 331:717–727, 1994.
10. Laine L, Cook D: Endoscopic ligation compared with sclerotherapy for treatment of esophageal variceal bleeding: A meta-analysis. Ann Intern Med 123:280–287, 1995.
11. Laine L: Acute and chronic gastrointestinal bleeding. Slesenger MH, Fordtran JS (eds): Gastrointestinal and Liver Disease: Pathophysiology/Diagnosis/Management, 6th ed. Philadelphia, W.B. Saunders, 1998, pp 198–219.
12. Mutlu GM, Mutlua EA, Factor P: GI complications in patients receiving mechanical ventilation. Chest 119:1222–1241, 2001.
13. Terdiman JP, Ostroff JW: Gastrointestinal bleeding in the hospitalized patient: A case-control study to assess risk factors, causes, and outcome. Am J Med 104:349–354, 1998.
14. Tryba M: Role of acid suppressants in intensive care medicine. Best Pract Res Clin Gastroenterol 15:447–461, 2001.

49. ACUTE PANCREATITIS

Mark W. Bowyer M.D.

1. What is acute pancreatitis?

Acute pancreatitis is an acute inflammatory condition of the pancreas that presents with abdominal pain and is usually associated with elevations of pancreatic enzymes in the blood. The clinical course can range from a mild disease to multiorgan failure and sepsis. Acute pancreatitis can be subcategorized as either edematous or as necrotizing pancreatitis. **Edematous pancreatitis** is characterized by the presence of interstitial edema of the pancreas and the presence of mild peripancreatic fat necrosis. **Necrotizing pancreatitis** is characterized by extensive parenchymal necrosis, areas of hemorrhage, and extensive peripancreatic and intrapancreatic fat necrosis.

2. Describe the expected course of acute pancreatitis.

The clinical course can range from a mild disease with complete recovery to a formidable process characterized by multiorgan failure, sepsis, and death.

3. What conditions cause acute pancreatitis?

Gallstones	45%
Alcohol	35%
Miscellaneous	10%
Idiopathic	10%

Variation in the frequency of different forms is quite marked from series to series and depends on the referral population. In some inner city centers, alcohol may account for more than 75% of cases. In general, the etiology of acute pancreatitis can be categorized as obstructive, toxin- or drug-induced, traumatic, metabolic, infectious, vascular, or miscellaneous.

4. What are the obstructive causes of pancreatitis?

Gallstones	Periampullary duodenal diverticula
Ampullary or pancreatic tumors	Choledochocele
Worms or foreign bodies	Hypertensive sphincter of Oddi
Pancreas divisum	

5. What are some of the toxins and drugs known to cause pancreatitis?

Toxins include ethyl alcohol, methyl alcohol, organophosphorus insecticides, and scorpion venom. More than 80 different drugs have been reported to cause pancreatitis. Many commonly used drugs, including acetaminophen, angiotensin-converting enzyme inhibitors, ergotamine, furosemide, tetracycline, aminosalicylic acid, corticosteroids, procainamide, thiazides, cimetidine, metronidazole, and ranitidine have been implicated. The drugs with the highest rates of pancreatitis include azathioprine and mercaptopurine (3–5%); didanosine (up to 23%); and pentamidine (4–22%).

6. What are the traumatic causes of pancreatitis?

Blunt trauma with disruption of the ductal system can result in acute pancreatitis. Iatrogenic trauma to the pancreas from endoscopic retrograde cholangiopancreatography, endoscopic sphincterotomy, and manometry of the sphincter of Oddi can also lead to pancreatitis.

7. What metabolic conditions can cause acute pancreatitis?

Hypertriglyceridemia (especially type V hyperlipoproteinemia) with levels in excess of 1000 mg/dl increases the risk of pancreatitis. Hypercalcemia has been associated with pancreatitis in rare cases; usually it is associated with hyperparathyroidism.

8. What other conditions have been implicated in the development of acute pancreatitis?

Parasites such as ascariasis and clonorchiasis and viral infections such as mumps, rubella, hepatitis, Epstein-Barr virus, and HIV have been implicated as etiologic factors for pancreatitis. Bacterial causes of pancreatitis include *Mycoplasma* species, *Campylobacter jejuni, Mycobacterium tuberculosis, Mycobacterium avium, Legionella* species, and leptospirosis. Other causes of acute pancreatitis include penetrating peptic ulcers, Crohn's disease, Reye's syndrome, cystic fibrosis, periarteritis nodosa, lupus, and malignant hypertension. Despite the multitude of known etiologic factors for acute pancreatitis, nearly 10% of the cases are called idiopathic.

9. Describe the pathophysiology of acute pancreatitis.

As evidenced by the multitude of etiologic factors, the process can be initiated by several different mechanisms. The resultant common pathway is premature activation of zymogen granules with initiation of the following cascade:

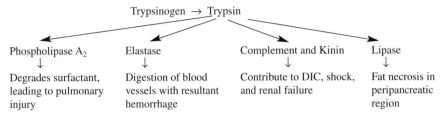

Trypsinogen → Trypsin

Phospholipase A₂	Elastase	Complement and Kinin	Lipase
↓	↓	↓	↓
Degrades surfactant, leading to pulmonary injury	Digestion of blood vessels with resultant hemorrhage	Contribute to DIC, shock, and renal failure	Fat necrosis in peripancreatic region

Ischemia of the organ appears to transform mild edematous pancreatitis into severe hemorrhagic or necrotizing forms of the disease. Increased deposition of fat in the peripancreatic region predisposes to more extensive necrosis; obesity is a major risk factor for severe pancreatitis. Necrotic pancreatic tissue becomes secondarily infected in 40–60% of cases.

10. Describe the clinical manifestations of acute pancreatitis.
Patients with acute pancreatitis typically complain of midepigastric pain that is constant and boring with radiation through to the back and associated with nausea and vomiting. In severe pancreatitis, hypotension and clinical signs of shock may be present secondary to fluid loss and the circulating mediators of inflammation.

11. What is the Grey-Turner sign?
The Grey-Turner sign is the flank discoloration that is classically associated with hemorrhagic pancreatitis.

12. What is Cullen's sign?
Cullen's sign refers to the periumbilical discoloration that may be present in hemorrhagic pancreatitis.

13. What laboratory tests aid in the diagnosis?
Serum amylase has been the most commonly used marker for acute pancreatitis. The first description of its measurement in pancreatitis was published in 1929. During the first 24 hours an elevated amylase level has a sensitivity of 81–84%. By the second day the sensitivity of amylase drops to 33%. The specificity of an elevated amylase level is low, because it also may be caused by perforated peptic ulcers, bowel infarctions, salivary gland trauma, renal failure, and macroamylasemia. Serum lipase is more specific than amylase and has a sensitivity of 85–100%; after four days it remains elevated in 90% of patients. Recent reports suggest that lipase is the more accurate test in acute pancreatitis, and some authors argue that obtaining both is not warranted. Collection of blood for measurement of white blood cell counts, glucose, lactate dehydrogenase, aspartate aminotransferase (AST), hematocrit, calcium, triglycerides, base deficit, and arterial blood gases may help to determine the severity and the prognosis of patients with any form of pancreatitis except the mildest cases.

14. What radiographic and imaging studies are useful?
Imaging techniques are crucial in confirming the diagnosis and providing clues to the cause of acute pancreatitis. The following modalities are useful:
Plain radiographs of the abdomen and chest should be obtained to rule out other conditions, such as a perforated viscus or a bowel infarction, that may simulate pancreatitis.
Ultrasonography remains highly useful (67% sensitivity, 100% specificity) in evaluating the biliary tract but is not useful for detecting the complications of acute pancreatitis. Ultrasound has limited ability to visualize the pancreas in the first 48 hours because of associated paralytic ileus.
Spiral contrast-enhanced computed tomography (CT) is the current method of choice for delineating the pancreas as well as determining the severity and many of the complications of pancreatitis. CT is also helpful for guiding percutaneous therapy.

Magnetic resonance imaging (MRI) can depict the presence and extent of necrosis and peripancreatic fluid collections as well as CT. MRI requires the administration of gadolinium (Gd) to detect necrosis. The fact that Gd is nontoxic in comparison with the iodinized contrast agents required for CT increases the attractiveness of MRI in some patients. CT retains the advantages of lower cost, greater availability, and ability to perform interventional procedures.

15. What methods are available to estimate the severity and prognosis of acute pancreatitis?

The natural history of acute pancreatitis ranges from a mild self-limiting process to a fulminant, rapidly lethal disease. Early identification of the severity of disease, therefore, is important to permit the appropriate application of monitoring and invasive therapeutic measures. Several clinical criteria systems have been developed, including Ranson's criteria, Glasgow criteria, and the APACHE II system. CT findings have also been used to estimate severity and have been correlated with mortality and complication rates. Ranson's criteria and the CT severity index are the most commonly used and are summarized below:

Ranson's Criteria

	NONBILIARY	BILIARY
At admission		
Age (yr)	> 55	> 70
White blood cells	> 16.0	> 18.0
Glucose	> 200	> 220
Lactate dehydrogenase	> 350	> 400
Aspartate aminotransferase	> 250	> 250
During 1st 48 hrs		
Fall in hematocrit	> 10	> 10
Rise in blood urea nitrogen	> 5	> 2
Calcium	< 8.0	< 8.0
Partial pressure of oxygen	<	...
Base deficit	> 4	> 5
Fluid sequestration	> 6l	> 4l

2 or less criteria (77%)	0.9% mortality
3–4 criteria (15%)	16% mortality
5–6 criteria (7%)	40% mortality
7–8 criteria (1%)	100% mortality

CT Severity Index

	POINTS
Grade of acute pancreatitis	
Normal pancreas	0
Pancreatic enlargement	1
Inflammation of pancreas and fat	2
1 fluid collection	3
≥ 2 fluid collections	4
Degree of necrosis	
No necrosis	0
One-third of pancreas	2
One-half of pancreas	4
> One-half of pancreas	6

0–3	Mortality = 3%, complication rate = 8%
4–6	Mortality = 6%, complication rate = 35%
7–10	Mortality = 17%, complication rate = 92%

16. What medical therapies are available for the treatment of acute pancreatitis? What works? What does not work?

The goals of medical therapy for acute pancreatitis are as follows:

1. **To limit the severity of pancreatic secretions.** It has been postulated that the inhibition of pancreatic secretions ameliorates the course of pancreatitis. The use of nasogastric suction has been found in recent controlled clinical trials *not* to be effective, although nasogastric suction may be helpful in a subset of patients with vomiting and abdominal distention. Premature resumption of oral feedings may cause reactivation of pancreatic inflammation; therefore, they should be withheld until pain, tenderness, fever, and leukocytosis resolve. Inhibition of pancreatic secretions by anticholinergics or somatostatin has failed to show significant benefit in controlled clinical trials. Several agents, including apoprotein, soybean trypsin inhibitor, camostat, and fresh frozen plasma, have been studied as inhibitors of pancreatic enzymes without clear benefit.

2. **To ameliorate complications by interrupting their pathogenesis.** Secondary bacterial infection occurs 40–60% of patients who develop necrotic pancreatic tissue. Thus, antibiotics traditionally have been recommended for the treatment of acute pancreatitis, although studies using antibiotics to prevent septic complications are sparse. A few controlled trials have begun to appear, however, and the evidence suggests that early antibiotic therapy (imipenem and cilastin) reduces the need for surgery and overall number of major organ complications in acute necrotizing pancreatitis. Close attention to hypovolemia and prevention of ischemia to the pancreas may help prevent mild pancreatitis from becoming more severe.

3. **To support the patient and treat the complications as they arise.** Currently the most important measures in the treatment of pancreatitis are supportive and symptomatic. Because pancreatitis is often associated with massive fluid shifts, monitoring and adequate replacement of intravascular fluid is essential. A central venous catheter and urethral catheter should be placed; if the patient has underlying cardiovascular disease, a pulmonary artery catheter may be needed for appropriate treatment. Most patients can be resuscitated with crystalloid, but colloid or blood may be needed. Hypokalemia is common, and potassium replacement is usually required. Hypocalcemia and hypomagnesemia may also occur and require replacement therapy. Because respiratory failure is a frequent feature of acute pancreatitis, serial arterial blood gases should be obtained with early intubation and positive end-expiratory pressure ventilation as indicated. Nutritional depletion is very common in acute pancreatitis, and nutritional support in the form of total parenteral nutrition should be used for patients with severe pancreatitis. The pain associated with acute pancreatitis may be severe, and intravenous narcotics may be required. Pulmonary embolism is a potential late complication in patients with pancreatitis; therefore, it is important to monitor fibrinogen levels and platelets. If a hypercoagulable state is demonstrated, heparin should be administered.

17. When is surgery indicated in the treatment of acute pancreatitis? What options are available?

The goals of surgery in the treatment of acute pancreatitis are as follows:

1. **To aid in diagnosis.** When the possibility of acute life-threatening extrapancreatic disease cannot be excluded by other means, diagnostic laparoscopy or celiotomy may be necessary.

2. **To limit pancreatic inflammation.** Surgical intervention is clearly indicated during the early phase of acute pancreatitis if life-threatening cholecystitis or cholangitis is present or cannot be excluded.

3. **To limit the pathogenesis of complications.** Lavage of the peritoneal cavity by surgically introduced catheters is frequently associated with dramatic improvement in cardiovascular, renal, and respiratory function. The efficacy of lavage has been attributed to removal of toxic materials in the peritoneal cavity. The incidence of late peripancreatic infection does not appear to be reduced with the use of lavage, and overall mortality is unchanged.

4. **To support the patient and treat complications.** Operative placement of a feeding jejunostomy can greatly simplify nutritional support. When pancreatic infection or abscess is confirmed (by needle aspiration) or strongly suspected, surgical debridement should be performed.

Surgical options include radical debridement and sump drainage with irrigation (14% hospital mortality in a series of 36 patients), or blunt debridement with packing of the pancreatic bed with repeat debridement at dressing changes (15% mortality in a series of 71 patients). Such patients are usually critically ill and require vigorous supportive care.

18. What are pancreatic pseudocysts?

Pancreatic pseudocysts are encapsulated collections of fluid with high enzyme concentrations that arise from the pancreas. The walls of the pseudocyst are formed by inflammatory fibrosis of peritoneal, mesenteric, and serosal membranes. The term *pseudocyst* denotes absence of an epithelial lining. Pseudocysts develop in about 2% of cases of acute pancreatitis. The cysts are single in 85% of cases and multiple in the remainder.

19. How should pancreatic pseudocysts be managed?

Asymptomatic pseudocysts require no specific treatment. Twenty-five to fifty percent of pseudocysts after acute pancreatitis resolve spontaneously. Recent data based on two retrospective studies suggest that pseudocysts of any size that remain asymptomatic require no treatment. Symptomatic pseudocysts typically are characterized by pain, fever, weight loss, tenderness, and a palpable mass. Symptomatic pseudocysts can be treated surgically (most common and time-honored approach), by interventional radiology (less successful), or by endoscopic cyst-gastrostomy or cyst-duodenoscopy.

20. What is the role of early endoscopic retrograde cholangiopancreatography (ERCP) and papillotomy in the treatment of acute biliary pancreatitis?

Fifteen years ago most endoscopists thought that ERCP was contraindicated in the acute phase of pancreatitis. In 1988 a randomized study reported by Neoptolemos et al. found that early ERCP with biliary decompression and stone removal reduced morbidity but not mortality in elderly patients in whom severe pancreatitis was predicted to develop. Based on subsequent randomized studies, Barkun made the following evidence-based recommendations:

1. Early ERCP (within 24–72 hours of onset of symptoms and admission) is safe in patients with a predicted severe episode of suspected acute biliary pancreatitis. Class B recommendation (fair evidence to support procedure) based on level 1 evidence.

2. Early ERCP (and sphincterotomy when bile duct stones are found) results in diminished biliary sepsis among patients with suspected biliary pancreatitis, especially those with a predicted severe attack. Diminished biliary sepsis, in turn, results in improved outcomes in this subgroup of patients. Class A (good evidence to support procedure) recommendation based on level 1 evidence.

3. Early ERCP (and sphincterotomy when common bile duct stones are found) results in decreased complication rates in patients with acute biliary pancreatitis and a predicted severe attack. Class A recommendation based on level 1 evidence.

4. At present, early ERCP should not be performed in patients with a predicted mild attack of acute pancreatitis of suspected biliary etiology. Class D recommendation (fair evidence that procedure should not be used) based on level 1 evidence.

BIBLIOGRAPHY

1. Banks PA: Practice guidelines in acute pancreatitis. Am J Gastroenterol 92: 377–386, 1997.
2. Barkun AN: Early endoscopic management of acute gallstone pancreatitis: An evidence-based review. J Gastrointest Surg 5:243–250, 2001.
3. Elmas N: The role of diagnostic radiology in pancreatitis. Eur J Radiol 38:120–132, 2001.
4. Golub R, Siddiqi F, Pohl D: Role of antibiotics in acute pancreatitis: A meta-analysis. J Gastrointest Surg 2:496–503, 1998.
5. McFadden W, Reber HA: Indications for surgery in severe acute pancreatitis. Int J Pancreatol 15:83–90, 1994.
6. Neoptolemos JP, Carr-Locke DL, London NJ, et al: Controlled trial of urgent endoscopic retrograde cholangiopancreatography and endoscopic sphincterotomy versus conservative treatment for acute pancreatitis due to gallstones. Lancet 2:979–983, 1988.

7. Nordback I, Sand J, Saaristo R, Paajan H: Early treatment with antibiotics reduces the need for surgery in acute necrotizing pancreatitis: A single-center randomized study. J Gastrointest Surg 5:113–120, 2001.
8. Ranson JHC: Acute pancreatitis. In Cameron JL (ed): Current Surgical Therapy, 5th ed. St. Louis, Mosby, 1995, pp 408–413.
9. Robinson PJA, Sheridan MB: Pancreatitis: Computed tomography and magnetic resonance imaging. Eur Radiol 10:401–408, 2000.
10. Steinburg W, Tenner S: Acute pancreatitis. N Engl J Med 330:1198–1210, 1994.
11. Vissers RJ, Abu-Laban RB, McHugh DF: Amylase and lipase in the emergency department evaluation of acute pancreatitis. J Emerg Med 17:1027–1037, 1999.

50. HEPATITIS AND CIRRHOSIS

Jon Perlstein, M.D., and Mark W. Bowyer, M.D.

1. What is hepatitis?

Hepatitis refers to any inflammatory process that involves liver parenchyma and may result in anything ranging from mere laboratory abnormalities to a fulminant illness with mortality. The most common etiologic factor is viral.

2. Which viruses are responsible?

Viral hepatitis may be caused by the A, B, C, D, and E hepatitis viruses; the Epstein-Barr virus (EBV); and cytomegalovirus (CMV). A non-A–E hepatitis virus, hepatitis G, has been recently described. In general, these viruses tend to cause similar clinical pictures ranging from asymptomatic to severe illness (rare).

3. What are the characteristics of hepatitis A?

The hepatitis A virus is an enterovirus of the family Picornaviridae, which causes an enterically transmitted disease acquired by ingestion of material that has been fecally contaminated. The virus passes through the stomach, replicates in the lower intestine, is transported to the liver, and begins to replicate in the cytoplasm. Cellular damage occurs as the body's immunologic defenses attempt to kill the virus.

The average incubation period to onset of symptoms is about 32 days but ranges between 3 and 6 weeks. Classically, there is a prodromal phase during which malaise, anorexia, epigastric or right upper quadrant pain, fever, rashes, diarrhea, and constipation are frequent complaints. The disease is usually recognized during the icteric phase, when dark urine and jaundice prompt patients to seek medical attention. Liver tests at this time reveal elevated transaminase and bilirubin levels, and the clinical diagnosis can be confirmed by detection of the IgM antibody to the virus.

The severity of the illness is age-related. Older adults tend to have worse symptoms than young adults. Most cases of acute hepatitis resolve rapidly over several weeks with complete clinical and biochemical recovery.

4. What are the characteristics of hepatitis B?

The hepatitis B virus (HBV) is the prototype of a new class of viruses, the Hepadnaviridae. Clinical expression of infection with HBV may range from a carrier state to fulminant hepatitis. In classic acute hepatitis B, the incubation period varies from 60 to 180 days. As with hepatitis A, there is a prodromal phase that in hepatitis B is more insidious and more prolonged, with arthritis and urticarial rash as additional symptoms. As in hepatitis A, symptoms tend to improve with the onset of jaundice. During the icteric phase, the bilirubin tends to rise less steeply than in hepatitis

A, but it reaches higher levels, and the jaundice lasts longer. There is a slower rise in aminotransferase levels, which peak much later than in hepatitis A.

Unlike hepatitis A, acute hepatitis B may become chronic hepatitis and cirrhosis. Patients may also have an asymptomatic infection without liver disease (healthy carriers).

HBV infection can be spread via parenteral transmission. Blood is the most effective vehicle for transmission, but the virus is present in other body fluids as well (e.g., saliva and semen). HBV infection is a common problem among intravenous drug abusers, homosexual men, and the sexual partners of infected patients. Vertical transmission may occur to infants from mothers who experience hepatitis B infection during the last trimester of pregnancy.

5. What laboratory tests are available for hepatitis B? How are they interpreted?

Sensitive immunoassays are available to measure the antigens associated with HBV and the antibodies it induces. The antigenic activity of the virus DNA core is designated HBc (core) Ag. The other surface coat of the virus has distinctive antigenicity and is designated HBsAg. These antigens evoke specific antibodies, and both constitute important immunologic markers of the infection and its course.

During a typical case of acute hepatitis B, HBsAg is first detected in blood during the incubation period, as early as 1 week after infection. The HBsAg level begins to decline after the onset of the illness and usually becomes undetectable within 3 months after exposure. The presence of HBsAg in serum indicates the potential for infectivity. Anti-HBc appears in the serum toward the end of the incubation period and persists during the acute illness and for several months to years thereafter. Anti-HBs is detected during convalescence (several weeks to months after disappearance of HBsAg) and persists for a prolonged period. A high titer of anti-HBs confirms immunity to HBV. Persistence of HBsAg is a sign of chronic hepatitis B.

6. What are the characteristics of hepatitis C?

Hepatitis C is the name given to this single-stranded RNA virus distantly related to the Flavivirus family. The hepatitis C virus is the major cause of posttransfusion, community-acquired, cryptogenic non-A, non-B hepatitis. Until the availability of serologic tests, it was responsible for 90–95% of all cases of posttransfusion hepatitis.

The incubation period to rise in aminotransferases is about 6–8 weeks. Symptoms are usually of moderate severity; 40–75% of cases are asymptomatic. Jaundice is uncommon (10%) and usually mild. There is a high rate of progression to chronic hepatitis and eventually cirrhosis. Early identification of infection is difficult. Alanine aminotransferase is more likely to be elevated than aspartate aminotransferase.

7. What laboratory test can detect the hepatitis C virus at the earliest point in the disease course?

Hepatitis C RNA can be detected by polymerase chain reaction (PCR) by 2 weeks after exposure.

8. What are the characteristics of hepatitis D?

Hepatitis D (or delta agent) is an incomplete RNA viral particle similar to plant viruses; it requires the presence of HBV for infection and replication to occur. Infection can occur only in HBsAg carriers exposed to the delta agent or in patients who are simultaneously infected with both HBV and hepatitis D. Acute simultaneous infection with both viruses may be associated with fulminant hepatitis. Chronic infection with hepatitis D is frequently associated with chronic active hepatitis or cirrhosis.

9. What is hepatitis E?

The hepatitis E virus produces a water-borne disease similar to but generally milder than hepatitis A. It may be transmitted by the fecal-oral route. It has an average incubation period of 40 days and is epidemic in a number of developing countries. Fulminant hepatitis may occur, especially among pregnant women, with a mortality rate as high as 20%.

10. What is hepatitis G?

Hepatitis G virus (HGV) is a unique virus that can be transmitted by blood. The association of hepatitis G with disease remains unclear, but it is estimated that approximately 0.3% of persons with acute viral hepatitis may be infected with HGV alone. Persistent infection with HGV appears to be quite prevalent in the general population; almost 2% of blood donors and 14–52% of patients with other types of viral hepatitis test positive for HGV RNA.

11. What is cholestatic hepatitis?

Chronic viral hepatitis or systemic inflammatory response syndrome (SIRS) may result in a cholestatic process diagnosed by jaundice, pruritus, elevated direct bilirubin, and elevated alkaline phosphatase. The etiology of this condition is canalicular dysfunction secondary to the viral infection and/or inflammatory response. Most episodes of cholestatic hepatitis are self-limited; however, one may need to rule out sources of extrahepatic biliary obstruction.

12. What is fulminant viral hepatitis?

Fulminant hepatitis occurs in about 1% of patients who have acute viral hepatitis requiring hospitalization. In fulminant hepatitis, massive hepatocellular necrosis occurs and is believed to be related to an abnormally rapid clearance of the viral antigens. Hepatitis B accounts for approximately 50% of cases, hepatitis C for about 45% and hepatitis A for about 5%. Fulminant hepatitis can also occur with a variety of hepatotoxic drugs and uncommon diseases. The end-result is fulminant hepatic failure (FHF). FHF is manifested by signs and symptoms of encephalopathy within 3–8 weeks after the onset of the illness. A profound coagulopathy occurs as a result of poor hepatic synthetic function and is best measured with the prothrombin time (PT). If the PT exceeds control by 10 seconds despite vitamin K supplementation, FHF has evolved. Renal failure, usually due to volume depletion and cerebral edema, is a frequent sequela of FHF.

13. What cardiovascular changes are associated with FHF? What is the treatment?

The typical cardiovascular changes associated with hepatic failure are decreased peripheral vascular resistance and increased cardiac output (hyperdynamic state). The increased cardiac output is believed to be a result of the opening of myocutaneous vascular shunts.

Pulmonary artery catheters are very useful in managing patients. Physiologically, the best method of treating the high cardiac output is by increasing peripheral vascular resistance. Dopamine and alpha-adrenergic agents can be used, but one must monitor for a tachyphylactic response and gastrointestinal bleeding. Clinical investigations are under way with the use of levodopa in an attempt to indirectly replete norepinephrine to the sympathetic nerve terminals.

14. What electrolyte disturbances are associated with FHF? What is the treatment?

Electrolyte disorders associated with cirrhosis and hepatic failure are commonly hyponatremia and hypokalemia. Hyponatremia is usually dilutional, secondary to a decrease in renal water excretion. Hypokalemia results from increased urinary excretion of potassium secondary to the influence of aldosterone and gastrointestinal losses.

These abnormalities are best treated with fluid and sodium restriction. The aldosterone antagonist spironolactone increases water loss more than sodium loss and also decreases renal potassium excretion. Combination therapy with furosemide and spironolactone can be used in refractory cases, but potassium levels must be monitored closely. The blood urea nitrogen (BUN) and creatinine must be monitored closely, and if any increase is noted, diuretic therapy should be discontinued to prevent a form of hepatorenal failure.

15. Describe the central nervous system changes seen with fulminant hepatitis. How are they treated?

Hepatic encephalopathy and cerebral edema are commonly seen with fulminant hepatitis and hepatic failure. The clinical features of hepatic encephalopathy are mental status changes, asterixis, precoma, and coma. The cause of the encephalopathy is believed to be the increased serum levels of ammonia, which indirectly results in an increased transport of amino acids across the blood-brain barrier.

The treatment of hepatic encephalopathy is based on reversing any precipitating factors and decreasing available amino acids for transport across the blood-brain barrier. If a specific medication is implicated, it should be discontinued. The primary treatment is catharsis with lactulose (15 ml 3 times/day) or magnesium citrate (240 ml/day), resulting in a lower stool pH and increased bacterial clearance. A reduction in the urease-producing bacteria via oral aminoglycosides (neomycin, 1gm 4 times/day) also aids treatment. Patients with hepatic encephalopathy need a reduction in dietary protein and do not tolerate standard protein formulations of total parenteral nutrition (TPN). TPN designed for patients with liver failure should contain fewer aromatic, neutral amino acids and more branched-chain amino acids. Such solutions are better tolerated, which is believed to be due to a decrease in available neutral amino acids as well as increased protein production and energy use via the branch-chained amino acids.

16. How is fulminant hepatitis treated?

No specific form of treatment other than orthotopic liver transplantation (OLT) has proved beneficial in fulminant hepatitis. The goal of current therapy is to sustain life and control hepatic failure over a period sufficient to allow hepatic regeneration before the patient dies of liver failure. Transplantation for fulminant hepatitis is still controversial. However, if OLT is considered, prompt surgical transplant consultation is critical: the worse the encephalopathy, the poorer the overall prognosis.

17. What is the prognosis for patients with fulminant hepatitis?

The overall survival rate of patients with fulminant hepatitis is 20–25%. Survival correlates best with the age of the patient and deepest level of encephalopathy reached. Over 50% of patients who reach only stage II encephalopathy survive. In contrast, survival for patients who progress to stage IV encephalopathy is only 20%.

18. What is chronic hepatitis?

Chronic hepatitis is defined as liver inflammation that persists for more than 6 months. There are two major variants: chronic persistent hepatitis and chronic active hepatitis. Chronic persistent hepatitis is a relapsing, remitting, benign, self-limited condition that is not associated with progressive liver damage and does not lead to liver failure or cirrhosis. Chronic active hepatitis is a vicious disease characterized by progressive destruction of hepatocytes over a span of years, with continued erosion of the hepatic functional reserve and eventual development of cirrhosis. It is estimated that about 5–10% of patients with acute hepatitis B and possibly as many as 33% of those with hepatitis C may develop chronic disease.

19. What are the nonviral causes of hepatitis?

Hepatic injury may be induced by a variety of chemical agents, drugs, and metabolic diseases. Drugs associated with chronic hepatitis or cirrhosis include acetaminophen, aspirin, chlorpromazine, dantrolene, ethanol, halothane, isoniazid, methyldopa, nitrofurantoin, propylthiouracil, and sulfonamides. Other hepatotoxins include carbon tetrachloride, phosphorus, tetracycline, chemotherapeutic agents, *Amanita phalloides* (mushroom toxin), and anabolic steroids. Metabolic diseases such as Wilson's disease, alpha$_1$-antitrypsin deficiency, and autoimmune hepatitis are associated with hepatitis and liver disease.

20. What is cirrhosis?

Cirrhosis is a diffuse process characterized by fibrosis and conversion of normal liver architecture into structurally abnormal nodules. The architectural disorganization of the liver is irreversible once established, and management is directed at both prevention of further liver cell damage and treatment of the complications.

21. What are the major causes of cirrhosis?

Alcohol is by far the most common cause of cirrhosis, accounting for 60–70% of cases. Chronic viral hepatitis, autoimmune hepatitis, primary biliary cirrhosis, primary sclerosing cholangitis, hemachromatosis, Wilson's disease, and idiopathic causes also lead to cirrhosis.

22. What are the major complications of cirrhosis?

Progressive liver cell damage and portal hypertension are sequelae of cirrhosis: they result in four major complications—ascites, spontaneous bacterial peritonitis, hepatic encephalopathy, and upper gastrointestinal bleeding—all of which may lead to admission to an intensive care unit.

23. How is cirrhotic ascites managed?

The initial management of cirrhotic ascites is conservative, emphasizing sodium restriction and bed rest. It is estimated that 10–20% of cirrhotic patients with ascites can be adequately treated this way. Patients who do not respond to conservative measures require diuretic therapy. Spironolactone is the agent of choice because of its physiologic action, potassium-sparing effects, and relative safety. Combination therapy with spironolactone and furosemide is used in patients who do not respond to spironolactone alone. In cases of diuretic-resistant ascites, therapeutic paracentesis should be considered, with possible albumin replacement. In truly unresponsive patients, the use of a peritoneovenous shunt should be considered, bearing in mind there is a high rate of complication (disseminated intravascular coagulation and sepsis) and no proven survival benefit with these devices.

24. How is primary spontaneous bacterial peritonitis (SBP) differentiated from secondary bacterial peritonitis?

The diagnosis of SBP is confirmed by ascitic fluid analysis. The key tests are cell count, total protein, lactate dehydrogenase, glucose, and Gram stain.

Fluid Test	Primary Bacterial Peritonitis	Secondary Bacterial Peritonitis
White blood cells (cells/mm^3)	> 500	> 500
Total protein (gm/dl)	< 1.0	> 1.0
Glucose (mg/dl)	> 50	< 50
Lactate dehydrogenase (U/L)	< 225	> 225
Gram stain	Monomicrobial	Polymicrobial

25. Define portal hypertension.

Portal hypertension is defined as portal venous pressure higher than 12 mmHg or a hepatic wedge venous pressure that exceeds the inferior vena cava pressure by more than 5 mmHg. Portal hypertension is classified as prehepatic, hepatic, or posthepatic according to the anatomic site of increased portal venous resistance. Cirrhosis is by far the most common cause of hepatic portal hypertension.

26. How is upper gastrointestinal tract bleeding associated with cirrhosis managed?

Approximately 70% of bleeding episodes in cirrhosis are due to variceal hemorrhage, but other causes such as gastritis, ulcer, and Mallory-Weiss tears should be kept in mind. Initial management is focused on volume resuscitation, correction of the coagulopathy, and reduction in portal venous pressure. Vasopressin was widely used to reduce portal pressure with high initial success rates. However, clinical trials have shown that somatostatin has similar results without the decreased coronary blood flow seen with vasopressin. Once the patient has been stabilized, endoscopy is performed to define the cause of bleeding. If bleeding is due to esophageal varices, injection sclerotherapy and/or banding becomes the preferred method of treatment and has a success rate of around 85% in arresting bleeding. If sclerotherapy is unsuccessful, a Sengstaken-Blakemore tube may be placed to tamponade bleeding, but the use of these tubes does not replace definitive therapy. If variceal bleeding continues, an operative portosystemic shunt (good risk patients only) or a transjugular intrahepatic portacaval shunt (TIPS) should be considered. An alternative approach is lower esophageal resection and/or esophagogastric devascularization (Sugiura procedure), which almost always stops the bleeding but is associated with a high mortality rate.

27. What is the role of orthotopic liver transplantation (OLT) in cirrhosis?
Liver transplantation has become the definitive treatment for end-stage cirrhosis. The one- and five-year survival rates are approximately 80% and 65%, respectively. The use of liver transplantation in patients with alcoholic cirrhosis is controversial. However, most transplant surgeons are willing to list the patients for transplantation if they prove that they abstain from alcohol and are currently participating in a rehabilitation course or group. The use of OLT for patients with hepatitis B or C is also controversial. However, with the use of hepatitis B immunoglobulin (HBIG), a reduction in the viral burden occurs, resulting in promising survival rates in patients with hepatitis B.

28. Does xenograft transplantation play a role in the treatment of FHF?
Several case reports in the recent literature describe heterotopically transplanting porcine livers to provide metabolic support prior to transplantation with a human liver. The majority of these cases were unsuccessful in providing hepatic function for longer than 36–48 hours secondary to acute rejection. Despite the removal of antipig antibodies by plasmapheresis and ex vivo en bloc perfusion of the donor pig kidneys, antibody and complement-mediated destruction of the xenografts occurred rapidly, resulting in graft-loss and worsening hepatic failure.

29. What advances have been made with regard to artificial liver support?
During the past few years, bioartificial liver support systems using hollow-fiber bioreactors, microcarrier cell culture techniques, and porcine hepatocytes have been transplanted in animals with acute liver failure and led to improved detoxification and synthetic function. Extracorporeal bioartificial liver systems using porcine hepatocytes have tested in vitro and shown to have cytochrome P450 activity, protein synthesis, and bilirubin conjugation. In vivo, these systems provided substantial metabolic support to the animals and improved neurologic function. With further research, bioartificial livers may become an effective bridge to orthotopic liver transplantation to patients awaiting available donor organs.

BIBLIOGRAPHY

1. Bain VG, Montero JL, de La Mata M: Bioartificial liver support. Can J Gastroenterol 15:313–318, 2001.
2. Blei AT, Cordoba J: Hepatic encephalopathy. The Practice Parameters Committee of the American College of Gastroenterology. Am J Gastroenterol 96:1968–1976, 2001.
3. Burroughs AK, Patch D: Transjugular intrahepatic portosystemic shunt. Semin Liver Dis 19:457, 1999.
4. Cardenas A, Gines P: Pathogenesis and treatment of fluid and electrolyte imbalance in cirrhosis. Semin Nephrol 21:308–316, 2001.
5. Garcia-Tsoa G: Current management of the complications of cirrhosis and portal hypertension: Variceal hemorrhage, ascites, and spontaneous bacterial peritonitis. Gastroenterology 120:726–748, 2001.
6. Gill RQ, Sterling RK: Acute liver failure. J Clin Gastroenterol 33(3):191–198, 2001.
7. Keeffe EB: Liver transplantation: Current status and novel approaches to liver replacement. Gastroenterology 120:749–762, 2001.
8. Lauer GM, Walker BD: Hepatitis C virus infection. N Engl J Med 345:41–52, 2001.
9. Lok AS, Heathcote EJ, Hoofnagle JH: Management of hepatitis B: 2000. Summary of a workshop. Gastroenterology 120:1828–1853, 2001.
10. Rahman T, Hodgson H: Clinical management of acute hepatic failure. Intens Care Med 27:467–476, 2001.
11. Walsh K, Alexander GJ: Update on chronic viral hepatitis. Postgrad Med J 77:498–505, 2001.

51. PERITONITIS

James P. Bonar, M.D., and Mark W. Bowyer, M.D.

1. What is the peritoneum?

The peritoneum is a highly evolved and specialized organ that functions to maintain the surface integrity of the intra-abdominal structures and to provide a smooth lubricated surface so that the intestines can move freely. The peritoneum is a serous membrane that, if flattened out, would cover an area of 1.7–2.2 square meters. It is composed of a monocellular layer of flattened mesothelial cells that rests on a thin layer of fibroelastic tissue.

2. What is the difference between the parietal and the visceral peritoneum?

The parietal peritoneum is the portion of the peritoneum that lines all of the abdominal cavity, covering the abdominal wall, diaphragm, and pelvis. The visceral peritoneum is the portion of the peritoneum that covers all the intra-abdominal viscera and mesenteries and is identical with the visceral serosa.

3. What features are unique to the peritoneum overlying the diaphragm?

The peritoneum overlying the diaphragm is interrupted by intracellular gaps called stomata, which serve as entrances into diaphragmatic lymphatic channels called lacunae. The lacunae ultimately drain into the substernal lymph nodes and then into the thoracic duct. In contrast to the nondiaphragmatic peritoneal surface, which behaves as a passive, semipermeable membrane allowing bidirectional exchange of water and electrolytes, the diaphragmatic stomata are capable of absorbing particulate matter, including bacteria.

4. Describe the mechanism by which contaminated peritoneal fluid is generally disseminated throughout the abdominal cavity.

The peritoneal fluid, contained within the peritoneal cavity, moves systematically toward the diaphragm as a function of the negative pressure beneath the diaphragm with each exhaled breath. The fluid is then cleared via the many lymphatic fenestrations on the diaphragmatic surface. Thus, the peritoneal cavity is in essence an enormous lymphocele that has direct contact with the lymphatic system via the thoracic duct.

5. How does the peritoneum normally deal with infection?

The peritoneum normally deals with an infection in three ways: (1) by direct absorption of bacteria into the lymphatic system via the stomata of the diaphragmatic peritoneum; (2) by local destruction of bacteria through phagocytosis by either resident macrophages or polymorphonuclear granulocytes attracted to the peritoneal cavity; and (3) by localization of the infection in the form of an abscess.

6. What is peritonitis?

The term *peritonitis* refers to a generalized or local inflammation of the mesenchymal cells lining the peritoneal cavity. Peritonitis has distinct phases, including contamination, dissemination, inflammation, and resolution or loculation. Inflammation may be initiated by a variety of etiologic insults with a resultant cascade of events that includes transudation of fluid, edema formation, and vascular congestion of the tissue layer immediately adjacent to the mesothelium. Classically peritonitis is a life-threatening process caused by visceral disruption that results from an intrinsic pathologic condition or external trauma.

7. Describe the clinical manifestations of classic peritonitis.

Abdominal tenderness is the hallmark of peritonitis; in fully developed cases, the tenderness is steady, unrelenting, and burning. Patients with generalized peritonitis suffer from diffuse tenderness and appear quite ill early in their clinical course. Typically they lie quietly, supine, and with knees flexed; breathing is shallow because any motion intensifies the abdominal pain. Voluntary guarding produces rigidity of the abdominal muscles, followed by spasm as the parietal peritoneum becomes inflamed. As the peritonitis advances, the reflex spasm may become so severe that boardlike abdominal rigidity is produced. Anorexia is common and frequently accompanied by nausea and vomiting. Patients often complain of chills and fever. Temperature elevation of a spiking nature is common; more ominously, hypothermia can be present. Tachycardia and diminished pulse pressure reflect early hypovolemia, and hypovolemic shock may occur rapidly as the peritonitis progresses. Increased tissue demands for oxygen and acidosis lead to tachypnea, which is characteristically shallow because deep respirations intensify the abdominal pain.

8. What is primary peritonitis?

Primary peritonitis is a diffuse microbiologic infection of the peritoneal cavity that occurs in the absence of a disruption of the gastrointestinal tract. Generally it is a consequence of peritoneal contamination from a remote source and without evidence of an intra-abdominal process. The peritonitis begins when microorganisms embed within the peritoneal cavity via hematogenous or lymphatic spread. Before the widespread use of antibiotics, primary peritonitis occurred most commonly in the pediatric population and was caused by *Streptococcus pneumoniae*. In adults, alcoholic cirrhosis and ascites are currently the most common underlying factors and represent a significant risk for morbidity and mortality. The ascites predisposes cirrhotic patients to infection because low complement and total protein levels impair bacterial opsonization. The pathogenesis also appears to include translocation of bacteria from the gut to mesenteric lymph nodes. Depressed reticuloendothelial phagocytic activity and deficient antibacterial activity in the ascitic fluid lead to infection.

9. What organisms are commonly associated with primary peritonitis?

In patients with cirrhosis, infections are often monomicrobial, with a predominance of enteric organisms, particularly *Escherichia coli*. Anaerobic organisms are uncommon, and polymicrobial infections occur in less than 10% of cases. In children, gram-positive organisms such as *S. pneumoniae* and group A streptococci prevail. Opportunistic organisms, including cytomegalovirus and *Mycobacterium tuberculosis*, are often found in immunocompromised patients.

10. How is spontaneous bacterial peritonitis (SBP) diagnosed?

The onset of clinical symptoms may be insidious, but jaundice, fever, encephalopathy, and abdominal pain or tenderness have a high prevalence. In contrast, about one-third or more of patients with SBP have no signs or symptoms directly referable to the abdomen. In such cases, deterioration of liver function, such as increasing encephalopathy, ascites, or jaundice, must lead to a suspicion of infection. In addition, temporary resistance to diuretics may be a sign of SBP. In the laboratory, the key to the diagnosis of SBP is examination of the ascitic fluid from a diagnostic paracentesis. The fluid should be examined for pH, lactate, glucose, protein, lactate dehydrogenase, and cell count with differential. Gram stain and cultures are also essential. An accurate method of culturing ascitic fluid is to place 10–20 ml into both aerobic and anaerobic blood culture bottles at the bedside to improve the sensitivity of the test. Overall, the best single predictor of infection is the absolute polymorphonuclear leukocyte (PMN) count. A PMN count > 500/mm^3 is highly suggestive of SBP; the patient should be treated as if it represented SBP, pending culture results. If the PMN count is > 1,000/mm^3, treatment for SBP should be continued regardless of culture results. A number of studies have concluded that the combination of an elevated PMN count (> 250/mm^3), a low pH (< 7.35), and an elevated lactate level (> 32 mg/dl) is highly predictive of SBP. In summary, the clinical spectrum of SBP ranges from a silent subclinical state to a severe and rapidly fatal illness.

11. How is SBP treated?

Empirical antimicrobial agents must be selected before culture results are available. Gram stain of the centrifuged ascites is the most useful test to guide the initial selection of an antimicrobial regimen. If the Gram stain is unrevealing or no organism is obvious, empirical treatment should cover a broad spectrum of pathogens. A literature review of 15 series involving 253 patients with SBP revealed that gram-negative bacilli caused 69% of cases. Of the gram-negative bacilli, *E. coli* was the most common (68%), followed by *Klebsiella* species (16%); smaller numbers of patients were infected with *Proteus, Pseudomonas*, and *Serratia* species. Gram-positive organisms were found in 30% of the cases, with *Streptococcus* species accounting for 86%. Anaerobes, including *Bacteroides* and *Clostridium* species, accounted for 5% of the pathogens. Based on these findings, the suggested initial empirical treatment is cefotaxime, 2.0 gm every 8 hours intravenously. Alternatively, ticarcillin/clavulanate, piperacillin/tazobactam, and ampicillin/sulbactam are also effective. Empirical therapy directed against anaerobes, *Pseudomonas* sp., and *Staphylococcus* sp. is not indicated unless these pathogens are suspected on clinical grounds or by Gram stain. In a randomized trial, five days of therapy was equivalent to 10 days in terms of mortality, cure rate, and recurrence. If the blood cultures are positive, a full 2 weeks of antimicrobial therapy is suggested. Antimicrobial therapy should be adjusted when results of culture and sensitivity testing become available.

12. What is secondary peritonitis?

Secondary bacterial peritonitis (classic peritonitis) is defined as a peritoneal infection that begins with perforation of a hollow viscus or transmural necrosis of the gastrointestinal tract, with subsequent contamination of the peritoneal cavity. It commonly occurs with trauma or other inflammatory processes, such as perforated appendicitis, perforated duodenal ulcer, or perforated sigmoid colon due to diverticulitis. Neoplastic processes also can cause gastrointestinal tract disruption through direct erosion or obstruction. Other entities that may lead to leakage of intestinal contents include volvulus, bowel obstructions due to adhesions, and postoperative anastomotic disruptions.

The diagnosis is usually made on clinical grounds, with the classic finding of abdominal pain associated with peritoneal signs, such as tenderness, guarding, and increased abdominal wall tone. Most patients look ill and have temperatures higher than 38°C (100.4° F). In cases of septic shock, however, the patient may be hypothermic. Radiographs may show free air under the diaphragm, suggesting perforation, or distended loops of bowel consistent with evidence of ileus. In patients in whom a history and physical exam may not be reliable (e.g., head-injured patients, paraplegics, elderly patients, or patients taking steroids), diagnostic peritoneal lavage (DPL) may be a useful method of determining the presence of peritonitis requiring surgery.

13. Which laboratory tests are helpful in diagnosing secondary peritonitis?

Leukocytosis greater than 11,000 cells/mm^3 with a left shift supports the clinical diagnosis of peritonitis. In contrast, leukopenia may be seen in the presence of overwhelming sepsis. DPL also may be used to determine the presence of peritonitis. The procedure is performed by instilling 1 L of warmed saline into the abdomen, followed by removal. The presence of > 500 white blood cells/mm^3 in the lavage fluid highly suggests the presence of intra-abdominal pathology. In addition, the finding of bile, pus, cloudy fluid, or a positive Gram stain is a clear indication for laparotomy. However, if the intra-abdominal pathology is well localized or if the patient is unable to mount a response, the lavage may produce a false-negative result.

14. How does Gram stain of peritoneal fluid help determine the cause of peritonitis?

Gram-positive cocci suggest the likelihood of SBP. Gram-negative rods suggest either primary or secondary peritonitis. Mixed flora suggest the likelihood of bowel perforation (secondary peritonitis).

15. Discuss the role of laparoscopy in secondary peritonitis.

Laparoscopy has become an important diagnostic tool, providing definitive diagnosis in over 90% of patients with peritonitis. Therapeutic strategies may change in upward of 10% of patients with preoperative diagnostic laparoscopy. The most common indication for laparoscopy is in young women with pelvic or right-sided abdominal pain. In this instance, the diagnosis of acute appendicitis vs. tubo-ovarian process can be made correctly. Peritonitis due to perforated peptic ulcers also has been diagnosed and repaired with the use of laparoscopy.

16. How does the level of perforation of the gastrointestinal tract affect the treatment of peritonitis?

Organisms responsible for peritonitis vary significantly depending on the level of perforation. Perforation of the upper gastrointestinal tract usually releases predominantly gram-positive organisms, whereas perforation of the distal small bowel or colon releases a mixture of aerobic (*E. coli, Proteus* sp., *Klebsiella* sp., and various streptococci and enterococci) and anaerobic bacteria (*Bacteroides fragilis*, peptococci, and peptostreptococci). Of interest, patients who have taken antacids or H_2 blockers often have a greater number of facultative gram-negative bacilli in their stomachs before perforation.

17. How should secondary peritonitis be managed?

The treatment of secondary peritonitis is primarily operative. The goals are to eliminate the source of contamination, to reduce the bacterial inoculum, and to prevent recurrent or persistent sepsis. Important aspects of perioperative care are fluid resuscitation and appropriate antibiotic therapy; all patients with peritonitis have some degree of hypovolemia. Infections in the peritoneal cavity are almost always polymicrobial and contain a mixture of aerobic and anaerobic organisms. The synergism of aerobic and anaerobic organisms is a major contributing factor to the pyogenic nature of intra-abdominal infections. Therefore, antibiotic treatment should be directed against both both aerobic and anaerobic bacteria, particularly gram-negative enteric bacteria (*E. coli*) and *B. fragilis*. Combination therapy with an aminoglycoside and an antianaerobic agent is a good choice; concerns with the use of aminoglycosides, however, include drug toxicity and attainment of adequate therapeutic levels. Suitable alternatives to aminoglycoside-based regimens include a third-generation cephalosporin and an antianaerobic agent or the combination of aztreonam and clindaymcin. In the intensive care unit, where resistant organisms may pose a problem, the empirical use of broad-spectrum antimicrobials (e.g., piperacillin-tazobactam, carbapenems, or a combination with aztreonam or a third-generation cephalosporin) is warranted. In addition, the combination of metronidazole and the quinolone ciprofloxacin was shown to have equivalent outcomes compared with monotherapy with imipenem-cilastatin in the treatment of secondary peritonitis.

18. What is tertiary peritonitis?

Patients who have prolonged hospital stays, often with multiple abdominal procedures, and who are unable to localize intra-abdominal infection because of either impaired host defenses or overwhelming infection may progress to persistent diffuse (tertiary) peritonitis. The clinical picture is occult sepsis without a well-defined focus of infection. In contrast to secondary peritonitis, tertiary peritonitis is associated with microbial flora such as *Staphylococcus. epidermidis*, *Pseudomonas aeruginosa, Candida* species, and enterococci rather than the common *E. coli* and *B. fragilis*. Despite aggressive management, progressive multisystem organ failure frequently develops; mortality rates > 60% have been reported.

19. Describe one technique that can facilitate management of tertiary peritonitis in critically ill septic patients.

In the open abdominal technique, propylene mesh is secured to the skin or abdominal fascia, and a zipper is fastened to the mesh. The peritoneal cavity is irrigated daily in the intensive care setting. The abdomen is temporarily closed with the zipper between irrigations.

20. What are the characteristics of an intraperitoneal abscess?

Intraperitoneal abscesses arise during resolution of generalized peritonitis and most commonly occur in the pelvis or subphrenic areas. These locations are a reflection of the anatomy of the peritoneum, which permits gravity-dependent flow of infected material into dependent cavities. Early symptoms may be vague but commonly include paralytic ileus, anorexia, abdominal distention, recurrent or persistent fever, chills, abdominal pain, and tachycardia. CT scanning and ultrasound have a diagnostic accuracy greater than 90%. Radionucleotide scans may be useful but have much lower specificity.

21. How should intraperitoneal abscesses be treated?

The three basic principles of management include (1) drainage of the abscess, (2) use of parenteral antibiotics, and (3) general care of patient status (i.e., correction of nutritional or metabolic derangements). Percutaneous drainage is the treatment of choice for most intra-abdominal abscesses and is successful in more than 85% of cases. Failure of percutaneous drainage requires open surgical drainage.

BIBLIOGRAPHY

1. Christou NV, Turgoun P, Wassef R, et al: Management of intra-abdominal infection: The case for intraoperative cultures and comprehensive broad-spectrum antibiotic coverage. Arch Surg 131:1193–1201, 1996.
2. Dalmau D, Layragues GP, Fenyves D, et al: Cefotaxime, desacetyl-cefotaxime, and bactericidal activity in spontaneous bacterial peritonitis. J Infect Dis 180:1597, 1999.
3. Farber MS, Abrams JH: Antibiotics for the acute abdomen. Surg Clin North Am 77:1395, 1997.
4. Fry DE: Prevention, diagnosis and management of infection. In Mattox KL, Feliciano DV, Moore EE (eds): Trauma, 4th ed. New York, McGraw-Hill, 2000, pp 349–372.
5. Maddaus MA, Ahrenholz D, Simmons RL: The biology of peritonitis and implications for treatment. Surg Clin North Am 68:431–443, 1988.
6. Navez B, d'Udekem Y, Cambier E, et al: Laparoscopy for management of nontraumatic acute abdomen. World J Surg 19:382, 1995.
7. Robertson GS, Wemyss-Holden SA, Maddern GJ: Laparoscopic repair of perforated peptic ulcers: The role of laparoscopy in generalized peritonitis. Ann R Coll Surg Engl 82:6, 2000.
8. Sawyer RG, Rosenlof LK, Adams RB, et al: Peritonitis in the 1990s: Changing pathogens and changing strategies in the critically ill patient. Am Surg 58:82, 1992.
9. Topley N, Liberek T, Davenport A, et al: Activation of inflammation and leukocyte recruitment into the peritoneal cavity. Kidney Int Suppl 56:S17–21, 1996.
10. Yang C-Y, Liaw Y-F, Chue C-M, et al: White count, pH, and lactate in ascites in the diagnosis of spontaenous bacterial peritonitis. Hepatology 5:85, 1985.
11. Yarze JC, Fritz HP, Herlihy KJ: Antibiotic prophylaxis for spontaneous bacterial peritonitis. Am J Gastroenterol 92:180, 1997.

VIII. Endocrinology

52. DIABETIC KETOACIDOSIS

Martina Schulte, M.D., and Philip S. Mehler, M.D.

1. What is diabetic ketoacidosis (DKA)?

DKA is an extremely serious metabolic complication of diabetes mellitus due to a state of relative or absolute insulin deficiency and a relative or absolute increase in counterregulatory hormones. It is characterized by the triad of acidosis, ketosis, and hyperglycemia.

2. Describe the pathophysiologic basis of DKA.

Insulin deficiency is the focal point of this disorder and causes both hyperglycemia and hyperketonemia. Under normal states, insulin ensures the storage of glucose as glucagon in the liver and free fatty acids as triglycerides in adipose tissue. With a deficiency of insulin, there are both increased hepatic glucose production through increased glycogenolysis and gluconeogenesis and decreased glucose utilization. The result is hyperglycemia.

The hyperketonemia is similarly due to a state of insulin deficiency. As a result of the depressed insulin level and the concomitantly elevated levels of catecholamines and other counterregulatory hormones, there is excessive production of free fatty acids from the breakdown of triglycerides. Free fatty acids are converted to ketone bodies in the liver. In addition, decreased ketone utilization contributes to the ketonemia.

3. Is DKA a complication of type 1 diabetes mellitus only?

Although DKA is generally considered a consequence of insulin deficiency that reflects the irreversible beta-cell damage seen in type 1 diabetes mellitus, studies have shown that DKA occurs in patients with type 2 diabetes mellitus as well. One study followed 21 adults who presented with DKA but had a subsequent course consistent with type 2 diabetes. The patients demonstrated insulin resistance in the presence of good glycemic control and had normal C-peptide levels. Another study looking at the occurrence of DKA in type 2 and newly diagnosed diabetic patients found that 26% of the patients with DKA had a history of type 2 diabetes. In addition, at 2 months after the DKA episode, 24% of the newly diagnosed and 8% of the patients with a history of type 2 diabetes were no longer taking insulin.

4. How is DKA diagnosed?

The combination of hyperglycemia, metabolic anion gap, and glycosuria with elevated blood ketones confirms the diagnsis of DKA. DKA is generally suspected from the history, especially in a known diabetic who presents with an acute illnes or a history of missed medications. Laboratory findings (see questions 7 and 8) can quickly confirm suspicion based on the history.

5. What are the common signs and symptoms of DKA?

Hyperglycemia is manifested by polyuria, polydipsia, polyphagia, lassitude, weight loss, and visual difficulties. The mental status ranges from lethargy to deep coma; 20% of patients present in a stuporous state. Nausea, vomiting, and abdominal pain, which are not usually due to definite intra-abdominal pathology, frequently complicate the early course of DKA. Acidosis is also responsible for one of the classic signs of DKA: Kussmaul breaths, which are long, deep, and sighing respirations made in an attempt to compensate for the metabolic acidosis by lowering arterial PCO_2. An odor of decaying apples or "Juicy Fruit" gum on the patient's breath, another positive sign of DKA, is due to acetone; the other ketoacids are odorless. In addition to hyperglycemia and hyperketonemia, there are other fluid and electrolyte disturbances. These are predominantly a result of hyperglycemia, which in turn causes glucosuria and, subsequently, osmotic diuresis with loss of electrolytes and concomitant volume depletion. In the average 70-kg man with established DKA, there is a 3–5 liter saline deficiency, a 300–500 mEq sodium deficiency, and a 150–250 mEq potassium deficiency. Further, the patient with DKA is often hypothermic because of the unavailability of substrate to generate heat.

6. What is the significance of abdominal pain in DKA?

Abdominal pain is commonly found in DKA. The definite cause is unknown, but gastric distention and stretching of the liver capsule have been offered as possible explanations for the pain, which is present approximately 20% of the time. Generally, the pain resolves promptly with treatment for DKA, but at the time of the initial evaluation, signs and symptoms indicative of an intraabdominal process should be pursued. Further, if abdominal signs and symptoms persist in spite of adequate treatment, one most definitely should consider underlying intraabdominal processes. This is especially true in patients over the age of 40 with DKA, since abdominal pain is likely to have an underlying cause in this group, such as pyelonephritis or appendicitis. Unexplained abdominal pain is more common in younger patients with severe DKA. The serum amylase is elevated approximately 75% of the time in DKA, but the cause is unknown. It is not specific for pancreatitis.

7. What are the usual laboratory findings in DKA?

DKA is characterized by hyperglycemia, acidemia of the increased anion gap type, bicarbonate level less than 15 mEq/L, and ketonemia, with positive values defined as greater than a 1:2 dilution. Hyperglycemia need not be impressive. Fifteen percent of patients with DKA have a glucose level less than 300 mg/dl. Also, although the majority of patients with DKA have an anion gap metabolic acidosis, there is a spectrum of different types of metabolic acidosis, ranging from purely anion gap to the nongap hyperchloremic type. The factor that determines which type of acidosis is present is linked with the patient's volume status on admission to the hospital. In addition, patients can present with a mixed acid-base problem, including coexistent metabolic acidosis, metabolic alkalosis, and respiratory alkalosis. An example of a mixed picture is the patients who presents with DKA and concomitant vomiting that produces volume contraction, along with severe abdominal pain and resultant hyperventilation.

8. What other laboratory abnormalities may be seen in DKA?

Hyponatremia is seen in more than half of patients with DKA. Usually it is in the form of pseudohyponatremia, which does not mean that the low-sodium concentration is incorrect. Nor does it necessarily indicate that there is low-serum osmolality, since hyperglycemia is also present. The usual correction fraction for this is that for each 100 mg/dl increase in the glucose level, the sodium concentration decreases by 1.6 mEq/L. Hypertriglyceridemia can also cause this phenomenon.

Potassium levels are also frequently abnormal. They can be either elevated or depressed, but in all patients total-body potassium is depleted. However, because of the transcellular shifts of potassium seen with insulin deficiency and acidosis, the initial potassium value can vary. Of substantial importance is the fact that during the course of therapy, the serum potassium level drops precipitously because of insulin therapy, correction of the acidosis, and increased urine output with intravenous fluid repletion. Thus, an initially "normal" serum potassium needs to be closely followed and repleted soon thereafter while treatment of the DKA ensues. A low potassium level on admission is an important finding, and potassium should be added to the first liter of fluids.

Lastly, as is the case with potassium, most patients with DKA are hyperphosphatemic on presentation to the hospital due to the effects of metabolic acidosis. In most patients, however, total-body phosphorus is depleted. This depletion is exacerbated by phosphorus moving into cells with treatment of the DKA. In DKA, the nadir is reached 2–3 days after admission to the hospital. However, in controlled studies, routine replacement has not been shown to be of benefit unless hypophosphatemia has been documented

9. Is the determination of serum ketone levels helpful in the treatment of patients with DKA?

Serum ketones should be determined once, at the outset, in any patients in whom DKA is suspected. In general, significant ketonemia is not present unless the serum ketones are positive at a dilution of 1:2 or greater. There are three blood ketones: betahydroxybutyrate, acetoacetate, and acetone. In DKA, the ratio of betahydroxybutyrate to acetoacetate is only mildly elevated. However, in some cases of DKA, the great majority of the ketones may exist as betahydroxy-butyrate, which is not picked up by the qualitative ketone measurements that detect only aceto-acetate. Thus, plasma ketones may be "falsely" low or negative. In fact, during successful therapy of DKA, these serum ketones may paradoxically rise or fail to fall, which is a result of the conversion of betahydroxybutyrate (not measured) to acetoacetate (measured) prior to its utilization. Serial ketone levels therefore can be misleading and are not recommended aside from the initial documentation of positivity.

10. How is DKA treated?

To avoid potential complications, meticulous attention to detail is essential. Insulin, fluids, and potassium supplementation are the cornerstones of therapy. The end point of insulin therapy is correction of acidemia and hyperglycemia. Unless insulin resistance is severe, rarely does the patient require insulin doses in excess of 5–10 u/hr. Until the mid-1970s, larger doses of insulin—40–100 u/hr—were used; currently, low-dose insulin therapy is the standard.

After rapid intravenous infusion of 5–10 u of regular insulin, begin an insulin drip at 2–4 u/hr, and measure the plasma glucose concentration 1 hour after staring the insulin infusion and at 1- to 2-hour intervals thereafter. If the glucose concentration is falling at a predictable rate of 75 mg/dl/hr, continue the drip at that rate. If the glucose concentration is unchanged or decreases only slightly, the patient is insulin-resistant, and infusion should be increased to 5–10 u/hr after another intravenous push of 5–10 u. Do not discontinue the insulin infusion if "hypoglycemia" (blood sugar less than 250 mg/dl) develops.

When this glucose level is reached, switch the intravenous fluids to ones containing glucose, and continue the infusion at the previous rate. Remember that it takes longer to clear the ketoacidosis (10–20 hours) than it does to correct the hypoglycemia (4–8 hours). Also, most diabetologists agree that at least the first 2–3 liters of fluids of should be in the form of isotonic saline to correct hypovolemia. Once this has been infused, hemodynamic considerations and attention to the serum sodium concentration should guide the choice of additional fluids.

11. Given that it may be misleading to follow serial ketone measurements during treatment of DKA, what is the best indicator of resolution of DKA?

The most reliable indicator of DKA resolution is the anion gap. Glucose corrects simply as a consequence of fluid repletion and thus cannot be relied on. Urinary ketones tend to remain detectable long after resolution of DKA. Therefore, they are also not good predictors of successful treatment. However, when the anion gap returns to normal, ketoacid production has ceased. Once the electrolytes demonstrate a normal anion gap, continue the insulin infusion for a few more hours to ensure that control has been achieved. After that, if the patient can eat, the patient's previous insulin regimen can be resinstituted (if known and if satisfactory), and the insulin infusion can be discontinued.

12. Why do most patients develop a hyperchloremic nongap acidosis after therapy for DKA?

Although several factors probably account for this finding, the most dominant factor is that renal threshold for ketones is quite low. Therefore, with volume expansion, excretion of ketones in the urine is increased. These excreted ketones are "bicarbonate equivalents," which limit the availability of substrate to regenerate bicarbonate. Approximately 75% of patients recovering from DKA develop a hyperchloremic metabolic acidosis, which resolves over 48–72 hours. Development of the hyperchloremic metabolic acidosis does not indicate that the insulin infusion has failed. For this reason, normalization of the gap rather than bicarbonate level is the key indicator for resolution of DKA.

13. What are the most common precipitants for development of DKA?

In most series, noncompliance with medication and infection are the most common precipitating events. Often no definable cause is found. Leukocytosis by itself is not a sensitive or specific indicator of infection in DKA because leukocyte counts in the 20,000 range are commonly seen in DKA due to stress and hemoconcentration. Recently, it has been shown that an elevated band count (10% or greater) is a sensitive and significant indicator of occult coexisting infection. Total leukocyte count, blood glucose, serum bicarbonate levels, and temperature have little value in predicting covert infection.

14. What are the major complications in DKA?

The mortality rate in DKA is in the range of 5–10%. Diabetics rarely die of ketoacidosis itself. Normally, death is attributable to associated medical conditions. Hypothermia and coma are negative prognostic signs. A few complications are potentially associated with the therapy of DKA. The major ones are hypoglycemia, hypokalemia, hypophosphatemia, and cerebral edema. With regard to the latter, if sudden coma develops 12–24 hours after starting therapy, particularly in a younger patient, increased intracranial pressure should be suspected. Most cases of cerebral edema occur in patients whose blood sugar is rapidly reduced ≤ 250 mg/dl. Multiple theories have been advanced to explain this phenomenon; the most plausible one involves unfavorable osmotic gradients that develop during therapy.

CONTROVERSY

15. What is the role of bicarbonate therapy in the treatment of DKA?

There is lack of complete agreement regarding the use of bicarbonate therapy in the treatment of DKA. Those in favor point to the deleterious side effects that acidosis causes on multiple organ systems, especially the effect on cardiac contractility and tissue perfusion. Arguments against the use of bicarbonate therapy are the potential for overshoot alkalosis, the development of paradoxical CNS acidosis, and the delayed improvement in ketosis.

Concern about the use of bicarbonate is its effect on a feedback control of endogenous acid production that is seen when increased ketoacid production reduces systemic pH and this, in turn, inhibits the rate of acid production. A small study in Japan looked at the rate of ketosis improvement in patients receiving bicarbonate as part of therapy for DKA and compared the results with control patients not receiving the alkali. The group receiving sodium bicarbonate had a 6-hour delay in the improvement of ketosis versus the control group. They also showed an increase in acetoacetate levels during alkali administration and an increase in 3-hydroxybutyrate after the alkali infusion completion. This study gives further credence to the argument against bicarbonate therapy, as it appears to have a negative effect on the metabolism and plasma levels of ketones.

The above studies make many clinicians believe that bicarbonate should not be used in DKA, at least not in patients with pH > 6.9. Some clinicians, however, argue that when the serum bicarbonate level is < 5 mEq/L, bicarbonate should be administered. Their argument is predicated on the fact that although more than 90% of ketoacidotic patients treated with only saline and insulin recover, a small fraction of patients dying from ketosis do so because of the deleterious hemodynamic effects of acidemia. These effects include myocardial dysfunction, arrhythmias, and antagonism of the effects of pressor-type compounds.

Ultimately, each case of DKA must be evaluated on an individual basis in terms of the use of bicarbonate. A prudent approach may be to use small quantities of bicarbonate therapy if respiratory compensation is at its limit and serum bicarbonate is of the order of 5 mE/q/L or less. In this scenario, any further diminution of the bicarbonate concentration would be associated with a severe decline in serum pH.

BIBLIOGRAPHY

1. Androgue HJ, Madias NE: Management of life-threatening acid-base disorders. N Engl J Med 338:26–34, 1998.
2. Androgue HJ, Wilson H, Boyd AE: Plasma acid base patterns in diabetic ketoacidosis. N Engl J Med 307:1603–1610, 1982.
3. Balasurbramanyam MD, Zern JW, Hyman DJ, Parlik V: New profiles of diabetic ketoacidosis. Arch Intern Med 159:669–675, 1997.
4. Fisher JN, Kitabchi AE: A randomized study of phosphate therapy in the treatment of DKA. J Clin Endocrinol Metab 57:177–180, 1983.
5. Israel RS: Diabetic ketoacidosis. Emerg Med Clin North Am 7:859–871, 1989.
6. Kitabehl AE, Murphy MB: Diabetic ketoacidosis and hyperosmolar hyperglycemic nonketotic coma coma. Med Clin North Am 72:1545–1563, 1988.
7. Musey VC, Lee JK, Crawford R, et al: Diabetes in urban African-Americans: Cessation of insulin is the major precipitating cause of diabetic ketoacidosis. Diabetes Care 18:483–489, 1995.
8. Okuda Y, Androgue HJ, Field JB, et al: Counterproductive effects of sodium bicarbonate in diabetic ketoacidosis. J Clin Endocrinol Metab 81:314–320, 1996.
9. Slovis CM, Mork EG, Bain RP: Diabetic ketoacidosis and infection. Am J Emerg Med 5:1–5, 1987.
10. Umpierrez GE, Kelly JP, Navarette SE, et al: Hyperglycemic crises in urban blacks. Arch Intern Med 157:669–675, 1997.

53. HYPEROSMOLAR NONKETOTIC COMA

Mary Chri Gray, M.D., and Philip S. Mehler, M.D.

1. What is hyperosmolar nonketotic coma (HNC)?

HNC is classically defined as plasma osmolarity > 350 mOsm/L, plasma glucose > 600 mg/dl, and lack of ketoacidosis in a diabetic patient with an altered level of consciousness. HNC is somewhat of a misnomer, because very few patients present with actual coma. Other names include hyperglycemic hyperosmolar syndrome (HHS) and nonketotic hypertonicity (NKH). Almost one-half of patients have a small increase in anion gap and mild metabolic acidosis. In one review of over 600 patients, approximately one-third had overlapping symptoms of diabetic ketoacidosis and hyperosmolar coma. The hallmark of this syndrome is hypertonicity with an increased effective osmolarity, calculated as $2 \times (Na^+ + K^+) + glucose/18$. Blood urea nitrogen (BUN) is not included because it is freely permeable across the cell membranes and does not contribute to an osmotic gradient, which results in flow of water from the intracellular to extracellular space.

2. Why do some diabetics present with diabetic ketoacidosis (DKA) and others with HNC?

The actual mechanism may be multifactorial. It had been thought that patients with HNC have enough endogenous insulin to suppress the release of free fatty acids but not enough to facilitate glucose transport and metabolism. However, it has been shown that insulin levels in DKA and HNC are similar, but the insulin counterregulatory hormones are increased to a lesser degree in HNC than in DKA.Glucagon, one of these hormones, is a potent force for the availability of free fatty acids and thus the development of ketone bodies with subsequent metabolic acidosis. This relative difference in glucagon may account for the difference in acidosis between the two syndromes. Another contributing factor is that hyperosmolarity decreases lipolysis with a resultant decrease in the availability of free fatty acids.

3. How does the presentation of HNC differ from that of DKA?

There are differences in the age of the patient, prior diagnosis of diabetes, duration of symptoms, extent of volume depletion, degree of hyperglycemia, and degree of acidosis. Patients with HNC are generally older with reported mean ages between 57 and 69 years. Up to two-thirds of patients with HNC have no previous diagnosis of diabetes. Patients with HNC have a more prolonged and insidious onset than those with DKA. The ketonemia and severe acidosis of DKA result in a more acute presentation. The prolonged prehospital phase with its ongoing osmotic diuresis results in a greater degree of volume loss and of hyperglycemia and hyperosmolarity than in DKA. In patients with HNC, significant changes in mental status are more common. The degree of mental stupor correlates with hyperosmolarity—not with acidosis. Finally, as stated above, the degree of acidosis is mild in HNC and cannot always be related to ketoanions.

4. Describe basic pathophysiology of HNC.

The central causative mechanism involves a hyperglycemia-induced osmotic diuresis and resultant dehydration. The hyperglycemia emanates from a commonly identified diabetogenic stressor, such as infection, which precipitates the onset of the syndrome. Hyperglycemic desensitization of the beta cells exhausts insulin reserves, and a state of peripheral resistance to the effects of insulin is induced. The resultant severe hyperglycemia, with average levels > 600 mg/dl, causes glycosuric diuresis, which, in turn, results in hypertonicity and dehydration. Although a substantial amount of sodium is lost through the kidney because of osmotic diuresis, the water loss is greater relative to the extracellular fluid. In this state of relatively low effective insulin, the glucose is primarily in the extracellular fluid, where it is osmotically active. The concentrations of intracellular and extracellular osmolarity are equalized. Such intracellular dehydration may be a prominent factor in producing central nervous system dysfunction. In response to this water shift, the serum sodium concentration falls by 1.6 mEq/L for every 100-mg rise in the serum glucose and produces the pseudohyponatremia commonly associated with hyperglycemia.

Additional pathophysiologic aberrations also are involved. The decrement in intravascular volume impairs renal function and causes the glomerular filtration rate (GFR) to fall. As this occurs, plasma glucose continues to rise. In addition, a problem with the thirst mechanism is seen in many patients with HNC. It is not mere coincidence that this syndrome is largely restricted to the infirm and neglected institutionalized patient who cannot recognize or respond to the need for water. Thus, the massive osmotic diuresis and its associated changes progress unabated until a change in mental status brings the patient to medical attention.

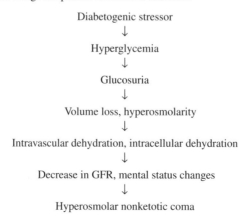

Diabetogenic stressor
↓
Hyperglycemia
↓
Glucosuria
↓
Volume loss, hyperosmolarity
↓
Intravascular dehydration, intracellular dehydration
↓
Decrease in GFR, mental status changes
↓
Hyperosmolar nonketotic coma

5. What are the main precipitants of HNC?

In contrast to DKA, in which a definable cause is often lacking, approximately one-half of patients with HNC have an associated illness that precipitated the syndrome. Infection, myocardial infarction, pancreatitis, gastrointestinal bleeding, hyperalimentation, and medications (e.g., thiazide diuretics, steroids, phenytoin) are the most frequently noted culprits. Presumably these stressors cause beta cell insufficiency in concert with peripheral insulin resistance and promote the development of profound hyperglycemia.

6. Describe the common clinical manifestations.

The history is characterized by insidious onset. Symptoms are often present for days to weeks before arrival at the hospital. The history is usually notable for complaints of progressive weakness, malaise, and perhaps hints of some possible precipitating events. There may be complaints of newly onset urinary incontinence secondary to the marked polyuria from the osmotic diuresis. Physical examination reveals substantial evidence of dehydration with tachycardia, hypotension, cool skin temperature, and decreased skin turgor. In contrast to DKA, there is usually no hypothermia. A depressed cognitive state ranging from profound stupor to mild clouding of the sensorium is present. In addition, focal neurologic abnormalities may be noted. With prompt and proper treatment, all of the neurologic abnormalities dissipate.

7. What laboratory findings are associated with HNC?

The average serum sodium is 140 mEq/L, despite the profound hyperglycemia, with a wide range of 119–188 mEq/L. In contrast to patients with DKA, initial hyperkalemia is distinctly uncommon. Given the osmotic diuresis, however, most patients have potassium depletion due to urinary potassium losses. The serum bicarbonate level is usually mildly depressed to a level of 17–19 mEq/L with a small increase in the anion gap that is somewhat difficult to explain. At one time, lactic acid was thought to be the cause; however, the more probable cause is accumulation of organic acids that remain undefined. Serum glucose usually exceeds 600 mg/dl, with values commonly in the 1,000 mg/dl range, and serum osmolality is > 320 mOsm/L. The serum osmolarity is calculated as follows:

$$2 \times (Na + K) + glucose/18 + BUN/2.8$$
$$(normal = 280–295 \text{ mOsm/L})$$

As stated above, the effective serum osmolarity does not include the BUN because it does not contribute to an osmotic gradient between intra- and extracellular spaces. Leukocytosis with a white blood cell count of 15,000–20,000 is frequently found, usually due to the effects of dehydration. Similarly, hemoconcentration results in a hematocrit in the range of 55–60%.

8. How is HNC treated?

The major aims of therapy for HNC are to reduce the hyperosmolarity, restore intravascular volume, and vigorously identify and treat any precipitating illness. Despite some controversy about what type of intravenous fluids to use, patients in a hyperosmolar state who are profoundly hypotensive and have orthostatic blood pressure changes clearly should receive normal saline initially to expand volume. In this instance, volume repletion should take precedence over all other considerations. Even with the use of normal saline, the hypertonic state will also correct, because the isotonic fluid is hypotonic relevant to the patient's osmolarity at that time. Once blood pressure has risen to an acceptable level and urine output is adequate, it is controversial whether to continue with normal saline or switch to a more hypotonic type of fluid.

The rate of correction is also controversial. Most clinicians believe that it should be achieved slowly over 24–48 hours. The water deficit in this setting can be calculated based on the "true" serum sodium concentration and on the assumption that 60% of the body's weight is water. For example, a body weight of 70 kg is multiplied by 0.6 to calculate total body water, which equals 42 liters. If the "true" serum sodium concentration is 154 mEq/L, the water needed to lower serum sodium to 140 can be calculated as follows:

$$42 * 154 \text{ mEq/L} = 140 \text{ mEq/L} * x$$
$$x = 46.2$$
$$46.2 \text{ L} - 42 \text{ L} = 4.2 \text{ L deficit}$$

Half of this 4.2-liter deficit should be replaced over the first 12 hours, and the remaining estimated deficit during the second 12 hours. A rate of decline in the serum osmolarity of 3 mOsm/hr is usually advocated. Faster correction may be associated with deleterious CNS changes, because as extracellular osmolarity is rapidly decreased, an osmotic gradient may develop between the brain and the plasma, which results in the movement of water into the brain, causing cerebral edema.

9. Discuss the role of insulin.

Given the fact that patients have been ill for 1–2 weeks before seeking medical care and are usually severely volume-depleted, a large amount of fluid is held in the intravascular space by the osmotic effect of glucose. Early reviews of HNC described many deaths among patients receiving insulin for the treatment of their condition. Presumably death was caused by rapidly progressive shock and hypotension concomitant with the rapid fall in blood glucose levels due to insulin. As insulin is given, glucose moves into cells, and fluid follows, causing a decrease in intravascular volume and possible vascular collapse. Glucose levels show a marked improvement with fluid replacement alone. *Insulin should be administered only after sufficient volume has been infused to replete intravascular volume.* If a continuous infusion of insulin is used, doses in the range of 0.5 U/hr to 1.0 U/hr are usually sufficient—less than that used in DKA.

10. What are the major potential complications of the treatment of HNC?

A number of complications have been reported, one of which is vascular occlusion, probably due to the combined effects of hypotension, dehydration, hemoconcentration, and resultant hyperviscosity rather than to a discreet, independent coagulopathy unique to HNC. The most common causes of death from HNC are vascular complications. Aggressive volume repletion should negate the propensity for vascular thrombosis. An additional hematologic complication is disseminated intravascular coagulation.

Cerebral edema, another dreaded complication of HNC, is actually quite rare. It is seen more often in younger patients with DKA. Its exact mechanism is unknown but may be related to a rapid shift of water into the brain (which has a higher effective osmolarity due to idiogenic osmoles) during treatment. A pH-sensitive sodium-acid exchange, which also responds to insulin, may cause a transport of sodium into the cell in exchange for acid, resulting in cell swelling. Another avoidable iatrogenic complication is the administration of insulin without adequate fluid resuscitation, as described above. Acute respiratory distress syndrome and rhabdomyolysis are two other serious complications that have been reported.

CONTROVERSY

11. Should patients receive hypertonic, hypotonic, or isotonic fluids?

Some clinicians prefer hypertonic electrolyte solutions, some prefer isotonic. Those who advocate isotonic fluids claim that use of hypotonic solutions causes cerebral edema, because water loss at the onset of the illness leads to formation of new intracellular particles called idiogenic osmoles. These particles protect brain cell volume. With a rapid fall in extracellular fluid osmolarity, water is osmotically drawn into the brain by the idiogenic osmoles. These osmotically active particles take a finite period to return to an osmotically inactive state. This school of thought, therefore, recommends hypertonic solutions, which are actually hypotonic in regard to the patient's hyperosmolar state.

Those who advocate hypotonic fluids base their argument on the deleterious potential of administration of excessive sodium and chloride. In addition, isotonic solutions do not remain hypotonic compared with the patient's serum, as the serum osmolarity decreases. The possibility of cerebral edema is dismissed as purely theoretical because it is an extremely rare complication of HNC. Also, if it were a real concern, one would expect it to occur more frequently in HNC than in DKA, but clinical experience indicates the exact opposite. Because mental status changes seem to correlate with the level of osmolarity, practitioners in the hypotonic camp advocate rapid reduction with a hypotonic fluid such as half-normal saline.

BIBLIOGRAPHY

1. Arieff AI: Cerebral edema complicating nonketotic hyperosmolar coma. Miner Electrolyte Metab 12(5–6):393–398, 1986.
2. Ennis EP, Stahl ESVB, Kreisberg RA: The hyperosmolar hyperglycemias syndrome. Diabetes Rev 2:115–126, 1994.
3. Lorber D: Nonketeotic hypertonicity in diabetes mellitus. Med Clin North Am 79:39–52, 1995.
4. Magee MF, Bhatt BA: Management of decompensated diabetes. Diabetic ketoacidosis and hyperglycemia hyperosmolar syndrome. Crit Care Clin 17:75–106, 2001.
5. Pope DW, Dansky D: Hyperosmolar hyperglycemic non-ketotic coma. Emerg Med Clin North Am 7:849–857, 1989.
6. Siperstein MD: Diabetic ketoacidosis and hyperosmolar coma. Endocrinol Metab Clin North Am 21:415–432, 1992.
7. Umpierrez GE, Khajavi M, Kitabchi AE: Diabetic ketoacidosis and hyperglycemic hyperosmolar nonketotic syndrome. Am J Med Sci 311:225–233, 1996.
8. Wachtel TJ, Tet-Mouradian LM, Goldman DL, et al: Hyperosmolarity and acidosis in diabetes mellitus. J Gen Intern Med 6:497–502, 1991.
9. Worthy IG: Hyperosmolar coma treated with intravenous sterile water. Arch Intern Med 146:945–947, 1986.

54. ADRENAL INSUFFICIENCY

Michael P. Young, M.D.

1. Is adrenal insufficiency common in ICU patients?

There is no agreed upon gold standard for confirming acute adrenal insufficiency in most ICU patients. The incidence of adrenal insufficiency in the ICU population is cited at 1–6% and, depending on the specific screening tests used to detect adrenal insufficiency, may be as high as 25–40 % for patients with severe sepsis and shock.

2. What are the main types of adrenal insufficiency seen in ICU patients?

1. **Chronic**
   - **Primary adrenal insufficiency** (Addison's disease): The major causes are autoimmune diseases (70%) and tuberculosis (10%). Rare causes include adrenal hemorrhage, adrenal metastasis, cytomegalovirus, HIV disease, amyloidosis, and sarcoidosis.
   - **Secondary adrenal insufficiency** is caused by inadequate production of adrenocorticotropic hormone (ACTH) due to chronic use of exogenous steroids (most common cause), hypopituitary state, or isolated ACTH deficiency.

2. **Acute adrenal crisis/ insufficiency** is characterized by an acute clinical presentation with profound hypotension, fever, and hypovolemia. Patients have very low cortisol levels (≤ 3 μg/dl).

3. **Relative adrenal insufficiency** is the most common and perplexing type of adrenal insufficiency seen in ICU patients. Patients with relative adrenal insufficiency may present with unexplained vasopressor dependency, unexplained development of multiple organ dysfunction, hypothermia, or inability to wean from mechanical ventilation. They have limited response to adrenal stimulation or lower-than-expected basal cortisol levels despite critical illness.

3. What are the clinical markers of acute adrenal insufficiency?

Various combinations of hypotension, tachycardia, severe hypovolemia, respiratory failure, nausea, vomiting, diarrhea, lethargy, and weakness are seen among patients with acute adrenal insufficiency. Patients with acute adrenal insufficiency due to chronic exogenous replacement may not initially exhibit hypotension since mineralocorticoid secretion may be intact until late-stage illness.

4. What laboratory abnormalities are associated with adrenal insufficiency?

The most common laboratory finding is hyponatremia. Low levels of chloride and bicarbonate and high levels of potassium are also frequent. Moderate eosinophilia, lymphocytosis, hypercalcemia, and hypoglycemia may also be seen.

5. How is adrenal insufficiency diagnosed?

Non-ICU patients. In a nonstressed patient, a random cortisol level > 20 µg/dl may rule out the diagnosis of adrenal insufficiency. A random cortisol level < 3 µg/dl confirms the diagnosis of adrenal insufficiency. In stresssed patients with intermediate cortisol levels, the diagnosis of adrenal insufficiency is made with one of the following stimulation tests:

- **ACTH stimulation test.** This is the test most often used to diagnose adrenal insufficiency. Cortisol levels are measured before and 30–60 minutes after a supraphysiologic dose of ACTH (250 µg). A normal response generates a poststimulation cortisol level ≥ 20 µg/dl.
- **Corticotropin-releasing hormone (CHR) stimulation.** CHR is given to stimulate cortisol levels. Unlike the ACTH stimulation test, CHR stimulation can rule out central adrenal insufficiency. A normal response generates a poststimulation cortisol level ≥ 20 µg/dl or a 30-60-minute rise in cortisol ≥ 7.
- **Low-dose (1-mg ACTH) stimulation.** This test may be able to detect adrenal atrophy associated with adrenal insufficiency. Because it is a newer test, there is no consensus on determining the lower level that equates with a normal cortisol response.

ICU patients: The positive and negative predictive values for provocative adrenal stimulation tests in critically ill patients are not known. Some authors recommend that, for critically ill patients (such as patients requiring vasopressors), adrenal stimulation tests are not indicated. Rather than undertaking stimulation tests, clinicians may check random cortisol levels. In the critically ill patient a cortisol level < 20 µg/dl may indicate adrenal insufficiency, and treatment with stress dose steroids may be indicated. If critically ill patients have intermediate random cortisol levels, clinicians may initiate an empirical course of stress-dose steroids. Without a clear clinical response after 1–2 days, the empirical steroids should be discontinued.

6. What is the differential diagnosis when patients present with clinical and laboratory findings consistent with acute adrenal insufficiency?

The clinical presentation of adrenal insufficiency is nonspecific. The clinical findings of hypotension, hypovolemia, tachycardia, fever, respiratory failure, abdominal pain, nausea, and vomiting are common findings in critically ill ICU patients. The routine laboratory findings found among patients with acute adrenal insufficiency are also common and nonspecific in the ICU population. Distinguishing between adrenal insufficiency and other causes of acute illnesses in the ICU requires a clinical index of suspicion and at least one of the following: (1) failure to respond adequately to an adrenal stimulation test, (2) inappropriately low basal cortisol levels, or (3) an unequivocal clinical response to empirical exogenous steroids.

7. What should we do when ICU patients have history of chronic steroid use?

The amount or duration of chronic steroid use required to clinically impair adrenal function is not well defined. Patients may become adrenally insufficient after taking the equivalent of 20 mg/day of prednisone for just 5 days. However, adrenal insufficiency is rare among patients taking steroids < 7 days. Patients may become adrenally insufficient after taking very-low-dose steroids for months to years (> 5 mg/day prednisone equivalent). Fearing life-threatening adrenal gland impairment, many physicians give "stress doses" (hydrocortisone, 300–400 mg/day or equivalent) to patients who receive chronic steroids on admission to the ICU. An increasing number of human and animal models have challenged the routine use of stress-dose steroids in the perioperative period for patientas taking chronic steroids. The ICU population receiving chronic steroids is less well studied. Some authors recommend that in ICU patients who have received chronic steroids and who present with systemic inflammatory response syndrome (SIRS) or hemodynamic compromise, a single cortisol level should be checked. If the cortisol level is < 20 µg/dl, the patient is considered to be adrenally insufficient. Treatment with stress-dose steroids during the acute illness should be initiated. Unfortunately, we lack clinical trials that permit clinicians to confidently withhold stress-dose steroids in critically ill ICU patients who have received chronic steroids despite having cortisol levels ≥ 20 µg/dl. In stable patients and unstressed ICU patients who have received chronic steroids, adrenal function may be tested with a short 250-µg ACTH stimulation test or with more sensitive tests, including the CRH stimulation or low-dose (1-µg) ACTH stimulation test.

8. What other ICU patients groups are at higher risk for adrenal insufficiency?
- **Patients with HIV disease.** The adrenal gland may be involved in > 50% of patients infected with HIV. However, because adrenal function requires < 20% of the gland to function, adrenal insufficiency in this population is uncommon (3%).
- **Patients with cancer.** Even when cancers metastasize to the adrenal gland, adrenal dysfunction is uncommon.
- **Patients with severe sepsis and septic shock.** Twenty five to 40% of patients with severe sepsis or septic shock show evidence of relative adrenal insufficiency.
- **High-risk postoperative patients.** Patients > 55 years old, patients undergoing major operations (e.g., coronary artery bypass grafting, abdominal aortic aneurysm repair, Whipple procedure), patients with multiple trauma, and postoperative patients requiring vasopressors or failing to wean from mechanical ventilation appear to be at higher risk for adrenal insufficiency.

9. What are the indicated therapies for ICU patients suspected to have adrenal insufficiency?
Fluid resuscitation. ICU patients with known or suspected adrenal insufficiency and ineffective arterial circulation require trials of vigorous fluid resuscitation. In patients who do not respond adequately to rapid boluses of isotonic fluid, vasopressors should be started and titrated to the lowest acceptable mean arterial pressure.

Steroid dosing in the ICU. When adrenal insufficiency is associated with hemodynamic compromise, stress doses of steroids should be administered intravenously as soon as possible. The dosing recommendations for adrenal insufficiency in the ICU are not evidence-based. In this setting administration of hydrocortisone, 300–400 mg day IV in 3 or 4 divided doses, is accepted practice (see table below).

Steroid duration in the ICU. For preexisting adrenal insufficiency, see the table below. For relative adrenal insufficiency associated with hypotension, the author recommends administration of stress-dose hydrocortisone (300 mg/day) for 72 hours. If the patient shows significant clinical improvement, the steroids may be tapered slowly over the next 5–7 days. If hypotension recurs, steroid dosing should return to the initial stress doses. If the patient restabilizes, a slower taper can be undertaken. When the diagnosis of adrenal insufficiency is equivocal in stressed patients (e.g., patients requiring vasopressors with random cortisol level of 15–25) and when there is no apparent clinical response to stress dose steroids after 24 hours, the steroids may be rapidly tapered off over the next 1–2 days.

Guidelines for Adrenal Supplementation Therapy

MEDICAL OR SURGICAL STRESS	CORTICOSTERIOD DOSAGE

Minor
  Inguinal hernia repair
  Colonoscopy
  Mild febrile illness
  Mild-to-moderate nausea/vomiting
	25 mg of hydrocortisone or 5 mg of methylprednisolone IV on day of procedure only

Table continued on following page

Guidelines for Adrenal Supplementation Therapy (Continued)

MEDICAL OR SURGICAL STRESS	CORTICOSTERIOD DOSAGE

Moderate
  Open cholecystectomy
  Hemicolectomy
  Significant febrile illness
  Pneumonia
  Severe gastroenteritis
	50–75 mg of hydrocortisone or 10–15 mg of methyl-
	  prednisolone IV on day of procedure
	Taper quickly over 1–2 days to usual dose

Severe
  Major cardiothoracic surgery
  Whipple procedure
  Liver resection
  Pancreatitis
	100–150 mg of hydrocortisone or 20–30 mg of methyl-
	  prednisolone on day of procedure
	Rapid taper to usual dose over next 1–2 days

Critically ill
  Sepsis-induced hypotension or shock
	50–100 mg of hydrocortisone IV every 6–8 hours or
	  0.18 mg/kg/hr as a continuous infusion + 50 μg/day
	  of fludrocortisone until shock is reversed
	May take several days to 1 week or more
	Then gradually taper, following vital signs and serum
	  sodium

From Coursin D, Wood K: Corticosteriod supplementation for adrenal insufficiency JAMA 287:236–240, 2002, with permission.

CONTROVERSY

10. Should stress-dose steroid supplementation be strongly considered in all patients with severe sepsis orseptic shock?

For: Nearly one-half of patients with severe sepsis or septic shock may have relative adrenal insufficiency. The mortality rate for such patients is 40–60%. Multiple animal models and human models indicate that adequate adrenal function is required to survive shock states. In addition, numerous case reports and case series describe dramatic clinical responses associated with steroid supplementation in critically ill patients with relative adrenal insufficiency. Thus, steroid supplementation for many, even most patients, with severe sepsis or sepsis shock makes sense, given the small risk of a short course of steroids.

Against: The most rigorous clinical trial to date indicated that steroids given to patients with septic shock did not reduce mortality rates. In fact, the steroid arm of this randomized, double-blinded study was associated with an increased rate of late infections. Thus, the "might-help, can't-hurt" argument for steroids in this setting is poorly supported. In addition, there is insufficient clinical research to understand the implication of relatively low cortisol levels or an inadequate response to cosyntropin stimulation for patients with severe sepsis or septic shock. Low cortisol levels and inadequate response to cosyntropin stimulation may be expressions only of severity of illness. Supplementation may only be treating disease markers rather than physiologic drivers of disease. Thus, administering supplemental steroids to patients with severe sepsis or septic shock probably creates additional risks without benefit to an already fragile group of patients.

BIBLIOGRAPHY

1. Brown CJ, Buie WD: Perioperative stress dose steroids: Do they make a difference? J Am Coll Surg 193:678–686, 2001.
2. Coursin DB, Wood KE: Corticosteriod supplementation for adrenal insufficiency. JAMA 287:236–240, 2002.
3. Krasner AS: Glucocorticoid-induced adrenal insufficiency. JAMA 282:671–676, 1999.
4. Lamberts WJ, Bruining HA, De Jong FH: Corticosteroid therapy in severe illness. N Engl J Med 337:1285–1292, 1997.

5. Loisa P, Rinne T, Kaukinen S: Adrenocortical function and multiple organ failure in severe sepsis. Acta
    Anaesthesiol Scand 46:145–151, 2002.
6. Mayo J, Collazos J, Martinez E, Ibarra S: Adrenal function in the human immunodeficieny virus-infected
    patient. Arch Intern Med 162:1095–1098, 2002.
7. Nieboer P, van de Werf TS, Beentjes JA, et al: Catecholamine dependency in a polytruama patient:
    Relative adrenal insufficiency? Intens Care Med 26:125–127, 2000.
8. Rivers EP, Gaspari M, Saad GA, et al: Adrenal insufficiency in high-risk surgical ICU patients. Chest
    119:889–896, 2001.
9. Ryndvall A: Plasma cortisol is often decreased in patients treated in an intensive care unit. Intens Care
    Med 26:545–551, 2000.
10. Schroeder S, Winchers M, Klingmuller D, et al: The hypothalamic-pituitary axis of patients with severe
    sepsis: Altered response to corticotropin-releasing hormone. Crit Care Med 29:310–316, 2001.
11. Shenker Y, Skatrud JB: Adrenal insufficiency in critically ill patients. Am J Respir Crit Care Med
    163:1520–1523, 2001.

55. THYROID DISEASE IN THE INTENSIVE CARE UNIT

Michael T. McDermott, M.D.

1. What is the euthyroid sick syndrome?

The euthyroid sick syndrome consists of a group of changes in serum thyroid hormone and thyroid-stimulating hormone (TSH) levels in patients with a variety of nonthyroidal illnesses, including infections, trauma, surgery, myocardial infarction, malignancies, inflammatory conditions, and starvation. This condition also is called the nonthyroidal illness syndrome. It results from changes in peripheral metabolism and transport of thyroid hormones induced by the nonthyroidal illness.

2. What hormone changes characterize the euthyroid sick syndrome?

Patients with mild-to-moderate nonthyroidal illnesses often develop low serum levels of total triiodothyronine (T_3) and free T_3. These changes result from decreased conversion of thyroxine (T_4) to T_3 by peripheral tissues, predominantly the liver. Serum TSH levels usually remain in the normal range.

With more severe nonthyroidal illnesses, serum T_3 levels may become very low; in addition, the total T_4 concentrations become depressed and the T_3 resin uptake (T_3RU) increases. These changes result from reduced binding of thyroid hormones to their transport proteins because of both impaired hepatic protein synthesis and circulating inhibitors of thyroid hormone-binding proteins. Free T_4 levels are more variable; they have been noted to be normal, increased, or decreased. Serum TSH levels remain normal or become slightly decreased at this stage.

When nonthyroidal illnesses resolve, thyroid hormone levels also return to normal. However, as hepatic protein synthesis improves and circulating inhibitors of thyroid hormone binding disappear, there may be a transient drop in serum free T_4 values with a resultant increase in serum TSH levels before complete normalization occurs.

3. How can euthyroid sick syndrome be distinguished from hypothyroidism?

In the euthyroid sick syndrome, serum T_3 is reduced proportionately more than T_4, the T_3RU is often high, and the TSH is normal or decreased. In primary hypothyroidism, serum T_4 is reduced proportionately more than T_3, the T_3RU is usually low, and the TSH is increased. Other tests also may be helpful. In the euthyroid sick syndrome, free T_4 is usually normal and reverse T_3 (RT_3) is increased; in hypothyroidism, both free T_4 and RT_3 are decreased.

4. Is the euthyroid sick syndrome an adaptive mechanism, or is it harmful?

Many experts consider the euthyroid sick syndrome an adaptive mechanism to reduce peripheral tissue energy expenditure during the nonthyroidal illness. Conversely, other argue that the alterations in circulating thyroid hormone levels may be harmful and accentuate the effects of the nonthyroidal illness. This issue is likely to remain controversial for years to come.

5. Should patients with the euthyroid sick syndrome be treated with thyroid hormone?

Management of patients with the euthyroid sick syndrome is highly controversial. Currently no convincing data demonstrate a recovery or survival benefit from treatment with either levothyroxine (LT$_4$) or liothyronine (LT$_3$). Experts continue to debate this issue and agree that large, prospective studies are needed. In the absence of more definitive data, thyroid hormone therapy cannot be recommended at this time.

6. Does the euthyroid sick syndrome have any prognostic significance?

The prognosis for recovery from critical nonthyroidal illness may be fairly well predicted from the severity of the reduction in serum levels of T$_3$ and T$_4$. Patients with extremely low serum T$_3$ levels have a very high mortality rate.

7. Are levels of thyroid hormone ever elevated in patients with nonthyroid diseases?

The serum T$_4$ may be transiently elevated in patients with acute psychiatric illnesses and in patients with various acute medical illnesses, such as hepatitis. The mechanisms underlying the elevations of T$_4$ are not well understood. This condition must be distinguished from true thyrotoxicosis.

8. What is thyroid storm?

Thyroid storm or crisis is a life-threatening condition characterized by an exaggeration of the manifestations of thyrotoxicosis. The mortality rate is currently about 20%.

9. How do patients develop thyroid storm?

Thyroid storm generally occurs in patients who have unrecognized or inadequately treated thyrotoxicosis and a superimposed precipitant event, such as thyroid surgery, nonthyroid surgery, infection, or trauma.

10. Describe the most common clinical manifestations of thyroid storm.

Fever (> 102° F) is the hallmark of thyroid storm. Tachycardia is usually present, and tachypnea is common, but blood pressure is variable. Cardiac arrhythmias, congestive heart failure, and ischemic heart disease may develop. Nausea, vomiting, diarrhea, and abdominal pain are frequent features. Central nervous system manifestations include hyperkinesis, psychosis, and coma. A goiter is a helpful finding but is not always present.

11. What laboratory abnormalities are seen in thyroid storm?

Serum T$_4$ and T$_3$, T$_3$RU, free T$_4$, and free T$_3$ are usually elevated, and serum thyrotropin (TSH) is undetectable. Other common laboratory abnormalities include anemia, leukocytosis, hyperglycemia, azotemia, hypercalcemia, and elevated liver-associated enzymes.

12. How is the diagnosis of thyroid storm made?

The diagnosis must be made on the basis of suspicious but nonspecific clinical findings. Serum thyroid hormone levels are always elevated; however, if the diagonis is strongly suspected, waiting for test results may cause a critical delay in the initiation of effective life-saving therapy. Furthermore, thyroid hormone levels alone cannot reliably distinguish patients with thyroid storm from those who have coincidental uncomplicated thyrotoxicosis. The above clinical features, therefore, are the key to diagnosis.

13. What other conditions may mimic thyroid storm?

Sepsis, pheochromocytoma, and malignant hyperthermia.

14. How should patients with thyroid storm be treated?

As soon as the diagnosis is made, measures should be taken to decrease thyroid hormone synthesis, to inhibit thyroid hormone release, to reduce the heart rate, to support the circulation, and to treat the precipitating condition. Specific medications include the following:

To decrease thyroid hormone synthesis
- Propylthiouracil (PTU), 200 mg every 4 hr (orally, rectally, or via nasogastric tube)
- Methimazole (Tapazole), 20 mg every 4 hr (orally, rectally, or via nasogastric tube)

To inhibit thyroid hormone release
- Sodium iodide (NaI), 1 gm over 24 hr intravenously
- Saturated solution of potassium iodide (SSKI), 5 drops every 8 hr orally
- Lugol's solution, 10 drops every 8 hr orally

To reduce heart rate
- Propranolol, 40–80 mg every 4–6 hr orally or 1–2 mg at 1 mg/min every 4–6 hr intravenously
- Esmolol, 0.25–0.50 mg/kg over 1 min intravenously, then 0.05–0.10 mg/kg/min infusion
- Diltiazem, 60–90 mg every 6–8 hr orally or 0.25 mg/kg over 2 min intravenously, then 10 mg/min infusion

To support the circulation
- Dexamethasone, 2 mg every 6 hr intravenously, *or*
- Hydrocortisone, 100 mg every 8 hr intravenously
- Intravenous fluids

15. What is myxedema coma?

Myxedema coma is a life-threatening condition characterized by an exaggeration of the symptoms of hypothyroidism. The estimated mortality rate is about 30%.

16. How do patients develop myxedema coma?

Myxedema coma usually occurs in elderly patients with untreated or inadequately treated hypothyroidism and a superimposed precipitating event. Precipitating events may include prolonged cold exposure, infection, trauma, surgery, myocardial infarction, congestive heart failure, pulmonary embolism, stroke, respiratory failure, gastrointestinal bleeding, and administration of various drugs, particularly those that have a depressive effect on the central nervous system.

17. Describe the most common clinical manifestations of myxedema coma.

Hypothermia, bradycardia, and hypoventilation are common; blood pressure, while generally reduced, is more variable. Pericardial, pleural, and peritoneal effusions are often found. An ileus is present in about two-thirds of patients, and acute urinary retention may also be seen. Central nervous system manifestations include seizures, stupor, and coma; deep tendon reflexes are either absent or exhibit a delayed relaxation phase. Typical hypothyroid changes of the skin and hair may be seen. A goiter, although often absent, is a helpful finding; a thyroidectomy scar may also be an important clue.

18. What laboratory abnormalities are seen in myxedema coma?

Serum T_4 and T_3, T_3RU, free T_4, and free T_3 are usually low, and TSH is significantly elevated. Other frequent abnormalities include anemia, hyponatremia, hypoglycemia, and elevated serum levels of cholesterol and creatine kinase (CK). Arterial blood gases usually reveal carbon dioxide retention and hypoxemia. The electrocardiogram often shows sinus bradycardia, various types and degrees of heart block, low voltage, and T-wave flattening.

19. How is the diagnosis of myxedema coma made?

The diagnosis must be made on clinical grounds based on the findings described above. Serum levels of thyroid hormones are reduced, and TSH is elevated. However, the delay involved in waiting for test results unnecessarily postpones the initiation of effective therapy.

20. How should patients with myxedema coma be treated?

As soon as the diagnosis is made, steps should be taken for rapid repletion of circulating thyroid hormone levels, replacement of glucocorticoids, support of vital functions, and treatment of the precipitating condition. Whether to use LT4, LT3, or a combination of both remains controversial and has not been settled by an adequate prospective evaluation. Specific medications include the following:

Rapid repletion of circulating thyroid hormones
- Levothyroxine (LT4), 300–500 µg over 5 min intravenously, then 50–100 µg/day orally or intravenously
- Liothyronine (LT3), 50–100 µg over 5 min intravenously, then LT4, 50–100 µg/day orally or intravenously
- LT4 plus LT3: LT4, 150–300 µg over 5 min intravenously, plus LT3, 10 µg over 5 min intravenously, then LT4, 50–100 µg/day orally or intravenously

Glucocorticoid replacement
- Hydrocortisone, 100 mg every 8 hr intravenously

Support of vital functions
- Oxygen
- Intravenous fluids
- Rewarming (blankets or central warming)
- Mechanical ventilation (if needed)

BIBLIOGRAPHY

1. Brent GA, Hershman JM: Thyroxine therapy in patients with severe nonthyroidal illnesses and low serum thyroxine concentration. J Clin Endocrinol Metab 63:1–8, 1986.
2. Brooks MH, Waldstein SS: Free thyroxine concentrations in thyroid storm. Ann Intern Med 93:694–697, 1980.
3. Burch HD, Wartofsky L: Life threatening thyrotoxicosis: Thyroid storm. Endocrinol Metab Clin North Am 22:263–278, 1993.
4. Camacho PM, Dwarkanathan A: Sick euthyroid syndrome: What to do when thyroid function tests are abnormal in critically ill patients. Postgrad Med 105:215–219, 1999.
5. Dillman WH: Thyroid storm. Curr Ther Endocrinol Metab 6:81–85, 1997.
6. Jordan RM: Myxedema coma. Pathophysiology, therapy, and factors affecting prognosis. Med Clin North Am 79:185–194, 1995.
7. McIver B, Gorman CA: Euthyroid sick syndrome: An overview. Thyroid 7:125–132, 1997.
8. Morley JE, Slag MF, Elson MK, Shafer RB: The interpretation of thyroid function tests in hospitalized patients. JAMA 249:2377–2379, 1983.
9. Nicoloff JT: Myxedema coma: A form of decompensated hypothyroidism. Endocrinol Metab Clin North Am 22:279–290, 1993.
10. Pittman CS, Zayed AA: Myxedema coma. Curr Ther Endocrinol Metab 6:98–101, 1997.
11. Simons RJ, Simon JM, Demers LM, Santen RJ: Thyroid dysfunction in elderly hospitalized patients: Effect of age and severity of illness. Arch Intern Med 150:1249–1253, 1990.
12. Tietgens ST, Leinung MC: Thyroid storm: Med Clin North Am 79:169–184, 1995.
13. Tsitouras PD: Myxedema coma. Clin Geriatr Med 11:251–258, 1995.
14. Yamamoto T, Fukuyama J, Fujioyoshi A: Factors associated with mortality of myxedema coma: Report of eight cases and literature survey. Thyroid 9:1167–1174, 1999.
15. Yeung S-CJ, Go R, Balasubramanyam A: Rectal administration of iodide and propylthiouracil in the treatment of thyroid storm. Thyroid 5:403–405, 1995.

56. HYPERCALCEMIC CRISIS

Jeanne Rozwadowski, M.D., and Marc-André Cornier, M.D.

1. What is hypercalcemia?

The usual range of total serum calcium is 8.1–10.5 mg/dl (2.0–2.6 mmol/L) in the setting of normal levels of serum proteins. Normal values for ionized calcium measurement, which is available in many laboratories, vary from 4.5 to 5.3 mg/dl (1.1–1.3 mmol/L). Hypercalcemia is defined as a calcium level that is elevated outside the normal range on at least three occasions. Serum calcium values between 10.6 and 10.9 mg/dl are often misleading and may not lead to detection of clinically significant disease, whereas values > 11.0 mg/dl are almost always indicative of disease. With the increased use of routine biochemical profile testing, hypercalcemia is found in up to 1.5% of patients.

2. Define hypercalcemic crisis.

Hypercalcemic crisis is a clinical diagnosis; therefore, no specific criteria are available. However, the accepted definition is a high serum calcium level, generally > 14 mg/dl, associated with acute signs and symptoms that can be attributed to hypercalcemia and that resolve with the lowering of calcium levels. Patients may manifest symptoms at variable levels of hypercalcemia, and the acuity of onset may be more important than the actual calcium level in contributing to the crisis. Patients tend to be volume-depleted and to have nausea and vomiting as well as metabolic encephalopathy. They also may have cardiac problems ranging from dysrhythmias to S-T segment depression, sinus arrest, and problems with atrioventricular conduction.

3. How do alterations in serum proteins affect total calcium levels?

Approximately 40–45% of serum calcium is protein-bound; the majority is bound to albumin. About 40–45% of calcium is free (ionized state), and 10% is complexed to cations such as phosphate, citrate, lactate, and bicarbonate. The level of circulating free calcium is the physiologically important value. In general, for every 1 gm/dl decrease or increase in serum albumin, total calcium is decreased or increased by 0.8 mg/dl, respectively, and should be "corrected" as such. A 1gm/dl increase or decrease in serum globulin results in an 0.16 mg increase or decrease in total calcium.

4. How do alterations in acid–base status affect total calcium levels?

Acid-base status also affects the protein binding of calcium. Acidosis reduces protein binding and therefore increases free calcium, whereas alkalosis increases protein binding and decreases free calcium. Hyperventilation (respiratory alkalosis) leads to perioral numbness and tingling—symptoms of hypocalcemia.

5. What conditions can falsely elevate a serum calcium level?

Any condition that raises serum protein levels can falsely elevate calcium levels. For example, high levels of protein can occur with excessive venous stasis during blood collection, and high levels of gammaglobulins or paraproteins can occur with multiple myeloma.

6. When should ionized calcium be measured?

If the patient's protein and acid–base status are normal, a total serum calcium measurement is probably adequate and appropriate. Total serum calcium is also less expensive and more reliable than ionized calcium. In the setting of altered protein and acid–base status, ideally a direct measurement of free, ionized calcium is preferable for the evaluation of hypercalcemia.

7. How is serum calcium regulated?

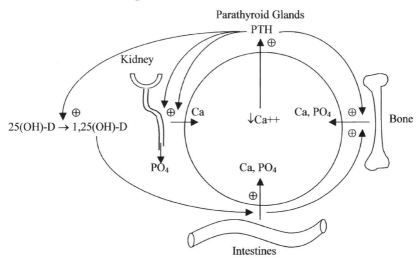

Summary of the basics of calcium (Ca) metabolism. Parathyroid hormone (PTH) increases serum calcium by stimulating bone resorption and distal renal tubular reabsorption. PTH also stimulates the renal conversion of 25-hydroxyvitamin D (25[OH]-D) to 1,25-dihydroxyvitamin D (1,25[OH]-D), which in turn increases intestinal absorption of calicum and phosphate (PO_4) and mobilization of calcium from bone. PTH affects phosphate by increasing its mobilization from bone and reducing its renal tubular reabsorption.

8. What are the signs and symptoms of hypercalcemia?

Signs and symptoms are frequently nonspecific but may include irritability, confusion, weakness, fatigue, anorexia, nausea, vomiting, constipation, photophobia, and polyuria. Severe hypercalcemia may be associated with CNS and cardiac depression and progressive stupor, coma, and shock. Hypercalcemia is associated with shortening of the Q-T interval, a prolonged P-R interval, and T-wave changeson EKG. Patients, especially those taking digitalis, may have cardiac arrhythmias. The hypercalcemic patient may manifest nephrolithiasis, nephrocalcinosis, peptic ulceration, or pancreatitis.

9. What is the differential diagnosis of hypercalcemia?

Over 90% of hypercalcemia can be explained by hyperparathyroidism (HPT) or malignancy. HPT is the more common diagnosis in the outpatient setting and is frequently detected on routine chemistry analyses. If HPT is diagnosed, the existence of multiple endocrine neoplasm type 1 or 2A should be considered. Malignancy is the more common culprit in the inpatient setting. The solid tumors associated with hypercalcemia are breast, lung, head and neck, renal, colon, and prostate.The associated hematologic malignancies are multiple myeloma, lymphoma, and leukemia. The other endocrine conditions that can cause hypercalcemia are hyperthyroidism, hypoadrenalism, vitamin D intoxication, and Paget's disease, especially in association with immobilization. Certain drugs also may cause hypercalcemiam such as lithium and thiazides. Vitamin A intoxication and ingestion of absorbable calcium-containing antacids (milk-alkalai syndrome) can cause hypercalcemia. Other causes include increased 1,25(OH)-D, which is associated with a variety of granulomatous diseases such as sarcoidosis, tuberculosis, and histoplasmosis. Hypercalcemia also can be seen in patients with kidney transplant, in the diuretic phase of renal failiure, in patients with benign familial hypocalciuric hypercalcemia, and in infancy as idiopathic hypercalcemia (Williams syndrome).

10. What are the most common causes of hypercalcemic crisis?

The most common cause is hypercalcemia of malignancy. In most—but not all—patients, the primary malignancy is known. HPT is a less frequent cause of hypercalcemic crisis. If parathyroid hormone levels are elevated, parathyroid carcinoma is a more likely cause than HPT.

11. What laboratory features suggest that hypercalcemia is PTH-mediated?

	PTH-mediated	*Non-PTH-mediated*
Calcium	< 13 mg/dl	> 14 mg/dl
Phosphate	Low	Low, normal, high
Chloride	> 104 mmol/L	< 100 mmol/L
Chlroid/phosphate	≥ 33	≤ 33
Intact PTH	High/normal	Low

12. What laboratory studies are important in the initial work-up of hypercalcemia?

The initial studies should include a serum metabolic panel (phosphate, magnesium, bicarbonate, chloride, creatinine, and albumin), a complete blood count, and an intact PTH (iPTH) level. If the iPTH is low, a PTH-related peptide (PTH-rp) level also should be measured (see question 14). Ideally, 24-hour calcium excretion also should be measured. When the diagnosis is not clear, 25(OH)-D and 1,24(OH)-D levels may be helpful.

13. How does a 24-hour calicum measurement help in the evaluation of hypercalcemic patients?

The 24-hour urine measurement helps to diagnose benign familial hypocalciuric hypocalcemia (FHH) and to distinguish it from HPT. FHH is an autosomal dominant condition with nearly complete penetrance; it is associated with decreased renal calcium clearance, normal-to-high serum PTH level, normal or low serum phosporus level, and mild hypermagnesemia. As the name suggests, FHH is a benign, asymptomatic condition that does not require therapy. In addition, a 24-hour calcium measurement helps to determine whether a hypercalcemic patients is at risk for developing kidney stones (levels > 400 mg/day).

14. Discuss the significance of PTH-related peptide.

PTH-rp is a humoral substance similar to PTH and shares about 70% of the same amino acid sequence. It binds to the PTH receptor and increases osteoclastic bone resorption and renal tubular calcium reabsorption; it also decreases renal phosphate uptake.

15. Define humoral hypocalcemia of malignancy (HHM).

HHM is the more common cause of hypercalcemia of malignancy. The malignant tumor produces a humoral substance that causes an increase in bone resorption, thus producing hypercalcemia. The less common cause of hypercalcemia of malignancy is local invasion of bone by the primary tumor.

16. What humoral factors are known to produce hypercalcemia?

About 80% of tumors causing hypercalcemia produce PTH-rp. Examples include the squamous cell cancers, breast cancer, and renal cell carcinoma. Cytokines, also called osteoclastic-activating factors (OAFs), stimulate bone resorption and cause hypercalcemia in some malignancies, such as lymphomas, myelomas, and metastases to bone. The OAFs include interleukins 1 and 6, tumor necrosis factor alpha, transforming growth factors alpha and beta, prostaglandin E_2, granulocyte-macrophage colony-stimulating factor, interferon, and lymphotoxin. Some lymphomas produce 1,25(OH)-D. Rare tumors (generally small cell lung and ovarian cancers) can produce native PTH.

17. What types of cancer are most likely to cause hypercalcemia?

The most common cancers that produce hypercalcemia are squamous cell carcinomas of the lung, esophagus, cervix, vulva, and head and neck. Lung cancers, both squamous cell and adenocarcinoma, account for about 35% of cancers causing hypercalcemia. Breast and renal cell carcinoma cause 20–25% and 10–15%, respectively. Head and neck squamous cell cancers account for about 10%, as do hematologic malignancies such as multiple myeloma and lymphoma. In rare cases, gastric, colon, colorectal, prostate, small cell lung, and ovarian cancers may cause hypercalcemia.

Most patients with hypercalcemia of malignancy have advanced disease and a known or easily identified primary tumor. The work-up for a patient with hypercalcemia of malignancy without a known primary tumor should be directed at searching for cancers that cause hypercalcemia.

18. What is the incidence of HPT? Are localization procedures useful?

Approximately 80–90% of patients with primary HPT have single parathyroid adenoma. Ten to 15% have hyperparathyroid hyperplasia. Less than 1% may have parathyroid carcinoma. Preoperative localization procedures add little to the initial evaluation of patients with HPT. The procedures lack both sensitivity and specificity in predicting the presence of the adenoma and are expensive. Localization is best done by an experienced surgeon, who in most cases removes the adenoma or identifies parathyroid hyperplasia.

19. Who should have surgery for primary HPT?

At the 1990 NIH Consensus Development Conference, the following indications for surgery were proposed:

1. Serum calcium > 11.4–12 mg/dl
2. Creatinine clearance reduced more than 30% for age in the absence of another cause
3. 24-hour urinary calcium > 400 mg
4. Any overt manifestation of primary HPT (nephrolithiasis, osteitis fibrosa cystica, classic neuromuscular diseases, previous episode of life-threatening hypercalcemia)
5. Bone mass reduced more than 2 SD compared with age-, gender-, and race-matched controls
6. Patients who request surgery or in whom long-term surveillance is unsuitable
7. Young patients (< 50 years of age)

20. Outline the initial therapy for hypercalcemic crisis.

1. Assess the patient. Does the patient really need urgent therapy? Assess the patient's prognosis and resuscitation status.

2. Ensure adequate hydration. Patients in hypercalcemic crisis are significantly volume-depleted. Normal saline (NS) is the solution of choice. The initial infusion rate should be rapid (200–300 ml/hr), and 4–10 L/day may be necessary. Of course, patients must be monitored carefully for fluid overload. The addition of potassium and/or magnesium to the infusate also may be necessary.

3. Add furosemide to NS. Be sure that the patient is adequately hydrated before using furosemide. For aggressive management, up to 80–100 mg every 1–2 hours can be used with close attention to fluid and electrolyte balance. For less urgent management, 40 mg every 4–6 hr can be used.

4. Administer intravenous biphosphonates. Pamidronate (Aredia), 90 mg infused over 24 hours, is the agent of choice. The infusion may be repeated in 7 days if necessary. Etidronate disodium (Didronel) also can be used at 7.5 mg/kg with at least 250 ml NS over 2 hours and repeated daily for 3–7 days.

5. Administer calcitonin, 4–8 IU/kg subcutaneously every 6–12 hours.

6. Consider glucocorticoids. The preferred agent is prednisone, 40-60 mg/day for 3–5 days.

7. Consider gallium nitrate, 100–200 mg/m² of body surface in 1,000 ml NS over 24 hours daily for 5 days. Avoid in patients with creatinine > 2.5 mg/dl.

8. Consider plicamycin, 25 mg/kg in 50 ml of D5W infused over 3 hours. This dose can be repeated daily for 3–4 days.

9. Consider dialysis.

10. Consider intravenous phosphate, given as 1,000 mg elemental phosphate (0.16 mM/kg) over 8–12 hr during each 24-hour period. *Caution:* Intravenous phosphate can cause hypotension and should be avoided in hyperphosphatemic patients. It is reserved for patients in whom all else has failed.

21. What is the most common mistake in the initial treatment of hypercalcemia?

Use of furosemide before intravascular volume has been repleted. Sodium and calcium excretion are coupled. Simply expanding the intravascular volume with saline induces a sodium diuresis associated with a resultant calcium diuresis. If the patient is volume-depleted, glomerular filtration is impaired, and sodium and calcium are reabsorbed in the proximal tubule. Using a loop diuretic in a volume-depleted patient increases sodium reabsorption and therefore limits calcium excretion and may actually worsen hypercalcemia.

22. What is the drug of choice in the acute treatment of hypercalcemic crisis?

Pamidronate, which is effective in 95% of patients and is safe and nontoxic. It works by impairing osteoclastic activity by binding to hydroxyapatite crystals. About 48 hours are required, however, before it has an effect on serum calcium. Calcitonin is useful in combination with pamidronate because it works quickly to reduce serum calcium levels by decreasing bone resorption and renal tubular reabsorption. Its effects last only about 48 hours, by which time pamidronate begins to work.

The other agents are not often used. Clinical experience with gallium nitrate is limited, and it should not be used without the guidance of an experienced endocrinologist. Glucocorticoids are useful in specific situations, such as hypercalcemia caused by a hematologic malignancy (myeloma or lymphoma) or by an excess of vitamin D (vitamin D intoxication or granulomatous diseases).

23. When is dialysis indicated?

Dialysis is indicated for patients refractory to treatment and patients with renal failure.

24. What are the options for chronic therapy?

1. Treat the primary cause of hypercalcemia, when possible.
2. Mobilize the patient.
3 Oral phosphates, 1–2 gm/day of elemental phosphate (e.g., K-Phos, 3 tablets 3 times/day orally), are useful if the serum phosphate level is not elevated.
4. Bisphosphantes: oral alendronate (Fosamax), 10 mg/day; oral risedronate (Actonel), 5 mg/day; oral etidronate (Didronel), 5–20 mg/kg/day; or intravenous pamidronate (Aredia), 30–90 mg as needed.
5. Mithramycin inhibits RNA synthesis of osteoclasts and may be used chronically or semiacutely. It is dosed at 25 µg/kg in 50 ml of D5W infused over 3 hours.
6. Glucocorticoids: 50–60 mg/day.

25. (a) What is the treatment of choice for a patient with a serum calcium of 13 mg/dl and minimal symptoms? (b) What if the serum calcium is 19 mg/dl and vital signs are stable, but mental status is altered?

(a) Start saline until volume is expanded, then add furosemide to promote calciuretic diuresis. Other therapies that may need to be added include calcitonin, steroids, and mithramycin. If the hypercalcemia is unresponsive, intravenous administration of pamidronate is the next choice.

(b) Saline and furosemide until volume is expanded, then add furosemide. This situation is more critical because of the mental status changes; thus, the prompt addition of a second-line therapy is necessary. A combination of calcitonin and pamidronate may be useful. Dialysis also may be necessary if the patient also has renal failure.

BIBLIOGRAPHY

1. Bilezikian JP: Management of acute hypercalcemia. N Engl J Med 326:1196–1203, 1992.
2. Centers for Disease Control Panel: Diagnosis and management of asymptomatic primary hyperparathyroidism: Consensus development conference statement. Ann Intern Med 114:593, 1991.
3. Edelson GW, Kleerekoper M: Hypercalcemic crisis. Med Clin North Am 79:79–92, 1995.

4. Mundy GR, Guise TA: Hypercalcemia of malignancy. Am J Med 103:134–145, 1997.
5. Nussbaum SR: Pathophysiology and measurement of severe hypercalcemia. Endocrinol Metab Clin North Am 22:343–361, 1993.
6. Ralston SH, Gallacher SJ, Patel U, et al: Cancer-associated hypercalcemia: Morbidity and mortality. Ann Intern Med 112:499, 1990.
7. Sanders LR: Hypercalcemia. In McDermott MT (ed): Endocrinology Secrets. Philadelphia, Hanley & Belfus, 1995, pp 71–80.
8. Watters J, Gerrard G, Dodwell D: The management of malignant hypercalcemia. Drugs 52:837–848, 1996.

IX. Hematology/Oncology

57. BLOOD PRODUCTS AND COAGULATION

David G.Burris, M.D., and Mark W. Bowyer, M.D.

1. What is the best fluid to treat shock due to acute blood loss?

Fresh whole blood, if it can be obtained, because it contains red cells for oxygen transport, coagulation factors, and platelets. It is usually not available because of its short storage life.

2. How long can blood be stored?

Forty-two days. Although up to 80% of the red cells are still viable after 42 days, the white cells and platelets are not, and clotting factors have minimal activity.

3. How is blood preserved?

Banked blood contains CAPD citrate to prevent coagulation and adenine, phosphate, and dextrose as energy sources for the cells. Blood is stored at 4–7°C to prevent bacterial growth.

4. What components of blood are available?

Packed red blood cells (PRBCs), fresh frozen plasma (FFP), cryoprecipitate, platelets, and white cell preparations.

5. What are PRBCs?

PRBCs remain after the centrifugation of whole blood and the removal of plasma . One unit of PRBCs raises the hemoglobin by 1 mg/dl or the hematocrit by an average of three points.

6. Discuss the indications for red cell transfusions in critically ill patients.

Red cell transfusions are used to maximize oxygen delivery to the tissues. The only absolute indications for transfusion are clinical evidence of tissue hypoxia or a hemoglobin level less than 7 mg/dl (hematocrit < 21). Patient age, chronic anemia, and coexisting disease that leads to tissue ischemia, including coronary artery disease, pulmonary insufficiency, and occlusive vascular disease, may require transfusion at higher hemoglobin levels.

7. What is the ideal hematocrit in critically ill patients?

Recent work suggests that survival may be impaired by transfusing patients to achieve an hematocrit greater than 25.

8. What is FFP?

FFP is plasma separated from the blood cells and placed immediately at or below –18° C to preserve the coagulation factors, which are labile. FFP contains fibrinogen; prothrombin; factors V, VII, VIII, IX, and XIII; antithrombin III; and proteins C and S.

9. List the the indications for FFP.

1. Coagulopathy due to a congenital deficiency, especially of factor II, V, VII, VIII, X, XI, or XIII.

2. Coagulopathy due to an acquired deficiency of multiple factors, such as severe liver disease, disseminated intravascular coagulation (DIC), or vitamin K depletion.

3. Dilutional coagulopathy in a massively transfused patient (more than one blood volume); monitor with coagulation studies and thrombelastography.

4. Reversal of warfarin effect (one unit of FFP decrease the prothrombin time by 2 seconds).

5. Treatment of antithrombin III deficiency.

10. What is cryoprecipitate?

Cryoprecipitate (cryo) is prepared from FFP by slow thawing at 4–6°C. Cryoprecipitate contains high concentrations of factor VIII, von Willebrand's factor, fibrinogen, and factor XIII.

11. List the indications for giving cryoprecipitate.

1. Hypofibrinogenemia (fibrinogen level less than 100 mg/dl)
2. Von Willebrand's disease
3. Hemophilia A (factor VIII deficiency)
4. Bleeding due to thrombolytic therapy

Cryoprecipitate can be used to promote hemostasis in a bleeding patient; in most circumstances, however, it is preferable to give FFP, which contains more of the essential clotting factors.

12. Define hemolytic transfusion reaction.

Hemolytic transfusion reactions occur when ABO- or Rh-mismatched blood is given. It may occur when as little as 10 ml of blood is infused; the reaction causes fulminant DIC and is associated with a mortality rate of about 35%. Significant morbidity also may occur; acute renal failure may result from acute tubular necrosis.

13. List the classic findings in hemolytic transfusion reaction.

Fever, chills, back or flank pain, chest pain, dyspnea, hypotension, oliguria, and hemoglobinuria. Intraoperatively this reaction may be heralded by sudden hemorrhage in a previously dry field.

14. How is a hemolytic transfusion reaction treated?

First and foremost, stop the transfusion. Support the patient with intravenous fluids, diuretics (mannitol), inotropes, plasma products, and monitoring in the intensive care unit (ICU).

15. What are the infectious risks of transfusion?

Although the risk depends on the prevalence of infection in the donating population, the overall risk of infection from a transfused unit is 1:30,000–1:150,000 for hepatitis C and 1:200,000–1:2,000,000 for human immunodeficiency virus (HIV). Transmission of cytomegalovirus (CMV) infection is the highest risk.

16. List common techniques of autologous transfusion.

1. **Preoperative autologous blood donation (PABD).** Blood is donated beginning 4–6 weeks before surgery, as frequently as every 3 days, and transfused postoperatively only as indicated.

2. **Acute normovolemic hemodilution (ANH).** Blood is withdrawn immediately before surgery, and intravascular volume is maintained intraoperatively by using crystalloid or colloid prior to surgical blood loss. The removed blood is transfused during or after surgery, as needed, to maintain the desired post-ANH hemoglobin concentration.

3. **Intraoperative blood salvage.** Blood is collected intraoperatively and centrifuged; red cells are washed and then reinfused.

17. What is the role of erythropoietin in critically ill patients?

ICU patients lose blood through repeated sampling, bleeding, drug reactions, and breakdown due to chronic illness. Previously patients were given transfusions. The use of erythropoietin in critically-ill patients has led to decreased blood transfusions and possibly increased survival.

18. Which blood substitutes may be used in critically ill patients?

1. **Perfluorochemical emulsions.** Fluoridation of hydrocarbons generates a biologically inert liquid with high oxygen solubility. Oxygen is dissolved in these solutions in a linear relationship to inspired oxygen. High levels of supplemental oxygen are required to provide clinically useful oxygen delivery. Newer formulations may overcome the adverse reactions and carry more oxygen. These products are not clinically available.

2. **Hemoglobin-based oxygen-carrying solutions.** The administration of free hemoglobin leads to nephrotoxicity and hypertension, mediated by nitric oxide scavenging. In addition, the administration of free hemoglobin results in an unfavorable oxygen dissociation curve.

Modifications of free-hemoglobin, including crosslinkage of the tetramer, conjugation with large molecules, polymerization, and liposome encapsulation, seem to resolve these problems. The hemoglobin for these solutions may be obtained from human, bovine, porcine, and bacteria (using recombinant techniques). A polymerized bovine solution has been approved for veterinary use in the U.S. and for human use in South Africa.

19. What is measured by prothrombin time (PT)?

PT assesses the activity of factor VII, which is involved in the extrinsic coagulation pathway only. It is prolonged in patients with liver disease and patients who are deficient in vitamin K.

20. What is measured by partial thromboplastin time (PTT)?

PTT assesses activities of the intrinsic coagulation pathway, which includes factors XII, XI, IX, and VIII. A prolonged PTT with a normal PT suggests an inherited defect in coagulation.

21. What is the most common inherited factor deficiency?

Hemophilia A, a deficiency of factor VIII (about 75%), followed by hemophilia B, a deficiency of factor IX (about 20%).

22. How does warfarin work?

Warfarin (Coumadin) inhibits the conversion of vitamin K to its active form. This inhibition interferes with the hepatic synthesis of vitamin K-dependent clotting factors II, VII, IX, and X. Warfarin primarily prolongs PT but may have an effect on PTT.

23. How does heparin work?

Heparin binds to and activates antithrombin III, which in turn inhibits several coagulation enzymes, including thrombin and activated factors X, XII, XI, and IX. The biologic half-life of heparin is 30–60 minutes; its effects can be reversed in 2–4 hours after an infusion is stopped. Heparin prolongs PTT.

24. What is low-molecular-weight heparin (LMWH)?

LMWH is a fragment produced by the chemical breakdown of heparin. It exerts its anticoagulant effect by binding with antithrombin III and inhibiting several coagulation enzymes. LMWH principally inhibits activated factor X.

25. What are the major differences between standard heparin and LMWH?

1. LMWH has a longer half-life and thus can be administered once daily.

2. LMWH gives a more predictable anticoagulant response at high doses and thus can be administered without monitoring (i.e., serial activated PTTs).

3. LMWH produces less bleeding complications than standard heparin at equivalent antithrombotic doses.

BIBLIOGRAPHY

1. Biopure Corporation: World's first oxygen therapeutic for human use approved in South Africa to treat acute anemia in surgery patients. www.biopure.com April 10, 2001.

 2. Cooper ES, et al: Practice parameter for the use of fresh-frozen plasma, cryoprecipitate, and platelets. JAMA 271:777, 1994.
 3. Coursin DB, Monk TG: Extreme normovolemic hemodilution: How low can you go and other alternatives to transfusion? Crit Care Med 29:908–909, 2001.
 4. Fakhry SM, Rutherford EJ, Sheldon GF: Hematologic principles in surgery. In Townsend CM, et al (eds): Sabiston Textbook of Surgery, 16th ed. Philadelphia, W.B. Saunders, 2001, pp 68-89.
 5. Goodnough LT, Brecher ME, Kanter MH, AuBuchon JP: Transfusion medicine. I: Blood transfusion. N Engl J Med 340:438–447, 1999.
 6. Herbert PC, Wells G, Blajchman MA, et al: A multicenter, randomized, controlled clinical trial of transfusion requirements in critical care. N Engl J Med 340:409-417, 1999
 7. Hess JR: Blood substitutes. Semin Hematol 33:369–378, 1996.
 8. Iperen CE, Gaillard CAMJ, Kraaijenhagen RJ, et al: Response of erythropoiesis and iron metabolism to recombinant human erythropoietin in intensive care unit patients. Crit Care Med 28:2773–2778, 2000.
 9. Kaufmann CR, Dwyer KM, Crews JD, et al: Usefulness of thrombelastography in assessment of trauma patient coagulation. J Trauma 42:716, 1997.
10. Litin SC, Gastineau DA: Current concepts in anticoagulant therapy. Mayo Clin Proc 70:266, 1995.

58. THROMBOCYTOPENIA AND PLATELETS

Hasan B. Alam, M.D., and Mark W. Bowyer, M.D.

1. What are the two principal functions of platelets in effecting hemostasis?

Platelets function to effect hemostasis by (1) formation of an initial platelet plug when exposed to subendothelial collagen and (2) by degranulation and secretion of proteins and catalysts for the clotting cascade. The initial platelet plug is a loose aggregation of platelets in an area of intimal injury and requires the presence of von Willebrand factor to form an adequate "plug." Heparin does not affect this primary hemostasis, which explains why hemostasis can occur in heparinized patients.

2. What is the most common congenital coagulation problem affecting platelet function?

Von Willebrand's (VW) disease. The absence of the VW factor disrupts the formation of platelet aggregates (see question 1).

3. How is thrombocytopenia defined?

A platelet count of less than 100,000 per cubic millimeter is considered to constitute thrombocytopenia, which is the most common platelet disorder in surgical patients.

4. What are the basic mechanisms causing thrombocytopenia?

It can be caused by decreased platelet production (marrow failure or replacement by cancerous cells or fibrosis), disordered platelet distribution/sequestration (hypersplenism), or increased platelet destruction (e.g., antibody-mediated destruction, prosthetic valves, extracorporeal bypass, disseminated intravascular coagulation [DIC]). These mechanisms can occur in isolation or in combination.

5. What is hypersplenism?

Hypersplenism refers only to excessive splenic function, which leads to accelerated destruction of the circulating cellular elements. Varying degrees of anemia, leukopenia, and thrombocytopenia will be present. Hypersplenism can occur in the absence of splenomegaly, as in chronic idiopathic thrombocytopenic purpura (ITP). If splenomegaly is present, the condition is called secondary hypersplenism.

6. What treatment options are available for patients with immune thrombocytopenic purpura (ITP)?

ITP is caused by IgG antibodies against the platelet glycoproteins (GPIIb/IIIa and GPIb/IX). Corticosteroids have long been the mainstay of therapy. Because of the side effects of long-term use, however, alternative therapies are commonly prescribed, including intravenous immunoglobulins (IVIG) and intravenous anti-D (IV anti-D). Both cause Fc receptor blockade as an important mechanism of acute platelet increase. IVIG works fast (within 24 hours) and can be used in Rh-negative and splenectomized patients, whereas IV anti-D causes a slower rate of platelet increase (within 72 hours) and is relatively ineffective in Rh-negative and splenectomized patients. IV anti-D is, however, effective in HIV-positive patients. Patients who initially respond to medical management but have a relapse within 1–3 months may be considered candidates for splenectomy. For refractory ITP combination chemotherapy (CHOP-like [cyclophosphamide, hydroxydaunomycin, Oncovin, prednisone]; vincristine, IVIG, solumedrol) is used initially, followed by maintenance therapy (e.g., combinations of steroids, danazol, azathioprine, mycophenolate mofetil, and cyclosporine).

7. How do you differentiate between thrombotic thrombocytopenic purpura (TTP) and hemolytic uremic syndrome (HUS)?

ITP and HUS share the following features: thrombocytopenia, hemolytic anemia, and thrombotic occlusions (mostly platelet plugs) in terminal arterioles and capillaries. Differentiating clinical features are the presence of focal neurologic symptoms in TTP and renal impairment in HUS. In addition, levels of plasma VW factor-cleaving protease are low in TTP and normal in HUD.

8. What is heparin-induced thrombocytopenia (HIT)?

Heparin continues to be the most common cause of drug-induced, antibody-mediated thrombocytopenia. The diagnosis must be considered in any patient who develops thrombocytopenia, has an unexplained fall in platelet count of 30–40%, or develops thrombotic complications 5–10 days after exposure to heparin. Two clinically distinct types of HIT have been described. HIT type I results in a mild reduction in platelet counts (usually > 100,000/mm^3) during the first few days of therapy and is thought to be related to a nonimmunologic platelet-aggregating effect of heparin. This effect may be seen in up to 28% of patients receiving either unfractionated (UF) or low-molecular-weight heparin (LMWH). HIT type II, which is immunologically mediated, is much less common (1–2%) and results in marked thrombocytopenia 5–10 days after the initiation of therapy. HIT type II may be associated with arterial and venous thrombosis in about one-half of patients. The onset is usually rapid (median time: 10.5 hours) in patients with recent exposure to heparin (within past 3 months). LMWH also has been associated with HIT type II, although less frequently than UF heparin. HIT with thrombotic complications has a mortality rate of 20%, and about 10% of patients require limb amputations.

9. How is HIT diagnosed?

A high index of suspicion is the key to early diagnosis, and in most patients the clinical presentation is highly suggestive. In complicated or unclear cases, laboratory tests can be done to support the diagnosis. Almost one-half of all patients with HIT have circulating antibodies to complexes composed of platelet factor 4 (PF4) and heparin. However, because most patients with circulating antibodies do not develop clinical HIT, screening of asymptomatic patients is not indicated. Two types of assays are available: functional assays and immunoassays. Functional assays measure heparin-dependent platelet activation by PF4-heparin antibodies in vitro. The [14]serotonin-release assay (STA) is considered the gold standard because of its positive predictive value of almost 100%; its negative predictive value, however, is about 20%. Immunoassays (e.g., enzyme-linked immunosorbent assay [ELISA]) measure the levels of antibodies in circulation, with a sensitivity of 93–97%, positive predictive value of 93–100%, specificity of 86–100%, and negative predictive value of 88–95%.

10. How is HIT treated?

Type I HIT requires no specific treatment; mild thrombocytopenia resolves even with the continuation of heparin. Type II HIT requires immediate withdrawal of all heparin. Because distinguishing between type I and type II can be difficult, the decision to stop heparin should be considered carefully on the basis of the clinical scenario. If continued anticoagulation is required, a vitamin K antagonist (warfarin) should be initiated. Until therapeutic levels of warfarin are achieved, an alternative, immediate-acting anticoagulant should be used. Newer agents for this purpose include:

Danaproid (low-molecular-weight glycosaminoglycan composed of heparin sulfate, dermatin sulfate, and chondroitin sulfate) acts primarily against factor Xa and has a limited antithrombin effect. Dose is titrated to keep anti-factor Xa levels between 0.5 and 0.8 U/ml. There is no antidote for bleeding.

Recombinant hirudin (lepirudin [Refludin]) is a 7-kDa peptide that acts directly on circulating and clot-bound thrombin. Anticoagulant effects last about 40 minutes. It is given as a slow bolus (0.4 mg/kg) followed by continuous infusion at 0.15 mg/kg to maintain activated partial thromboplastin time (aPPT) between 1.5 and 2.5 times baseline.

Argatroban is a 509-dalton, arginine-based direct thrombin inhibitor that inhibits both soluble and clot-bound thrombin. Its half-life is 10.2–46.2 minutes, and steady-state activity is achieved within 1–2 hours of continuous infusion. The dose is adjusted to keep aPTT between 1.5 and 3 times baseline (maximal dose: 10 gm/kg/min).

11. Does sepsis contribute to thrombocytopenia?

Thrombocytopenia, probably immune-mediated, is associated with sepsis. Treatment of the cause of sepsis restores the platelet count to normal.

12. Discuss some causes of platelet dysfunction in the ICU.

The principal causes of platelet dysfunction and thrombocytopenia in the ICU are drug side effects, uremia, and sepsis. Antibiotics, nitrates, local anesthetics, alpha- and beta-adrenergic blockers, xanthine derivatives, diuretics, H_2 receptor blockers, and dextran are examples of drugs that can impair platelet activity. Uremia, also a common condition among ICU patients, is an important cause of platelet dysfunction.

13. What are the indications for platelet transfusion?

The platelet count that should serve as a trigger for platelet transfusion has evolved over the past two decades. Although somewhat controversial, the following threshold levels have been proposed in the literature:

- Bleeding prophylaxis in a stable oncologic patient: $10,000/m^3$ (formerly $< 20,000/mm^{3)}$
- Lumbar puncture in a leukemic patient: $10,000/mm^3$
- Stable HIT: $10,000/mm^3$
- Bone marrow aspiration: $20,000/mm^3$
- Gastrointestinal endoscopy in patients with cancer: $20,000–40,000/mm^3$
- DIC: $20,000–50,000/mm^3$
- Fiberoptic bronchoscopy: $20,000–50,000/m^3$
- Major surgery: $50,000/mm^3$
- Thrombocytopenia secondary to massive transfusion: $50,000/mm^3$
- Invasive procedures in patients with cirrhosis: $50,000/mm^3$
- Cardiopulmonary bypass: $50,000–60,000/mm^3$
- Neurosurgical procedures: $100,000/mm^3$
- Thrombocytopenia and bleeding (intracerebral, gastrointestinal, genitourinary, or retinal hemorrhage): $100,000/mm^3$

There is no specific count at which bleeding is completely prevented. In addition to the count, quality and function of platelets are also important. However, life-threatening bleeds can occur with platelet counts $< 5,000/mm^3$ and spontaneous bleeding with counts $< 10,000–20,000/mm^3$.

14. How does aspirin affect platelet function?
Aspirin irreversibly inhibits platelet cyclo-oxygenase, resulting in a functional platelet defect that persists for the duration of the platelet's life span (8–9 days). The optimal dose of aspirin required to decrease morbidity and mortality from atherosclerotic disease is yet to be determined.

15. What laboratory test measures platelet function?
The bleeding time is a sensitive measurement of platelet function.

16. How are platelet disorders managed?
The patient's drug regimen should be carefully scrutinized to eliminate or substitute medications implicated in thrombocytopenia. Platelet transfusion may be required. Uremia-associated thrombocytopenia can be treated with hemodialysis. Cryoprecipitate, 1-desamino-8-D-arginine vasopressin (DDAVP), and conjugated estrogens also have been used with good results.

BIBLIOGRAPHY

1. AuBuchon JP: Platelet transfusion therapy. Clin Lab Med 16:797–816, 1996.
2. Chong BH, Eisbacher M: Pathology and laboratory testing of heparin-induced thrombocytopenia. Semin Hematol 35(4):3–8, 1998.
3. Eisenstaedt RS: Transfusion therapy: Blood components and transfusion complications. In Rippe JM, et al (eds): Intensive Care Medicine, 3rd ed., Boston, Little Brown, 1996, pp 1414–1420.
4. Fuse I: Disorders of platelet function. Crit Rev Oncol Hematol 22:1–25, 1996.
5. Goldstein KH, Abramson N: Efficient diagnosis of thrombocytopenia. Am Fam Physician 53:915–920, 1995.
6. Green RM: Treatment of heparin-induced thrombocytopenia and thrombosis. Semin Vasc Surg 9:292–295, 1996.
7. Hussein MA, Hoeltge GA: Platelet transfusion therapy for medical and surgical patients. Cleve Clin J Med 63:245–250, 1996.
8. Lipsett PA, Perler BA: The use of blood products for surgical bleeding. Semin Vasc Surg 9:347–353, 1996.
9. McCrae KR, Bussel JB, Mannucci PM, et al: Platelets: An update on diagnosis and management of thrombocytopenic disorders. Hematology (Am Soc Hematol Educ Progr) 1:282–305, 2001.
10. National Institutes of Health: Platelet transfusion therapy. NIH Consensus Statement 6(7):1–6, 1986.
11. Rebulla P: Platelet transfusion trigger in difficult patients. Transfus Clin Biol 8:249–254, 2001.

59. DISSEMINATED INTRAVASCULAR COAGULATION

Jonathan Rosenberg, M.D., and Julie Hambleton, M.D.

1. What is disseminated intravascular coagulation (DIC)?
DIC is not a disease entity in itself but a dynamic process involving clotting activation, thrombin generation, consumption of coagulation factors, deposition of fibrin, and fibrinolysis. Both excessive thrombin and plasmin can be produced; therefore, both thrombosis and bleeding can be seen simultaneously.

2. What are the various forms of DIC?
DIC can be acute and fulminant in conditions such as amniotic fluid embolism and meningococcemia or chronic, subtle, and asymptomatic in conditions such as malignancy and collagen vascular disease. Consumption of clotting factors can occur systemically throughout the entire vascular system, or it can be localized within hemangiomas, aortic aneurysms, and renal allografts undergoing rejection.

3. What characterizes acute and chronic DIC?

In **acute DIC**, thromboplastic material (endogenous or exogenous) is released suddenly into the vascular system. As a result, the delicate balance between coagulation factors and the fibrinolytic system/anticoagulant factors is disturbed. Coagulation factors are consumed, and the fibrinolytic system is activated, leading to major bleeding. Microvascular thrombosis causes tissue ischemia and dysfunction. Both bleeding and clotting may be observed at the same time.

In **chronic DIC**, coagulation activation is compensated by increased coagulation factor and platelet production as well as increased activity of the fibrinolytic system. The clinical presentation of chronic DIC is quite variable. Both mild bleeding and macrovascular thromboses (deep venous thrombosis, arterial emboli) may occur, but microvascular thrombosis leading to organ damage is unusual. Chronic DIC may present solely with laboratory abnormalities without clinical sequelae.

4. In critical care, which conditions are associated with DIC?

Any condition that produces damage or disruption of vascular endothelium or that releases damaged or necrotic tissue into the bloodstream can be the trigger for DIC. Classically, obstetric complications, sepsis, injuries (especially brain and crush injuries), shock, hypoxia, burns, vasculitis, transfusion reactions, anaphylaxis, immune complex diseases, and treatment of malignancies such as acute promyelocytic leukemia are among the dozens of causes of acute DIC.

5. What are some of the common causes of chronic DIC?

Malignancies—especially disseminated prostate cancer, mucin-producing adenocarcinomas, and acute promyelocytic leukemia—can be associated with chronic DIC. Vascular disorders such as giant hemangiomas, aortic aneurysms, and valvular heart disease can produce local consumption with systemic signs of DIC. Some obstetric complications, such as eclampsia and retained dead-fetus syndrome, produce chronic DIC. Other associated conditions include acute myocardial infarction, peripheral vascular disease, paroxysmal nocturnal hemoglobinuria, polycythemia vera, myeloid metaplasia, autoimmune diseases, glomerulonephritis, sarcoidosis, amyloidosis, diabetes, hyperlipoproteinemias, and liver disease. At any time, the balance may shift and an acute process may emerge.

6. What are the clinical signs of acute and chronic DIC?

In **acute DIC,** microvascular thrombi may predominate. Skin, kidneys, and lungs are the major targets, but brain, gastrointestinal tract, liver, heart, and pancreas also are commonly affected. Acral cyanosis, delirium, coma, oliguria, azotemia, hypoxia, dyspnea, and ulceration reflect tissue ischemia. Frank necrosis of tissue may lead to skin necrosis, gangrene, cerebral infarction, renal cortical necrosis, and pulmonary and bowel infarction. If bleeding predominates, petechiae and ecchymoses appear, and skin puncture sites ooze. Genitourinary, pulmonary, gastrointestinal, and intracranial hemorrhage can follow.

In **chronic DIC**, the bleeding may be milder. Mucous membranes and puncture sites oozing as well as petechiae and ecchymoses may predominate. Both venous and arterial thromboembolic disease also may develop. Chronic compensated DIC may be clinically silent and evident only as abnormal lab values.

7. What lab values characterize DIC in the acute and chronic forms?

In **acute DIC**, prothrombin time (PT), activated partial thromboplastin time (aPTT), and thrombin time are prolonged. Platelet count and fibrinogen are often decreased. Levels of fibrin/fibrinogen degradation products (FDPs) and D-dimers may be elevated.

The **chronic or compensated form** shows a more variable pattern. Changes similar to acute DIC are seen but often are less severe. In many cases, however, PT and aPTT may be normal or "supernormal" because the presence of activated factors affects in vitro tests. Fibrinogen may be normal or elevated as an acute-phase reactant. Platelets may be normal or slightly depressed. FDPs and D-dimer levels should be elevated in nearly every case. Numerous other specialized coagulation tests become abnormal with DIC but are not commonly available.

8. What clues are present in the peripheral smear for DIC?

A blood smear from a patient with DIC may show red cell fragments (schistocytes), poly-chromatophilia, leukocytosis with a left shift, and moderate-to-severe thrombocytopenia. Schistocytes are present in 90% of patients with chronic DIC but in only 50% of patients with acute DIC. An abnormal peripheral smear with some or all of the above features is suggestive but not diagnostic of DIC.

9. What laboratory abnormalities may confound the diagnosis of DIC?

Fibrinogen is an acute-phase reactant and may be normal or elevated in a variety of inflamma-tory states that accompany severe illness. As a result, it is not always a reliable marker of con-sumption. Following the trend of fibrinogen levels over time may indicate the presence of a consumptive process. Coexisting liver disease may make the diagnosis more difficult (see below).

10. Is it possible to make the diagnosis of DIC in the setting of advanced liver disease?

The liver produces the majority of coagulation factors. Impaired liver synthetic function pre-vents replenishment of depleted clotting factors. Poor reticuloendothelial clearance in the liver of FDPs and activated clotting factors can lead to elevated levels of FDPs and D-dimers as well as prolonged PT. Fibrinogen is produced by the liver and may be decreased in patients with liver disease. Furthermore, thrombocytopenia is common in liver disease. As a result, DIC is often in-distinguishable from advanced liver disease. However, laboratory abnormalities in liver disease tend to be fairly stable, whereas in DIC they progressively worsen over time.

11. Discuss the treatment of DIC.

In both acute and chronic DIC, initial therapy is directed toward the underlying cause. Hemodynamic support is critical in acute fulminant DIC. More specific tools, depending on the cause of DIC, include evacuation of the uterus in women with dead-fetus syndrome, antibiotics in patients with infection, and anticancer therapy in patients with malignancy. If the inciting event cannot be reversed or if a prolonged recovery time is expected after reversal, therapy may be needed for the DIC process to prevent further thromboses and bleeding.

Many authors urge stopping the consumption process with intravenous or subcutaneous he-parin before replacing specific coagulation components (fresh frozen plasma, cryoprecipitate, platelets), although this approach must be considered carefully in the bleeding patient. If bleeding continues after consumption is controlled and hemostatic factors are replaced to satisfactory levels, some authors recommend antifibrinolytic therapy with epsilon-aminocaproic acid. Its use is controversial and potentially hazardous, because blocking fibrinolysis may accelerate microvascu-lar clotting. In chronic DIC, hemorrhage is not usually life threatening, but thrombosis may be a serious complication. Anticoagulation may or may not be appropriate during treatment of the un-derlying triggering event. Subcutaneous heparin, oral anticoagulants, and antiplatelet agents (as-pirin, dipyridamole) have had variable success. Blood component therapy is rarely needed.

12. How is the efficacy of DIC therapy evaluated?

With adequate liver function, fibrinogen levels should rise and FDP levels should fall within 3–6 hours after therapy is initiated. Improvement in platelets, PT, and aPTT may vary with re-placement efforts and endogenous production rates of the various elements. Thrombotic and bleeding phenomena should gradually cease. Heparin therapy may be initiated as follows:

1. Institute heparin at 7.5 U/kg/hr IV.

2. One or two hours later, transfuse platelets to reach a count of 50, and give cryoprecipitate to reach a fibrinogen level of 150 (one unit should increase fibrinogen by 5–10 mg/dl).

3. Measure platelet and fibrinogen levels 30–60 minutes after transfusion.

4. Repeat determinations every 2–4 hours.

5. If adequate counts and levels cannot be attained or counts and levels fall, increase heparin by 2.5 U/kg/hr.

6. Repeat sequence of evaluation.

An alternative approach includes waiting 4 hours after initiation of aggressive therapy for the underlying cause of DIC. If parameters do not stabilize or improve, begin heparin subcutaneously at a dose of 80 U/kg every 4–6 hours).

CONTROVERSIES

13. Is heparin really indicated in DIC?

Few well-designed, objective studies have addressed this question. Most authors agree that termination of the inciting event is the most desirable approach to the treatment of DIC. When the causes of DIC are more difficult to control, heparin may be used to blunt the consequences of ongoing DIC. Some believe that heparin is indicated for amniotic fluid embolism, severe transfusion reactions, macrovascular thromboses, prevention of DIC with treatment of promyelocytic leukemia, retained fetus syndrome, purpura fulminans, septic abortion, heat stroke, and septicemia. Others believe that it is of no help in sepsis, shock, or obstetric complications. Its use in patients with renal or hepatic failure, extensive vascular damage, severe thrombocytopenia, or hypofibrinogenemia is hazardous. Most authors agree, however, that when heparin is used in DIC, careful monitoring of the patient and lab parameters is essential.

14. What dose of heparin is effective?

Full-dose heparin is used for embolic events and major vessel occlusion. The dose necessary to control microvascular thromboses and to stop consumption remains controversial. Some authors recommend full-dose heparin; others believe that low-dose heparin (400–500 U/hr intravenously or 80 U/kg every 4–6 hr subcutaneously) may suffice to prevent new thromboses at the microvascular level. The dose of heparin can be titrated to achieve therapeutic efficacy. There is also a lower risk of hemorrhage with lower dosing levels. Intravenous heparin allows better moment-to-moment control than subcutaneous heparin. Whatever method is chosen, the clinical situation, fibrinogen, D-dimer, and FDP levels along with platelet counts should be monitored for stabilization or improvement.

15. What information does D-dimer add to FDP levels?

In the DIC process, fibrin is generated, then digested by plasmin. FDP levels are believed to be the most sensitive test for the combined result of thrombin and plasmin activation. FDP measures the products of both fibrinogen and fibrin degradation. The D-dimer test detects elevated levels of fragments of crosslinked fibrin. It specifically shows that thrombin has been produced, causing the crosslinking of fibrin clot via activated factor XIII and that fibrinolysis has occurred via plasmin action. D-dimer is elevated in over 90% of confirmed DIC cases and is specific for fibrin degradation. It is a confirmatory test for interpreting elevated FDP.

16. What therapies are under evaluation for patients with DIC?

DIC in sepsis is a major cause of morbidity and mortality. Recent work with recombinant activated protein C in patients with severe sepsis and evidence of DIC showed a nearly 20% relative survival advantage at 28 days. Bleeding during infusion of the drug was the major adverse event. Recombinant activated protein C, however, has not yet been approved by the Food and Drug Administration. High-dose antithrombin III concentrates show no survival advantage in patients with severe sepsis due to infection. Another promising agent is recombinant nematode anticoagulant protein C2, an inhibitor of the Xa complex.

BIBLIOGRAPHY

1. Baker WF: Clinical aspects of disseminated intravascular coagulation: A clinician's point of view. Semin Thromb Hemost 15:1–57, 1989.
2. Bick RL: Disseminated intravascular coagulation: Objective clinical and laboratory diagnosis, treatment, and assessment of therapeutic response. Semin Thromb Hemost 22:69–88, 1996.
3. Bernard GR, et al: Efficacy and safety of recombinant human activated protein C for severe sepsis. N Engl J Med 344:699–709, 2001.

4. Beulter E, Lechtman MD, Collier BS, Kipps TJ (eds): Williams' Hematology, 5th ed. New York, McGraw-Hill, 1995.
5. Cembrowski GS, Griffin JH, Mosher DF: Diagnostic efficacy of six plasma proteins in evaluating consumptive coagulopathies. Arch Intern Med 146:1997–2002, 1989.
6. Feinstein DI: Treatment of disseminated intravascular coagulation. Semin Thromb Hemost 14:351–362, 1988.
7. Fourrier F, Chopin C, Huart J, et al: Double blind, placebo-controlled trial of antithrombin III concentrates in septic shock with disseminated intravascular coagulation. Chest 104:882–888, 1993.
8. Fuse S, Tomita H, Yoshida M, et al: High dose of intravenous antithrombin III without heparin in the treatment of disseminated intravascular coagulation and organ failure in four children. Am J Hematol 53:18–21, 1996.
9. Goad KE, Gralnick HR: Coagulation disorders in cancer. Hematol Oncol Clin North Am 10:457–484, 1996.
10. Humphries JE: Transfusion therapy in acquired coagulopathies. Hematol Oncol Clin North Am 8:1181–1201, 1994.
11. Levi M, Ten Cate H: Disseminated intravascular coagulation. N Engl J Med 341:586–592, 1999.
12. Richey ME, Gilstrap LC, Ramin SM: Management of disseminated intravascular coagulopathy. Clin Obstet Gynecol 38:514–520, 1995.
13. Warren BL, et al: High-dose antithrombin III for severe sepsis: A randomized controlled trial. JAMA 286:1869–1878, 2001.

60. SICKLE CELL DISEASE

Kathryn L. Hassell, M.D.

1. What is sickle cell disease?

The term *sickle cell disease* refers to a group of inherited hemoglobinopathies in which abnormal beta-hemoglobin chains are produced. They occur when one beta-globin gene has the sickle cell mutation (valine is substituted for glutamic acid in the sixth position of the beta chain) and the other beta-globin gene is abnormal. People who carry one hemoglobin S gene and one normal gene have **sickle cell trait (HbAS)**. They do not have sickle cell disease, although concentrating defects in the kidney, occasional hematuria, and, less commonly, papillary necrosis and splenic infarction at high altitude may occur.

Patients with two hemoglobin S genes have **sickle cell anemia (HbSS)**, which is characterized by hemolytic anemia with baseline elevations in reticulocyte count and indirect bilirubin as well as episodic painful ischemic events due to sickling of red blood cells with occlusion of small blood vessels by adherent and/or deformed cells. Even in the absence of pain, chronic organ damage often occurs, especially in the spleen, lungs, kidneys, retina, and femoral and humeral heads.

Patients who have one hemoglobin S gene and one hemoglobin C gene have **HgbSC disease**, which usually is associated with milder anemia, fewer painful episodes, and less chronic organ injury than sickle cell anemia.

Patients with one gene for hemoglobin S and one gene with a mutation for beta-thalassemia have **HbSβ° or HbSβ⁺ thalassemia**. HbSβ° thalassemia clinically resembles sickle cell anemia in severity. HbSβ⁺ thalassemia is usually less severe, with mild anemia, relatively fewer painful episodes, and less chronic organ injury compared with sickle cell anemia. The mean corpuscular volume (MCV) is low in both forms, reflecting the thalassemic component.

When sickle cells are exposed to extreme conditions, such as hypoxia or osmotic changes (e.g., dehydration), the sickle hemoglobin can polymerize, and the red cell assumes a sickled shape, which occludes small vessels and can cause acute and chronic organ damage. Even without sickling, however, red blood cells express increased adhesion molecules and adhere to vascular endothelium, resulting in vascular injury and chronic organ damage.

2. How is sickle cell disease diagnosed?

Sickle cell disease is diagnosed by hemoglobin electrophoresis. Because of the differences in charges, hemoglobin S and other abnormal hemoglobins migrate differently from normal hemoglobin A. Use of "sickle cell prep," which detects the presence of hemoglobin S, cannot distinguish among sickle cell trait (AS), sickle cell anemia (SS), HgbSC disease, HbSβ° thalassemia, or HbSβ$^+$ thalassemia, because it it does not quantitate the amount of sickle hemoglobin or detect other abnormal hemoglobins.

3. What evaluation should be done for patients presenting with a painful sickle cell crisis?

A painful crisis, characterized in many patients by diffuse pain in the back, abdomen, or extremities, may be triggered by a precipitating event, which should be corrected to prevent further vasoocclusion. Extremes of temperature and heavy physical exertion may predispose to crises; dehydration can occur easily with poor oral intake or excessive fluid losses due to the renal concentrating defect induced by chronic ischemia to the renal medulla. Infections may precipitate a painful crisis. Despite thorough evaluation, however, the precipitating event of some crises cannot be determined.

Evaluation should include careful history-taking and a thorough physical examination with attention to possible sites of infection. Laboratory studies should include complete blood count with a reticulocyte count to confirm that the patient is producing red blood cells in response to the increased destruction of sickled cells. Baseline chemistry testing should be done to determine hepatic and renal function. Cultures of urine, sputum, and blood, followed by empirical antibiotic coverage, should be done in the setting of fever. A chest x-ray is useful in patients with hypoxia, a history of pulmonary disease, or pulmonary signs or symptoms.

4. What infections are common in sickle cell disease?

Because most patients with sickle cell anemia (HbSS) and HbSβ° thalassemia have an infarcted spleen by age 3 or 4 years, they are susceptible to encapsulated organisms, including *Haemophilus influenzae, Streptococcus pneumoniae,* and *Neisseria meningitidis.* Pyelonephritis is also common, is often associated with bacteremia, and predisposes to sickling with subsequent papillary necrosis. Osteomyelitis can also develop and is most commonly caused by staphylococci, although the incidence of osteomyelitis due to *Salmonella* species is increased in sickle cell patients compared with other patients.

5. How are painful sickle cell crises treated?

The usual approach to painful crisis includes intravenous fluids to attain and maintain adequate, but not excessive, hydration. Supplemental oxygen by nasal cannula is given to reverse any hypoxia that may precipitate red cell adhesion and sickling. Parenteral analgesics, usually morphine sulfate, are given intravenously on a fixed schedule (not as needed) until the pain has subsided enough to use oral analgesics. Evidence of infection (positive urinalysis or cultures) is treated appropriately, and in the setting of fever, empirical intravenous antibiotic coverage is recommended.

6. Define acute chest syndrome.

Acute chest syndrome (ACS) may develop in the setting of an acute painful crisis and is characterized by chest pain, fever, increasing hypoxia, and, ultimately, development of pulmonary infiltrates on chest x-ray. It may occur in the setting of pneumonia but is probably pathophysiologically distinct and represents leaky vascular endothelium and ischemia of the lung due to sickled and/or adherent red blood cells. Studies have demonstrated that ACS is more commonly associated with infection in children and with pulmonary fat emboli in adults. Pulmonary embolism (not associated with sickle cell disease) may be an appropriate consideration; if present, it should be treated with anticoagulation. Otherwise, heparin has not been shown to be an effective therapy for ACS. Treatment may involve simple red blood cell transfusion or red blood cell exchange transfusion (see below) to remove sickled blood and arrest the process. Because it is often difficult to differentiate between worsening pneumonia and ACS, intravenous antibiotics should be given.

7. What is aplastic crisis?

Aplastic crisis is characterized by a rapid fall in hemoglobin associated with few or no reticulocytes and indicating a failure of the bone marrow to respond to increased cell turnover. Folate deficiency can occur in the setting of chronic hemolytic anemia if the patient does not take supplemental folate, and this may precipitate an aplastic crisis. Parvovirus (B19) has been associated with bone marrow suppression and subsequent aplastic crisis; other viral infections or severe bacterial infections may also suppress the bone marrow. Treatment of aplastic crisis becomes necessary when the hematocrit becomes dangerously low. Packed red blood cells are given to support an adequate hematocrit until bone marrow suppression is resolved, folate is repleted, and the reticulocyte count improves.

8. What is splenic sequestration?

Splenic sequestration usually does not occur in adults with HbSS or HbSβ° thalassemia because the spleen has infarcted by age 3 or 4 years. In HbSC disease or HbSβ+ thalassemia, however, the disease is relatively mild and splenic function can be preserved into adulthood. Splenic sequestration is characterized by rapid, painful enlargement of the spleen, with rapid falls in hemoglobin and occasionally platelets due to sickling and sudden intravascular pooling of blood in the spleen. In adults, the sequestration is often relatively mild, with only a 1–2 gm/dl drop in hemoglobin; transfusion is rarely required for support. On rare occasions, the spleen may become so massive and/or necrotic that splenectomy is required.

9. What cerebrovascular complications can occur with sickle cell disease?

Stroke may affect as many as 6–12% of patients with sickle cell anemia (HbSS) or HbSβ° thalassemia in childhood or young adulthood. In children, strokes tend to be thrombotic in nature, whereas adults tend to have hemorrhagic strokes. These strokes are usually due to large-vessel disease, and abnormal vessels may be seen on angiogram or magnetic resonance imaging in some cases. Acute management involves red blood cell exchange transfusion to remove sickle red blood cells and enhance oxygen-carrying capacity. Simple blood transfusions are not recommended because blood viscosity may be increased with increased hematocrit if sickled cells are not removed. Hyperventilation should be avoided, and anticonvulsants are sometimes needed, since seizures can occur during acute infarction.

10. What other acute complications may develop with sickle cell disease?

Intrahepatic sickling can occur, with rapid rises in liver enzymes, a fall in hemoglobin due to sequestration in the liver, and, in severe cases, an extreme rise in conjugated bilirubin and prothrombin time, indicating acute liver failure. Acute renal failure, in the absence of sepsis or other systemic illness, is relatively uncommon. Acute multiorgan failure syndrome, characterized by acute pulmonary, hepatic, and renal failure, can occur but may be rapidly reversed with exchange or simple transfusion. Priapism can occur with or without systemic painful crisis. Gallstones are very common due to chronic hyperbilirubinemia and may cause acute cholecystitis or common bile duct obstruction. Acute myocardial infarction is not more common in patients with sickle cell disease than in the general population; however, pulmonary hypertension, probably due to chronic lung injury by sickle red blood cells, is thought to be the leading cause of death in adult patients with sickle cell disease.

11. What are the surgical risks for patients with sickle cell disease?

Patients with sickle cell anemia (HbSS) or HbSβ° who undergo general anesthesia may be at increased risk for development of acute painful crisis and ACS. Simple transfusion therapy, with a goal of reducing the percentage of sickle hemoglobin to 60%, was as effective as exchange transfusion (with < 30% HgbS) in preventing perioperative complications in a recent randomized trial in sickle cell anemia. Patients should be carefully monitored for hypoxia, with a minimum of 50% oxygen in combination with the anesthetic agent, to avoid precipitation of red cell sickling. Adequate hydration should be carefully maintained.

12. Discuss the role of acute transfusion in sickle cell disease.

Packed red blood cell transfusions are indicated in the setting of severe anemia with hemo-dynamic instability, severe hypoxia, or acute end-organ injury. The final hematocrit after transfu-sion should not exceed a value > 30% because blood viscosity will increase at higher values. In patients with a baseline hematocrit > 30%, transfusion therapy should result in a return to base-line hematocrit. If life-threatening events such as acute stroke, acute liver failure, ACS, acute pri-apism, or arterial hypoxia syndrome develop, red blood cell exchange transfusion should be considered, especially if the hematocrit has not fallen significantly below baseline values. Most commonly, an apheresis instrument can be used in an automated exchange procedure through a double-lumen dialysis catheter. Alternatively, aliquots of blood are removed through an arterial or venous line and replaced with whole blood or "reconstituted" packed red blood cells. In all cases of transfusion, an effort should be made to match transfused units to minor antigens on the patient's red blood cells (minor antigen match); otherwise, sickle cell patients tend to rapidly de-velop multiple alloantibodies, making future cross-matching difficult.

13. Discuss the role of hydroxyurea (Hydrea) in the treatment of sickle cell disease.

In some patients with sickle cell disease, there is persistent production of hemoglobin F (fetal hemoglobin). These patients have been observed to have a milder form of sickle cell disease. Hydroxyurea therapy is associated with increased production of hemoglobin F in sickle cell pa-tients. A placebo-controlled trial of hydroxyurea in adults with severe sickle cell anemia (HbSS) or HbSβ° thalassemia demonstrated a 50% reduction in pain events and ACS. This study suggests that hydroxyurea may offer benefits to adults with sickle cell anemia (HbSS) or HbSβ° thalassemia who have frequent pain events or recurrent ACS. However, it has not been shown to offer protection against stroke or chronic organ injury or to have benefits in other forms of sickle cell disease.

CONTROVERSIES

14. Is pulse oximetry reliable in sickle cell patients?

Noninvasive assessment of oxygen saturation can be done using a pulse oximeter, with good correlation to measured saturation by arterial blood gas. It has recently been noted, however, that in patients with sickle cell disease pulse oximetry may be off by as much as ± 4% compared with measured oxygen saturation by blood gas, especially in those with hemoglobins of less than 11 gm/dl. If there is doubt about hypoxia, an arterial blood gas analysis is indicated.

15. What is the role of bone marrow transplant in sickle cell disease?

Allogeneic bone marrow transplant has been successfully performed in children with severe sickle cell disease using matched sibling bone marrow or cord blood. Appropriate selection of candidates for transplant, application to adult patients, and the role of unrelated donors or mini-allogeneic transplantation have yet to be determined.

BIBLIOGRAPHY

1. Ataga K, Orringer E: Renal abnormalities in sickle cell disease. Am J Hematol 63:205, 2000.
2. Castro O, Finke-Castro H, Coats D: Improved method for automated red cell exchange in sickle cell dis-ease. J Clin Apheresis 3:93, 1986.
3 Charache S, Barton FB, Moore RD, et al: Hydroxyurea and sickle cell anemia. Clinical utility of a myelo-suppressive "switching" agent. The Multicenter Study of Hydroxyurea in Sickle Cell Anemia. Medicine 75:300, 1996.
4. Charache S, Lubin B, Reid CD: Management and therapy of sickle cell disease. NIH Publication No. 95-2117, 1995.
5 Comber JT, Lopez BL: Evaluation of pulse oximetry in sickle cell anemia patients presenting to the emer-gency department in acute vasooclussive crisis. Am J Emerg Med 14:16, 1996.
6. Deneberg BS, Criner G, Jones R, Spann J: Cardiac function in sickle cell anemia. Am J Cardiol 51:1674, 1985.
7. Hassell KL, Eckman JR, Lane PA: Acute multiorgan failure syndrome: A potentially catastrophic com-plication of severe sickle cell pain episodes. Am J Med 96:155, 1994.

8. Krauss J, Freant L, Lee J: Gastrointestinal pathology in sickle cell disease. Ann Clin Lab Sci 28:19, 1998.
9. Prohovnik I, Pavlakis SG, Pionelli S, et al: Cerebral hyperemia, stroke and transfusion in sickle cell disease. Neurology 34:344, 1989.
10. Vichinsky EP, Haberkern CM, Neumayr L, et al: A comparison of conservative and aggressive transfusion regimens in the perioperative management of sickle cell disease. The Preoperative Transfusion in Sickle Cell Disease Study Group. N Engl J Med 333:206, 1995.
10. Vichinsky EP, Neumayr L, Earles A, et al: Causes and outcomes of the acute chest syndrome in sickle cell disease. National Acute Chest Syndrome Study Group. N Engl J Med 342:1955, 2000.
11. Walter MC: Bone marrow transplantation for sickle cell disease: Where do we go from here? J Pediatr Hematol Oncol 21:467, 1999.

61. ONCOLOGIC EMERGENCIES

Deborah R. Cook, M.D., and William Eng Lee, M.D.

1. List important oncologic emergencies.
- Spinal cord compression
- Hypercalcemia
- Superior vena cava syndrome
- Tumor lysis
- Neutropenic fever
- Malignant pericardial effusion

2. Why is it important to identify and treat spinal cord compression quickly?
A delay in treatment of only a few hours may lead to irreversible neurologic damage.

3. What are the common clinical features of acute epidural spinal cord compression?
In more than 90% of patients, progressive axial or radicular pain precedes the diagnosis by days or months. It can mimic the symptoms of degenerative joint disease; however, the discomfort can occur at any level, is commonly aggravated by percussion of the spinal column, and is not relieved by recumbency. Sixty to 85% of patients with an epidural compression also report motor weakness. Other findings include autonomic dysfunction such as urinary retention, constipation, and sensory loss.

4. Which cancers commonly cause epidural spinal cord compression?
In adults, breast, lung, and prostate cancers account for more than 60%. In children, the most common cancers are sarcomas, neuroblastoma, and lymphoma.

5. Which imaging studies are helpful in making the diagnosis?
Radiographs: If vertebral body metastases are present, the chance of epidural disease is greater than 60%. However, false-negative radiographs are seen in 10–17% of patients with epidural spinal cord compression.
Bone scan: More sensitive than plain radiographs in detecting metastatic disease to the vertebral body. Bone scans are generally negative in multiple myeloma.
Computed tomography (CT) myelogram and magnetic resonance imaging (MRI): MRI and CT myelography are superior to plain films, bone scans, and CT as diagnostic imaging methods. Advantages of MRI include the following: (1) the entire thecal sac can be imaged, regardless of spinal block; (2) it is not contraindicated in patients with large brain metastases, thrombocytopenia, or coagulopathy; and (3) it is less invasive than a myelogram.

6. Discuss the treatment options for epidural spinal cord compression.
Corticosteroids: Dosing should begin immediately for optimal pain reduction and to improve neurologic symptoms. Dexamethasone, 10–100 mg, is administered as an intravenous

bolus, followed by 2–24 mg 4 times/day. The larger doses are reserved for patients with more profound neurologic findings.

Radiation: The definitive treatment consists of radiation therapy.

Surgery: Laminectomy or anterior decompression should be reserved for patients with spinal instability, uncertain diagnoses, epidural compression in areas of prior radiation, or progressive neurologic compromise despite steroids and radiation therapy.

7. List the three major mechanisms by which malignancy causes hypercalcemia.
1. Osteolytic metastases with local release of cytokines
2. Tumor secretion of parathyroid hormone (PTH)-related protein
3. Tumor production of 1,25-dihydroxyvitamin D (calcitriol)

8. What types of cancers are commonly associated with hypercalcemia?
Squamous cell cancers such as non-small cell lung, head and neck, esophageal, and cervical cancers can produce PTH-like peptides. Lymphoma, multiple myeloma, and hypernephromas can release other hormonal factors which contribute to hypercalcemia. Breast cancers and non-small cell lung carcinoma can cause hypercalcemia by direct bone metastases. Hodgkin's and some non-Hodgkin's lymphomas may produce calcitriol.

9. List the available therapies for hypercalcemia.
1. Intravenous hydration with isotonic saline (2.5–4 L are given in the first 24 hours to increase renal clearance of calcium).
2. Loop diuretics such as furosemide enhance the calciuric effects of volume expansion. Thiazide diuretics are absolutely contraindicated because they increase distal tubular reabsorption of calcium.
3. Biphosphonates such as pamidronate and zoledronic acid inhibit the function and viability of osteoclasts. They also bind to hydroxyapatite in bone and inhibit the breakdown and release of calcium.
4. Calcitonin inhibits bone resorption and increases renal excretion of calcium. Its onset of action is rapid but short-lived.
5. Plicamycin (mithramycin) inhibits RNA synthesis in the osteoclasts. It is rarely used, however, because of significant side effects, including hepatotoxicity, renal dysfunction, and GI distress as well as thrombocytopenia.
6. Gallium nitrate binds to and decreases the dissolution of the hydroxyapatite crystals in bone.

10. What are the causes of superior vena cava (SVC) syndrome?
1. Malignant intrathoracic tumors. Extrinsic compression of the SVC by mediastinal malignancy accounts for up to 85% of the cases of SVC syndrome. Primary lung cancer (generally small cell or squamous cell carcinoma) or lymphoma are the most common histologic types. Other malignancies that may cause SVC compression include thymic tumors, breast cancer, testicular cancer, and metastatic disease from carcinoma of unknown primary site.
2. Fibrosing mediastinitis
3. Thrombosis, primary or secondary to instrumentation or indwelling catheters
4. Granulomatous disease of mediastinal lymph nodes
5. Idiopathic causes

11. What are the clinical manifestations of SVC syndrome?
Symptoms commonly consist of swelling of the face, trunk, and/or upper extremities; dyspnea; dysphagia; chest pain; and cough. Some patients complain of neurologic symptoms such as dizziness, vision changes, or syncope. Physical findings include facial edema, plethora, distended neck veins, and distention of the superficial veins of the chest wall and anterior abdominal wall. Signs of airway obstruction or increased intracranial pressure such as tachypnea, stridor, lethargy, or papilledema require prompt initiation of treatment.

12. How is the diagnosis of SVC syndrome made?
It is based on the clinical manifestations, although chest x-ray findings support the diagnosis in 80% of cases. Diagnosis may be obtained via sputum cytology, pleural fluid cytology, lymph node biopsy, bronchoscopy, mediastinoscopy, or thoracotomy.

13. Describe the treatment for SVC syndrome.
Accurate diagnosis of the underlying cause is important before treatment is initiated. Mediastinal irradiation is the therapy for most cases of SVC syndrome due to malignancy. Over 75% of patients respond within 3 weeks. Chemotherapy should be the initial mode of treatment in patients with SVC syndrome due to small cell lung carcinoma or lymphoma. The role of anticoagulation in treatment of SVC syndrome is controversial.

14. Define tumor lysis syndrome.
Tumor lysis syndrome refers to a group of metabolic complications that may occur after treatment of neoplastic disorders. Findings usually include hyperphosphatemia, hyperkalemia, hyperuricemia, and hypocalcemia (due to precipitation of calcium phosphate). The syndrome can occur 1–5 days after significant malignant cell lysis due to chemotherapy. In severe cases, acute renal failure, cardiac arrhythmias, or convulsion may ensue.

15. What are the risk factors for tumor lysis syndrome?
The major risk factor is a large tumor burden with a rapidly proliferating tumor that is highly responsive to chemotherapy. Examples include non-Hodgkin's lymphoma, acute lymphoblastic leukemia, chronic myelogenous leukemia in blast crises, and Burkitt's lymphoma. Other predisposing factors are dehydration, obstructive uropathy, renal insufficiency, and increased levels of lactate dehydrogenase or uric acid before initiation of chemotherapy.

16. Describe the treatment for tumor lysis syndrome.
The best treatment is prevention. Patients about to receive chemotherapy or radiation for a malignancy with rapid cell turnover should be pretreated with allopurinol and intravenous hydration to maintain a high urine output. Sodium bicarbonate infusion may worsen the symptoms of hypocalcemia. Hemodialysis to remove excessive circulating uric acid may be required in patients in whom diuresis cannot be induced. Frequent monitoring of blood urea nitrogen, creatinine, uric acid, calcium, phosphate, and potassium levels is required to detect metabolic aberrations.

17. What are the predisposing factors for infection in cancer patients?
Patients with cancer are "compromised hosts" at risk for infection due to the underlying malignancy and as a result of anticancer therapy. Risk factors for infection include defects in cellular and humoral immunity, disruption of mucosal and skin integrity, tumor-related obstruction, granulocytopenia, and iatrogenic procedures.

18. What is the major source of infection?
The patient's endogenous flora.

19. Describe the evaluation of febrile, neutropenic patients.
A careful history and physical exam should include evaluation of all potential mucosal and epithelial portals of entry. The sinuses, oral cavity, and perirectal areas are important sources of infection in neutropenic patients. Any indwelling venous catheters should be inspected and palpated. The laboratory evaluation should include Gram stain and cultures of blood, urine, sputum, throat, stool, and other available fluids. Lumbar puncture should be performed if CNS infection is suspected. Chest x-rays should always be obtained along with radiologic evaluation of the paranasal sinuses, abdomen, and other sites as clinically indicated. Neutropenic patients with cancer who are at low risk for developing severe infections or life-threatening complications may be candidates for outpatient treatment with parenteral or oral antibiotics.

20. Describe the treatment for fever in neutropenic patients.

After cultures have been obtained, empirical broad-spectrum antibiotic coverage should be initiated promptly. Acceptable regimens include (1) aminoglycoside and antipseudomonal beta-lactam; (2) vancomycin, aminoglycoside, and antipseudomonal beta-lactam; and (3) monotherapy with a third-generation cephalosporin, carbapenem, or quinolone. Most important are the necessary modifications to the initial regimen as dictated by the clinical course of the patient, the isolation of organisms, and persistence of febrile neutropenia. Modifications may include adding coverage for anaerobic, viral, and/or fungal infections. If infection from an indwelling catheter is suspected, vancomycin should be added to cover methicillin-resistant staphylococci.

21. What are the common clinical features of a malignant pericardial effusion?

Acute-onset dyspnea, orthopnea, cough, chest discomfort, jugular venous distention, hepatomegaly, and edema. If the effusion develops slowly, symptoms may be minimal.

22. What are the most common cancers that involve the pericardium?

Carcinomas of the lung and breast, melanoma, and the lymphomas.

23. What is the treatment for malignant pericardial effusion?

Pericardiocentesis: Performed immediately, it can be lifesaving as well as diagnostic.

Chemotherapy and radiation: Most effective in cancers that are sensitive.

Intrapericardial instillation: Use of sclerosing agents such as tetracycline, bleomycin, and radionuclides can prevent reaccumulation of the effusion.

Indwelling pericardial catheters: Can be placed with local anesthesia and has lower morbidity.

Surgery: Surgical creation of a pericardial window; pericardiectomy.

BIBLIOGRAPHY

1. Brigden ML: Hematologic and oncoloic emergencies. Postgrad Med 109:143–163, 2001.
2. Byrne TN: Spinal cord compression from epidural metastases. N Engl J Med 327:614–619, 1992.
3. Cascino TL: Neurologic complications of systemic cancer. Med Clin North Am 77:265–278, 1993.
4. Flombaum CD: Metabolic emergencies in the cancer patient. Semin Oncol 27:322–334, 2000.
5. Harvey HA: The management of hypercalcemia of malignancy. Support Care Cancer 3:123–129, 1995.
6. Hughes WT, Armstrong D, Bodey GP, et al: 1997 guidelines for the use of antimicrobial agents in neutropenic patients with unexplained fever. Infectious Diseases Society of America. Clin Infect Dis 25:551–573, 1997.
7. Kalemkerian GP, Darwish B, Varterasian ML: Tumor lysis syndrome in small cell carcinoma and other solid tumors. Am J Med 103:363–367, 1997.
8. Loblaw DA, Laperriere NJ: Emergency treatment of malignant extradural spinal cord compression: An evidence-based guideline. J Clin Oncol 16:1613–1624, 1998.
9. Major PP, Coleman RE: Zoledronic acid in the treatment of hypercalcemia of malignancy: Results of the International Clinical Development Program. Semin Oncol 28:17–24, 2001.
10. Markman M: Diagnosis and management of superior vena cava syndrome. Cleve Clin J Med 66:59–61, 1999.
11. Pizzo PA: Management of fever in patients with cancer and treatment-induced neutropenia. N Engl J Med 328:1323–1332, 1993.
12. Vaitkus PT, Hermann HC, LeWinter MM: Treatment of malignant pericardial effusion. JAMA 272:59–64, 1994.

X. Rheumatology

62. RHEUMATOLOGIC DISEASES IN THE ICU

Danny C. Williams, M.D., F.R.C.P.C., F.A.C.P., F.A.C.R.

1. What is the differential diagnosis for acute, inflammatory arthritis occurring in the critical care setting?

Differential Diagnosis for Acute, Inflammatory Arthritis

MONOARTHRITIS (SINGLE JOINT)*		POLYARTHRITIS (MULTIPLE JOINTS)*	
Septic arthritis	Septic prosthetic joint	Infective endocarditis	Psoriatic arthritis
Crystalline arthritis	Neuropathic joint	Viral arthritis	Systemic vasculitis
Traumatic arthritis	Steroid injection	Gonococcal arthritis	Serum sickness
Hemarthrosis	synovitis	Reactive arthritis	Sickle-cell disease
Osteonecrosis	Iatrogenic infection	Rheumatoid arthritis	Pancreatitis
		Systemic lupus erythematosus	Cancer
		Enteropathic arthritis	Sarcoid

* Classification of these disorders by the number of involved joints reflects their most common pattern of clinical presentation.

2. When evaluating articular pain in a patient, what physical features can differentiate inflammatory arthritis from bursitis, tendinitis, or cellulitis?

*Feature**	*Arthritis*	*Bursitis*	*Tendinitis*	*Cellulitis*
Erythema	Often	Often	Seldom	Always
Warmth	Often	Often	Seldom	Always
Swelling	Global	Focal	Linear	Focal
Subjective pain	Global	Focal	Focal	Focal
Joint-line tenderness	Always	None	None	None
Joint stress pain	Always	None	None	None
Joint flexion deformity	Often	Seldom	Seldom	None
Loss of range	Global	Partial	Partial	None
Active range of motion	Limited	Limited	Limited	Normal
Passive range of motion	Limited	Normal	Normal	Normal
Effusion	Often	Often	Seldom	None
Crepitance	Often	Seldom	Seldom	Seldom
Skin-fold tenderness	Seldom	Seldom	Seldom	Always

* In absence of nonsteroidal anti-inflammatory drugs (NSAIDs) or corticosteroids.

True arthritis is usually present if there is evidence of articular inflammation, joint capsule distension (effusion), tenderness at the joint margins, and equal limitation of active and passive range. **Caution:** Arthritis, bursitis, tendinitis, and cellulitis may coexist.

3. What are the indications for arthrocentesis?

Diagnostic	Therapeutic
Septic arthritis*	Pus drainage
Crystalline arthritis	Crystal depletion
Hemarthrosis	Blood removal
Inflammatory vs. non-inflammatory arthritis	Effusion-induced joint pain
	Effusion-induced functional impairment
	Corticosteroid injection

* The primary consideration for performing any joint tap is to rule out infection as a cause of arthritis. An undiagnosed septic arthritis can lead to rapid (2–14 days), irreversible joint destruction and also provide a reservoir for dissemination of systemic infection in critically ill patients. Note that a red, hot joint indicates septic arthritis, until proven otherwise.

4. How do you perform arthrocentesis of the knee?

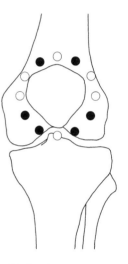

In the critical care setting, the knee is a frequent target of arthritis. Thus, proficiency in knee arthrocentesis is essential. The joint space can be accessed at one of six points circumscribing the patella (see figure). Visualizing the patella as a clock face is helpful. Large suprapatellar compartment effusions should be aspirated at the 11- or 1-o'clock position, with the knee in slight flexion. If the lateral or medial approach (8- or 4-o'clock) is used, simultaneous compression of the suprapatellar compartment may enhance synovial fluid collection. The inferior approach (7- or 5-o'clock) is performed with the knee flexed at 90°. The "key to the knee" is placing the needle underneath a "relaxed" patella.

General guidelines are as follows:
- Go where the joint capsule appears maximally distended
- Indent the skin with a retracted, ballpoint pen tip to mark the entry site
- Prepare and maintain a sterile field
- Use sufficient local anesthesia (e.g., 1% lidocaine without epinephrine)
- Use an 18–21-gauge, long needle (larger bore for large or viscous effusions)
- Never penetrate abnormal skin (e.g., cellulitis) to tap a joint
- Continuously aspirate from the entry point to the effusion
- Drain the joint dry

5. What studies are essential in synovial fluid analysis?

The three Cs: Culture, Cell Count, and Crystals.

Culture and Gram stain: Infection is the most important diagnostic issue in acute arthritis. Gram stain and routine culture should be performed on all synovial fluid samples, including those from patients with known rheumatic disease. A positive Gram stain can direct initial antibiotic selection. Additionally, therapeutic response can be monitored by Gram staining serially obtained synovial fluid specimens. Special stains and cultures (e.g., mycobacteria, fungi, and viruses) are reserved for unusual cases, such as an immunocompromised patient presenting with chronic monarthritis. The recovery rate of microbes from synovial fluid in nongonococcal, bacterial arthritis typically exceeds 95%, in contrast to gonococcal arthritis, where recovery is only 30%. In "reactive" arthritis, viable organisms are not recovered; the infection (e.g., *Salmonella* enteritis) is extra-articular.

Cell count and differential: The cell count can reveal the underlying nature of an acute arthritis. Synovial effusions are classified as being noninflammatory, inflammatory, or purulent (see below). In general, large leukocyte counts with polymorphonuclear (PMN) predominance suggest acute infection. However, considerable overlap may exist between "septic" cell counts and those of crystalline arthritis or connective tissue diseases. Likewise, the assumption that "low leukocyte counts exclude infection" is faulty; trust the culture!

Feature	Noninflammatory	Inflammatory	Purulent
WBC/mm^3	200–2000	2000–75,000	Often > 100,000
PMNs	< 25%	> 50%	> 75%
Prototypic disorder	Osteoarthritis	Rheumatoid arthritis	Septic joint

WBC = total white blood cells (leukocytes).

As with the Gram stain, serial assessment of leukocyte quantity and type can gauge therapeutic efficacy. Lack of improvement in leukocyte parameters usually indicates treatment failure or a loculated effusion.

Crystals: Crystal identification (monosodium urate or calcium pyrophosphate) can be diagnostic (gout or pseudogout); however, crystals do not exclude the possibility of concurrent infection.

6. Describe the management of acute septic arthritis.

Acute septic arthritis in the critical care setting occurs primarily in elderly patients with pre-existing joint abnormalities (e.g., arthritis, prosthetic joints) and chronic disease (e.g., cancer, cirrhosis, diabetes, renal failure). Extra-articular sources of bacteremia, such as the skin (e.g., indwelling catheters, decubitus ulcers), gastrointestinal tract, genitourinary tract, lungs, and intravenous drug abuse, account for most joint infections. On rare occasions, penetrating trauma, arthroscopy, corticosteroid joint injections, and osteomyelitis can cause septic arthritis by direct bacterial inoculation. Acute septic arthritis is best managed by following the **three Es**: Establish, Eradicate, and Evacuate.

Establish the infection. Diagnostic arthrocentesis is the procedure of choice for identifying the organism(s) responsible for septic arthritis. In most cases, only one joint is affected—usually the knee. However, if polyarticular involvement is apparent, all suspicious joints should be tapped to increase the probability of a positive Gram stain and culture. Recovery of the infectious organism(s) may be enhanced by directly injecting some of the synovial fluid into blood culture bottles. In rare instances, it may be necessary to biopsy the synovium to recover an organism. Blood cultures should *always* be obtained as well as other cultures indicated by the clinical presentation. *Pearl: Staphylococcus aureus* accounts for the majority of nongonococcal joint infections.

Eradicate the infection. Clinical features (e.g., urinary tract infection, pneumonia) and the synovial fluid Gram stain should direct the initial antibiotic choice. Gram-positive organisms are treated with penicillinase-resistant penicillins or first-generation cephalosporins. If methicillin-resistant staphylococci are suspected (e.g., intravenous drug abuse, hemodialysis), vancomycin is indicated. Third-generation cephalosporins or broad-spectrum penicillins with or without aminoglycosides or quinolones are used for gram-negative coverage. With a negative Gram stain, the preceding antibiotics used in combination provide the best coverage while awaiting results of the synovial fluid culture. The culture and sensitivity results should dictate the final antibiotic regimen. Most nongonococcal septic arthritis infections require at least 2 weeks of intravenous antibiotics followed by an additional 2–4 weeks of oral therapy. *Pearl:* A negative Gram stain or the presence of gout crystals in the synovial fluid does not exclude septic arthritis.

Evacuate the infection. The presence of nonviable bacteria or bacterial antigens within a joint may provoke an inflammatory response severe enough to cause irreparable damage. Thus, antibiotics alone are not sufficient treatment for septic arthritis. Bacteria and inflammatory products should be evacuated from an infected joint by serial arthrocentesis, arthroscopy, or open surgical drainage. Serial arthrocentesis is best performed on a "willing" patient with an accessible, noncomplicated joint.

Other measures. An additional component in the management of septic arthritis is immobilization of the affected joint in a neutral position for a few days. Immobilization should be followed by gentle range-of-motion and strengthening exercises once the joint inflammation subsides. Although nonsteroidal anti-inflammatory drugs (NSAIDs) and corticosteroids have been shown to reduce joint damage in animal models of septic arthritis, they are not yet recommended in the initial treatment of joint infection in humans. The early administration of anti-inflammatory medications may conceal an ongoing infection. Plain radiographs of the affected joint are usually obtained to rule out osteomyelitis and as a baseline study of joint architecture. Other than effusion, early radiographs of septic joints are usually devoid of diagnostic features.

7. **What is the best procedure for clearing a septic joint?**

There are three options for evacuating the contents of a septic joint: serial arthrocentesis, arthroscopy, and open surgical drainage. The best method remains controversial and depends on multiple factors, including synovial fluid viscosity, bacterial virulence, joint architecture, patient compliance, and operator performance. Closed-needle aspiration is the traditional procedure for clearing infection from accessible, uncomplicated joints. In general, arthrocentesis and synovial fluid analysis are performed at least once daily for 4–7 days while the patient is taking appropriate antibiotics. Orthopedic consultation is indicated if there is no interim improvement in the physical exam or Gram stain and cell count of the synovial fluid. Surgical consultation also should be obtained in the following situations:

- Delayed diagnosis (> 1 week)
- Difficult arthrocentesis (viscous, debris-laden synovial fluid)
- Difficult joints (hip, sacroiliac, shoulder, sternoclavicular, wrist)
- Damaged joints (arthritis, prostheses, trauma)
- Osteomyelitis
- Patient preference

8. **What clinical features, other than arthritis, are suggestive of connective tissue disease?**

The diagnosis of connective tissue disorders is largely dependent upon the history and physical exam. Laboratory investigations (e.g., antinuclear antibodies) should be obtained to confirm a presumptive diagnosis. The following select list of clinical features may indicate an underlying connective tissue disorder, especially when several organ systems are involved simultaneously.

Clinical Features that May Indicate an Underlying Connective Tissue Disorder

Cardiac	Genitourinary	Neurologic	Pulmonary
Dysrhythmias	Urethritis	Cognitive dysfunction	Pleuritis
Pericarditis	Ulceration	Altered behavior	Pneumonitis
Valvular disease	Testicular pain	Altered consciousness	Interstitial fibrosis
Myocarditis	Recurrent fetal loss	Seizure	Hemorrhage
		Stroke	Hypertension
Cutaneous	**Hematologic**	Peripheral neuropathy	Embolism
Alopecia	Anemia	Aseptic meningitis	
Facial rash	Hemolysis		**Renal**
Livedo reticularis	Leukopenia	**Ocular**	Glomerulonephritis
Palpable purpura	Leukocytosis	Xerophthalmia	Tubular acidosis
Calcinosis	Thrombocytosis	Episcleritis	Nephrolithiasis
Sclerosis	Thrombocytopenia	Scleritis	
Subcutaneous nodules		Iritis	**Systemic**
Erythema nodosum	**Lymphoreticular**	Visual loss	Fever
Psoriasis	Adenopathy		Fatigue
Pyoderma	Splenomegaly	**Oral**	Cachexia
		Xerostomia	
Enteric	**Musculoskeletal**	Ulceration	**Vascular**
Dysphagia/reflux	Arthralgia	Parotid swelling	Acute hypertension
Malabsorption	Articular deformity	Telangiectasia	Raynaud's phenomenon
Peritonitis	Tenosynovitis		Acral cyanosis
Hepatitis	Myalgia		Thrombosis
Pancreatitis	Muscle weakness		
Colitis			
Bowel infarction			

9. When does an elevated erythrocyte sedimentation rate (ESR) reflect an underlying connective tissue disorder?

The ESR is a nonspecific test (Westergren method preferred) for systemic inflammation. ESR elevation typically results from cytokine-induced hepatic synthesis of acute-phase reactants, in particular fibrinogen. However, some noninflammatory factors such as advanced age, female gender, and pregnancy, can also cause elevation of the ESR. The ESR can be helpful in evaluation of numerous rheumatic diseases, but it is not diagnostic. Even when extreme ESR elevations are encountered ($\geq$ 100 mm/hr), infection is more likely (35%) than connective tissue disease (25%). Thus, when an elevated ESR is obtained in a critical care patient, the diagnosis of a connective tissue disorder still depends on the presence of characteristic clinical features (see above). The ESR is perhaps most useful in serial assessment of ongoing disease activity in disorders such as rheumatoid arthritis, polymyalgia rheumatica, and giant cell arteritis.

The "upper limit of normal" ESR value for most patients can be calculated by the following formulas:

$$\text{ESR}_{(male)} = \text{age} \div 2 \qquad \text{ESR}_{(female)} = (\text{age} + 10) \div 2$$

The platelet count (thrombocytosis) can be used as a crude substitute for ESR; platelets act as "acute-phase reactant" cells.

10. What laboratory evaluations are useful in the diagnosis of connective tissue diseases?

There are no screening tests for the diagnosis of connective tissue disorders. Because of their lack of specificity, positive serologic tests in the absence of supporting clinical features usually result in misdiagnoses. Serologic evaluation of patients with suspected autoimmune disease should proceed in three stages: systemic inflammation determination, autoantibody identification, and supplemental testing.

Systemic inflammation determination: A routine CBC (complete blood count) and ESR are usually adequate to demonstrate systemic inflammation. CBC abnormalities typically include leukocytosis, a normocytic/normochromic anemia, and thrombocytosis. Additional laboratory indicators of systemic inflammation may include:

↑ C-reactive protein (CRP)*	↑ C3 (third component of complement)
↑ Fibrinogen	↑ Ferritin
↑ Haptoglobin	↓ Albumin
↑ Gamma globulins	↓ Transferrin

* CRP is more specific, but more expensive than ESR.

Autoantibody identification: Serum autoantibodies (e.g., antinuclear antibodies) may help confirm a particular connective tissue disorder, but should not be used to screen for rheumatic disease. The most frequently used autoantibody tests for suspected rheumatic disease are rheumatoid factor (anti-IgG antibody) and antinuclear antibody (ANA). In autoimmune disease, a positive ANA indicates the presence of specific nuclear antigens which can usually be identified by an "ANA profile" (see below). Autoantibodies may also be directed against cellular antigens in the cytoplasm and cell-surface membrane. Common disease associations with specific autoantibodies are listed below.

Autoantibody	Disorder (% Positive)
Rheumatoid factor	Rheumatoid arthritis (85%)
ANA profile:	
• Anti-dsDNA (double-stranded DNA)	Systemic lupus erythematosus (60%)
• Anti-Sm (Smith antigen)	Systemic lupus erythematosus (30%)
• Anti-SS-A	Sjögren's syndrome (60%)
• Anti-SS-B	Sjögren's syndrome (40%)
• Anti-RNP	Mixed connective tissue disease (95%)
Anti-Scl-70	Diffuse scleroderma (30%)

Table continued on following page

Autoantibody	*Disorder (% Positive)*
Anti-centromere	Limited scleroderma (90%)
Anti-histone	Drug-induced lupus (90%)
Anti-Jo-1	Polymyositis (20%)
Anti-neutrophilic cytoplasmic antibody (ANCA)	Wegener's granulomatosis (90%)
Anti-phospholipid	Antiphospholipid antibody syndrome (100%)

- A positive ANA is suggestive of an autoimmune disorder only if the pretest probability is high.
- A negative ANA virtually excludes active systemic lupus erythematosus.
- Antibody overlap is common (e.g., a patient with lupus may simultaneously have dsDNA, SS-A, histone, rheumatoid factor, and phospholipid antibodies).
- Autoantibodies may be seen in non-connective tissue disorders (e.g., rheumatoid factor in subacute bacterial endocarditis) and normal individuals.

Supplemental testing: Ancillary tests for connective tissue disorders assess disease mechanisms, tissue damage, and disease activity. The following investigations may be useful in the diagnosis and management of some patients with connective tissue disease.

Diagnostic Tests for Connective Tissue Disorders

DISORDER	TEST
Immune complex disease	Complement (C3, C4)
Hemolysis	Coombs' test
Myositis	Creatine kinase
Nephritis	Urinalysis and creatinine
Thrombosis	Lupus anticoagulant or anticardiolipin antibody
Vasculitis	Hepatitis profile or cryoglobulins

- Hypocomplementemia and high-titer, dsDNA antibodies are associated with active systemic lupus erythematosus; in particular, active lupus nephritis.

11. **When does an elevated serum creatine kinase (CK) indicate inflammatory muscle disease?**
An increased CK in conjunction with symmetric muscle weakness is suggestive of an autoimmune, inflammatory myopathy. However, in the critical care setting, the following causes of an elevated CK should also merit consideration:
- Myocardial injury: ischemia, infarction, myocarditis or surgery
- Muscle trauma: ischemia, crush injury, biopsy, or intramuscular injections
- Drug-induced: ethanol, corticosteroids, lipid-lowering agents, cimetidine, cocaine, opiates, benzodiazepines, barbiturates, or zidovudine
- Infectious myositis: bacterial, viral, mycobacterial, fungal, or parasitic
- Endocrine disorders: hypothyroidism or hypoparathyroidism
- Central nervous system injury: ischemia or trauma
- Miscellaneous disorders: seizures, hemolysis, malignant hyperthermia, muscular dystrophy, motor neuron disease, or peripheral neuropathy

Autoimmune muscle inflammation may occur independently (polymyositis), with rash (dermatomyositis), in "overlap" syndromes (e.g., mixed connective tissue disease), or in association with cancer. The core features of polymyositis typically include neck flexor and proximal limb girdle weakness, infrequent myalgias, and elevated serum muscle enzymes. Other organ systems may become involved, such as the gastrointestinal tract (dysphagia), the lungs (interstitial lung disease), the heart (myocarditis), the joints (arthritis), and the blood vessels (Raynaud's phenomenon). The diagnosis is established by performing electromyography with subsequent biopsy of the abnormal muscle. Additional serum proteins which can also reflect muscle damage include the aminotransferases, lactate dehydrogenase, aldolase, and myoglobin.

Among muscle proteins, CK is the most sensitive indicator of muscle injury, whereas aspartate aminotransferase (AST) is the most specific for actual muscle inflammation.

12. What clinical features suggest that a thrombotic event is due to the antiphospholipid syndrome (APS)?

Clinical Features

Major manifestations
  Recurrent thromboses (venous > arterial; usually lower limb deep venous thrombosis or stroke)
  Multiple miscarriages (3rd > 2nd > 1st trimester)
  Low-grade thrombocytopenia (70,000–100,000 platelets/mm^3)
  Anionic phospholipid and/or β_2-glycoprotein-I or prothrombin antibodies
Other manifestations
  Cutaneous: Livedo reticularis, superficial thrombophlebitis, acral ischemic necrosis, or splinter hemorrhages
  Neurologic: Seizure, chorea, multi-infarct dementia, transverse myelitis, or migraines
  Cardiac: Valvular disease (vegetations), myocardial infarction, or cardiomyopathy
  Pulmonary: Embolism, hypertension, or intra-alveolar hemorrhage
  Skeletal: Osteonecrosis

The APS can occur as an independent disorder (primary APS) or in association with another connective tissue disease (e.g., the "lupus anticoagulant" of systemic lupus erythematosus). Though most thromboses are focal, a "catastrophic" variant of the APS may occur with rampant vascular occlusion and multiple organ failure.

Phospholipid antibodies are usually detected by one or more of the following investigations:
  • False-positive serologic test for syphilis (Venereal Disease Research Laboratory [VDRL] test)
  • Prolonged activated partial thromboplastin time (PTT) which **does not** correct with added (1:1 dilution) normal plasma, but **does** correct with added phospholipid.
  • Prolonged Russell viper venom time
  • Positive anticardiolipin antibody (high titer IgG)
  Caution: Some infections or drugs may also induce phospholipid antibodies.

13. How do connective tissue disorders commonly affect the lungs?

Effects of Connective Tissue Disorders on Lungs

DISORDER	PLEURITIS	PNEUMONITIS	NODULES	FIBROSIS	HEMORRHAGE	↑ BP	EMBOLI
RA	•		•	•			
SLE	•	•		•	•	•	•
DIL	•	•					
Sjögren's syndrome	•			•			
MCTD	•	•		•	•	•	
PM/DM		•		•			
PSS		•		•			
CREST				•		•	
APS					•	?	•
Wegener's granulomatosis	•	•	•	•	•		
CSS	•	•	•	•			

RA = rheumatoid arthritis, SLE = systemic lupus erythematosus, DIL = drug-induced lupus, MCTD = mixed connective tissue disease, PM/DM = polymyositis/dermatomyositis, PSS = diffuse scleroderma, CREST = limited scleroderma, APA = antiphospholipid syndrome, CSS = Churg-Strauss syndrome, and ↑ BP = pulmonary hypertension.

14. How do you differentiate acute lupus pneumonitis from an infectious pneumonia?
Acute lupus pneumonitis is characterized by sudden dyspnea, cough with occasional sputum, fever, tachypnea, pleural irritation, infrequent hemoptysis, and hypoxemia. Chest radiographs usually reveal bibasilar infiltrates with pleural effusions; however, unilateral involvement can occur. The white blood cell count is typically normal, though this may be misleading; most patients (> 50%) with active SLE are leukopenic. Although acute lupus pneumonitis typically occurs in patients with systemically active disease, it is uncommon. A patient with lupus with the above features is more likely to have a bacterial, viral, mycobacterial, or *Pneumocystis carinii* infection. Furthermore, pharmacologic agents such as NSAIDs, methotrexate, azathioprine, chlorambucil, and cyclophosphamide may cause a toxic pneumonitis clinically indistinguishable from acute lupus pneumonitis. The diagnosis is one of exclusion and is made after sputum cultures, bronchoalveolar lavage, and lung biopsy offer no evidence of infection. There is no tissue-specific abnormality which can establish the diagnosis. The initial treatment consists of high-dose corticosteroids (1–2 mg/kg prednisone equivalent per day).

15. What special precautions should be taken when intubating a patient with rheumatoid arthritis?
Cervical spine disease is a common manifestation of rheumatoid arthritis, primarily affecting the C1–C2 articulation. Furthermore, 30% of patients with advanced, erosive arthritis will have radiographic evidence of atlantoaxial subluxation (> 3 mm between the C1 arch and the C2 odontoid process). These patients are at risk for spinal cord compression when subjected to manipulative procedures such as endotracheal intubation, even in the absence of symptoms. The following list identifies features upon which a pre-intubation, cervical spine radiograph (with lateral flexion views) should be obtained.
• Physically deforming rheumatoid arthritis
• Rheumatoid arthritis duration > 3 years
• Long-term corticosteroid use
• Osteoporosis risk factors
• Intractable neck pain
• Prior cervical spine subluxation
• Clinical evidence of cervical myelopathy
An anesthesiologist should be present for emergent intubations (without radiographs) or if clinical and/or radiographic findings of atlantoaxial subluxation are present.
Caution: Cricoarytenoid joint arthritis may also complicate endotracheal intubation.

16. How can acral necrosis be avoided in a patient with Raynaud's phenomenon?
Raynaud's phenomenon is a stress-induced (e.g., cold temperature), vascular disorder characterized by episodic, reversible ischemia of the extremities. The triphasic color response (white → blue → red) results from vasospastic alterations (ischemia → stasis → hyperemia) of acral blood flow. The following factors may precipitate sustained, acral ischemia with resulting necrosis in patients with significant Raynaud's phenomenon.
• Cold stress (including subnormal body core temperature)
• Emotional stress
• Hypoperfusion
• Pharmacologic agents: β-blockers
                                    Sympathomimetic drugs (α-agonists)
                                    Ergot alkaloids
The initial management of Raynaud's phenomenon consists of providing warmth to the extremities, maintaining acral perfusion, and reducing psychological stress. Vasodilators (e.g., nifedipine) and/or sympatholytic agents (e.g., prazosin) are indicated for patients with intolerable symptoms or atrophic, acral skin. Topical 2% nitroglycerin applied for 20 minutes, three times a day to affected digits may improve refractory cases. A daily 325 mg aspirin may be effective for patients with a concurrent, occlusive vasculopathy (e.g., scleroderma).

17. Which connective tissue disorders have cardiac manifestations?

Cardiac Manifestations of Connective Tissue Disorders

DISORDER	PERICARDITIS	MYOCARDITIS	VALVULAR DISEASE	CONDUCTION DEFECTS	CAD
RA	•	•	Nodules		
AS	•		Aortitis (AI)	AVB	
Lyme				AVB	
ARF	•	•	•		
SLE	•	•	Libman-Sacks endocarditis		•
DIL	•				
NLS				AVB	
MCTD	•	•		AVB	
PM/DM		•		AVB	
PSS		Fibrosis		SVT/VT	
APS			•	AVB	•
Kawasaki's disease		•			Aneurysms
Takayasu's arteritis		•	AI		•
Marfan's syndrome			MVP/AI/MR		

AS = ankylosing spondylitis, ARF = acute rheumatic fever, NLS = neonatal lupus syndrome, CAD = coronary artery disease, AVB = atrioventricular block, AI = aortic insufficiency, MVP = mitral valve prolapse, MR = mitral regurgitation, and SVT/VT = supraventricular/ventricular tachycardia.

18. Describe the initial treatment of acute flares of rheumatoid arthritis.

Manifestation	Initial Treatment*
Keratoconjunctivitis sicca	Hydroxymethylcellulose drops or ointment
Acute synovitis (monarthritis)	Intra-articular steroid injection
Acute synovitis (polyarthritis)	NSAID (if no risk factors) *and/or* 10–20 mg prednisone equivalent per day
Acute pleuritis	NSAID (if no risk factors) *and/or* ≤ 15 mg prednisone equivalent per day
Acute pleuritis (with large pleural effusions)	≤ 0.5 mg/kg prednisone equivalent per day
Acute pericarditis	NSAID (if no risk factors) *and/or* ≤ 0.5 mg/kg prednisone equivalent per day

* Only if infection is ruled out or covered with appropriate antibiotics.

Disease-modifying agents (e.g., methotrexate) have no role in the management of acute rheumatoid flares, except in the rare instance of severe vasculitis.

Physiotherapy is a valuable, but often overlooked adjunct to the management of inflammatory arthritis.

19. How do you manage an acute exacerbation of connective tissue disease?

A critical care patient with connective tissue disease is likely to have dysfunction or failure of one or more organ systems. Thus, the traditional approach to the pharmacologic treatment of an acute flare is frequently restricted by the risk of further toxicity. An example would be the withholding of NSAIDs in a patient suffering from congestive heart failure, renal insufficiency, hepatic dysfunction, gastrointestinal hemorrhage, and/or thrombocytopenia. Other issues which can limit treatment options are limited routes of drug administration, drug interactions, drug hypersensitivity, pregnancy, wound healing, infection, and level of patient consciousness. In most patients, acute management will involve the administration of some form of corticosteroid. However, corticosteroids are to be avoided in scleroderma, septic arthritis, osteonecrosis, Raynaud's phenomenon, and fibromyalgia. Corticosteroids are not innocuous; they promote impaired wound healing, hyperglycemia, risk of infection, fluid retention, hypokalemia, adrenal insufficiency, and neuropsychiatric disturbances. Life-threatening disease (e.g., systemic vasculitis) will often require the concomitant administration of a cytotoxic agent, such as cyclophosphamide.

20. When and how are "pulse" corticosteroids used?

Pulse corticosteroids are reserved for life-threatening manifestations of rheumatic disease when rapid suppression of systemic inflammation is needed. Acute episodes of systemic vasculitis, lupus cerebritis, and lupus pneumonitis are usually treated with pulse corticosteroids. The pulse typically consists of 1 gm/day of methylprednisolone given intravenously for 3 days. The safest approach to administering such a large dose is to infuse it *slowly* as 250 mg every 6 hours. Adverse reactions may include transient flushing, headache, increased blood pressure, and acute psychosis. It may be prudent to monitor serum electrolytes and blood glucose in patients at risk for hypokalemia and hyperglycemia. Patients with concurrent infection should be placed on antibiotics before receiving any corticosteroids. Arrhythmias, myocardial infarction, and sudden death have been reported in patients with preexisting cardiovascular disease; thus, telemetry is recommended for such patients. In addition, all recipients of pulse therapy are at risk for developing osteonecrosis (avascular necrosis).

21. Describe the initial treatment of acute flares of systemic lupus erythematosus.

Manifestation	Initial Treatment*
Fever	NSAID (no risk factors) *and/or* ≤ 15 mg prednisone equivalent per day
Acute dermatitis (mild)	Topical corticosteroid
Acute dermatitis (moderate)	≤ 20 mg prednisone equivalent per day
Acute polyarthritis	NSAID (no risk factors) *and/or* 10–20 mg prednisone equivalent per day
Acute myositis	0.5–1 mg/kg prednisone equivalent per day
Acute serositis[†] (mild–moderate)	NSAID (no risk factors) *and/or* ≤ 15 mg prednisone equivalent per day
Acute serositis[†] (moderate–severe)	0.5–1 mg/kg prednisone equivalent per day
Acute myocarditis (with congestive heart failure)	1 mg/kg prednisone equivalent per day
Acute nephritis (new onset) (active urine sediment/proteinuria)	1 mg/kg prednisone equivalent per day
Acute cerebritis (with seizures/↓ mental status)	1 gm methylprednisolone per day for 3 days (*plus* anticonvulsants) *followed by* 1 mg/kg prednisone equivalent per day
Acute thrombosis (with phospholipid antibody)	Anticoagulation (Heparin → warfarin, keep INR 3–4)
Acute thrombocytopenia or hemolytic anemia (moderate)	0.5–1 mg/kg prednisone equivalent per day
Acute thrombocytopenia or hemolytic anemia (life-threatening)	1 gm methylprednisolone per day for 3 days *followed by* 1 mg/kg prednisone equivalent per day *and/or* 1–2 gm/kg IV gamma-globulin for 1–5 days
Acute vasculitis (cutaneous)	≤ 0.5 mg/kg prednisone equivalent per day
Acute vasculitis (systemic)	1 gm methylprednisolone per day for 3 days *followed by* 1 mg/kg prednisone equivalent per day

* Only if infection is ruled out or covered with appropriate antibiotics.
[†] Acute serositis includes pleuritis, pericarditis, and/or peritonitis.
INR = international normalization ratio.

- Ibuprofen may cause aseptic meningitis in SLE patients.
- Avoid sulfonamides in SLE patients; they may induce a disease flare or hypersensitivity reaction.
- Divided, daily doses of corticosteroids are more potent than single daily doses; however, the potential for toxicity is greater.

22. How do you manage an acute gout attack?

Acute gouty arthritis frequently occurs in hospitalized patients. Predisposing factors include acute illness, pre-admission alcohol consumption, trauma, surgery, and medications such as diuretics, antimycobacterial agents, and low-dose aspirin. Most gout attacks are monarticular (90%) and commonly affect the first metatarsophalangeal joint (podagra), the mid-foot, or ankle. Occasionally the arthritis is accompanied by a low-grade fever and/or leukocytosis. Polyarticular gout presentations with systemic features can be confusing and mimic other types of inflammatory arthritis. Thus, the critical component of gout management is arthrocentesis, by which monosodium urate crystals can be detected and infection ruled out. As with other connective tissue disorders, comorbid conditions may complicate the pharmacologic treatment of patients with acute gout.

Manifestation	*Treatment*	
	ENTERAL ACCESS	PARENTERAL ACCESS
Acute monarthritis (uncomplicated)	NSAID[†] *and/or* colchicine 0.6 mg[‡] *or* intra-articular steroid *or* prednisone 30 mg/day (taper over 2 weeks)	Intra-articular steroid *or* triamcinolone 60 mg IM (single dose) *or* IV methylprednisolone[§]
Acute monarthritis (complicated*)	Intra-articular steroid *or* prednisone 30 mg/day (taper over 2 weeks)	Intra-articular steroid *or* triamcinolone 60 mg IM (single dose) *or* IV methylprednisolone
Acute polyarthritis (uncomplicated)	NSAID *and/or* colchicine 0.6 mg *or* prednisone 30 mg/day (taper over 2 weeks)	Triamcinolone 60 mg IM (single dose) or IV methylprednisolone
Acute polyarthritis (complicated)	Prednisone 30 mg/day (taper over 2 weeks)	Triamcinolone 60 mg IM (single dose) or IV methylprednisolone

* Complicated—designation for patients with impaired organ function at risk for NSAID or colchicine toxicity.
[†] NSAID—prototype: indomethacin 200 mg/day × 2 days, then 150 mg/day tapered according to symptoms.
[‡] Colchicine 0.6 mg is given as one tablet PO 2 times/day → 3 times/day to minimize gastrointestinal distress. Intravenous colchicine is not recommended.
[§] IV methylprednisolone is given as 30 mg/day tapered over 2 weeks.

Note: Allopurinol and probenicid should not be used in acute gout attacks.

23. When evaluating back pain, what features are suggestive of a serious disorder?

In the general population, the etiology of back pain is often idiopathic (85% of all cases) and usually attributed to "mechanical" factors. Regardless, most patients (75%) will have resolution of their symptoms within a month of onset. Back pain in the critical care patient may portend a greater problem, however, than that resulting from an uncomfortable bed. The following features are associated with potentially serious causes of back pain.

- Acute, severe pain without obvious cause
- Pain unresponsive to rest or positional change
- Unrelenting nocturnal pain
- Significant trauma
- Sensorimotor deficit
- Pain worse with Valsalva maneuvers
- Bowel or bladder dysfunction
- Pain radiation into both lower limbs

- Constitutional symptoms
- First onset under 30 years old or over 50
- Prolonged morning stiffness
- Peripheral synovitis
- Immunosuppression or prolonged corticosteroid use
- Prior cancer
- Osteoporosis risk factors

BIBLIOGRAPHY

1. Bohlmeyer TJ, Wu AHB, Perryman MB: Evaluation of laboratory tests as a guide to diagnosis and therapy of myositis. Rheum Dis Clin North Am 20:845–856, 1994.
2. Espinoza LR (ed): Infectious arthritis. Rheum Dis Clin North Am 24:2, 1998.
3. Klippel JH, Dieppe PA (eds): Rheumatology, 2nd ed. London, Mosby, 1998.
4. McCune WJ (ed): Systemic lupus erythematosus. Rheum Dis Clin North Am 20:1, 1994.
5. Polly HF, Hunder GG: Rheumatologic Interviewing and Physical Examination of the Joints, 2nd ed. Philadelphia, W.B. Saunders, 1978.
6. Ruddy S, Harris ED, Sledge CB (eds): Kelley's Textbook of Rheumatology, 6th ed. Philadelphia, W.B. Saunders, 2001.
7. Sorokin R: Management of the patient with rheumatic diseases going to surgery. Med Clin North Am 77:453–464, 1993.
8. Wallace DJ, Hahn BH (eds): Dubois' Lupus Erythematosus, 5th ed. Baltimore, Williams & Wilkins, 1997.
9. Weisman MH, Weinblatt ME (eds): Treatment of the Rheumatic Diseases. Philadelphia, W.B. Saunders, 1995.
10. Wiedemann HP, Matthay RA: Pulmonary manifestations of the collagen vascular diseases. Clin Chest Med 10:677–722, 1989.
11. West SG (ed): Rheumatology Secrets, 1st ed. Philadelphia, Hanley & Belfus, 1997.

XI. Neurology

63. COMA

Adrian A. Jarquin-Valdivia, M.D., and David Bonovich, M.D.

1. Define coma.

Coma is a pathologic condition in which the patient is unconscious and appears to be asleep. The patient is incapable of responding and is unaware of either external stimuli or inner needs. A patient in a coma is unable to interact with his or her environment.

2. Which anatomic structures must be malfunctioning to produce coma?

Coma is caused by either bilateral cerebral hemispheric dysfunction or injury to the reticular activating system (RAS).

3. What can we deduce about the cause of coma by understanding its anatomy?

Cerebral hemispheric or brainstem RAS dysfunction may result from structural or metabolic lesions. Structural lesions of the RAS are usually associated with focal neurologic signs because of its anatomic location in the brainstem, adjacent to multiple cranial nerves and ascending and descending tracts. A structural lesion must be large to affect both cerebral hemispheres and produce coma. In the absence of focal neurologic signs, coma is usually the result of a global toxic or metabolic suppression of the cerebral hemispheres and/or the RAS.

4. What are the initial steps in managing a patient with coma?

First, the ABCs (airway, breathing, and circulation) should be addressed. Oxygen should be administered via facemask, and vascular access should be obtained. If the patient does not have a secure airway, intubation should be performed. If, after a history is obtained and a physical and neurologic exam performed, the cause of coma is uncertain, empirical therapy for reversible causes such as Wernicke's encephalopathy and narcotic overdose should be initiated with thiamine and naloxone. A bedside blood glucose determination should be performed; if hypoglycemia is present, D50W should be administered.

5. Describe the diagnostic approach to comatose patients.

It is important to have a systematic approach to coma. The history as obtained from relatives, friends, or paramedics may reveal an obvious cause such as drug or alcohol overdose, sepsis, or abnormalities of glucose metabolism. The general physical examination, beginning with vital signs and proceeding in a systematic manner to include the head, eyes, ears, nose, and throat as well as the lungs, heart, abdomen, extremities, and skin, may help to identify infectious causes, respiratory or cardiac disorders, or liver failure, especially in patients with chronic liver disease. Careful attention should be given to evaluation of the skin and mucous membranes for needle marks or signs of emboli and to the ocular fundi for evidence of papilledema, which suggests increased intracranial pressure. Assessment of the vital signs may suggest an infectious cause or respiratory disorder. The neck should be examined for nuchal rigidity, which suggests the possibility of meningeal irritation. A rectal examination should assess the stool for blood. Although a full neurologic exam may not be possible, one can test brainstem reflexes and look for evidence of focal motor abnormalities as well as reflex asymmetry, including plantar response. A description of the respiratory pattern should be noted.

6. Match the following clinical signs with the cause of coma with which it is associated.

1. Purpuritic rash	A. Basilar skull fracture
2. Battle sign	B. Atropine poisoning
3. Bilateral, large, fixed pupils	C. Meningitis
4. Unilateral, large, fixed pupil	D. Third-nerve palsy suggesting
5. Nuchal rigidity and fever	temporal lobe herniation
6. Gynecomastia, spider angiomata	E. Anoxic encephalopathy
7. Bilateral, pinpoint pupils	F. Locked-in syndrome
8. Unilateral chemosis and proptosis	G. Chronic liver disease
9. Myoclonus	H. Narcotic overdose
10. Quadriplegia, loss of lower cranial	I. Meningococcemia
nerve function, but retained vertical	J. Diabetic ketoacidosis
eye movements	K. Fat embolism
11. Malnourished, extraocular palsies	L. Wernicke's encephalopathy
12. Long bone fractures, petechiae	

Answers: 1, I; 2, A; 3, B; 4, D; 5, C; 6, G; 7, H; 8, J; 9, E; 10, F; 11, L; 12, K.

A purpuritic rash should suggest meningococcemia. Battle sign (a bluish discoloration behind the ear associated with basilar skull fracture), cerebrospinal fluid (CSF) rhinorrhea, or other signs of facial trauma should suggest head trauma as the cause of coma. Bilateral fixed unreactive pupils should suggest atropine or scopolamine overdose. A unilateral, fixed, dilated pupil should suggest a third-nerve palsy secondary to temporal lobe herniation but has been seen in psychiatric patients who put atropine-like drugs in one eye. Nuchal rigidity should suggest meningitis or subarachnoid hemorrhage. Gynecomastia and spider angiomas are associated with chronic liver disease and suggest liver failure and alcohol as possible causes for coma. Bilateral pinpoint pupils are commonly seen in narcotic overdose. A bloody nasal discharge with unilateral chemosis should suggest mucormycosis which is associated with diabetic ketoacidosis. Myoclonus is typical of metabolic encephalopathies, especially anoxia. A pontine infarction can give rise to a condition in which a patient cannot communicate by movement or speech and therefore appears to be in coma, a condition known as the "locked-in syndrome." Such patients are awake and alert and can usually communicate by vertical eye movements. Wernicke's encephalopathy can present as sudden coma; the common denominator is malnutrition, not alcoholism. A few days after long bone fractures, confusion leading to coma may develop, with hypoxemia and the characteristic petechial rash of fat emnbolism.

7. How does the finding of a new focal abnormality on neurologic examination affect the management of a comatose patient?

Focal neurologic abnormalities generally indicate a structural central nervous system (CNS) lesion such as tumor, abscess, infarct, or hemorrhage. Focal metabolic failure may be seen in hypoglycemia or Wernicke's encephalopathy. Imaging with computed tomography (CT) or magnetic resonance imaging (MRI) should be considered mandatory early in the management of such patients to exclude lesions that may require aggressive medical and/or surgical intervention and to assess prognosis.

8. Does a nonfocal neurologic exam exclude a mass as the cause of coma?

No. Although most cases of coma with a nonfocal neurologic exam are due to toxic-metabolic causes, bilateral subdural hematomas, subarachnoid hemorrhages, hydrocephalus (communicating or noncommunicating), trauma with diffuse axonal injury (DAI), or lesions involving the bilateral frontal lobes may not show any gross focal abnormalities on neurologic testing.

9. What initial laboratory evaluations should be performed in coma of uncertain etiology?

A drug screen (both urine and blood) and blood alcohol level, complete blood count, serum electrolytes, glucose, calcium, phosphate, magnesium, creatinine, blood urea nitrogen, and liver and thyroid function tests should be ordered. An arterial blood gas analysis is mandatory, and cultures of blood, urine, and sputum should be obtained if infection is likely. An initial electrocardiogram should be obtained. A CT scan of the head should be performed if the cause is not obvious or if focal signs are present on neurologic exam. A lumbar puncture should be performed if a primary CNS infection is likely, but only after the presence of a CNS mass has been excluded.

10. Describe the approach to the comatose trauma patient.

Although the general approach is similar, the likelihood of a structural cause of coma is high in trauma patients. Traumatic causes of coma include subdural or epidural hematomas, focal intracerebral hemorrhage with mass effect and midline shift, bilateral contusions, and DAI. Consideration also must be given to other causes, such as brainstem infarction, hypertensive hemorrhage, hypoxia, hypo- or hyperglycemia, drug or alcohol ingestion, or a primary CNS mass lesion, such as abscess or tumor. If the patient has focal signs on exam, such as a third-nerve palsy, immediate neuroimaging with a CT scan and neurocritical care or neurosurgical consultation are indicated.

11. What are the common causes of coma in a medical ICU?

Most cases of coma in a medical-surgical (nontrauma) ICU are toxic-metabolic and are often multifactorial. Once the effects of sedatives and paralytics have been considered, sepsis, hypotension, hypoxia, hypothermia, acid-base disorders, glucose and electrolyte abnormalities, and the side effects of medications are common causes. Hepatic and uremic failure often contribute to coma. Primary CNS infections such as meningitis or encephalitis are less common but need to be considered in the appropriate setting. If a severe coagulopathy is present, intracranial hemorrhage and subdural hematomas should be excluded. Focal signs on exam suggest a structural lesion such as a CNS infarction, tumor, or abscess and should be evaluated with a CT or MRI scan. If no obvious cause for coma is apparent, an electroencephalogram is indicated to exclude nonconvulsive status epilepticus.

12. What other conditions may mimic coma?

- "Locked-in" syndrome: caused by extensive pontine damage. Patients can move their eyes vertically but are incapable of any other movement or response.
- Guillain-Barré syndrome: an acute peripheral nerve disorder characterized by ascending weakness that, when extensive, can cause a state of de-efferentation in which the patient is not in a coma but cannot move.
- Botulism: an acute intoxication with the toxin of *Clostridium botulinum*, characterized by a descending pattern of weakness. Patients initially experience extraocular and pharyngeal muscle weakness (with diplopia, dysarthria, and dysphagia) that quickly progresses to diffuse weakness.
- Critical illness neuromyopathies and acute tetraplegic myopathy: entities seen in the critical care setting that, if extensive, can induce profound weakness and numbness.
- Catatonia: a rare psychiatric manifestation of severe depression, characterized by the finding of waxy flexibility on physical exam and no history of anatomic, toxic, or metabolic brain insult. It may improve with electroconvulsive therapy.
- Psychogenic: on rare occasions a coma-like state can be part of a psychosomatic disorder. It can diagnosed by careful history and physical exam, including oculocaloric testing.

BIBLIOGRAPHY

1. Alguire PC: Rapid evaluation of comatose patients. Postgrad Med 87:223–228, 1990.
2. Casado J, Serrano A: Coma in Pediatrics: Diagnosis and Treatment. Madrid, Ediciones D'az de Santos SA, 1997.
3. Goetz CG, Pappert EJ: Textbook of Clinical Neurology. Philadelphia, Saunders, 1999.
4. Kelly BJ: Clinical assessment of the nervous system. In Tobin MJ (ed): Principles and Practice of Intensive Care Monitoring. New York, McGraw-Hill, Inc., 1998.
5. Kleeman CR: Metabolic coma. Kidney Int 36:1142–1158, 1989.
6. Mercer WN, Childa NL: Coma, vegetative state, and the minimally conscious state: Diagnosis and management. Neurologist 5:186–193, 1999.
7. Plum F, Posner J: The Diagnosis of Stupor and Coma, 3rd ed. Philadelphia, F.A. Davis, 1980.

64. BRAIN DEATH

Adrian A. Jarquin-Valdivia, M.D., and David Bonovich, M.D.

1. What is brain death?

Brain death was first described by Mollaret and Goulon in 1959 as "coma dépassé." Technologic advancements in medicine have enabled physicians to keep the body functioning despite a nonfunctioning brain. The advent of successful organ transplantation in the early 1960s and the need for donor organs resulted in the need to define brain death both medically and legally. This need led to the publication of the Harvard criteria in 1968. Subsequent modifications include more stringent guidelines for the determination of apnea, recognition of persistent spinal reflexes in brain death, and additional tests to confirm the absence of brain function. The President's Commission for the Study of Ethical Problems in Medicine, Biomedical, and Behavioral Research (1981) introduced the Uniform Determination of Death Act, which defines death as follows: "1. The irreversible cessation of circulatory and respiratory functions, or 2. The irreversible cessation of all functions of the entire brain, including the brainstem."

2. What are the current guidelines for the determination of brain death?

The diagnosis of brain death is clinical; it is based on certain prerequisites (establishing the cause and excluding reversible causes) and clinical signs. It requires the written documentation of two licensed physicians.

  1. **Cessation of cerebral function.** This diagnosis requires clinical evidence of a state of deep coma (Glasgow Coma Scale score of 3). The patient must be unreceptive and unresponsive to noxious stimuli. True decerebrate or decorticate posturing is not consistent with the diagnosis of brain death. In some circumstances it is preferable to perform one or more confirmatory tests.

  2. **Cessation of brainstem function.** This diagnosis requires the lack of brainstem reflexes, including the absence of pupillary, corneal, jaw, gag, cough, swallowing, grimacing, and yawning reflexes and any kind of spontaneous or inducible extraocular movements combined with the persistence of apnea despite adequate stimulus to breathe ($pCO_2 > 60$). If brainstem reflexes cannot be clinically evaluated with certainty (as in severe facial trauma), confirmatory tests are recommended. In the absence of confirmatory tests, the patient should be observed continuously in an intensive care setting for 12 hours. If anoxic damage is suspected, observation for 24 hours is recommended. The absence of cerebral blood flow as confirmed by cerebral angiography is the only measure of cerebral function that does not require additional clinical observation and laboratory evaluation to confirm the diagnosis of brain death.

3. When can a patient be declared brain dead?

Concise reviews by Pitts (1984) and Wijdicks (2001) and the Consensus Statement by the American Academy of Neurology (1995) summarized the current criteria for brain death as follows:

  1. **The cause of brain injury must be known.** The cause of brain injury can be determined clinically through careful history and physical exam. Laboratory studies, such as blood counts, coagulation studies, electrolytes, blood gases, serum and urine toxicology, and cerebrospinal fluid analysis, help establish the cause. In general, however, diagnostic imaging studies are used to produce convincing evidence of irreversible brain damage. CT, MRI, and, in some cases, cerebral angiography are performed to confirm the cause of brain injury.

  2. **Metabolic and toxic central nevous system (CNS) depression must be excluded.** Reversible causes of apparent brain death must be ruled out and documented in the chart. These include pharmacologic agents such as barbiturates, benzodiazepines, and neuromuscular blockade;

endogenous metabolic disorders, such as severe hepatic encephalopathy, hyperosmolar coma, hyponatremia, and uremia; severe systemic hypotension with a concomitant decrease in cerebral blood flow; and hypothermia. Loss of thermoregulation is often associated with brain death. Normothermia (> 32° C) must be restored before the determination of brain death.

3. **There must be no demonstrable brain function.** The diagnosis of brain death requires that there be no evidence of brain function. The patient must be unresponsive without spontaneous movement, response to pain, or brainstem function. The possibility of neuromuscular blockade by pharmacologic agents must be ruled out by history and/or the application of a peripheral nerve stimulator. The possibility of the locked-in state should be ruled out by instructing the patient, while the eyelids are open, to move the eyes up, down, and to the sides.

4. How is the cessation of brainstem function demonstrated?

The absence of brainstem function is demonstrated by the absence of brainstem reflexes and the presence of apnea. Tests for brainstem function include:

1. **Pupillary response to light:** the pupils in brain death are fixed and midposition to dilated (5–8 mm in size), without response to light. Pupillary findings in critically ill or comatose patients include the following:

Small, reactive: metabolic or sedative drugs (e.g., atropinics, adrenergics.)

Unilateral fixed, dilated: cranial nerve (CN) III palsy (transtentorial herniation).

2. **Doll's eyes,** or oculocephalic reflex: tests midbrain, pontine, and medullary function. In a comatose patient with an intact brainstem, the eyes lag behind when the head is turned suddenly to one side. This lag in eye movement is not present in brainstem injury. The reflex is not present in conscious patients. This maneuver is to be done only when stability of the cervical spine is ensured.

3. **Cold calorics,** or the oculovestibular reflex: tests midbrain, pontine, and medullary function. This reflex persists even after the oculocephalic reflex has disappeared; thus, it is important in patients who lack an oculocephalic response. The test is performed by irrigating intact and unobstructed external ear canals (one at a time, 5 minutes between each side) with 50 ml of iced water while both eyes are held open. The normal reflex results in nystagmus, with the fast component away from the side of stimulation. If the communication of the intact brainstem with the telencephalon has been lost, the eyes will deviate tonically toward the irrigated side, without the production of nystagmus. Extensive brainstem injury, or brain death, results in the absence of all eye movements.

4. **Medullary function.** Lack of medullary function is demonstrated by the absence of the cough and gag reflexes, but the most reliable marker of medullary death is the cessation of spontaneous respirations as demonstrated by the performance of an apnea test.

5. How is an apnea test performed?

To demonstrate apnea, one must provide the injured brainstem with an adequate stimulus to breathe. In the apnea test, the arterial tension of carbon dioxide provides the stimulus. The minimum level of pCO_2 required to demonstrate apnea in the severely injured or "dead" brain is a matter of debate in the literature, but minimal levels of 44–60 torr have been recommended.

Guidelines for Apnea Testing

---

1. Ventilate for at least 20 minutes to produce a normal pCO_2 (37–40 torr) and hyperoxia with an FIO_2 of 1.00 before disconnection from the ventilator.

2. After disconnection from mechanical evaluation, maintain 100% O_2 flow to endotracheal tube by T-piece. The American Academy of Neurology also suggests using a cannula through the endotracheal tube at the level of the carina with 10 L/min of oxygen for the duration of the test.

3. Continue apnea for 5–10 min or until hypoxia, hypotension, or ventricular arrhythmias result. The carbon dioxide level in blood will rise at a rate of 2–4 torr/min.

4. Follow pCO_2 by arterial blood gas measurements to document a final $pCO_2 > 60$ torr, an increase in $pCO_2 > 20$ torr, or a pH < 7.24.

---

6. Are spinal reflexes absent in brain death?

No. The current guidelines recognize the persistence of spinal reflexes in brain death; approximately 75% of patients with documented brain death exhibit spinal reflexes. Deep tendon spinal reflexes are often present.

7. What are the indications for the use of confirmatory tests in brain death?

Confirmatory tests are not required in brain death and do not supersede clinical criteria. They can be considered in patients with an indeterminant apnea test, hypercapnia, severe obesity (which makes detection of respiratory movement difficult), severe congestive heart failure and/or hemodynamic instability, and severe facial trauma (which makes examination of the face and eyes difficult or impossible). Confirmatory tests may aid in the transplantation of organs.

8. What are the accepted confirmatory tests for brain death?

There are two types of confirmatory tests: those that document loss of bioelectrical activity (electroencephalogram [EEG], sensory-evoked potential [SEP], brainstem auditory-evoked response [BAER]) and those that document loss of blood flow (pancerebral angiography, scintigraphy, transcranial Doppler).

Contrast angiography. This invasive technique requires catheterization via the femoral or axillary arteries. A definitive test requires visualization of both extracranial carotid and vertebrobasilar systems. A positive test is one in which "no flow" is identified within the cranial vault. Typically, the dye column tapers symmetrically with nonfilling of the cervical carotids (pseudo-occlusion) or an abrupt block at the cranial base. This is in marked contrast to the bilateral filling of the external carotid system. The vertebral vessels disappear at the atlanto-occipital junction. Occasionally, the basilar can be seen against the clivus. There is no visualization of the venous phase. This test may endanger the patient because it requires transport to the angiography suite and administration of contrast.

Radionucleotide cerebral imaging. This is a noninvasive, simple, and safe method of measuring cerebral blood flow. Portable gamma cameras allow bedside exams to be completed in 15 minutes. The test requires an IV bolus of sodium pertechnetate technetium 99m (15–21 mCi/adult) or 99mTc-labeled hexamethyl propyleneamine oxime, followed by anterior images recorded every 3 seconds for a total of 60 seconds. Counts attributable to the external carotid system are eliminated by subtraction techniques or a tourniquet placed around the forehead to eliminate scalp flow. With normal cerebral blood flow, sequential images show activity over the common carotid arteries—anterior and middle cerebral arteries—capillaries—sagittal sinus—internal jugular bilaterally. Occasionally, the scalp veins drain into the sagittal sinus, resulting in minimal late sagittal sinus activity in the absence of identifiable arterial activity.

Transcranial Doppler. This emerging technology is the easiest and fastest test to perform and does not require transport of the patient from the intensive care unit. Documentation of oscillating flow or systolic spikes is typical of brain death. These findings need to be demonstrated on two different occasions 30 minute apart. There are no reports of clinically brain-dead children or adults who "survive" after demonstration of such transcranial patterns. The examination includes bilateral extracranial vessels (common carotid arteries, internal carotid arteries, and vertebral arteries) and any bilateral intracranial arteries and is repeated in 30 minutes. In approximately 15% of patients, this test cannot be done, particularly in older patients. Ventricular drains or skull defects (e.g., craniectomies, neonatal status) that preclude an increase in intracranial pressure interfere with the reliability of the test.

9. What is the role of EEG in the diagnosis of brain death?

The EEG is an accepted confirmatory test for brain death. Published guidelines[2] include such factors as electrode positions, time of recording, and impedance settings. Factors that may result in an isoelectric EEG that is indistinguishable from brain death include **hypothermia** that produces a transient, reversible electroencephalographic silence (ECS). Therefore, a central temperature of at least 32°C (90°F) is required before determination of brain death by EEG.

Cardiovascular shock may result in reversible ECS. In this case, loss of electrical activity is secondary to decreased cerebral perfusion resulting from systemic hypotension. Electrical activity may be restored by increasing systemic blood pressure. Therefore, a systemic blood pressure of at least 80 mmHg is prerequisite to the diagnosis of brain death by EEG. **Barbiturate coma** or toxic levels of other CNS depressant drugs (benzodiazepines, trichlorethylene) may also result in ECS; therefore, the possibility of drug overdose must be ruled out by careful history and/or appropriate toxicology screen if the EEG is to reliably diagnose brain death. Most CNS depressant drugs do not produce the clinical criteria necessary for the diagnosis of brain death because of their effect on pupil size (most produce small pupils). Exceptions include scopolamine and glutethimide, which produce large pupils.

10. Discuss the role of BAER in the diagnosis of brain death.

In brain death, the brainstem and auditory short-latency responses are absent. The observation that all BAER components after wave I or II are absent in brain death but preserved in toxic and metabolic disorders suggests that BAER may be useful in evaluating patients in whom coma of toxic etiology is suspected (in particular, barbiturate coma is known to produce an isoelectric EEG).

11. What are the cardiac manifestations of brain death?

Despite aggressive cardiovascular support, patients determined to be brain dead progress to cardiovascular collapse within 1 week. In fact, most die within 2 days after the diagnosis of brain death. Heart-rate variability is lost (loss of vagal function) as well as heart-rate response to atropine-like drugs. The electrocardiographic changes associated with the initial stage of brain death include widening of the QRS complex (Osborn waves), prolongation of the QT segment, and nonspecific ST changes.

More advanced stages of brain death are marked by bradycardia, followed by conduction abnormalities, including atrioventricular block and interventricular conduction delays. Atrial fibrillation is relatively common in the terminal stages of brain death, with atrial activity often continuing after the cessation of ventricular complexes.

12. Is it possible to predict which comatose patients will progress to brain death?

It is not possible to determine with confidence which comatose patients will progress to brain death, even though several studies have identified clinical parameters associated with poor neurologic outcome. The best predictors of neurologic outcome are the Glasgow Coma Scale score at presentation and the level of brainstem function observed within the first 24 hours after presentation. The lack of pupillary response to light or corneal reflexes on initial exam is a very poor prognostic sign. By 72 hours after cerebral insult, the motor response to pain increases in predictive value; absent or posturing response to pain is associated with poor neurologic recovery.

BIBLIOGRAPHY

1. American Academy of Neurology, Quality Standards Subcommittee: Practice parameters for determining brain death in adults (summary statement). Neurology 47:309–310, 1995.
2. American Electroencephalographic Society: Guideline three: Minimum technical standards for EEG recording in suspected cerebral death. J Clin Neurophysiol 11:10–13, 1994.
3. Chatrian G: Electrophysiologic evaluation of brain death: A critical appraisal. In Aminoff MJ: Electrodiagnosis in Clinical Neurology. New York, Churchill Livingstone, 1986, pp 669–736.
4. Ducrocq X, Hassler W, Moritake K, et al: Consensus opinion on diagnosis of cerebral circulatory arrest using Doppler-sonography. Task Force Group on Cerebral Death of the Neurosonology Research Group of the World Federation on Neurology. J Neurol Sci 159:145–150, 1998.
5. Freitas J, Azevedo E, Teixeira J, et al: Heart rate variability as an assessment of brain death. Transplant Proc 32:2584–2585, 2000.
6. Goldie WP, et al: Brainstem auditory and short latency somatosensory evoked responses in brain death. Neurology 31:248–256, 1981.
7. Haupt WF, Rudolf J: European brain death codes: A comparison of national guidelines. J Neurol 246:432–437, 1999.

8. Jenkins DH, Reilly PM, Schwab W: Improving the approach to organ transplantation: A review. World J Surg 23:644–649, 1999.
9. Lam AM: Neurophysiologic monitoring. In Newfield P, Cotrell JE (eds): Handbook of Neuroanesthesia. Philadelphia, Lippincott Williams & Wilkins, 1999, pp 34–52.
10. Pitts LH: Determination of brain death. West J Med 140:628–631, 1984.
11. Schwartz J, et al: Radionucleotide cerebral imaging confirming brain death. JAMA 249:246–247, 1983.
12. Tsai SH, et al: Cerebral radionucleotide angiography: Its application in the diagnosis of brain death. JAMA 248:591–592, 1982.
13. Walker A: Cerebral Death. Baltimore, Urban and Schwartzenberg, 1985.
14. Wijdicks EF: The diagnosis of brain death. N Engl J Med 344:1244–1246, 2001.

65. STATUS EPILEPTICUS

David C. Bonovich, M.D.

1. Define status epilepticus.

The World Health Organization defines status epilepticus (SE) as "a condition characterized by an epileptic seizure that is sufficiently prolonged or repeated at sufficiently brief intervals so as to produce an unvarying and enduring epileptic condition." In the clinical setting SE may be defined as seizure activity lasting 30 minutes or intermittent seizure activity for 30 minutes or more during which consciousness is not regained.

2. What are the different types of SE? How do they present?

SE is best divided into three categories: convulsive status epilepticus (CSE), nonconvulsive status epilepticus (NCSE), and partial status epilepticus (PSE). Although only CSE is life-threatening, all forms of status may result in serious disability. SE also can be divided into seizures that involve the whole brain (CSE and NCSE) and seizures that involve only part of the brain (PSE). Seizures invovling the whole brain may be subdivided into those associated with obvious motor movement (CSE) and those not associated with obvious motor involvement (NCSE).

CSE is the most serious type of SE. Seizures are characterized by rhythmic shaking of the limbs and body, tongue biting, and loss of consciousness. As the duration of the seizures increases, the movements may become reduced, sometimes to eye fluttering, although generalized electricity activity continues in the brain. Although the diagnosis of CSE is obvious in most cases, the differential diagnosis includes rigors associated with fever and sepsis, myoclonic jerks, and pseudo-status epilecticus (seizures of psychogenic origin not associated with electrical discharges from the brain).

NCSE may be more difficult to diagnose. Although there is no generally accepted classification of NCSE, two major types are recognized: partial complex and petit mal. In partial complex SE, alteration of consciousness lasts more than 30 minutes because of abnormal cortical electrical activity. Generalized tonic-clonic motor activity is absent, but stereotypical movements such as lip smacking, chewing, or picking at one's clothes may occur. The patient may be misdiagnosed as intoxicated or as having a psychiatric disorder. Petit mal SE is often difficult to distinguish from partial complex SE, except with electroencephalographic (EEG) recordings. Patients appear lethargic but may be able to answer simple questions slowly. Eye blinking may be present, but automatisms are less common than in partial complex SE.

Continuous PSE consists merely of persistent focal motor seizures that last longer than 30 minutes and do not impair consciousness.

3. What are the most common causes of CSE?

Cessation of antiepileptic drugs, withdrawal from alcohol, drug overdose, and cerebrovascular disease are the most common causes of CSE. Approximately 50% of adults with CSE have no previous history of epilepsy. Many of these presentations occur in the setting of acute neurologic illnesses such as stroke. Other causes include electrolyte imbalances, head injury, toxic effects of drugs, hypoxic-ischemic insults, brain tumors, central nervous system (CNS) infection, and renal failure. In about 15% of patients, no cause can be found.

4. Why is urgent treatment of CSE a medical necessity?
The electrophysiologic progression of CSE is divided into five stages: (1) discrete seizure activity, (2) merging of seizure activity, (3), continuous electrical discharge, (4) intermittent suppression of seizure activity, and (5) periodic epileptiform discharges. Prolonged CSE also is associated with systemic distrubances. An initial increase in minute ventilation gives way to hypoventilation and apnea. Pulmonary vascular resistance may become elevated, and in some cases pulmonary edema may develop. Aspiration is common. Arrhythmias may be seen in up to 60% of patients with prolonged SE. Hyperthermia may result from catecholamine release and prolonged vigorous muscle activity. In addition, lactic acidosis and other metabolic disturbances may develop.

Sound experimental data suggest that permanent cell damage occurs in several cortical and subcortical locations after 60 minutes of convulsive status. In addition, clinical studies have shown that the longer CSE continues, the more difficult it is to control, and the greater the incidence of neurologic sequelae. Thus, it is important to recognize and treat CSE early and aggressively before such complications develop.

5. What are the most important initial steps when faced with a patient with CSE?
As always, the ABCs (airways, breathing, and circulation) must be addressed immediately. Supplemental oxygen should be applied, and a secure intravenous (IV) line should be started. If an adequate airway and ventilation are not present, an endotracheal tube should be inserted, and ventilation should be assisted. If neuromuscular blockade is to be used for intubation, a short-acting agent is recommended to avoid obscuring clinical seizure activity. A 0.9% sodium chloride solution should be the initial IV fluid infused, because it can be used to treat hypotension if it occurs and is compatible with IV phenytoin or fosphenytoin. Liberal hydration with normal saline (200 ml/hr) should be started to minimize the risk of renal failure from rhabdomyolysis and to prevent dehydration.

6. Which tests should be ordered immediately for a patient presenting with CSE?
A complete blood count, anticonvulsant levels, serum electrolytes, glucose, serum osmolarity, blood urea nitrogen, creatinine, calcium, magnesium and phosphate, a drug screen, blood alcohol level, and arterial blood gas analysis should be ordered immediately.

7. Once the ABCs have been addressed, what are the next steps in managing a patient with CSE?
The following approach is intended only as a guideline. Individual circumstances may dictate different therapies. Although seizures must persist for 30 minutes to be classified as SE, one should not wait until 30 minutes have passed before initiating therapy. Once IV access has been secured, thiamine (100 mg IV) should be administered, followed by 50 ml of 50% dextrose solution if bedside glucose testing revealed hypoglycemia. Lorazepam, 0.10 mg/kg, should be given at a rate no faster than 2 mg/minute and in 4-mg doses to a maximal adult dose of 10 mg. Simultaneously, a loading dose of fosphenytoin should be administered at a rate of 100 mg/min. Fosphenytoin is a water-soluble form of phenytoin and lacks the propylene glycol vehicle that has been implicated in the hypotension and cardiac arrhythmias sometimes seen during traditional IV phenytoin loading. Fosphenytoin is expressed as phenytoin equivalents; thus, the loading dose is the same as for phenytoin (18 mg/kg). If fosphenytoin is unavailable, phenytoin (18–20 mg/kg given at a rate no faster than 50 mg/min or 25 mg/min in the elderly) should be infused. Over 80% of cases of CSE are controlled by the combination of lorazepam and a phenytoin preparation.

If seizures persist after initial fosphenytoin loading, an additional 5 mg/kg of fosphenytoin (or phenytoin if it is the only form available) should be given. If this dose is ineffective, tracheal intubation, if not already secured, is indicated because the cardiorespiratory depressant effects of barbiturates (the next drug to be added) and benzodiazepines are additive. In addition, many of patients experience hypotension as barbiturates or further benzodiazepines are administered and require IV hydration and blood pressure support with inotropes such as dopamine.

The optimal treatment of refractory cases of CSE not responsive to phenytoin and lorazepam is an area of ongoing debate. If not already involved, a neurologist who is an expert in SE should be consulted.

Traditionally, phenobarbital (15- to 20-mg/kg loading dose) has been recommended as the next medication, given at a rate no faster than 50–100 mg/min until the full dose was given or the seizures stopped. Phenobarbital loading is followed by a maintenance dose of 1–4 mg/kg/day. If phenobarbital load fails to stop the seizures, many physicians now recommend pentobarbital or midazolam. Pentobarbital is administered as a loading dose of 2–8 mg/kg over 2 minutes, followed by a maintenance dose of 0.5–5 mg/kg/hr until the seizures stop clinically or burst suppression is reached on the EEG. Alternatively, a loading dose of midazolam (10 mg over 3–5 minutes), followed by a maintenance dose of 0.05–0.4 mg/kg/hr, can be used until the EEG is free of seizures.

If these steps are unsuccessful, lidocaine, 2 mg/kg over 5 minutes followed by a drip of 3 mg/kg/hr for no more than 12 hours, may be used. Lidocaine should not be used in patients with heart or liver failure or patients with cardiac arrhythmias or bundle-branch blocks. General anesthesia with an inhalational agent such as isoflurane can also be considered if the above measures are unsuccessful. Propofol recently has been used for refractory CSE. Its mechanism of action is still unclear. The loading dose of 1 mg/kg is repeated every 5 minutes until seizure activity is suppressed. A maintenance dose of 2–10 mg/kg/hr is then used. An IV preparation of valproic acid has been developed, and animal data suggest that it may be effective in CSE, although it has not been approved by the Food and Drug Administration.

8. What factors should be taken into account in determining which neuromuscular blockers (NMBs) should be administered to a patient with CSE if these agents are necessary?

NMBs at times may be desirable to help reduce the metabolic derangements and hyperthermia resulting from prolonged vigorous muscle contraction. All NMBs cause profound muscle weakness, but agents vary greatly in duration of action. If neuromuscular blockade is necessary and continuous EEG recording is *not* being performed, a single dose of a short-acting, nondepolarizing agent should be administered; it is impossible to ascertain clinically whether seizure activity is continuing in the presence of neuromuscular blockade. Anticonvulsant treatment should continue as outlined earlier, and EEG monitoring should be strongly considered. If a long-acting agent is used or if multiple doses of a short-acting agent are given, continuous EEG monitoring is mandatory to prevent unrecognized SE. All patients receiving NMBs should be intubated.

9. What steps are appropriate after the seizures are controlled?

Once the seizures are controlled, it is important to establish the etiology of the SE. Appropriate blood work and cultures should be ordered. Imaging with CT or MRI should be done as soon as possible to rule out structural CNS causes. Lumbar puncture may help to rule out CNS infections and subarachnoid hemorrhage. Empirical antibiotics should be started if an infectious etiology is suspected, and maintenance doses of anticonvulsants should be administered and adjusted based on serum levels.

10. Does fever or cerebrospinal fluid (CSF) pleocytosis always indicate an infectious etiology of CSE?

Most patients with CSE exhibit an increase in body temperature, which in rare cases may progress to extremes (up to 107°F) even in the absence of an infectious etiology. In addition, mild pleocytosis of peripheral blood and CSF may occur in such patients. Although fever and pleocytosis of blood and CSF may be the result of CSE, it is imperative not to attribute these findings to the effect of repeated seizures until all other possibilities have been excluded. In general, empirical coverage for infectious etiologies (until all cultures are negative) is preferable to undertreatment of a serious infection.

BIBLIOGRAPHY

1. Aminoff MJ, Simon RP: Status epilepticus: Causes, clinical features and consequences in 98 patients. Am J Med 69:657–666, 1980.
2. Chapman MG, Smith M, Hirsch NP: Status epilepticus. Anaesthesia 56:648–659, 2001.
3. Crawford TO, Mitchell WG, Snodgrass SR: Lorazepam in childhood status epilepticus and serial seizures: Effectiveness and tachyphylaxis. Neurology 37:190–195, 1987.
4. Leppik IE: Status epilepticus. Neurol Clin 4:633–643, 1986.
5. Provencio JJ, Bleck TP, Conners AF: Critical care neurology. Am J Respir Crit Care Med 164:341–345, 2001.
6. Uthman BM, Wilder BJ: Emergency management of seizures: An overview. Epilepsia 30(Suppl 2): S33–S37, 1989.
7. Wijdicks EFM: The Clinical Practice of Critical Care Neurology. Philadelphia, Lippincott-Raven, 1997.
8. Wilder BJ (ed): The use of parenteral antiepileptic drugs and the role of fosphenytoin. Neurology 46 (Suppl 1):S1–S28, 1996.

66. CEREBRAL ANEURYSMS

David Palestrant, M.D., and David Bonovich, M.D.

1. What is the incidence of subarachnoid hemorrhage (SAH) from ruptured intracranial aneurysms?

The incidence is estimated at 6–28 per 100,000 population.

2. What is the incidence of asymptomatic intracranial aneurysm?

Autopsy studies have shown a prevalence of about 2% in the general population. The risk of hemorrhage from previously unruptured aneurysm is believed to be about 1% annually; however, precise figures are not known.

3. What are the major types of intracranial aneurysms?

Saccular aneurysms: by far the most common aneurysmal type and cause of subarachnoid hemorrhage.

Mycotic aneurysms: 1–5% of intracerebral aneurysms result from septic embolization due to valvular vegetations in patients with bacterial endocarditis. Mycotic aneurysms typically appear about 4–5 weeks after an acute embolic event. They usually are found in the distal middle cerebral artery circulation, although 10% are found more proximally. Mycotic aneurysms usually resolve with adequate antibiotic therapy but occasionally require endovascular or surgical correction. Streptococci are the most common pathogen.

Traumatic aneurysms: although true traumatic aneurysms are rare, false aneurysms are more common. False aneurysms result from the complete disruption of the vessel wall with resulting clot formation. Traumatic aneurysms may be found in association with skull fractures.

Fusiform aneurysms: caused by dilated tortuous vessels that may rupture, dissect, or form thrombi that embolize distally. The pathology of fusiform aneurysms appears to be distinct from the pathology of both atherosclerosis and saccular aneurysms.

4. What are the risk factors for developing saccular aneurysms?

Both congenital and acquired factors are involved. Approximately 6.7% of all cerebral aneurysms occur in families; familial aneurysms typically present earlier than nonfamilial aneurysms. Aneurysms also are associated with arteriovenous malformations (AVMs); they have been noted on the feeding vessels in approximately 7% of patients. Other nonmodifiable risk factors include autosomal dominant polycystic kidney disease (2% of patients), neurofibromatosis type I, and connective tissue disorders such as Ehlers-Danlos type IV, fibromuscular dysplasia, and Marfan syndrome. Approximately 16% of patients with polycystic kidney disease develop intracranial aneurysms. The exact pathologic cause of saccular aneurysms has not been clearly elucidated, but they tend to occur at bifurcations of major cerebral vessels where flow pressures are highest.

5. What are the risk factors for intracranial aneurysmal rupture?

Rupture occurs most frequently between 40 and 60 years of age with a peak frequency between 55 and 60 years of age. Family history of SAH is an important predisposing factor; 5–10% of patients have a positive family history. In most studies, women appear to be at higher risk than men, and there is a slightly higher incidence during pregnancy. Size of the aneurysm is also important; larger aneurysms are more likely to rupture than smaller ones (2% of aneurysms < 5 mm in diameter vs. > 40% of aneurysms between 6 and 10 mm in diameter. Aneurysms > 3 mm are thought to be at increased risk for rupture.

6. Besides aneurysms, what are the other causes of SAH?

Arterial dissection: Dissections are disruptions of the arterial wall in which blood flows into the intima, creating a false lumen. When they involve the vertebral arteries, they may present with SAH or embolic storke and often are associated with lower cranial nerve palsies and brainstem infarctions. Anterior circulation dissections also may occur, but SAH associated with anterior circulation dissections is decidedly rare.

Cerebral AVMs: Occasionally SAH is seen without the normal pattern of intracerebral hemorrhage. In such cases, a concomitant saccular aneurysm must be excluded.

Pituitary apoplexy: Patients usually present with a sudden headache along with deterioration of visual acuity. Eye movement abnormalities and deterioration in level of consciousness also may be seen. Magnetic resonance imaging (MRI) or computed tomography (CT) usually indicates the pituitary as the source.

Perimesencephalic SAH (so-called angionegative SAH): The subarachnoid blood is isolated anterior to the pons. The diagnosis is confirmed by excluding an aneurysm with angiography or CT angiography. The risk for rebleeding is low, and prognosis is good. Patients do not develop the dangerous sequelae seen in aneurysmal SAH.

Head trauma: SAH is common in head trauma.

7. What are the signs and symptoms of intracranial aneurysmal rupture?

The most pathognomonic presentation includes an explosive headache, nausea, vomiting, neck stiffness, and photophobia, possibly associated with loss of consciousness. Focal neurologic deficits are sometimes evident at presentation; one of the most common is a third nerve palsy in association with posterior communicating artery aneurysms. Abducens palsies are also seen and thought to be related to increased intracranial pressure and possibly to brainstem herniation as a result of traction on the nerve. Depending on location, other neurologic deficits are also seen, including motor and sensory deficits, visual loss, and loss of brainstem reflexes.

Signs and Symptoms of Subarachnoid Hemorrhage

SYMPTOMS OF SUBARACHNOID HEMORRHAGE	SIGNS OF SUBARACHNOID HEMORRHAGE
Sudden, severe headache	Neck stiffness
Nausea and vomiting	Brudzinski's, Kernig's sign
Dizziness	Fever
Vertigo	Hypertension
Fatigue	Blurred vision
Diplopia	Oculomotor paralysis
Photophobia	Hemiparesis
	Confusion and/or agitation
	Coma

From Smith R, Miller J: Pathophysiology and clinical evaluation of subarachnoid hemorrhage. In Youmans JR (ed): Neurological Surgery, 3rd ed. Philadelphia, W.B. Saunders, 1990, with permission.

Systemic signs associated with SAH include cardiac arrhythmias and ischemia. These cardiovascular signs are well described in the literature and are generally attributed to norepinephrine release. Cardiac arrhythmias are most common in the first 48 hours. Systemic hypertension and bradycardia may be seen as manifestations of increased intracranial pressure. Aspiration pneumonia and pulmonary edema are the most common pulmonary manifestations. The latter is thought to be due to left ventricular failure resulting in increased pulmonary capillary hydrostatic pressure. Neurogenic pulmonary edema can develop rapidly after subarachnoid hemorrhage and is also felt to be secondary to norepinephrine release, leading to increased capillary permeability.

8. What is a sentinel bleed? Why is it significant?

A sentinel bleed is an initial minor bleed or "leak" from a cerebral aneurysm. It is considered a minor bleed because, although it results in a severe headache, it may go unrecognized or may be misdiagnosed (as a migraine headache, for instance). It is important to recognize sentinel bleeds because they often serve as warning sings of subsequent catastrophic events. Proper recognition and care may affect mortality. The mortality rate from unruptured aneurysms identified by sentinel bleeds is reported to be lower than that from aneurysmal bleeds that are not preceded by warning leaks (28.9% v.s 43.2%).

9. How is SAH diagnosed?

CT scans of the brain, if performed within 24 hours of rupture, have a sensitivity of about 90%. In addition, CT scanning can give valuable information about the amount and location of hematomas or subarachnoid blood, the presence of ventricular blood, and the size of the ventricles. If the CT is negative for the presence of subarachnoid blood, a lumbar puncture is indicated. It may be difficult to distinguish subarachnoid blood from a traumatic tap, and the presence of xanthochromia on lumbar puncture is the most sensitive distinguishing measure. Xanthochromia can be detected by about 4 hours after a subarachnoid hemorrhage and remains up to 3 weeks afterwards. Traumatic taps are also evident by the clearing of blood with the serial collection of a number of tubes (usually only three tubes are needed).

10. What factors are associated with poor prognosis after rupture of an intracranial aneurysm?

The amount of blood, older age, posterior circulation aneurysms, and early development of hydrocephalus. The degree of meningeal irritation, level of consciousness, and the presence of focal motor deficits can be used to identify patients who are at increased risk of perioperative death. Under these criteria, patients are grouped into five grades.

Classic Presentation and Prognosis for Ruptured Cerebral Aneurysm

GRADE	CRITERIA	ESTIMATED PERIOPERATIVE MORTALITY (%)
I	Asymptomatic or minimal headache and slight nuchal rigidity	0–5
II	Moderate-to-severe headache, no nuchal rigidity other than cranial nerve palsy	2–10
III	Drowsiness, confusion, or mild focal deficit	10–15
IV	Stupor, moderate to severe hemiparesis, possible early decerebrate rigidity and vegetative disturbances	60–70
V	Deep coma, decerebrate rigidity, moribund appearance	70–100

Adapted from Peerless SJ.[21] Grades according to Hunt and Hess.[11]

11. What are the major complications of ruptured intracranial aneurysms?

Global cerebral ischemia, rebleeding, acute hydrocephalus, vasospasm, and hyponatremia.

12. What causes global cerebral ischemia?

Inadequate cerebral perfusion as the intracranial pressure rises aove the arterial pressure. It often occurs at the time of SAH and results in the high mortality rate at presentation. It is also the reason that many high-grade patients cannot be saved despite arriving at the hospital alive.

13. What percentage of patients rebleed? What is their prognosis?

Up to 15% of patients rebleed in the first day, and 35–40% rebleed over the next 4 weeks if the aneurysm remains unsecured. Rebleeding is associated with a further 50% mortality rate.

14. What invasive and noninvasive measures can be used to prevent rebleeding?

A single randomized clinical trial demonstrated no difference in terms of overall outcome between early and late surgical intervention, with the important exception that patients who were alert on admission generally did better with early surgery. In most large centers earlier intervention is now preferred. No randomized studies have evaluated early endovascular coiling. ICU management issues include keeping the patient calm and pain-free, avoiding severe hypertension before the aneurysm is secured, and ensuring adequate cerebral perfusion.

15. How is hydrocephalus managed?

With urgent ventricular drain placement. In the first 24 hours, patients should be monitored closely for gradual obtundation, slow pupillary responses to light, and downward deviation of the eyes. A ventricular drain (EVD) should be placed urgently in patients who present with a grade 3 or greater hemorrhage.

16. When does cerebral vasospasm develop? What are its consequences?

Vasospasm may occur in as many as 60–75% of patients following SAH. It occurs between days 4 and 21 with the peak incidence between days 5 and 9. Vasospasm rarely starts after day 12. It may result in further neurologic devastation due to ischemic strokes.

17. How is vasospasm diagnosed?

Vasospasm may be diagnosed clinically by the appearance of neurologic deficits that cannot be explained by other causes such as hydrocephalus, rebleeding, or metabolic derangements. Transcranial Doppler (TCD) is a useful noninvasive tool for the diagnosis of vasospasm. Spasm is indicated by elevated flow velocities on TCD. Angiographically, vasospasm can be demonstrated by the narrowing of large arteries passing through the subarachnoid space. About 30% of angiographically apparent vasospasm is clinically significant.

18. Describe the treatment of cerebral vasospasm.

Treatment involves the prevention or reversal of arterial spasm and minimization of the ischemia that results from the spasm. Strategies include the following:

1. **Calcium channel blockers (CCBs).** Because of their effect on smooth muscle relaxation, CCBs have been investigated as a means of preventing vasospasm in multiple clinical trials. Oral nimodipine has been shown to reduce poor outcome after SAH but did not protect against secondary ischemia. This finding implies another effect of the drug—potentially a neuroprotective effect. Other CCBs have shown a reduction in secondary ischemia, but no change in outcome. Nimodipine has become the standard of care in many centers because of its effect on outcome.

2. **Hemodynamic therapy.** So-called triple-H therapy (hypervolemia, hemodilution, and hypertension) has been the cornerstone of vasospasm management. Hypervolemic therapy is often used in an attempt to augment cerebral blood flow, but recent reviews and studies have found little eivdence to support this practice. Arterial hypertension is believed to have its effect by maximizing cerebral perfusion pressure, thereby increasing blood flow to the brain.

3. **Percutaneous transluminal angioplasty and papaverine therapy.** These strategies are used in an attempt to open narrowed vessels. Although their efficacy has not been demonstrated in randomized, controlled trials, several large observational series have demonstrated marked clinical

improvement as well as angiographically sustained dilation of cerebral blood vessels following angioplasty. However, balloon angioplasty is mainly of benefit in dilating more proximal areas of vasospasm. Papaverine is a potent vasodilator that has also shown benefit. Its major limitation is that its effect is transient; treatment may have to be repeated as frequently as every 24 hours.

19. What causes hyponatremia? How is it best managed?

In the past, hyponatremia has been attributed to the syndrome of inappropriate antidiuretic hormone (SIADH); recently, however, it has been associated more with natriuresis and hypovolemia, referred to as cerebral salt wasting (CSW). The exact cause of CSW has not been determined, although several natriuretic factors have been studied. Treatment involves maintaining adequate volume and supplementing sodium by mouth or intravenously. The hyponatremia is usually mild to moderate; only rarely does the sodium level drop below 120 mmol/L.

20. How is CSW distinguished from SIADH?

Both conditions present with hyponatremia, decreased plasma osmolarity, and inappropriately high urine osmolarity. The distinguishing features are that CSW is a state of decreased effective arterial blood volume, whereas SIADH is a state of normal effective arterial blood volume. CSW is treated by volume and sodium replacement and SIADH by fluid restriction.

21. Describe the operative repair of cerebral aneurysms.

Several different surgical methods are used to repair cerebral aneurysms:

1. **Clipping:** The most effective of all the surgical techniques, clipping involves the dissection of the neck of the aneurysmal sac and the placement of a clip at the origin of the neck from the feeder vessel.

2. **Trapping:** This technique involves permanently occluding the vessel proximally and distally to the aneurysm and relies on the presence of adequate collateral blood flow to the affected area.

3. **Proximal ligation:** This technique involves ligation of the feeder artery to reduce blood flow through the aneurysm. The subsequent decrease in blood flow and transmural pressure results in thrombosis and/or obliteration of the aneurysmal sac. As with trapping, this technique is restricted to specific cases in which collateral blood flow is sufficient to prevent subsequent ischemic damage.

4. **Wrapping:** Reinforcement of the aneurysmal wall with synthetic material (e.g., Gelfoam) prevents further enlargement of the sac.

22. What nonoperative alternative treatments are available?

At selected centers, a viable alternative to surgical clipping is endovascular coiling performed by an interventional radiologist. With the use of detachable coils placed in the aneurysmal lumen, intraluminal thrombosis rates of up to 85% have been reported. No head-to-head studies have compared surgical and endovascular techniques, but multiple observational series and a retrospective study have indicated that endovascular coiling is probably comparable to surgical techniques.

BIBLIOGRAPHY

1. Allen GS, et al: Cerebral arterial spasm—a controlled trial of nimodipine in patients with subarachnoid hemorrhage. N Engl J Med 308:619–624, 1983.
2. Awad I, Carter P, et al: Clinical vasospasm after subarachnoid hemorrhage: Response to hypervolemic hemodilution and arterial hypertension. Stroke 18:365–372, 1987.
3. Cascasco A, et al: Selective endovascular treatment of 71 intracranial aneurysms with platinum coils. J Neurosurg 79:3–10, 1993.
4. Disney L, Weir B, Petruk K: Effect on management mortality of a deliberate policy of early operation on supratentorial aneurysms. Neurosurgery 20:695–701, 1987.
5. Elliot JP, Newell DW, Lam DJ, et al: Comparison of balloon angioplasty and papaverine infusion for the treatment of vasospasm following aneurysmal subarachnoid hemorrhage. J Neurosurg 88:277–284, 1998.

6. Espinosa F, Weir B, Noseworthy T: Nonoperative treatment of subarachnoid hemorrhage. In Youmens JR (ed): Neurological Surgery, 3rd ed. Philadelphia, W.B. Saunders, 1990, pp 1661–1668.
7. Feigin VL, Rinkel G, van Gign J: Circulatory volume expansion for aneurysmal SAH. Cochrane Database Syst Rev 2000.
8. Feigin VL, Rinkel GJ, Algfa A, et al: Calcium antagonists for aneurysmal subarachnoid hemorrhage. Cochrane Database Syst Rev 2000
9. Firlik A: Effect of transluminal angioplasty on cerebral blood flow in management of symptomatic vasospasm following aneurysmal SAH. J Neurosurg 86:830–839, 1997.
10. Higashida R, et al: Endovascular treatment of intracranial aneurysms with a new silicone microballoon device: Technical considerations and indications for therapy. Radiology 174:687–691, 1990.
11. Hunt W, Hess R: Surgical risk as related to time of intervention in the repair of intracranial aneurysms. J Neurosurg 28:14–20, 1968.
12. Kassell NF, et al: Cerebral vasospasm following aneurysmal subarachnoid hemorrhage. Stroke 16:562–572, 1985.
13. Kassell N, Boarini DJ: Patients with ruptured aneurysms: Pre- and postoperative management. In Wilkens RH, Rengachary SS (eds): Neurosurgery. New York, McGraw-Hill, 1985, pp 1367–1371.
14. Kassell N, et al: The international cooperative study on the timing of aneurysm surgery. Part I: Overall management results. J Neurosurg 73:18–36, 1990.
15. Kassell N, et al: The international cooperative study on the timing of aneurysm surgery. Part II: Surgical results. J Neurosurg 73:37–47, 1990.
16. Mee E, et al: Controlled study of nimodipine in aneurysm patients treated early after subarachnoid hemorrhage. Neurosurgery 22:484–490, 1988.
17. Miller J, Diringer M: Management of aneurysmal subarachnoid hemorrhage. Neurol Clin 13:451–478, 1995.
18. Nakatomi H: Clinicopathological study of intracranial fusiform and dolichoectatic aneurysms. Stroke 31:896–900, 2000.
19. Newell D, et al: Angioplasty for the treatment of symptomatic vasospasm following subarachnoid hemorrhage. J Neurosurg 71:654–659, 1989.
20. Palmer BF: Hyponatremia in a neurosurgical patient: Syndrome of inappropriate antidiuretic hormone secretion versus cerebral salt wasting. Nephrol Dial Transplant 15:262–268, 2000.
21. Peerless SJ: Intracranial aneurysms. In Newfield P, Cottrell J (ed): Handbook of Neuroanesthesia. 1983, pp 173–183.
22. Smith R, Miller J: Pathophysiology and clinical evaluation of subarachnoid hemorrhage. In Youmans JR (ed): Neurological Surgery, 3rd ed. Philadelphia, W.B. Saunders, 1990, pp 1644–1660.
23. Van Gijn J, Rinkel GJ: Subarachnoid hemorrhage: Diagnosis, causes, and management. Brain 124:249–278, 2001.
24. Vermeulen M, Lindsay KW, van Gijn J: Subarachnoid hemorrhage. Philadelphia, W.B. Saunders, 1992, pp 1–13.
25. Weir B: Intracranial aneurysms and subarachnoid hemorrhage: An overview. In Wilkens RH, Rengachary SS (eds): Neurosurgery. New York, McGraw-Hill, 1985, pp 1308–1329.
26. Whitfield PC: Timing of surgery for aneurysmal subarachnoid haemorrhage. Cochrane Database Syst Rev 2001.
27. Wijdicks EFM: Acid-base disorders, hypertonic and hypotonic states. In Wijdicks EFM (ed): The Clinical Practice of Critical Care Neurology. Philadelphia, Lippincott-Raven, 1997, pp 368–370.

67. STROKE

David Bonovich, M.D.

1. Define ischemic stroke.

A stroke results from a disruption in blood flow to the brain. Ischemia is defined as hypoemia, a decrease in the delivery of oxygen and glucose to a target organ—in this case, the brain. In the brain ischemia may be characterized as global (as in cardiac arrest) or focal (involving a specific vessel or a specific group of vessels in the brain); embolic or thrombotic; and large-vessel (involving one of the major blood vessels of the brain) or small-vessel (involving one of the small penetrating vessels of the brain).

2. What are the major risk factors for thrombotic cerebral infarction?

Hypertension is by far the most significant factor. The increased risk is proportional to the degree of hypertension. Age is also a risk factor: the incidence of cerebral infarction increases with age and is 1.3 times higher in men than in women. Other risk factors include diabetes, coronary artery disease, congestive heart failure, atrial fibrillation, and left ventricular hypertrophy. Obesity, hypercholesterolemia, and hyperlipidemia are risk factors in as much as they are risk factors for atherosclerotic disease.

3. What are the major risk factors for embolic cerebral infarction?

Embolic cerebral events are usually of cardiac origin. Major risk factors include ischemic heart disease with mural thrombus; cardiac arrhythmia, especially atrial fibrillation; prosthetic cardiac valves; rheumatic heart disease; structural valvular abnormalities, such as mitral stenosis; and bacterial endocarditis. Atrial fibrillation alone, without evidence of rheumatic heart disease, increases the risk of stroke by approximately fivefold. Elderly patients incur the greatest risk from atrial fibrillation, as the proportion of strokes due to this arrhythmia increases with age. Atheroscleroses of the aorta, carotid arteries, and vertebral arteries are also risk factors.

4. Does drug abuse predispose patients to stroke?

Drug abuse has emerged as a significant risk factor leading to stroke in young patients. At least one study has shown drug abuse to be the most frequently identified potential risk factor among stroke patients under the age of 35.

5. What is the normal value for cerebral blood flow?

In normal adults, cerebral blood flow is approximately 55 ml/100 gm of brain tissue/min, or 15% of normal cardiac output. When blood flow decreases to < 20 ml/100 mg/min, evoked potentials are lost and the electroencephalogram (EEG) becomes isoelectric. When blood flow decreases to < 15 ml/100 mg/min and is not quickly restored, irreversible brain injury occurs.

6. Describe the blood supply to the brain.

Four arteries carry blood to the brain. They are the two internal carotid arteries anteriorly and the two vertebral arteries posteriorly. The internal carotid arteries arise from the common carotid arteries. The left common carotid artery is a branch of the left subclavian artery; the right carotid artery arises from the right brachiocephalic trunk. Each common carotid artery bifurcates at the angle of the jaw, into external and internal branches. The internal carotid arteries supply the optic nerves, the retina, and the majority of the cerebral hemispheres (the frontal, parietal, and anterior temporal lobes).

Branches of the carotid artery include (1) ophthalmic artery, (2) posterior communicating artery, (3) anterior choriodal artery, (4) anterior cerebral artery, and (5) middle cerebral artery.

The posterior circulation is fed by two vertebral arteries. The right and left vertebral arteries arise from the subclavian arteries bilaterally and enter the posterior fossa through the foramen magnum. They give rise to the posterior inferior cerebellar artery and the anterior and posterior spinal arteries before merging to form the basilar artery at the level of the pontomedullary junction. The vertebrobasilar system supplies the cervical cord, brainstem, medial and posterior temporal lobes, and occipital lobes.

The posterior cerebral artery (PCA) supplies the occipital lobes. In a majority of patients (70%), this artery originates from the bifurcation of the basilar artery. In 95% of the cases, one or both PCAs arise from the basilar artery, whereas in the remaining 5% the posterior cerebral arteries arise from the internal carotid artery bilaterally.

Major branches of the basilar artery include (1) labyrinthine artery to the middle ear, (2) superior cerebellar artery, (3) posterior cerebral artery, and (4) anterior inferior cerebellar artery (AICA).

7. Describe the circle of Willis.

The vertebrobasilar system is joined to the carotid system by an anastomotic ring. The anterior and posterior communicating arteries link the anterior/posterior and the left/right hemispheric circulations. Four arteries compose the circle: posterior communicating artery, posterior cerebral artery bilaterally, anterior communicating artery, and anterior cerebral artery bilaterally.

8. Describe the clinical presentation of the large vascular ischemic stroke.

The neurologic presentation of patients suffering an ischemic cerebral event depends on the location and size of the infarct. Carotid artery infarction generally results in unilateral symptoms; vertebrobasilar system infarction may result in bilateral symptoms.

Carotid artery occlusion results in contralateral hemiparesis, hemihypesthesia, homonymous hemianopia, agnosia, and, if the dominant hemisphere is affected, global aphasia. Some patients (15%) exhibit an ipsilateral Horner's syndrome. Often the size of the infarct results in marked cerebral edema, and the patient may become obtunded or in coma. Most carotid occlusions are thrombotic. Transient ischemic episodes precede major carotid artery occlusions approximately 50% of the time. Some patients with complete carotid occlusion may have few if any neurologic deficits because collateral blood flow via the circle of Willis may allow sufficient blood flow to prevent ischemia.

Middle cerebral artery ischemia may result in a clinical picture similar to that of carotid artery occlusion. In acute carotid stenosis (e.g., an atherosclerotic blood vessel that progresses to complete closure) and carotid artery dissection, emboli may travel to the middle cerebral artery, leading to ischemia in the middle cerebral artery territory. Such ischemia typically results in motor dysfunction that affects the face and upper extremity but spares the leg. Branch occlusions result in fewer deficits. Speech and language function may be affected because the middle cerebral artery supplies the speech and language centers of the brain (in the left hemisphere in the vast majority of people).

Anterior cerebral artery ischemia is much less common. It results in contralateral motor dysfunction that affects the leg more than the arm and face.

Basilar artery occlusion results in bilateral cranial nerve palsies and quadriparesis. If the infarction includes the reticular activating system in the brainstem, the patient presents in coma. It is possible, however, for the high midbrain level reticular activating system to be spared, while motor pathways are affected. This complete loss of motor function in an awake patient is commonly referred to as locked-in syndrome. Other symptoms of ischemia to the basilar artery include vertigo, ataxia, and diplopia.

Unilateral vertebral artery occlusion may result in ischemia of the lateral medulla (if the posterior inferior cerebellar artery is involved). Ischemia of the spinothalamic tracts results in ipsilateral ataxia, facial hypesthesia, and contralateral loss of pain and temperature below the face. Loss of function of the ninth and tenth cranial nerves results in dysphagia and hoarseness. Horner's syndrome may also occur ipsilateral to the lesion. This syndrome is commonly referred to as the lateral medullary syndrome or Wallenberg's syndrome.

9. What is a lacunar infarct?

Lacuna is Latin for a small pit or hollow cavity. Cerebral lacunes refer to multiple small infarcts resulting from occlusion of the small penetrating branches (50–150 microns in diameter) of the major cerebral vessel. The infarcted brain tissue softens and decays, leaving small cavities (1–3 mm in diameter) that are evident at autopsy. Lacunes produce a variety of sensory and motor symptoms, depending on their location. Multiple lacunes may result in loss of intellectual capacity with impairment of recent memory. In some cases, severe dementia may result. There are four classic lunar syndromes:

1. **Pure motor hemiparesis:** weakness that equally affects the face, arm, and leg on one side of the body, with preservation of sensory, intellectual, and speech function.

2. **Pure hemisensory loss:** loss of sensation on one side of the body, with preservation of motor, intellectual, and speech function.

3. **Dysarthria–clumsy hand syndrome:** weakness predominantly of the hand and dysarthric (slurred) speech.

4. **Ataxia–hemiparesis:** ataxia and weakness involving the face, arm, and leg on one side of the body, with a superimposed ataxia. The coordination difficulties are in excess of what would be expected in pure motor hemiparesis.

10. What is a watershed or border-zone infarct?

A watershed or border-zone infarct refers to an area of focal cerebral ischemia resulting from decreased perfusion pressure. Watershed infarcts typically occur bilaterally in boundary zones between major vascular beds such as the middle cerebral artery and the posterior cerebral artery. Bilateral watershed infarcts usually are due to systemic hypotension. Unilateral border-zone infarcts may be associated with ipsilateral large vessel stenosis.

11. Discuss the treatment of acute ischemic stroke.

Stroke prevention through risk factor modification, antiplatelet agents, and warfarin anticoagulation in atrial fibrillation has favorably affected the incidence of new events. However, effective treatment of stroke in the acute setting has proved a more difficult task.

In 1995, the use of intravenous thrombolytic therapy with tissue plasminogen activator (rt-PA) was shown to improve outcome in patients suffering from acute stroke if therapy could be initiated within 3 hours from onset of symptoms. Other trials using intravenous rt-PA have not proved successful mainly because of the time windows (up to 5 hours from symptom onset). More recently the use of intra-arterial prourokinase has shown benefit in treating middle cerebral artery occlusion if treatment can be initiated within 6 hours from symptom onset. Studies are under way to investigate combination therapy with intravenous rt-PA followed by intra-arterial rt-PT to determine whether additional benefit over the use of either therapy alone is possible. The goal is to reestablish blood flow before tissue death. The major complication of thrombolytic therapy is intracerebral hemorrhage. In the 1995 study, rates of hemorrhage in patients receiving rt-PA were in the range of 6%, whereas patients not receiving rt-PA had a hemorrhage rate of 0.6%.

The use of antiplatelet agents in the acute setting has been shown to give a small but statistically significant benefit, and the combination of aspirin with rt-PA also has shown benefit in terms of reperfusion, although the risk of hemorrhage may be increased.

The use of heparin in the setting of acute stroke has been a topic of debate for many years. Its use is based on the concept of clot propagation or recurrent embolism from a cardiac or vascular source as a cause of neurologic deterioration in stroke. Anticoagulation has shown benefit in lowering the incidence of stroke in patients with atrial fibrillation. However, its use in the treatment of acute ischemic stroke remains controversial.

Treatment modalities other than thrombolytic therapy are also being investigated. Glutamate has been shown to be the major mediator of cell death in ischemic stroke models. The effects of glutamate are mediated by glutamate receptors, which are voltage-sensitive calcium channels. Unfortunately, none of the studies looking at drugs that block these channels have shown benefit. Other studies investigating neuroprotective agents also have failed to show clinical benefit.

Other treatment considerations include the avoidance of acute reductions in blood pressure. Because the blood flow around areas of infarcted brain is already low, further reducing the blood flow by lowering blood pressure can result in an extension of the area of infarction. As a result, higher blood pressures are generally desirable in the setting of acute stroke, and vigorous attempts to lower blood pressure should be avoided. The use of sedative medications in the setting of acute stroke should also be minimized, because their use may interfere with the clinician's ability to follow serial neurologic exams.

Finally, routine care considerations—such as range-of-motion exercises for limbs rendered immobile or weak as a result of the stroke; prevention of aspiration, pulmonary emboli, and skin breakdown; and nutritional support—are also important.

12. Describe hypertensive encephalopathy.

This term refers to an encephalopathy characterized by headache, nausea, vomiting, visual disturbances, seizures, confusion, and coma in the setting of severe hypertension. One theory suggests that the rapid rise in blood pressure is accompanied by loss of cerebral autoregulation, producing areas of focal vasospasm and ischemia together with areas of cerebral vasodilation and increased flow. Cerebral edema is a common but not constant feature. Causes are related to age and include (1) acute glomerulonephritis (children and adolescents), (2) chronic glomerulonephritis (young adults), (3) eclampsia (child-bearing women), and (4) malignant hypertension (patients older than 30–40 years). The only consistent sign is systemic hypertension. Papilledema is almost always present, and its absence should cast some doubt on the diagnosis.

13. What is a TIA?

A transient ischemic attack (TIA) is a reversible ischemic episode that does not result in infarction or permanent deficit. The attacks, by definition, must completely resolve within 24 hours; most will resolve within 1 hour. Carotid TIAs are associated with carotid atheromatous disease. Ischemia in the carotid distribution results in deficits in the ipsilateral visual field or contralateral sensorimotor function. Visual and hemispheric symptoms typically do not occur simultaneously. **Amaurosis fugax** refers to the transient ipsilateral monocular blindness resulting from a TIA. Transient hemispheric attacks refer to ischemia in the region of the middle cerebral artery with focal motor and sensory deficits in the contralateral arm and hand.

14. What is the significance of carotid artery stenosis?

Carotid stenosis may result in cerebral ischemia, presenting as TIAs or, in more severe cases, as stroke. Ischemia is most often the result of atherosclerotic microembolism rather than distal infarction secondary to stenosis.

15. What is subclavian steal syndrome?

This syndrome refers to symptoms of vertebrobasilar insufficiency that arise in association with exercise, particularly of the arms. It reflects the diversion (or steal) of blood from the vertebral artery to the brachial artery. When the vasodilation that accompanies exercise is coupled with a proximal subclavian or innominate artery stenosis, blood may flow retrograde through the vertebral artery to fill the dilated vascular pool in the arm. This syndrome is confirmed when symptoms are associated with a decreased blood pressure in one arm and an ipsilateral supraclavicular bruit. It is more common on the left than on the right.

BIBLIOGRAPHY

1. Adams RD, Victor M: Cerebrovascular disease. In Adams RD, Victor M (eds): Principles of Neurology, 4th ed. New York, McGraw-Hill, 1989, pp 617–691.
2. Bannister R: Disorders of the cerebral circulation. In Brain's Clinical Neurology, 6th ed. London, Oxford University Press, 1985, p 285.
3. Barnett HJ: Cerebral ischemia and infarction. In Wyngaarden J, Smith L (eds): Cecil Textbook of Medicine. Philadelphia, W.B. Saunders, 1988, pp 2162–2163.
4. Brott TG, Haley EC, Levy DE, et al: Urgent therapy for stroke. I. Pilot study of tissue plasminogen activator administered within 90 minutes. Stroke 23:632–640, 1992.
5. Devuyst G, Bogousslavsky J: Clinical trial update: Neuroprotection against acute ischaemic stroke. Curr Opin Neurol 12:73–79, 1999.
6. Dunbabin W, Sandercock PAG: Preventing stroke by modification of risk factors. Stroke 21:36–39, 1990.
7. Furlan A, Higashida R, Wechsler L, et al: Intra-arterial prourokinase for acute ischemic stroke. The PROACT II study: A randomized controlled trial. Prolyse in Acute Cerebral Thromboembolism. JAMA 282:2003–2011, 1999.
8. Gress DR: Stroke: Revolution in therapy. West J Med 161:288–291, 1994.
9. Group TNr-PSS: Tissue plasminogen activator for acute ischemic stroke. N Engl J Med 333:1581–1587, 1995.
10. Hacke W, Kasate M, Fieschi C, et al: Intravenous thrombolysis with recombinant tissue plasminogen activator for acute hemispheric stroke: The European cooperative acute stroke study (ECASS). JAMA 274:1017–1025, 1995.
11. Haley EC, Levy DE, Brott TG, et al: Urgent therapy for stroke. Part II. Pilot study of tissue plasminogen activator administered 91–180 minutes from onset. Stroke 23:641–645, 1992.
12. Kaku D, Lowenstein D: Emergence of recreational drug use as a major risk factor for stroke in young adults. Ann Intern Med 113:821–827, 1990.
13. Liebeskind DS, Kasner SE: Neuroprotection for ischaemic stroke: An unattainable goal? CNS Drugs 15:165–174, 2001.
14. Lutsep HL, Clark WM: Neuroprotection in acute ischaemic stroke: Current status and future poential. Drugs R D 1:3–8, 1999.
15. Rowland LP: Merrit's Textbook of Neurology, 8th ed. Philadelphia, Lea & Febiger, 1989.

16. Schellinger PD, Fiebach JB, Mohr A, et al: Throbolytic therapy for ischemic stroke: A review. Part I: Intravenous trhombolysis. Crit Care Med 29:1812–1819, 2001.
17. Schellinger PD, Fiebach JB, Mohr A, et al: Thrombolytic therapy for ischemic stroke: A review. Part II: Intra-arterial thrombolysis, vertebrobasilar stroke, phase IV trials, and stroke imaging. Crit Care Med 29:1819–1825, 2001.
18. Slivka A, Levy D: Natural history of progressive ischemic stroke in a population treated with heparin. Stroke 15:980–989, 1984.

68. LANDRY-GUILLAIN-BARRÉ SYNDROME

David C. Bonovich, M.D., and Brian J. Kelly, M.D.

1. What is the Landry-Guillain-Barré syndrome?

The Landry-Guillain-Barré syndrome (LGBS) is an acute or subacute polyradiculoneuropathy characterized by immune-mediated demyelination. LGBS affects all ages.

2. What factors may predispose a patient to LGBS?

Although cause and effect have never been proved, LGBS recently has been associated with cytomegalovirus, Epstein-Barr virus, and bacterial infections with *Campylobacter jejuni*. Up to 50% of patients have suffered a recent respiratory or gastrointestinal infection. An additional 15% have had a recent vaccination. Of all the vaccinations studied, only the 1976–1977 swine flu vaccine was associated with a statistically significant increase in incidence of LGBS, possibly secondary to contamination of the vaccine with the P2-myelin protein from the chick embryos from which the vaccine was made.

3. Describe the pathology of LGBS. How does it explain the typical clinical features of LGBS?

There are two forms: a demyelinating form (more common) and an axonal form. The prognosis is better for the demyelinating form than for the axonal form. The primary pathologic process in the **demyelinating form** is segmental demyelination of the peripheral nerves due to an autoimmune process that is both humorally and cell mediated. Because the primary process is a loss of myelin, the peripheral nerves that are most heavily myelinated (i.e., motor and joint-position sensory nerves) are more severely affected than unmyelinated or lightly myelinated nerves (i.e., nerves that mediate pain and temperature sensation). The **axonal form** is associated with wallerian degeneration, minimal lymphocytic response, and no demyelination or inflammation. The node of Ranvier appears to be the target of attack in the axonal form, and associations with elevated IgG, GMI, and *C. jejuni* have been described.

4. What are the typical features of LGBS?

The initial symptoms of LGBS are usually paresthesias in the distal extremities and pain or stiffness in the proximal limbs, followed quickly by progressive weakness of the limbs, trunk, and cranial muscles. The weakness most frequently begins in the legs and spreads in an ascending fashion, although other patterns of disease progression have been described. Patients lose their reflexes early in the course of the disease. It is usually symmetrical but does not have to be so.

Respiratory function is often compromised by involvement of the phrenic and intercostal nerves. Patients may develop autonomic dysfunction characterized by wide fluctuations in heart rate and blood pressure. There have been reports of cardiac arrest as a result of autonomic instability. Cranial nerve deficits occur and may affect speech or swallowing. Vibratory sensation and proprioception are usually severely impaired, whereas pinprick and temperature sensation are often normal.

5. What is the differential diagnosis of subacutely evolving, generalized motor weakness?

Spinal cord injury	Tick paralysis
Toxins (hexacarbon, lead, thallium, or organophosphate intoxication)	Diphtheritic polyneuropathy
	Vasculitic polyneuropathy
Poliomyelitis	Lambert-Eaton myasthenic syndrome
Botulism	Dermatomyositis
Porphyria	Carcinomatous meningitis
Myasthenia gravis	Saxitoxin poisoning
Periodic paralysis	

6. How is the diagnosis of LGBS confirmed?

The diagnosis may be made predominantly on clinical grounds. LGBS typically presents as an ascending weakness with absent reflexes. Lumbar puncture also may be helpful. The typical pattern is an acellular spinal fluid with greatly increased protein and normal glucose. In some cases, however, the increase in protein may not begin until well into the course of the illness.

7. What is the typical clinical time course for LGBS?

The usual course is divided into three phases:

1. Initial period: characterized by deterioration of strength; lasts between 1 and 3 weeks.

2. Plateau phase: characterized by a stable or minimally changing exam; lasts from several days to several weeks.

3. Recovery phase: the beginning of remyelination, characterized by slowly improving strength; lasts from several weeks to several months (as long as it takes for remyelination of damaged nerves).

8. What are the mortality and morbidity rates of LGBS?

The mortality rate is 2–5%. Most deaths result from secondary complications, such as sepsis secondary to pulmonary and urinary infections; pulmonary emboli; delayed treatment of respiratory failure; and dysautonomias. These complications can be minimized by excellent medical and nursing care in the intensive care unit (ICU).

9. Which patients with LGBS require ICU observation?

Any patient with evidence of respiratory muscle or bulbar muscle weakness should be transferred to the ICU for observation. Similarly, patients who show evidence of significant autonomic dysfunction or rapidly progressive generalized weakness should be followed closely in the ICU.

10. What percentage of patients require respiratory support with a mechanical ventilator?

Between 10% and 23% of patients with LGBS eventually require mechanical ventilation.

11. What is the best way to follow respiratory function in a patient with a neuromuscular disease such as LGBS?

Frequent bedside pulmonary function testing is the best method of assessing and following respiratory function. Measurements of vital capacity and maximum inspiratory and expiratory pressures give good indications of developing weakness in the respiratory muscles. Observation of respiratory patterns—whether the patient uses accessory muscles to breathe, respiratory rate, and how high the patient can count during one inspiration—also may be helpful. Arterial blood gas determinations frequently remain normal until respiratory failure is severe; therefore, such measurements lead to a false sense of security regarding respiratory status.

12. When should patients with LGBS be intubated?

This issue is controversial, and several factors need to be taken into account. Respiratory failure is due to a combination of respiratory muscle insufficiency, which leads to hypercapnic respiratory failure, and pneumonia secondary to an inability to cough adequately or protect the airway. Clinically, neuromuscular respiratory failure is characterized by rapid, shallow breathing, restlessness, sweating, staccato speech, increased accessory muscle use, tachycardia, and the presence of an abdominal paradox. The following are general guidelines for intubation:

1. When the vital capacity becomes less than 15 ml/kg of body weight
2. When the maximum inspiratory pressure is less than –25 to –30 cmH$_2$O
3. When patients have such severe bulbar weakness that they cannot handle secretions or protect their airway
4. When patients can no longer maintain normal pCO$_2$ and pH on arterial blood gas determination (often a very late sign)

The rapidity of disease progression also should be considered. The more rapidly evolving the motor weakness, the more aggressive the clinician should be regarding early intubation.

13. If a neuromuscular blocker is needed to facilitate intubation, which one should be used?

Succinylcholine has been associated with hyperkalemia-induced cardiac arrest due to the massive release of potassium from denervated muscle cells in paralyzed patients. This risk is greatest in patients with longstanding paralysis, but its use should be considered contraindicated in all patients with LGBS. Therefore, a nondepolarizing muscle relaxant such as vecuronium, atracurium, or cisatracurium should be used whenever possible.

14. Which patients with LGBS experience dysautonomias?

Autonomic nervous system dysfunction is usually present if the disease is severe enough to require mechanical ventilation. Dysautonomias result from either excessive or insufficient sympathetic and parasympathetic activity. In addition, a wide variety of arrhythmias can occur and may be a major cause of mortality. Treatment of dysautnomias consists of hydration and other supportive measures, such as avoiding changes in position and using stool softeners to prevent straining-induced vagal stimulation. If drugs are necessary to treat dysautnomias or arrhythmias, small doses of short-acting, titratable agents are recommended.

15. Are there any effective treatments for the neurologic injury associated with LGBS?

Until 1978 treatment of LGBS was largely supportive. Since then it has been demonstrated that plasma exchange (removing 50 ml/kg of plasma in each of five sessions on alternating days and replacing it with 5% albumin) is effective in shortening the course of the disease. The beneficial effects of plasma exchange are greatest when it is begun within 2 weeks of disease onset. In addition, high-dose intravenous immunoglobulin (IVIG) (0.4 gm/kg/day for 5 days) have been shown to be equally effective in reducing the number of ventilator days and length of time until the patient can walk.

IVIG is easier to administer and less costly than plasma exchange, but several small series suggested that its use was associated with a higher relapse rate than plasma exchange. A recent large study, however, found IVIG and plasma exchange to be equally effective with no difference in outcome at 48 weeks. Given the potential for serious complications associated with plasma exchange (many related to central line placement and line complications), IVIG is recommended as the initial treatment for LGBS. IVIG is contraindicated in patients with IgA deficiency and known anaphylaxis to blood products. Such patients should be treated with plasma exchange.

16. What is the prognosis in acute LGBS?

Most patients experience excellent recovery in muscle function with time, often returning to normal. A small percentage of patients are left with various degrees of persistent weakness. In other patients, reflexes remain absent.

17. Are there any ICU issues unique to LGBS?

In addition to the obvious need for meticulous pulmonary and nutritional support, special care should be taken to avoid pressure palsies of the arms and the legs. All patients require deep venous thrombosis prophylaxis with intermittent pneumatic compression devices or subcutaneous heparin, and adequate pain control. In addition, patients with LGBS are usually completely alert yet often cannot communicate because of intubation and paralysis. Therefore, patients should be allowed to communicate their needs and concerns whenever possible. They may require tremendous emotional support and judicious use of anxiolytics.

BIBLIOGRAPHY

1. Ashbury AK: Diagnostic considerations of Guillain-Barré syndrome. Ann Neurol 9(Suppl):1–15, 1981.
2. Chowdry D, Arora A: Axonal Guillain-Barré syndrome: A critical review. Acta Neurol Scand 103:267–277, 2001.
3. Feldman JM: Cardiac arrest after succinylcholine administration in a pregnant patient recovered from Guillain-Barré syndrome. Anesthesiology 72:942–944, 1990.
4. Guillain-Barré Study Group: Plasmapheresis and acute Guillain-Barré syndrome. Neurology 35: 1096–1103, 1985.
5. Kokontis L, Gutmann L: Current treatment of neuromuscular disease. Arch Neurol 57:939–943, ◆◆◆◆.
6. Koski CL: Guillain-Barré syndrome. Neurol Clin 2:355–366, 1984.
7. Plasma Exchange/Sandoglobulin Guillain-Barré Syndrome Trial Study Group: Randomized trial of plasma exchange, intravenous immunoglobulin, and combined treatments in Guillain-Barré syndrome. Lancet 349:225–230, 1997.
8. Prineas JW: Pathology of the Guillain-Barré syndrome. Ann Neurol 9(Suppl):6–9, 1981.
9. Provencio JJ, Bleck TP, Conners AF: Critical care neurology. Am J Respir Crit Care Med 164:341–345, 2001.
10. Wijdicks EFM: The Clinical Practice of Critical Care Neurology. Philadelphia, Lippincott-Raven, 1997.

69. MYASTHENIA GRAVIS

David C. Bonovich, M.D., and Brian J. Kelly, M.D.

1. Define myasthenia gravis.

Myasthenia gravis (MG) is an autoimmune disorder of neuromuscular transmission manifested by weakness and fatigability of voluntary skeletal muscle. The major characteristic is faituging of the skeletal muscle with repeated or continuous activity. There are two forms: ocular MG, in which the weakness is confined to the extraocular muscles, and a generalized form that affects ocular and facial muscles as well as muscles of the trunk.

2. What are the ages of peak incidence of MG?

MG may begin at any age, but it is more prevalent in women (female-to-male ratio: 4:1). Women tend to develop the disease at a younger age than men.The peak incidence for women is between 10 and 40 years of age; for men, between 50 and 70 years of age.

3. What are the usual clinical features of MG?

MG is characterized clinically by fluctuating weakness that has a predilection for the extraocular and bulbar muscles. Most patients have prominent ptosis, with or without opthalmoparesis, dysphagia, and dsyarthria (less common).

4. Describe the pathophysiology of MG.

MG is an autoimmune disease. The target antigen is the nicotinic acetylcholine receptor (AchR) in the postsynaptic membrane of the neuromuscular junction. AchR antibodies may be identifiable in the serum of about 85% of patients. This antibody response results in a marked decrease in the number of functyional AchRs, causing faulty neuromuscular transmission.

5. What other conditions are associated with MG?

Disorders of the thymus are common in patients with MG. Up to 70% of myasthenics have evidence of lymphoid follicle hyperplasia in the thymus, and up to 15% harbor a thymoma. Other types of autoimmune disorders associated with MG include thyroid disorders, pernicious anemia, Addison's disease, diabetes mellitus, lupus erythematosus, rheumatoid arthritis, and polymyositis.

6. How is the diagnosis of MG confirmed?

Clinical findings of fluctuating weakness with a predilection for the extraocular and bulbar muscles strongly suggest the diagnosis. In some patients, however, the diagnosis may not be clear from the history and clinical exam alone, especially early in the course of the disease. The response to edrophonium (Tensilon), a short-acting acetylcholinesterase inhibitor, may be especially helpful in diagnosing MG. Administration of edrophonium increases the concentration of acetylcholine in the neuromuscular junction. The Tensilon test should not be performed unless the clinician is clear about the specific muscles to be tested. The standard dose is 10 mg, but a test dose of 1–2 mg (0.1–0.2 ml) should be given first because rare patients are sensitive to Tensilon and may develop marked bradycardia and/or bronchospasm. If the test dose is tolerated, the remaining 8 mg may be given.

In addition, electrophysiologic testing can be quite helpful in diagnosing MG. The use of repetitive-simtulation electromyography (EMG) is especially useful for patients who test negative for AchR antibodies.

7. How is MG differentiated from Lambert-Eaton myasthenic syndrome (LEMS)?

LEMS is a rare condition in which antibodies are formed against voltage-gated calicum channels, resulting in impaired ability of the presynaptic cells to release acetylcholine. Although MG and LEMS have some common clinical features, LEMS does not involve extraocular muscles; thus, ptosis and diplopia, which are very common in MG, do not occur. In addition, repetitive nerve stimulation (particularly at high frequencies) in LEMS demonstrates an increase in the size of the muscle response.

8. What is the most serious complication of MG?

Fatal respiratory failure can result from severe involvement of the respiratory muscles. Respiratory failure can also result from pulmonary aspiration due to difficulty in swallowing and protecting the upper airway secondary to bulbar weakness.

9. What is the best way to assess respiratory function in patients with MG?

As with other neuromuscular diseases, rapid, shallow breathing and paradoxical abdominal movement suggest impending respiratory failure. Hypoxia, hypercapnia, and respiratory acidosis may not occur until late in the disease. Thus, frequent evaluation of respiratory function using vital capacity and mean inspiratory force is the best way to follow at-risk patients with MG and other neuromuscular diseases that affect the respiratory muscles.

10. Which two conditions can cause rapidly progressive weakness and respiratory failure in a patient with MG?

Myasthenic crisis is a severe, life-threatening worsening of MG. It occurs more commonly in pateints with severe bulbar weakness after physical stress, such as upper respiratory infection or surgery, and is characterized by profound weakness and respiratory failure.

Myasthenic crisis must be differentiated from **cholinergic crisis**, in which an overdose of acetylcholinesterase inhibitors results in profound weakness due to continuous depolarization of the postsynaptic membrane, which in turn results in a depolarizing type of neuromuscular blockade. In general, cholinergic crisis causes other symptoms, such as excessive salivation, cramps, diarrhea, and blurred vision. There is also a history of a marked increase in pyridostigmine use. A small dose of edrophonium often differentiates the two conditions, as it usually causes significant improvement in myasthenic crisis but worsens cholinergic crisis. This test should be performed only when emergency airway management is available, because it can cause severe respiratory failure in patients with cholinergic crisis.

11. How is MG managed?

Medical management usually involves the use of long-acting acetylcholinesterase inhibitors such as pyridostigmine (Mestinon). Mestinon significantly improves neuromuscular function in patients with MG. Steroids and other immunosuppressive agents also may be helpful. Azothioprine, methotrexate, cyclosporine, and mycophenolate are believed to be effective.

Thymectomy is often beneficial, with clinical improvement in about 80% of patients. It should be considered especially in patients with generalized MG. Plasma exchange and IVIG are often used in patients with severe exacerbations and can be highly effective in these settings. Immunoadsorption, a new therapy in which plasma exchange is used in conjunction with a resin that adsorbs acetylcholine receptor antibodies, should be considered in patients with severe myasthenic crisis.

12. What conditions or agents can exacerbate MG?

Infection from any source, fever, delivery, and surgical or emotional stresses can worsen MG and may result in myasthenic crisis. Aminoglycoside and polymyxin antibiotics, beta blockers, quinidine, and procainamide, as well as several antidepressants and anticonvulsants ,have been found to worsen MG. Steroids (which are often used to treat MG) can result in a transient worsening of MG in the first few days of therapy, possibly by adversely affecting the balance of various T-lymphocyte subgroups.

13. How should a patient in myasthenic crisis be treated?

Myasthenic crisis is defined by the need for respiratory assistance. When a patient is believed to be at risk for developing respiratory embarrassment and begins to have difficulty in swallowing (placing the patient at risk for aspiration), he or she should be moved to the ICU. When vital capacity falls below 15 ml/kg of body weight or when the patient cannot handle secretions, he or she should be intubated and supported with mechanical ventilation. The goals therapy should be to reduce the work of breathing, to determine the underlying reason for development of myasthenic crisis, and to restore adequate respiratory and bulbar function.

1. During the initial 24–48 hours after intubation, settings for mechanical ventilation should be focused on allowing the ventilator to assume most of the control of breathing; thus, a volume control mode with continuous mandatory ventilation should be considered.

2. A vigorous search for any underlying infection should be initiated, and careful attention should be given to proper pulmonary toilet.

3. Careful attention also should be given to the prevention of venous thrombosis. Measures should include the application of sequential compression devices and/or the use of subcutaneous heparin or low-molecular-weight heparin.

4. All anticholinesterase medications should be stopped for 48–72 hours. Often a drug holiday restores responsiveness to medications later and may help with secretion management.

5. Either plasma exchange or IVIG therapy should be initiated as soon as possible after intubation to hasten neuromuscular recovery. Mestinon may be restarted after several days of plasma exchange, with the dose gradually increased based on clinical response.

6. If there is no response to plasma exchange or IVIG after 5 days, consider adding prednisone (1 mg/kg/day).

14. What factors should be considered perioperatively in a myasthenic patient undergoing thymectomy?

The most important goal is to optimize respiratory muscle function preoperatively. Plasma exchange or IVIG, and sometimes steroids, are used to accomplish this goal. The dose of Mestinon should be reduced as much as possible without compromising respiratory function, because patients may become more sensitive to its effects postoperatively. If the patient was taking steroids preoperatively, stress doses of steroids should be given in the perioperative period. Extubation should not be considered until all of the effects of the inhalational agents used for anesthesia have fully dissipated and it is clear that respiratory function is adequate. It is better to be conservative in the decision to extubate the patient. After extubation, respiratory function should be followed closely, and the patient should be observed for signs of fatigue.

BIBLIOGRAPHY

1. Adams SL, Mathews J, Grammer LC: Drugs that may exacerbate myasthenia gravis. Ann Emerg Med 13:532–538, 1984.
2. Arsura EL, Bick A, Brunner NG, et al: High-dose intravenous immunoglobulin in the management of myasthenia gravis. Arch Intern Med 146:1365–1368, 1986.
3. Berrouschot J, Baumann I, Kalishewski P, et al: Therapy of myasthenic crisis. Crit Care Med 25:1228–1235, 1997.
4. Engel AG: Myasthenia gravis and myasthenic syndromes. Ann Neurol 16:519–534, 1984.
5. Fenichel GM: Myasthenia gravis. Pediatr Ann 18:432–438, 1989.
6. Gajdos P, Chevret S, Clair B, et al: Clinical trial of plasma exchange and high-dose intravenous immunoglobulin in myasthenia gravis. Myasthenia Gravis Clinical Study Group. Ann Neurol 41:789–796, 1997.
7. Galdi AP: Diagnosis and Management of Muscle Disease. New York, SP Medical and Scientific Books, 1984, pp 54–72.
8. Grob D, Simpson D, Mitsumoto H, et al: Treatment of myasthenia gravis by immunoadsorption of plasma. Neurology 45:338–344, 1995.
9. Palace J, Vincent A, Beeson D: Myasthenia gravis: Diagnostic and management dilemmas. Curr Opin Neurol 14:583–589, 2001.
10. Provencio JJ, Bleck T, Conners AF: Critical care neurology. Am J Respir Crit Care Med 164:341–345, 2001.
11. Rowland LP: Controversies about the treatment of myasthenia gravis. J Neurol Neurosurg Psychiatry 43:659–694, 1980.
12. Seybold ME: Myasthenia gravis: A clinical and basic science review. JAMA 250:2516–2521, 1983.
13. Weschler AS, Olanow CW: Myasthenia gravis. Surg Clin North Am 60:931–945, 1980.

70. ALCOHOL WITHDRAWAL

Jill A. Rebuck, Pharm.D., B.C.P.S.

1. Which patients are most at risk for alcohol withdrawal?

Alcohol withdrawal is often observed after elective surgery or emergent admission. Any patient with a history of significant, prolonged alcohol intake who exhibits tachycardia, hypertension, hyperreflexia, tremor, anxiety, irritability, hallucinations, seizures, delirium, nausea, or vomiting may be displaying signs and symptoms of alcohol withdrawal. The individual response to alcohol withdrawal varies, and patients may exhibit only a few signs and symptoms. Alcohol withdrawal, therefore, should be considered in all patients with a history of long-standing alcohol consumption.

2. Describe the time course for development of delirium tremens.

Delirium tremens (DTs) is a life-threatening syndrome marked by severe neuronal hyperexcitation. Usually it presents 3–5 days after cessation of alcohol intake, but symptoms may appear much later (after 1–2 weeks of hospitalization). The typical duration is less than 1 week.

3. What is the incidence of delirium tremens?

DTs occur in approximately 5% of hospitalized alcoholics. The mortality rate ranges from 1% to 15%.

4. Which class of medications should be used to treat alcohol withdrawal?

Benzodiazepines are the most effective therapy because of reduction of symptom severity, decreased incidence of delirium, and reduction of seizure activity.

5. What is the benzodiazepine of choice for treatment of alcohol withdrawal in the ICU?

Lorazepam is the most commonly used benzodiazepine in the ICU for acute treatment because of its relatively short half-life, lack of active metabolites, and capability for either intravenous bolus dosing or continuous infusion. On transfer to a step-down unit within the hospital, longer-acting benzodiazepines, such as diazepam or chlordiazepoxide, are preferred.

6. Should propofol be considered for refractory DTs?

Propofol is an alquilphenol with a mechanism of action similar to that of ethanol; it affects both glutamate and gamma aminobutyric acid (GABA) receptors within the central nervous system. If a patient is refractory to high-dose benzodiazepines (> 20 mg/hr), a propofol infusion may be considered in intubated patients as an alternative strategy to control severe DTs. Propofol should be closely titrated, and dosages should be decreased as clinical status improves.

7. What adjunctive therapies may be useful for treatment of alcohol withdrawal?

Beta blockers, clonidine, and carbamazepine are adjunctive therapies that improve withdrawal severity. However, their effect on seizures and delirium are less well studied. Beta blockers have no anticonvulsant activity and may be associated with delirium. Clonidine may be most beneficial in patients with elevated blood pressure and heart rate. Carbamazepine has less central nervous system depressant activity but a high frequency of side effects (dizziness, nausea, vomiting, rash, pruritus). None of these adjunctive agents should be used in place of benzodiazepine therapy but as add-on therapy when indicated.

8. In patients at risk for alcohol withdrawal, should treatment be initiated on a symptom-triggered or fixed-schedule basis?

Studies suggest that symptom-triggered therapy is preferred because of lower total benzodiazepine requirements and shorter duration of treatment compared with fixed-schedule therapy. The data, however, are derived from patients in non-ICU settings, such as inpatient detoxification units. Thus, as-needed vs. scheduled benzodiazepine therapy remains controversial in ICU patients because multiple signs and symptoms may be masked by the increased severity of illness and unresponsiveness of many critically ill patients.

9. When is haloperidol considered as part of the treatment regimen?

Haloperidol is the preferred agent for treatment of delirium in adult ICU patients. Patients should be monitored closely for QT prolongation or arrhythmias, and therapy should be discontinued if adverse effects appear. Therapy typically includes 2–5 mg intravenously every 6 hours. Patients also should be monitored for extrapyramidal side effects, and low-dose anticholinergic therapy should be initiated if necessary. Because haloperidol alters the seizure threshold, it should be administered with caution.

10. What are the clinical differences between short- vs. long-acting benzodiazepines for alcohol withdrawal?

Shorter-acting agents have the advantage of less oversedation and easier titration to effect in acutely ill patients. Advantages of longer-acting agents include less potential for addiction as well as more sustained therapeutic effect; the risk of oversedation, however, must not be ignored.

11. What simple questionnaire helps to assess the risk of alcohol withdrawal symptoms?

The **CAGE** questionnaire, which consists of four questions:
1. Have you felt you should cut down on your alcohol consumption?
2. Have people annoyed you by criticizing your drinking?
3. Have you felt guilty about your drinking?

4. Have you ever had a drink first thing in the morning (**eye**-opener) to steady your nerves or get rid of a hangover?

Patients who answer "yes" to any of these question should be monitored, and those who answer "yes" to three or more questions are at high risk of alcohol withdrawal symptoms.

12. How often do seizures occur in relation to withdrawal of alcohol use?

Between 2% and 5% of alcoholics experience withdrawal seizures, which are usually generalized. Seizure typically occur within 48 hours of the last drink but may occur at any time within the first week of withdrawal. Patients with a history of previous detoxifications or non–alcohol-related admissions are at increased risk for development of withdrawal seizures (known as the "kindling effect"). The kindling hypothesis states that every withdrawal episode acts as an irritative phenomenon to the brain, and the accumulation of several alcohol withdrawal episodes tends to lower the seizure threshold.

13. Do alcohol withdrawal clinical pathways improve care?

Clinical pathways are useful in the inpatient hospital setting to screen and identify patients at risk of developing withdrawal symptoms and to treat the symptoms appropriately. They often are used for patients in whom alcohol withdrawal is a secondary diagnosis revealed by a risk screening tool, such as a substance abuse assessment questionnaire. Pathways also have the advantage of facilitating intervention for the underlying alcoholism after discharge. The Clinical Institute Withdrawal Assessment for Alcohol, revised (CIWA-Ar) scale, a validated, reliable measure of the current severity of alcohol withdrawal, consists of 10 items: nausea and vomiting, tremor, autonomic hyperactivity, anxiety, agitation, tactile disturbances, auditory disturbances, visual disturbances, headache, and disorientation. Although this scale is useful for communicative patients who can answer questions, the ICU patient with multiple comorbidities may not be able to respond because of sedation, mechanical ventilation, and related issues. However, all patients at risk must be monitored closely for symptoms of alcohol withdrawal.

BIBLIOGRAPHY

1. Beresford TP, et al: Comparison of CAGE questionnaire and computer-assisted laboratory profiles in screening for covert alcoholism. Lancet 336:482–485, 1990.
2. Erstad BL, et al: Management of alcohol withdrawal. Am J Health-Syst Pharm 52:697–709, 1995.
3. Mayo-Smith M, et al: Pharmacological management of alcohol withdrawal: A meta-analysis and evidence-based practice guideline. JAMA 278:144–151, 1997.
4. McCowan C, et al: Refractory delirium tremens treated with propofol: A case series. Crit Care Med 28:1781–1784, 2000.
5. Saitz R, et al: Individualized treatment for alcohol withdrawal: A randomized double-blind controlled trial. JAMA 272:519–523, 1994.
6. Schumacher L, et al: Identifying patients "at risk" for alcohol withdrawal syndrome and a treatment protocol. J Neurosci Nurs 32:158–163, 2000.

71. HEAD TRAUMA

David Palestrant, M.D., and David Bonovich, M.D.

1. Where does head trauma rank as a cause of death in the United States?

Traumatic brain injury (TBI) ranks second to stroke as a cause of death from neurologic disorders. In the U.S. alone, approximately 1.6 million people suffer head injuries each year; 270,000 require hospitalization; 52,00 die; and 80,000 suffer neurologic disability. Severe head injury is the leading cause of neurologic disability in the U.S.

2. What are the leading causes of head trauma?

Motor vehicle crashes 49%; falls 28%; all others 23%. Worldwide, motor vehicle crashes are the leading cause of TBI-related death in young people, and falls are the leading cause in people over 65 years of age.

3. What is the mortality rate associated with severe head trauma?

Mortality and morbidity rates are related to increased intracranial pressure (ICP). For patients with severe TBI and ICP < 20 mmHg, the mortality rate is about 20%; for those with ICP > 20 mmHg, the mortality rate is close to 50%. For patients with severe TBI and ICP > 40 mmHg, the mortality rate approaches 75%; for patients with ICP > 60 mmHg, the mortality rate approaches 100%.

4. What factors are important in predicting outcome from severe head trauma?

Factors associated with a poor neurologic outcome include:
- Intracranial hematoma
- Increasing age
- Abnormal motor response
- Impaired or absent pupillary response to light on initial exam
- Early systemic insults: hypotension, hypercarbia, and/or hypoxemia

5. What is the Glasgow coma scale? Why is it important?

Developed in 1974 by the neurosurgical department at the University of Glasgow, the scale was an attempt to standardize the assessment of the depth and duration of impaired consciousness and coma, particularly in the setting of trauma. The scale is based on eye opening, verbal responses, and motor responses. Of these, motor response is the most sensitive and correlates best with neurologic outcome. A score of 15 is possible in a completely awake and oriented patient. A score < 8 indicates significant brain injury and the possible need for airway protection.

Eye opening

Spontaneous	4
To speech	3
To pain	2
None	1

Best verbal response

Oriented	5
Confused	4
Inappropriate	3
Incomprehensible	2
None	1

Motor response

Obeys commands	6
Localizes pain	5
Withdraws from pain	4
Flexes to pain	3
Extends to pain	2
None	1

6. What is the significance of primary versus secondary head injury?

Primary injury occurs at the time of impact. A primary injury may result in contusion, laceration, and/or axonal injury. It cannot be treated directly, because there is no treatment for the sudden mechanical disruption of brain tissue.

Secondary brain injury refers to the evolution of brain injury after impact. It is the leading cause of hospital death. Hypoxia and hypotension are the most common causes of secondary brain injury. Hypotension, defined as a single systolic blood pressure measurement below 90 mmHg, may be associated with a doubling of the mortality rate and an increase in morbidity of patients with TBI. Other causes of secondary injury include intracranial hematomas (subdural, epidural, and parenchymal) and generalized cerebral edema, which results in elevated ICP. .

Since primary brain injury cannot be treated directly, the brain must be protected from secondary injury and elevated ICP to provide an optimal environment for spontaneous recovery.

7. What are the important considerations for intubating patients with head trauma?

1. Associated cervical spine fractures occur in 5–10% of head-injured patients. This often depends on the mechanism of injury (motor vehicle crashes, fall > gunshot wound). Care should be taken to avoid hyperextension of the neck at the time of intubation. Awake intubation, axial traction, and/or cricothyrotomy are appropriate options in head-injured patients.

2. Patients are considered to have "full stomachs" and should undergo awake intubation or rapid-sequence induction to avoid possible aspiration of stomach contents.

3. Patients with associated traumatic injuries are often hypovolemic, and care should be taken in administering induction drugs to avoid hypotension.

4. Care should be taken to avoid coughing and straining on the endotracheal tube, both of which result in a marked increase in intracranial pressure (ICP).

5. Associated maxillofacial and neck injuries should be noted, because they may increase the difficulty of intubation.

6. Nasal intubations are contraindicated in patients with basilar skull and/or Le Fort fractures.

8. What clues suggest the presence of a basilar skull fracture?

Basilar skull fractures result in hemotympanum, ecchymosis over the mastoid area (Battle's sign), and/or periorbital ecchymosis (raccoon's eyes).

9. What percentage of adult head-injured patients develop intracranial hematoma?

About 40% of head-injured patients develop intracranial hematoma as a result of head injuries. Of these, an estimated 40% are intracerebral, 20% are subdural, and another 20% are epidural.

10. Why is intracranial hematoma significant?

Immediate surgical intervention is imperative if patients are to survive. In a review of 82 severely head-injured patients with significant intracranial hemorrhage (> 5 mm midline shift or hemorrhagic contusion > 2 cm on CT scan), early surgical evacuation was shown to have a remarkable impact on survival. Patients taken to surgery more than 4 hours after injury had a 90% mortality rate. Evacuation of subdural hematomas within 2 hours after injury may decrease mortality rates by up to 70%.

11. How does head trauma affect ICP?

Head trauma can result in increased ICP. The cranial vault encloses a fixed space occupied by brain, cerebrospinal fluid (CSF), and blood. To maintain normal ICP, a change in any one of these constituents must be accompanied by a compensatory change in at least one of the other two. The brain is able to offer only minimal compensation. In head trauma, an increase in mass due to cerebral edema or hematoma must be accompanied by an increase in venous outflow and/or CSF volume to maintain normal ICP. Physiologic compensatory mechanisms include the displacement and absorption of CSF together with spontaneous hyperventilation, which decreases cerebral blood volume. If these mechanisms do not provide adequate compensation, the result is a rise in ICP. This fact is demonstrated by the intracranial compliance curve shown below. This pressure-volume curve (see figure below) demonstrates a "critical" volume (the knee in the curve), above which compensatory mechanisms are not effective in the noncompliant cranium.

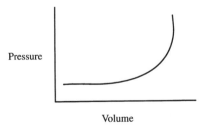

Pressure

Volume

12. What are the mechanisms by which head injury elevates intracranial pressure?

• Increased mass secondary to intracranial hematoma formation
• Cerebral edema secondary to disruption of cell membranes, and blood brain barrier
• Increased blood volume secondary to loss of autoregulation
• Increased CSF volume secondary to obstruction to flow by edema or clot formation

13. What is the significance of elevated intracranial pressure?

The elevation in ICP without an equivalent rise in systemic mean arterial pressure (MAP) results in a decrease in the cerebral perfusion pressure and the risk of brain ischemia.

$$CPP = MAP - ICP$$

Ideally, an arterial line should be placed at the time of ICP monitor placement. This line allows accurate moment-to-moment measurement of the systemic MAP and calculation of CPP. The calculation of CPP requires that both transducers be placed at the level of the external auditory canal. A normal ICP is < 10 mmHg. An elevation in ICP > 20 mmHg in a resting patient for more than a few minutes may be associated with a significant increase in morbidity. An ICP > 40 mmHg is considered life threatening. A normal CPP is approximately 80–90 mmHg. The basic concept is that when CPP is below the lower limit of pressure autoregulation, cerebral blood flow becomes dependent on the CPP. Previously a CPP > 60 mmHg was considered adequate to prevent brain ischemia. Currently, however, the minimal CPP in patients with TBI is controversial.

14. How is ICP monitored?

The three commonly used methods to monitor ICP are the intraventricular catheter, the subarachnoid screw, and the epidural transducer. See reference 16 for the detailed descriptions of each method. Most authorities now believe that, whenever feasible, an intraventricular catheter should be placed so that ICP can be monitored; at the same time, CSF may be removed to treat elevations in ICP.

15. What are plateau waves?

In 1960 Lumberg published observations of variations in ICP in 143 patients. He demonstrated that ICP may rise to very high levels and that increased ICP cannot be reliably predicted on clincal grounds alone. He also demontrated the variability of ICP waves over time and described three specific patterns of variation:

A waves are periods of extremely elevated ICP (50–100 mmHg) that last 5–20 minutes. They may be superimposed on an elevated baseline and also may be associated with a marked decrease in CPP. A waves are also called **plateau waves**.

B waves are high-frequency oscillations (0.5–2/min) that result in pressures between 0 and 50 mmHg. Although they are not always pathologic, they often progress to A waves.

C waves are small rhythmic oscillations in pressure at a frequency of 4–8/min. They are associated with ICP measurements of 0–20 mmHg and are considered normal.

16. Which patients should be monitored for increased ICP?

A review of 207 head-injured patients by Narayan et al. in 1982 suggested that two groups of patients should be routinely monitored: (1) those with abnormal CT scans on admission (high-density lesion consistent with hemorrhage or low-density lesion consistent with contusion) and (2) those with normal CT scans who demonstrate two or more of the following adverse features on admission: (a) systolic blood pressure < 90 mmHg, (b) age > 40 years, and (c) unilateral or bilateral motor posturing. Patients who are not routinely monitored should have a repeat CT head scan at 12–24 hours. This study showed that 96% of patients with normal CT scans and fewer than two adverse features had normal ICPs throughout their ICU course, whereas 53–63% of patients with abnormal CT scans developed elevated ICP.

17. What are the essentials of management of head-injured patients?

1. Management and protection of the airway.
2. Controlled ventilation to maintain normal or slightly lower pCO_2.
3. Appropriate triage to early surgery (< 4 hr after injury).
4. Maintenance of cerebral blood flow.
5. Treatment of elevated intracranial pressure.

6. Evaluation and treatment of secondary systemic disorders:
   Gastrointestinal bleeding
   Disseminated intravascular coagulopathy
   Neurogenic pulmonary edema
   Endocrine abnormalities (diabetes insipidus, syndrome of inappropriate antidiuretic hormone)
   Hypotension secondary to hemorrhagic or spinal shock
   Hypoxemia secondary to chest trauma or aspiration

18. Describe the treatment for elevated ICP.
1. Elevation of the head of the bed to > 20° to enhance venous drainage.
2. Hyperventilation to a pCO_2 of 25–30 mmHg, for short periods in the acute setting.
3. Mannitol, 0.5–1.0 gm/kg emergently, then dose every 1–3 hours to maintain a serum osmolarity > 295 < 315 mOsm.
4. Furosemide, 0.5 mg/kg, may be used in an attempt to reduce CSF production, but caution is necessary to avoid dehydration.
5. Drainage of CSF from ventriculostomy catheter (most effective in obstructive hydrocephalus, least effective in diffuse edema with narrowed ventricles).
6. Surgical decompression to remove hematoma or necrotic injured brain.
7. Attention to head positioning to avoid jugular venous compression and obstruction to the cranial venous outflow tract.
8. Pentobarbital coma may be useful in hemodynamically stable patients with refractory intracranial hypertension.
9. Seizure prophylaxis may be considered to prevent the increase in ICP associated with seizures.

19. How does hyperventilation decrease ICP?
Hyperventilation decreases ICP by producing cerebral vasoconstriction and a resultant decrease in cerebral blood flow (CBF). There is a relatively linear relationship between pCO_2 of 20–80 mmHg and CBF.

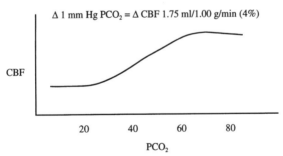

$\Delta 1$ mm Hg $PCO_2 = \Delta$ CBF 1.75 ml/1.00 g/min (4%)

CBF

20   40   60   80

PCO_2

This effect is mediated through acute alterations in cerebral interstitial fluid pH; therefore, it generally becomes less effective after 48–72 hours. Currently, hyperventilation is used to bring ICP under control in the acute setting before other decreasing measures can be introduced. If used prophylactically and for long periods, the vasoconstrictive effects of hyperventilation may cause ischemia and worsen outcome. Thus, most authorities recommend that hyperventilation be used only for the acute short-term management of increased ICP.

20. How does mannitol decrease ICP?
Brain tissue has slightly higher osmolarity than blood, with a gradient of approximately 3 mOsm/L maintained by the blood-brain barrier. Mannitol is an osmotically active agent that reverses this osmotic gradient and shifts water from the brain to the blood. An increase in blood osmolarity by 10 mOsm/L removes 100–150 ml of water from the brain.

Hyperosmolar treatment of elevated ICP increases the normal serum Osm of 290 to 300–315 mOsm/L. An Osm < 300 is ineffective; > 315 results in renal and neurologic dysfunction.

21. Discuss the role of barbiturates in the treatment of head injury.

Barbiturates result in a decrease in the cerebral metabolic rate that may result in a decrease in cerebral blood flow requirements and theoretically should work to lower ICP. They may be effective in lowering ICP and decreasing mortality in the setting of refractory elevation of ICP. However, no data support the prophylactic use of barbiturates. If used, barbiturates must be titrated with caution in head-injured patients, because they result in systemic hypotension that, if not adequately treated, results in a detrimental decrease in CPP.

22. Is there a role for steroids in the treatment of head injury?

Steroids are not useful in the treatment of head injury. No data indicate an improved outcome or suggest that they lower ICP in the setting of head injury.

23. What is the effect of PEEP on head-injured patients?

PEEP, or positive end-expiratory pressure, increases intrathoracic pressure and thus may cause a decrease in venous outflow from the cranial vault and a decrease in venous return to the heart. The result may be an increase in ICP, a decrease in cardiac output (hypotension), and a subsequent decrease in CPP. The effect of a given increment of PEEP is unpredictable, although levels < 10 cmH$_2$O probably do not seem to have a significant effect on ICP.

24. Should dextrose-containing solutions be avoided in head trauma patients?

Infusion of dextrose-containing solutions, especially 5% dextrose and water, is contraindicated in the acute treatment of the neurotrauma patient. Sugar and water pass freely into the brain cells, and once inside the sugar is metabolized, leaving free water behind and causing the cell to swell and cerebral edema to worsen. Normal saline with an osmolarity of 308 mOsm/L is the preferred crystalloid for use in head injury.

BIBLIOGRAPHY

1. Andrews BT: The intensive care management of patients with head injury. In Andrews BT (ed): Neurosurgical Intensive Care. New York, McGraw-Hill, 1993, pp 227–242.
2. Becker D, Miller JD, Ward JD, et al: The outcome from severe head injury with early diagnosis and intensive management. J Neurosurg 47:491–502, 1977.
3. Braakman R, Schouten HJA, Blaauw-van Dishoeck M, et al: Megadose steroids in severe head injury: Results of a prospective double-blind clinical trial. J Neurosurg 58:326–330, 1983.
4. Brain Trauma Foundation: Guidelines for the management of severe head injury. J Neurotrauma 13:639–734, 1996.
5. Cooper C, Stirt J: Monitoring. In Sperry R, Stirt J, Stone D: Manual of Neuroanesthesia. Philadelphia, B.C. Decker, 1989.
6. Duffy K, Becker D: State of the art management of closed head injury. J Crit Care Med 3:291–302, 1988.
7. Eisenberg H, Frankowski R, Constant C, et al: High dose barbiturate control of elevated intracranial pressure in patients with head injury. J Neurosurg 69:15–23, 1988.
8. Ghajar J: Traumatic brain injury. Lancet 356:923–929, 2000.
9. Gunnar W, et al: Head injury and hemorrhagic shock: Studies of the blood-brain barrier and intracranial pressure after resuscitation with normal saline solution, 35 saline solution, and dextran 40. Surgery 103:398–407, 1988.
10. Heffner J, Sahn S: Controlled hyperventilation in patients with intracranial hypertension. Arch Int Med 143:765–769, 1983.
11. Jennett B, Teasdale G, Braakman R, et al: Prognosis of patients with severe head injury. Neurosurgery 4:283–288, 1979.
12. Kalsbeek W, Mclaurin R: The national head and spinal cord injury survey: Major findings. J Neurosurg 53:s19–s31, 1980.
13. Marshall L, Smith R, Shapiro H: The outcome with aggressive treatment in severe head injuries. I. The significance of intracranial pressure monitoring. J Neurosurg 50:20–25, 1979.
14. Miller J, Becker D, Ward J, et al: Significance of intracranial hypertension in severe head injury. J Neurosurg 47:503–516, 1977.

15. Miller J, Becker D, Ward J, et al: Significance of intracranial hypertension in severe head injury. J Neurosrug 47:503–516, 1977.
16. Miller J, Butterworth J, Gudeman S, et al: Further experience in the management of severe head injury. J Neurosurg 54:289–299, 1977.
17. Narayan R, Kishore P, Becker DP, et al: Intracranial pressure: To monitor or not to monitor? J Neurosurg 56:650–659, 1982.
18. Robertson C: Management of cerebral perfusion after traumatic brain injury. Anesthesiology 95:513–1517, 2001.
19. Seelig J, Becker D, Miller JD, et al: Traumatic acute subdural hematoma: Major mortality reduction in comatose treated within four hours. N Engl J Med 304:1511–1517, 1981.
20. Sokoll M: Monitoring intracranial pressure. In Blitt C: Monitoring in Anesthesia and Critical Care Medicine. New York, Churchill Livingstone, 1985, pp 413–425.

XII. Pharmacology

72. DIURETICS

Teresa E. Wagner, M.D., and Lynn M. Schnapp, M.D.

1. What are the common indications for use of diuretics?
- Hypertension
- Edematous states, including congestive heart failure, nephrotic syndrome, ascites (use of loop diuretics, thiazides, or potassium-sparing diuretics)
- Hyperkalemia (use of loop diuretics)
- Hypercalcemia (use of loop diuretics)
- Nephrolithiasis associated with hypercalciuria (use of thiazide diuretics)

2. List the metabolic effects of the commonly used diuretics.

	Thiazides	*Loop Diuretics*	*Potassium-sparing Diuretics*
Serum uric acid	↑	↑	±
Serum glucose	↑	↑	±
Serum lipids	↑	↑/±	±
Serum potassium	↓	↓	↑
Serum sodium	↓	↓	↓
Serum magnesium	↓	↓	↑
Serum calcium	↑*	↓	±

* Only in patients with preexisting hypercalcemia.

3. List the clinical consequences of the metabolic effects of diuretics.
1. Subsequent increase in serum uric acid levels may precipitate an acute gouty attack
2. Effect on glucose metabolism can result in decreased control of established diabetes (i.e., hyperglycemia and increased insulin resistance)
3. Induction of a hyperosmolar, nonketotic diabetic syndrome in patients with no preexisting diabetes (rare)
4. Mild hyponatremia is also a common side effect and does not usually require therapy; however, life-threatening hyponatremia (Na < 100 mEq/L) is a potential but rare complication.
5. Hypokalemia may predispose to the development of:
   - Cardiac arrhythmias
   - Exacerbation of hypertension
   - Renal failure
   - Increased incidence of cerebrovascular disease

4. Describe the effect of diuretics on lipid profile.
Although diuretics are widely prescribed as first-step agents for the treatment of hypertension and congestive heart failure, several studies have shown that they have deleterious effects on the serum lipid profile. Diuretic use can result in increased levels of triglycerides, very-low-density lipoproptein (VLDL), total cholesterol, and low-density lipoprotein (LDL). Diuretics

can directly increase insulin secretion and leads to hypersecretion of the counterregulatory hormones (cortisol, growth hormone, and catecholamines). Insulin is known to stimulate triglyceride sythesis, whereas catecholamines increase hepatic cholesterol production.

5. Define diuretic resistance and diuretic tolerance.

A patient is considered **diuretic-resistant** when an optimal diuretic response cannot be obtained by using conventional doses. A patient is considered **diuretic-tolerant** when increased amounts of drug are needed over time to produce equivalent effects.

6. Describe the mechanism responsible for resistance to chronic loop diuretic therapy.

Persistent blockade of solute resorption at the thick ascending limb of the loop of Henle floods the distal nephron with increased amounts of sodium. In turn, the distal nephron undergoes hypertrophy and increases its sodium resorptive capacity. Thus, chronic administration of loop diuretics leads to a progressively diminishing response.

7. A 52-year-old man with cirrhosis due to hepatitis C is admitted to the MICU for evaluation for liver transplantation. He required chronic furosemide therapy at 40 mg/day for his edematous state. Since admission his weight has increased, and he has developed a positive fluid balance despite continuous administration of his regular dose of furosemide. How can diuretic resistance and tolerance be overcome?

Assuming that the patient is receiving the appropriate medication, several options are available. The dose of oral furosemide may be increased, or the route of administration may be changed to intravenous boluses or a continuous infusion. Alternatively, a different class of diuretic may be added for synergy. The distal nephron, which undergoes hypertrophy in response to chronic loop diuretic therapy, remains highly sensitive to thiazide diuretics. This is the basis for the observed synergy between furosemide and metolazone.

8. Estimate the "safe" maximal dose of furosemide in patients with chronic renal insufficiency.

Decreased renal function leads to a concomitant decrease in the renal clearance of loop diuretics, resulting in less delivery of the drug to the urinary site of action. In patients with normal renal function, approximately 50% of an IV dose of furosemide reaches the tubules. In patients with severe renal insufficiency, only about 10% of the same dose reaches the tubules. In patients with normal renal function, 40 mg of furosemide IV is required to obtain a maximal response. In patients with severe renal insufficiency, a fivefold increase (e.g., 200 mg IV) is required to obtain a similar response. In a patient with severe renal insufficiency who has not responded to this calculated IV dose of furosemide, further increases in dosage are unlikely to result in additional benefit but may increase the risk of toxicity (e.g., ototoxicity).

9. What are the advantages of continuous infusion compared with intravenous boluses of loop diuretics?

Continuous intravenous infusion of loop diuretics appears to result in increased urine volume and sodium excretion compared with intermittent intravenous boluses. In addition, the risk of ototoxicity is decreased. After a loading dose, a furosemide drip can be initiated at 10–20 mg/hr, depending on renal function. If diuresis is insufficient or not sustained, a second loading dose can be administered, followed by a doubling of the drip rate. Further increases in infusion rate should take into account risk of toxicity.

10. How do diuretics affect the short-term outcome in patients with chronic heart failure?

Diuretics, at appropriate doses, can relieve vascular congestion and the associated pulmonary and peripheral edema, thereby providing both symptomatic relief (e.g., shortness of breath) and improvement in the quality of life. However, excessive diuresis can cause fatigue, hypotension, and azotemia.

11. Does diuretic therapy reduce the mortality due to chronic heart failure?

Yes. The addition of low-dose spironolactone (12.5–25 mg/day) to standard (angiotensin-converting enzyme [ACE] inhibitor, loop diuretic, dogoxin, and low-dose beta blocker) reduces morbidity and mortality in patients with severe heart failure. Its cardioprotective effect may be secondary to decreased myocardial fibrosis by inhibiting collagen formation and and to decreased sodium retention by aldosterone receptor blockade.

12. What are the effects of diuretics on morbidity and mortality in the treatment of hypertension?

Long-term diuretic therapy (low-dose thiazide diuretic) results in decreased progression of hypertension, reversal of left ventricular hypertrophy, prevention of congestive heart failure, and reduction in the incidence of and mortality from strokes and coronary heart disease.

13. How does dopamine affect renal dysfunction in critically ill patients?

It is common practice in medical intensive care units to use low-dose dopamine infusions (approximately 2 µg/kg/min) to facilitate urine output in patients developing renal dysfunction. Although low-dose dopamine may result in increased urine output by decreasing renal vascular resistance, it does not prevent the development of acute renal failure.

14. Are diuretics useful in preventing contrast-induced nephropathy in patients with chronic renal insufficiency?

No. Diuretics are not helpful in preventing contrast-induced nephropathy and in fact may be harmful. The best preventive measure is intravenous hydration plus acetylcysteine, 600 mg orally twice daily on the day preceding and on the day of contrast administration. Mannitol, dopamine, and atrial natriuretic peptide do not prevent contrast-induced nephropathy.

15. Does coadministration of diuretics with albumin help to achieve increased diuresis in patients with cirrhosis or other causes of hypoalbuminemia?

Clinical studies have shown conflicting results, and this topic remains controversial. A randomized crossover study found no improved efficacy with albumin and furosemide compared with furosemide alone in patients with cirrhosis and ascites.

BIBLIOGRAPHY

1. Bellomo R, Chapman M, Finfer S, et al: Low-dose dopamine in patients with early renal dyfunction: A placebo-controlled randomized trial. Australian and New Zealand Intensive Care Society (ANZICS) Clinical Trials Group. Lancet 356:2139–2143, 2000.
2. Brater DC: Diuretic therapy. N Engl J Med 339:387–395, 1998.
3. Chalasani N, Gorski JC, Horlander JC, et al: Effects of albumin/furosemide mixtures on responses to furosemide in hypoalbuminuric patients. J Am Soc Nephrol 12:1010–1016, 2001.
4. Cohn JN: The management of chronic heart failure. N Engl J Med 335(7):490–498, 1996.
5. Conger JD: Interventions in clinical acute renal failure: What are the data? Am J Kidney Dis 26:565–576, 1995.
6. Dormans TPJ, van Meyel JJM, Gerlag PGG, et al: Diuretic efficacy of high dose furosemide in severe heart failure: Bolus injection versus continuous infusion. J Am Coll Cardiol 28:376–382, 1996.
7. Madu EC, Reddy RC, Madu AN, et al: Review: The effects of antihypertensive agents on serum lipids. Am J Med Sci 312:76–84, 1996.
8. Pitt B, Zannad F, Remme WJ, et al: The effect of spironolactone on morbidity and mortality in patients with severe heart failure. N Engl J Med 341:709–717, 1999.
9. Tepel M, van der Giet m, Schwarzfeld C, et al: Prevention of radiographic-contrast-agent-induced reductions in renal function by acetylcysteine. N Engl J Med 343:180–184, 2000.
10. Ramsay LE, Yeo WW, Jackson RR: Metabolic effects of diuretics. Cardiology 84(Suppl 2):48–56, 1994.

73. INOTROPIC AND VASOPRESSOR DRUGS

Richard H. Savel, M.D., and Michael A. Gropper, M.D., Ph.D.

1. What are the indications for the use of inotropic and vasopressor drugs?

Inotropes and vasopressors are typically used when there is evidence of inadequate perfusion of vital tissues during the course of various pathologic conditions: distributive shock due to sepsis, anaphylaxis, or spinal cord injury; cardiogenic shock due to myocardial infarction, cardiac injury, or valvular dysfunction; and extracardiac obstructive shock resulting from massive pulmonary emboli, pericardial tamponade, constrictive pericarditis, severe pulmonary vascular disease, or, rarely, coarctation of the aorta. Evidence of inadequate perfusion may be overt, as in cardiovascular collapse, or it may be more subtle, indicative of regional maldistribution of organ blood flow with failure to perfuse and maintain individual organ function. Vasoactive drugs may be indicated either to restore overall cardiovascular status or to improve perfusion to various regional vascular beds. In adults, vasopressors are typically indicated when systolic blood pressure is less than 90 mmHg.

2. What pressors and inotropic drugs are available? What are their mechanisms of action?

Various drugs that act primarily by stimulating adrenergic receptors are available. Alpha-adrenergic agonists mediate peripheral vasoconstriction, beta-1 adrenergic agonists augment cardiac output and heart rate, beta-2 agonists induce bronchodilation and mediate peripheral vasodilation, and dopaminergic agonists induce dilation of the renal and mesenteric circulations. Some vasoactive drugs work by directly activating adrenergic receptors; others work, at least in part, through the indirect release of endogenous intraneuronal stores of catecholamines. This distinction may be important in a few specific clinical situations and should be kept in mind when selecting a vasoactive drug or in gauging the efficacy of a drug in a particular clinical situation (see below).

Epinephrine is a direct-acting, naturally occurring alpha, beta-1, and beta-2 agonist with some differential activity at the various receptors based on dose. At doses of 1–2 μg/min, epinephrine is primarily a beta agonist and would be expected to cause vasodilation and increased stroke volume and heart rate. At 2–10 μg/min, it has both beta and alpha effects, although beta effects again predominate, and at doses > 10 μg/min, alpha agonist effects predominate and cause vasoconstriction.

Norepinephrine is a direct-acting, naturally occurring alpha agonist with some beta-1 and virtually no beta-2 activity. It has inotropic effects at doses of 1–2 μg/min and at higher doses is the most potent and dependable vasoconstricting agent available. It also is a venoconstrictor and can increase venous return.

Dobutamine is a direct-acting, synthetic beta-1 agonist with some beta-2 agonist activity; it acts primarily as an inotrope. Dobutamine causes less tachycardia than isoproterenol, epinephrine, or dopamine and also may decrease both systemic and pulmonary vascular resistance, thereby causing some hypotension, particularly if intravascular volume is low.

Dopamine is a synthetic catecholamine with both direct and indirect agonist activity at alpha, beta-1, and dopaminergic receptors. It has well-characterized differential activity at these receptor subtypes based on dose, which dictates its dose-dependent functional effects. At 0.5–2 μg/kg/min, dopamine activates dopaminergic receptors. This induces regional vasodilation of the renal and mesenteric circulation leading to increases in renal and gut blood flow. In addition to its dopaminergic effects on the renal vasculature, dopamine also acts as a natriuretic hormone by diminishing sodium reabsorption through dopaminergic effects in the distal tubule and collecting ducts. Coexisting therapy with haloperidol or phenothiazines may blunt these dopaminergic effects. At 2–5 μg/kg/min, dopamine activates both dopaminergic as well as beta-1 receptors. At 5–10 μg/kg/min, it is primarily a beta-1 agonist. At doses above 10 μg/kg/min, dopamine also activates alpha receptors. Above 20 μg/kg/min, the alpha effect is the predominant effect of dopamine. Because of its indirect activity, dopamine may have an unpredictable response in patients receiving monoamine oxidase (MAO) inhibitors, tricyclic antidepressants, or cocaine, and it should either not be used or be used with caution in these patients due to possible induction of a hyperadrenergic state. Dopamine also can inhibit insulin secretion and may contribute to hyperglycemia in some patients.

Metaraminol is a synthetic, direct alpha agonist that also has a substantial indirect mechanism of action. It is also taken up by nerve terminals and may serve as a false neurotransmitter. This may partially explain the tendency of patients to develop tolerance or tachyphylaxis to this drug over time. It is less dependable as a vasoconstrictor than either norepinephrine or phenylephrine and is no longer widely used.

Phenylephrine is a synthetic, direct-acting alpha agonist with virtually no beta agonist activity. As such it has less potential to induce arrhythmias or increase myocardial oxygen demand than drugs with beta agonist activity.

Three other inotropic agents are available that do not activate adrenergic receptors. **Amrinone** inhibits the enzyme phosphodiesterase, thereby increasing cyclic adenosine monophosphate (cAMP) in cardiac myocytes and smooth muscle cells. The result is marked augmentation of stroke volume with little increase in heart rate as well as peripheral vasodilation. This drug is most useful in patients with a severe cardiogenic hypoperfusion state. **Glucagon** is a polypeptide hormone that binds to nonadrenergic surface receptors and activates adenylate cyclase, thereby increasing cAMP. Glucagon appears to be most useful in treating hypoperfusion states induced by or complicated by beta adrenergic blockade. **Vasopressin**, a peptide hormone, is a potent vasoconstrictor that acts directly on the vasopressin receptor. It recently has been used for hypotension in septic shock and has been added to the indicated drugs for Advanced Cardiac Life Support.

3. What pharmacologic principles must be considered in choosing or judging the efficacy of a particular vasoactive substance?

Because most of these drugs work via activation of adrenergic receptors, the number of receptors in an individual patient obviously affects the performance of the drug. Adrenergic receptors tend to be upregulated following chronic adrenergic blockade and downregulated in states of adrenergic excess or with chronic beta-adrenergic treatment, as in patients with airflow limitation due to asthma or emphysema. Furthermore, since some of these drugs work by indirectly releasing endogenous intraneuronal stores of catecholamines, the state of these intraneuronal stores also is important. The concomitant use of drugs, such as tricyclic antidepressants or cocaine, that inhibit the reuptake of norepinephrine at nerve terminals or of drugs that cause accumulations of norepinephrine at nerve terminals (MAO inhibitors) will obviously affect the performance of indirectly acting vasoactive substances. Receptor affinity and efficacy also are important considerations in judging response to a vasoactive drug. Elderly patients, for example, have increased norepinephrine release with stress, which suggests possible decreased adrenoreceptor function with age. Hypoxia and acidosis are both known to decrease adrenergic receptor affinity, while vascular sensitivity to norepinephrine is increased in the presence of jaundice and hyperlipidemia. Thus a variety of exogenous and endogenous factors may act to either increase or decrease the expected response to a given vasoactive drug and should always be considered in the selection of these compounds.

4. What drugs should be chosen for a given clinical situation, and over what concentrations should they be used?

Vasoactive drugs should be used after careful consideration of the particular hemodynamic state in each individual patient and only after intravascular volume status has been restored to an adequate level. Once intravascular volume has been restored (pulmonary capillary wedge pressure 12–18 cmH_2O or central venous pressure 5–15 cmH_2O) but perfusion is still judged to be inadequate, the selection of appropriate pharmacologic support should be based on the ability of the drug to correct or augment the hemodynamic deficit present. If the problem is believed to be inadequate cardiac output, the drug chosen should have prominent activity at beta-1 receptors and little effect at alpha receptors that increase afterload and further reduce stroke volume. If the perfusion deficit is due to marked reductions in peripheral vascular resistance, then a drug that increases resistance (an alpha agonist) should be used. The hemodynamic picture is often more complex than those presented above, or other special considerations (e.g., oliguria, underlying ischemic heart disease, arrhythmias) may exist and further complicate the decision-making process.

In general, **epinephrine** is useful in patients with severe reductions in cardiac output in whom the arrhythmogenicity and marked augmentation in heart rate and myocardial oxygen consumption that occur with this drug are not limiting factors. Epinephrine is the drug of choice for anaphylactic shock, due to its activity at beta-1 and beta-2 receptors, and it can also be used in cases of refractory septic shock, due to its ability to activate both beta and alpha receptors at high dose. The usual dosage range is 2–20 µg/min.

Dopamine is most often relied upon to reverse hypotension and maintain vital organ perfusion in the setting of hypoperfusion due to reduced cardiac output. It does so with less increase in myocardial oxygen consumption than epinephrine but tends to cause more tachycardia than dobutamine in this setting, and unlike dobutamine, usually increases rather than decreases pulmonary capillary wedge pressures. This effect may be undesired in the patient with high baseline wedge pressures in whom further increases may precipitate pulmonary edema. The dopaminergic effects which promote renal vasodilation and natriuresis have led to the frequent use of low-dose or "renal dose" dopamine, both to increase urine output and to preserve renal function in oliguric patients at risk for the development of acute tubular necrosis. Although dopamine can increase urine output and renal blood flow, there is at present no clear clinical or experimental evidence to support a renal protective effect of dopamine in this setting. One recent trial compared the effects of fluid repletion with saline alone to saline plus renal dose dopamine and found no difference in renal function between the two groups. Other uncontrolled studies have suggested only modest protective effects of renal dose dopamine in combination with loop diuretics in oliguric patients within 48 hours of an ischemic insult. Thus, the widespread use of low-dose dopamine as a renal sparing agent may need to be reassessed based on current knowledge. If it is to be used it probably needs to be begun early following the insult and discontinued if substantial diuresis or improvement in renal function is not observed. Dopamine at higher concentrations (alpha agonist range > 15 µg/kg/min) also is useful in cases of reduced systemic vascular resistance but may be less reliable than norepinephrine or phenylephrine in this setting.

Norepinephrine is used to restore overall cardiovascular status in cases of reduced systemic vascular resistance and should be the drug of choice when a direct-acting adrenergic agonist is needed (tricyclic overdose, cocaine overdose). Because of the excessive vasoconstriction noted with this agent, this drug often is used with dopamine at low dose in an attempt to preserve renal and mesenteric blood flow. Norepinephrine is the pressor of choice for septic shock at doses of 1–24 µg/min.

Dobutamine should be used when reduced cardiac output is considered the cause of the perfusion deficit, and it should not be considered the sole therapy if the decrease in output is accompanied by a significant decrease in mean arterial pressure. This is because dobutamine may cause further reductions in both preload and afterload and further reduce mean arterial pressure. However, if both mean arterial pressure and intravascular filling are near normal, a recent study suggests that dobutamine may be more effective than dopamine in enhancing forward flow and in distributing the flow to improve tissue oxygenation. Dobutamine is used at a dose of 2–20 µg/kg/min.

Phenylephrine is used to increase systemic vascular resistance in patients who cannot tolerate any further myocardial stimulation (arrhythmias, angina). It should be given initially at 100–180 µg/min and then adjusted to desired blood pressure. This agent is also useful for septic shock.

Inotropes and Vasopressors

DRUG	RECEPTOR PROFILE	CLINICAL ACTIVITY		DOSE
		Cardiac	*Peripheral*	
Dopamine	DA_1, DA_2 agonist	++ Chronotropism	+ Renal, mesenteric	1–4 µg/kg/min
	β_1 agonist	++ Inotropism	artery dilation	(renal dose)
	β_2 agonist		+ Vasodilation	2–20 µg/kg/min
	α agonist			(vasoconstriction
				at higher doses)

Table continued on following page

Inotropes and Vasopressors (Continued)

DRUG	RECEPTOR PROFILE	CLINICAL ACTIVITY		DOSE
		Cardiac	*Peripheral*	
Dobutamine	β_1 agonist β_2 agonist	+ Chronotropism +++ Inotropism	+ Vasodilation	1–20 μg/min
Epinephrine	β_1 agonist β_2 agonist α agonist	+++ Chronotropism +++ Inotropism	++ Vasoconstriction	1–20 μg/min
Norepinephrine	α_1 agonist β_2 agonist	++ Inotropism ++ Chronotropism	+++ Vasoconstriction	2–20 μg/min
Phenylephrine	α agonist	No effect	++ Vasoconstriction	2–100 μg/min
Amrinone	PDE_{II} inhibitor	+ Chronotropism +++ Inotropism	Vasodilation	0.75 mg/kg over 5 min, then 5–15 μg/kg/min

5. What parameters should be followed to assess the adequacy of response to a particular vasoactive substance?

The general guidelines to determine the adequacy of success in treatment of shock states include maintenance of mean arterial pressure > 60 mmHg with evidence of adequate regional blood flow to various vital organs. The means of assessing the adequacy of regional tissue perfusion, however, are not ideal, and the best parameters to follow continue to be debated. However, clinical evidence of adequate regional perfusion is always available, and the level of sensorium, urine output, and skin color and temperature are good crude estimates of regional blood flow to brain, kidney, and skin, respectively. Some investigators advocate the use of overall estimates of oxygen transport to assess tissue perfusion. Shoemaker and coworkers use vasoactive drugs along with fluids and blood products to maintain a cardiac index > 4.5 L/min/m², oxygen delivery > 600 ml/min/m², and oxygen consumption > 170 ml/min/m² during the first 2–3 days postoperatively in critically ill surgical patients and have demonstrated improved survival if these parameters can be achieved. However, interventions aimed at achieving Shoemaker's supraphysiologic goals of cardiac index, DO_2 and VO_2, have not reduced morbidity or mortality rates in critically ill patients when intervention was begun after admission to the ICU. However, one recent study using goal-directed therapy for septic shock found an improvement in mortality rate when attempts were made to keep central venous oxygen saturation above 70% and the interventions took place very early in the hospital course. Finally, blood lactate levels also serve as an overall marker of tissue hypoxia or underperfusion. A decrease in blood lactate with treatment is a crude marker of improvement in regional blood flow to underperfused vascular beds. A failure to decrease or an increase in lactate levels with adequate blood pressure suggests that regional tissue hypoxia is ongoing and that further attempts to augment oxygen delivery or redistribute blood flow should be attempted.

6. What are the complications of these drugs?

The major adverse effects are related to excessive alpha- or beta-adrenergic stimulation. Although vasoconstriction may be needed to increase mean arterial pressure above a critical level, further vasoconstriction may worsen regional blood flow and cause further tissue hypoxia. The minimum dose of vasopressor (alpha agonist) that brings mean arterial pressure above 60 mmHg should be used, and excessive vasoconstriction should be avoided. Unopposed vasoconstriction is also a potential problem with local extravasation of vasopressors. Peripheral infiltration of intravenous-fluid-containing vasopressors can produce local tissue gangrene if unrecognized or left untreated. Central venous access should be used to deliver vasopressors whenever possible. If peripheral tissue infiltration with a vasopressor does occur, the area should be infiltrated with 5–10 mg of phentolamine (alpha blocker) diluted in 10 cc normal saline to counter the alpha-mediated vasoconstriction. Constriction of pulmonary vessels may cause ventilation perfusion mismatch and actually worsen oxygenation and oxygen delivery. Blood gases should be monitored frequently when beginning therapy with vasoactive drugs, and measures to correct worsening hypoxemia embarked upon so that oxygen delivery is not impaired. The other major complications to be watched for when using vasopressors and inotropes are cardiac in origin. These drugs have the potential to induce a variety of lethal arrhythmias and to markedly increase myocardial oxygen demand. In the patient with limited coronary perfusion, such an increase in oxygen demand can induce cardiac ischemia or infarction.

7. What is the best drug for treatment of septic shock? Are any new drugs available?

Some evidence suggests that norepinephrine should be used as the first-line agent in septic shock. The mortality rate in patients receiving norepinephrine was 62% compared with 82% in patients treated with other vasopressors. These data refute concerns about deleterious vasoconstriction and increased mortality associated with norepinephrine. Further randomized studies are needed to confirm this finding.

Animal models have revealed a deficiency of vasopressin in septic and cardiogenic shock that can be reversed by continuous infusion of the drug. Vasopressin mediates vasoconstriction via V1 receptors on vascular smooth muscle, whereas its antidiuretic effect is mediated via V2 receptors in the renal collecting duct system. Increased vasopressin levels are associated with a reduced need for other vasopressors. The new cardiopulmonary resuscitation guidelines recommend vasopressin at a dose of 40 U intravenously as an equivalent to epinephrine, 1 mg intravenously, for treatment of ventricular fibrillation. Studies have shown that vasopressin infusions of 0.01–0.04 U/min in patients with septic shock lead to increased urine output and decreased pulmonary vascular resistance. Infusions > 0.04 U/min may lead to adverse events. The human studies have been small and focused on physiologic endpoints rather than clinical coutcomes. For these reasons and because of the potential adverse side effects of vasopressin, clinical use in sepsis cannot be recommended until large controlled clinical trials are performed.

BIBLIOGRAPHY

1. Duke GJ, Bersten AD: Dopamine and renal salvage in the critically ill patient. Anesth Intensive Care 20:277–287, 1992.
2. Fenwick JC, Dodek PM, Ronco JJ, et al: Increased concentrations of plasma lactate predict patholgoic dependence of oxygen consumption on oxygen delivery in patients with adult respiratory distress syndrome. J Crit Care 5:81–86, 1990.
3. Gattinoni L, Brazzi L, Pelosi P, et al and the SVO_2 collaborative group: A trial of goal-oriented hemodynamic therapy in critically ill patients. N Engl J Med 333:1025–1032, 1995.
4. Hesselvik JF, Brodin B: Low dose norepinephrine in patients with septic shock and oliguria: Effects on afterload, urine flow, and oxygen transport. Crit Care Med 17:179–180, 1989.
5. Higgins TL, Chernow B: Pharmacotherapy of circulatory shock. Dis Month, June 1987, pp 313–361.
6. Holmes CL, Patel BM, Russel JA, Walley KR: Physiology of vasopressin relevant to management of septic shock. Chest 120:989–1002, 2001.
7. King EG, Chin WDN: Shock: An overview of pathophysiology and general treatment goals. Crit care Clin 1:547–561, 1985.
8. Larach DR, Kofke WA: Cardiovascular drugs. In Kofke WA, Levy JH (eds): Postoperative Critical Care Procedures of the Massachusetts General Hospital. Boston, Little, Brown, 1986, pp 464-522.
9. Lollgren H, Drexler H: Use of inotropes in the critical care setting. Crit Care Med 18:S56–S60, 1990.
10. Martin C, Viviand X, Leone M, Thirion X: Effects of norepinephrine on the outcome of septic shock. Crit Care Med 28:2758–2765, 2000.
11. Parrillo JE: Septic shock in humans: Clinical evaluation, pathogenesis, and therapeutic approach. In Shoemaker WC, et al: Textbook of Critical Care, 3rd ed. Philadelphia, W.B. Saunders, 1995.
12. Peters JI, Utset OM: Vasopressors in shock management: Choosing and using wisely. J Crit Illness 4:62–68, 1989.
13. Rivers E, Nguyen B, Havstad S, et al: Early goal-directed therapy in the treatment of severe sepsis and septic shock. N Engl J Med 345:1368–1377, 2001.
14. Schaer GL, Fink MP, Parillo JE: Norepinephrine alone versus norepinephrine plus low-dose dopamine: Enhanced renal blood flow with combination pressor therapy. Crit Care Med 13:492–496, 1985.

15. Shoemaker WC, Appel PL, Kram HB: Oxygen transport measurements to evaluate tissue perfusion and titrate therapy: Dobutamine and dopamine effects. Crit Care Med 19:672–688, 1991.
16. Shoemaker WC, Kram HB, Appel PL: Therapy of shock based on pathophysiology, monitoring, and outcome prediction. Crit Care Med 18:S19–S25, 1990.
17. Sibbald WJ, Calvin JE, Holliday RL, Driedger AA: Concepts in the pharmacologic and nonpharmacologic support of cardiovascular function in critically ill surgical patients. Surg Clin North Am 63:455–482, 1983.
18. Vernon DD, Banner W, Garrett JS, Dean JM: Efficacy of dopamine and norepinephrine for treatment of hemodynamic compromise in amitriptyline intoxication. Crit Care Med 19:544–549, 1991.
19. Wheeler AP, Bernard GR: Treating patients with severe sepsis. N Engl J Med 340:207–214, 1999.
20. Zaloga GP, Delacey W, Holmboe E, Chernow B: Glucagon reversal of hypotension in a case of anaphylactoid shock. Ann Intern Med 105:65–66, 1986.

74. VASODILATORS

Wanda C. Miller-Hance, M.D.

1. What are the effects of vasodilating agents?

The primary effects of vasodilators are relaxation of vascular smooth muscle and increasing the diameter of veins (capacitance vessels), arterioles (resistance vessels), and arteries (conduit vessels). Secondary effects of these agents include a reduction in cardiac preload (venodilators) and/or cardiac afterload (arteriolar dilators).

2. How are vasodilators classified?

Vasodilators are classified as either venous or arterial, although most agents exhibit activity on both vascular beds. Vasodilators also are classified according to their mechanisms of action.

3. What are the clinical indications for the use of vasodilators?

Vasodilating compounds are effective in the treatment of hypertension, acute pulmonary edema, and chronic congestive heart failure. In addition, they are used as adjuncts in the elective lowering of arterial blood pressure during anesthesia and surgery (controlled hypotension) in order to provide better operating conditions and to minimize surgical blood loss.

4. What parameters should be followed to assess the adequacy of response to a particular vasoactive substance?

Although the main effect of vasodilators is a reduction in preload and/or afterload, the net effect is critically dependent on the baseline hemodynamic state, particularly ventricular function and peripheral circulation. The potency of these agents requires frequent blood pressure assessments (in many cases via invasive monitoring) in addition to administration via mechanical infusion devices.

5. What are the most commonly used vasodilators? Describe their mechanisms of action and clinical indications for their use.

Nitrovasodilators

Nitric oxide is a naturally occurring potent vasodilator released by the endothelium. This compound plays a critical role in regulating vascular smooth muscle tone. The selective vasodilating effect of inhaled nitric oxide on the pulmonary circulation has proved to be beneficial in the treatment of pulmonary hypertensive conditions. This agent may also have clinical applications in improving oxygenation in patients with acute respiratory distress syndrome.

Sodium nitroprusside is a potent, rapidly acting agent with an extremely short half-life that acts on arterial and venous vascular smooth muscles. This drug is classified as a nitrovasodilator, producing its biologic effect via the release of nitric oxide. The hemodynamic effects of sodium nitroprusside are primarily afterload reduction by arterial vasodilation and preload reduction by increasing venous capacitance. These effects are typically associated with a reflex increase in heart rate and cardiac output. Sodium nitroprusside is used extensively in the management of hypertensive emergencies, acute valvular regurgitation, low cardiac output states, and congestive heart failure. The aqueous solution of sodium nitroprusside is photosensitive and should be protected from light.

Nitroglycerin causes nonspecific vascular smooth muscle relaxation, with predominant venous over arterial dilation. Its mechanism of action is presumably similar to that of sodium nitroprusside. Nitroglycerin increases venous capacitance and decreases venous return, affects preload more than afterload, and reduces myocardial oxygen consumption. Heart rate is unchanged or minimally increased. Effects on cardiac vasculature include redistribution of coronary blood flow to ischemic areas of the subendocardium and relief of coronary spasm. Noncardiac effects include decreases in platelet aggregation, dilation of cerebral vessels and potential increases in intracranial pressure, decreases in renal blood flow in relation to systemic arterial pressure, and dilation of pulmonary vessels. Clinical indications include ischemic heart disease, hypertension, and ventricular failure. Nitroglycerin is metabolized in the liver by glutathione reductase. The nitrate ion, a metabolic product, may oxidize hemoglobin to methemoglobin. Significant methemoglobinemia is rare and can be treated with methylene blue (1–2 mg/kg intravenously over 5 minutes). Chronic administration of long-acting forms may lead to tolerance in arterial vessels but not in the venous vessels.

Adrenergic-blocking agents

Prazosin is a relatively selective postsynaptic alpha-1 receptor blocker that lowers blood pressure by decreasing systemic vascular resistance. Therapeutic uses include treatment of essential hypertension, decrease of afterload in patients with congestive heart failure, and preoperative preparation of patients with pheochromocytoma.

Phentolamine is a direct-acting agent producing competitive alpha-adrenergic receptor blockade (alpha-1 and alpha-2). Alpha-1 antagonism and direct smooth muscle relaxation account for the peripheral vasodilation and the fall in arterial blood pressure. The extent of the hemodynamic response to alpha receptor blockade is proportionate to the degree of existing sympathetic tone. Phentolamine is particularly useful in the treatment of conditions associated with excessive alpha stimulation (e.g., pheochromocytoma) and for local infiltration to limit tissue injury that may result from the accidental extravasation of an alpha agonist (e.g., norepinephrine).

Beta-blocking drugs are typically administered for heart rate control and less frequently used for blood pressure management. Among beta-blockers, **labetalol** is the most commonly used drug for blood pressure reduction. Labetalol is a selective alpha-1 antagonist and a nonselective beta-adrenergic receptor antagonist. The ratio of alpha to beta blockade following intravenous administration is estimated to be approximately 1:7. The combination of alpha and beta blockade is responsible for a reduction in peripheral vascular resistance and arterial blood pressure without associated reflex tachycardia. A number of other beta-adrenergic antagonists are available for the treatment of hypertension, including **atenolol, metoprolol, acebutalol,** and **carvedilol.**

Calcium channel antagonists

These organic compounds block calcium influx through slow channels. The use of these agents is generally associated with afterload reduction, negative inotropism, decreases in sinoatrial node automaticity and atrioventricular conduction, and systemic and coronary vasodilation. They generally reduce myocardial oxygen demand by decreasing afterload and improve oxygen supply by increasing coronary blood flow. **Nifedipine** has potent effects on systemic blood pressure making it a widely used agent for the nonparenteral prompt treatment of hypertension. Unlike **verapamil** and **diltiazem**, nifedipine has fewer effects on cardiac contractility, making it a more suitable agent in patients with ventricular dysfunction.

Ganglionic blocking agents

Trimethaphan has powerful effects as a ganglionic blocking agent. The blockade of acetylcholine receptors in autonomic ganglia in addition to direct smooth muscle relaxation and histamine release account for the effects of this drug in lowering arterial blood pressure. This agent has a fast onset but its duration of action exceeds that of sodium nitroprusside. Trimethaphan decreases arterial blood pressure by arteriolar and venous dilation. In contrast to many other peripheral vasodilators, trimethaphan is not associated with cerebral vasodilation.

Postoperative neurologic assessment may be complicated by drug-induced mydriasis and cyclopegia. This drug may be useful in the setting of a dissecting aortic aneurysm.

Central alpha-2 agonists

Clonidine is a centrally acting alpha agonist that stimulates alpha-2 receptors in the depressor area of the vasomotor center leading to inhibition of sympathetic outflow. This results in alterations in the release of neurotransmitters, decreases in heart rate, arterial blood pressure, cardiac output, and peripheral vascular resistance. Nonhemodynamic effects of clonidine therapy include sedation, analgesia, and suppression of the signs and symptoms of opioid withdrawal.

Direct vasodilators

Hydralazine is a potent, direct-acting vasodilator that causes smooth muscle relaxation of arteriolar resistance vessels with minimal to no effect on venous capacitance. Its mechanism of action may be related to interference with calcium utilization or activation of guanylyl cyclase. The onset of action is relatively slow, typically seen within 10–20 min, with the antihypertensive effect usually lasting about 2–4 hr. The decreases in peripheral vascular resistance and fall in arterial blood pressure are frequently accompanied by reflex tachycardia. In addition to increasing myocardial contractility and cardiac output, hydralazine acts as a potent cerebral vasodilator and abolishes cerebral autoregulation. Renal blood flow is usually maintained. Hydralazine is particularly effective in the treatment of pregnancy-induced hypertension. The drug undergoes acetylation and hydroxylation in the bowel and/or liver. **Minoxidil** is also a potent arteriolar vasodilator with hemodynamic effects quite similar to those of hydralazine. It dilates primarily arterioles and has little effect on capacitance vessels. The precise mechanism for the vasodilatory action of minoxidil is unknown. Pharmacologic effects include an adrenergically mediated increase in myocardial contractility and cardiac output.

Angiotensin-converting enzyme (ACE) inhibitors

ACE inhibitors may produce favorable hemodynamics in patients with congestive heart failure. **Captopril** was the first drug in this class to be widely used for lowering of blood pressure. Several other agents are now available (**enalapril, lisinopril, quinapril, ramipril, benazepril**). ACE inhibitors are very useful for the treatment of hypertension and ischemic heart disease. In patients with diabetes, ACE inhibitors appear to slow the development of diabetic glomerulopathy.

Angiotensin II-receptor antagonists

Various agents with angiotensin II antagonistic properties have been introduced recently for clinical use in patients with hypertension. Examples include **losartan, candesartan, irbesartan,** and **valsartan**. These agents prevent the effects of angiotensin II, relax smooth muscle, and promote vasodilation.

Opioids

Morphine sulphate has been traditionally used in the treatment of pulmonary edema. Besides its narcotic effect, an important part of its action is a reduction in both afterload and preload. This reduction in vascular tone is secondary to a decrease in central sympathetic outflow or splanchnic pooling.

6. What clinical effects are associated with vasodilator therapy?

In addition to improving hemodynamics, vasodilators are also considered to improve exercise tolerance and quality of life.

7. What toxicity is associated with nitric oxide?

The administration of nitric oxide at low concentrations (0.1–50 parts per million) is generally considered safe. Pulmonary toxicity can occur at levels that exceed 50 parts per million. Nitric oxide is a known atmospheric pollutant. Methemoglobinemia is a significant complication of inhaled nitric oxide that requires intermittent analysis of blood methemoglobin levels.

8. What are the most common adverse effects/complications of vasodilators?

The most common untoward effect of vasodilators is an exaggeration of their hypotensive effects, leading to coronary, cerebral, and systemic hypoperfusion. The most common adverse effects may be grouped according to class of agents:

Nitrovasodilators: hypotension, flushing, headache, dizziness, nausea, vomiting, cyanide/thiocyanide toxicity (sodium nitroprusside), decreases in arterial oxygen saturation, methemoglobinemia.

Adrenergic-blocking agents: orthostatic hypotension (alpha- and beta-blockers), paradoxical hypertension, bradycardia, flushing, nausea, itching, tingling of the scalp, precipitation of asthma or congestive heart failure, hypoglycemia and a reduction in exercise capacity (labetalol).

Calcium channel antagonists: cardiac depression, bradycardia, conduction system blockade (verapamil, diltiazem) and peripheral edema (nifedipine).

Ganglionic blocking agents: postural hypotension, mydriasis, histamine release, noncompetitive inhibition of pseudocholinesterase and the development of tachyphylaxis with continued use (trimethaphan).

Central alpha-2 agonists: postural hypotension, sedation, dry mouth and the potential for rebound hypertension associated with abrupt discontinuation of the drug (clonidine).

Direct vasodilators: postural hypotension, reflex tachycardia, sodium and fluid retention, lupus erythematosus-like syndrome (hydralazine), pleural and pericardial effusion and pulmonary hypertension (minoxidil), hypertrichosis (minoxidil).

ACE inhibitors: postural hypotension, renal dysfunction, hyperkalemia, taste disturbances, bone marrow suppression, cough and angioedema.

Angiotensin II-receptor antagonists: hypotension, hyperkalemia in patients who have renal disease or take potassium supplements or potassium-sparing agents.

9. Discuss the metabolism of sodium nitroprusside.

After parenteral injection sodium nitroprusside enters red blood cells, where it may receive an electron transfer from the iron of oxyhemoglobin, resulting in an unstable nitroprusside radical and methemoglobin. The nitroprusside radical spontaneously breaks down into five cyanide moieties.

The cyanide ions can be involved in one of three possible reactions: binding with methemoglobin to form cyanmethemoglobin; converting to thiocyanate in the liver or kidneys; or combining to inactivate cytochrome oxidase as a terminal toxic event. This last reaction is responsible for acute cyanide toxicity suggested by restlessness, mental confusion, and hyperreflexia, characterized by acute resistance to the hypotensive effects of increasing doses of sodium nitroprusside (tachyphylaxis), metabolic acidosis, cyanosis, increased venous oxygen content (due to the inability to metabolize oxygen), and cardiac dysrhythmias. The best confirmatory test for nitroprusside toxicity is a blood cyanide level. Doses that avoid toxicity are not firmly precisely established; however, recommended doses should not exceed 0.5 mg/kg/hr.

10. How is cyanide toxicity treated?

Cyanide toxicity is the result of cytochrome oxidase poisoning and the inhibition of oxidative phosphorylation, leading to cytotoxic hypoxia. This condition is treated by discontinuation of the sodium nitroprusside infusion and administration of 100% oxygen. The pharmacologic treatment is targeted at reversal of the cyanide binding to the cytochrome system by administration of sodium thiosulfate (150 mg/kg over 15 min). Sodium thiosulfate reacts with cyanide to form thiocyanate, which is then excreted by the kidneys. Thiocyanate toxicity, although rare, can occur in patients with renal dysfunction and results in symptoms of fatigue, anorexia, nausea, seizures, tremor, disorientation, and psychotic behavior.

Severe cyanide toxicity may also necessitate the use of amyl nitrite or 3% sodium nitrate (5 mg/kg IV over 5 min). These two compounds may cause the accumulation of methemoglobin, which competes with cytochrome oxidase for the cyanide ion to form inactive cyanmethemoglobin. Hydroxycobalamin (which complexes circulating cyanide to form vitamin B12) is proposed by some as the treatment of choice for nitroprusside toxicity.

11. List contraindications to sodium nitroprusside therapy and conditions requiring special precautions.

Contraindications include hepatic failure (due to inability to detoxify cyanide), leber's optic atrophy and tobacco amblyopia (both disorders of cyanide metabolism), hypothyroidism (condition may be exacerbated), and vitamin B12 deficiency (due to reduced cyanide metabolism).

Conditions requiring special precautions include renal failure (due to inability to metabolize thiocyanate), aortic stenosis (limited ability to increase cardiac output), hypertrophic cardiomyopathy (drug may exacerbate left ventricular outflow tract gradient), conditions associated with decreased intracranial compliance (drug may increase intracranial pressure), and eclampsia (fetal effects not clearly defined). Nitroprusside may worsen arterial hypoxemia in patients with obstructive lung disease by interfering with pulmonary vasoconstriction and promoting ventilation-to-perfusion mismatching.

BIBLIOGRAPHY

1. Furberg CD, Yusuf S: Effect of vasodilators on survival in chronic congestive heart failure. Am J Cardiol 62:41–45, 1988.
2. Gascho JA, Zelis R: Arteriolar and venous vasodilators in congestive heart failure. In Singh BN, Dzau VJ, Vanhoutee PM, Woosley RL (eds): Cardiovascular Pharmacology and Therapeutics. New York, Churchill Livingstone, 1994, pp 815–826.
3. Hardman JG, Limbirg LE: The Pharmacologic Basis of Therapeutics, 10th ed. New York, McGraw-Hill, 2001.
4. Harrison DG, Bates JN: The nitrovasodilators: New ideas about old drugs. Circulation 87:1461–1467, 1993.
5. Murphy J, Lavie CJ, Bresnahan DR: Nitroprusside. In Messerli FH (ed): Cardiovascular Drug Therapy. Philadelphia, W.B. Saunders, 1996, pp 858–864.
6. Mueller RL, Scheidt S: Nitroglycerin. In Messerli FH (ed): Cardiovascular Drug Therapy. Philadelphia, W.B. Saunders, 1996, pp 865–875.
7. Parmley WW: Vasodilator drugs in the treatment of heart failure. In Parmley WW, Chatterjee K (eds): Cardiology: Physiology, Pharmacology, Diagnosis. Philadelphia, Lippincott-Raven, 1996, pp 1–18.

75. PHARMACOTHERAPY FOR TACHYCARDIA IN THE CRITICALLY ILL PATIENT

Wanda C. Miller-Hance, M.D.

1. How are antiarrhythmic agents classified? Describe the electrophysiologic effects of these drugs.

Antiarrhythmic drugs exert blocking actions predominantly on sodium, potassium, and calcium channels, and beta adrenoreceptors. These pharmacologic agents are generally classified according to their presumed mechanism of action. Various approaches have been proposed in the classification of antiarrhythmic drug therapy, each of these schemes with defined strengths and weaknesses. The drug classification system described by Vaughan Williams (see table below) and modified over the years is one frequently used and may be helpful in predicting the response of a particular dysrhythmia to a specific agent.

Classification of Antiarrhythmic Drugs

CLASS OF ACTION	DRUGS
Class I: Local anesthetic properties by competitive inhibition of the fast sodium channel. Drugs may be subclassified into IA, IB, and IC categories.	
IA Agents: Moderately depress phase zero upstroke of the action potential, slow conduction and prolong repolarization. Effectively slow conduction in atria, ventricles, and accessory connections.	Quinidine Procainamide Disopyramide

Table continued on following page

Classification of Antiarrhythmic Drugs (Continued)

CLASS OF ACTION	DRUGS
Class I *(continued)*	
IB Agents: Shorten action potential duration and result in minimal alteration of conduction. These agents are usually not effective in the treatment of supraventricular tachycardia.	Lidocaine Mexiletine Tocainide Phenytoin
IC Agents: Significantly depress phase zero upstroke, with marked slowing of conduction but impart little change in refractoriness.	Flecainide Encainide Propafenone
Class II: Beta-adrenergic receptor blockers. Antiarrhythmic effects result from slowing conduction and decreasing automaticity, particularly in the sinoatrial (SA) and atrioventricular (AV) nodes.	Propranolol Esmolol Metoprolol
Class III: Primarily prolong the action potential with resultant prolongation of refractoriness.	Amiodarone Bretylium Sotalol Ibutilide
Class IV: Calcium channel antagonists with predominant sites of action in the SA and AV nodes.	Verapamil Diltiazem

2. Describe the most common adverse effects of antiarrhythmic drug therapy.

All antiarrhythmic drugs have associated side effects and the potential for causing significant toxicity (see table below). Adverse effects may relate to excessive dosages and plasma concentrations, resulting in both cardiovascular and noncardiovascular toxicity, or may be unrelated to plasma concentrations (idiopathic). Cardiovascular side effects are primarily hemodynamic or electrophysiologic. The majority of the antiarrhythmic agents are associated with negative inotropic properties, manifested most frequently in patients with moderate to severely impaired left ventricular function. These agents may also lead to drug-induced or drug-aggravated cardiac dysrhythmias (proarrhythmic effect). Numerous noncardiovascular side effects of these drugs have also been documented.

Major Adverse Effects of Antiarrhythmic Drugs

	DRUG	ADVERSE EFFECTS
Class IA	Quinidine	GI (nausea, vomiting, anorexia, diarrhea), thrombocytopenia, fever, proarrhythmia, drug interactions (e.g., digoxin)
	Procainamide	Lupus-like syndrome, negative inotropic effects, hypotension, AV block, agranulocytosis
	Disopyramide	Anticholinergic side effects (dry mouth, urinary retention), left ventricular (LV) failure
Class IB	Lidocaine	CNS (paresthesias, tremor, confusion, seizures), GI (nausea, vomiting), drug interactions (propranolol, tocainide)
	Mexiletine	CNS (tremor, dizziness, diplopia) and GI (nausea)
	Tocainide	Interstitial pneumonitis, agranulocytosis
	Phenytoin	Hypotension, CNS (nystagmus, ataxia, stupor), blood dyscrasias, hepatitis
Class IC	Flecainide	CNS, GI, proarrhythmia, LV failure
	Encainide	CNS (dizziness, diplopia, paresthesia), proarrhythmia
	Propafenone	GI (nausea), CNS (dizziness), proarrhythmia
Class II	Propranolol	Hypotension, bradycardia, AV block, bronchospasm, hypoglycemia, LV failure
	Esmolol	Hypotension, negative inotropic effects
	Metoprolol	Bradycardia, hypotension, LV failure

Table continued on following page

Major Adverse Effects of Antiarrhythmic Drugs (Continued)

	DRUG	ADVERSE EFFECTS
Class III	Amiodarone	GI (nausea, vomiting), pulmonary fibrosis, hypothyroidism, skin discoloration, corneal microdeposits
	Bretylium	GI, hypotension
	Sotalol	Hypotension, bradycardia, proarrhythmia, LV failure, fatigue, dizziness, dyspnea
	Ibutilide	Hypotension, congestive heart failure, proarrhythmia
Class IV	Verapamil	Bradycardia, sinus arrest, negative inotropic effects, exacerbation of heart failure
	Diltiazem	Hypotension, worsening of LV failure, bradyarrhythmias

GI, gastrointestinal; CNS, central nervous system.

3. What are the important initial steps in the evaluation of patients with tachycardia?

The following issues should be considered in the initial evaluation of a patient with tachycardia: clinical condition (stable vs. unstable), presence of serious signs or symptoms, and whether signs and symptoms are related to the rhythm disturbance. In unstable patients with signs and symptoms related to tachycardia, immediate cardioversion should be considered.

4. How are supraventricular tachydysrhythmias (SVTs) classified?

SVTs originate from cardiac tissue above the level of the ventricular myocardium. A clinically useful SVT classification outline proposes three general categories: sinus tachycardia, AV node-independent tachycardias, and AV node-dependent tachycardias. Sinus tachycardia is defined by a rate greater than 100 beats/min and generally has a gradual onset and termination. This tachycardia may represent a physiologic response (e.g., secondary to anemia, fever, or hypovolemia) or may be nonphysiologic (secondary to acute myocardial ischemia or severe congestive heart failure). Sinus tachycardia rarely requires pharmacologic treatment and main efforts should address correction of any underlying abnormality. AV node-independent tachycardias are atrial rhythm disturbances not influenced by AV node conduction block (e.g., atrial flutter, atrial fibrillation, atrial tachycardia, and premature atrial contractions), whereas AV node-dependent tachyarrhythmias (AV node reentry, AV reentry, nonparoxysmal junctional tachycardia) rely on AV node conduction or AV junction automaticity for maintenance of the tachycardia.

5. What information is useful in the evaluation of patients with SVTs?

Valuable tools in the evaluation of SVT mechanisms which allow for successful management of dysrhythmia include the medical history, careful cardiac examination, high-quality 12-lead electrocardiogram (including a rhythm strip) obtained during the acute rhythm disturbance, and in some cases echocardiography. Particular clues to consider in the differential diagnosis of SVT include the pattern of dysrhythmia onset and termination, the QRS morphology and duration, the pattern of ventricular response to the tachycardia, the p-wave morphology during SVT, and the response to vagal maneuvers or specific drugs.

6. Discuss the pharmacology of adenosine and its role in the therapy of SVTs.

Adenosine, a purine agonist, is the drug of choice for acute treatment of SVT. To terminate the tachycardia a bolus of adenosine is rapidly injected intravenously, preferably into a central vein, at doses of 6–12 mg. Transient sinus slowing or AV nodal block results because of the drug's extremely short half-life (less than 10 seconds). This effect is mediated via the activation of the A_1 adenosine receptor.

Adenosine is of benefit in the diagnosis of atrial tachycardias and may also be useful in the differentiation of wide QRS tachycardias. Side effects are transient, generally well tolerated, and most frequently include dyspnea and flushing. Cardiac side effects include sinus pauses, sinus bradycardia, sinus tachycardia, and AV block.

7. Discuss the pharmacologic therapy of atrial fibrillation.

Atrial fibrillation is a common dysrhythmia characterized by irregular, disorganized atrial depolarizations which result in ineffective atrial systole and an irregular ventricular response. In addition to hemodynamic compromise which may be life-threatening, detrimental effects of this rhythm disturbance may include an increased risk of atrial thrombotic phenomenon and potential for systemic arterial embolization. Goals in the treatment of this dysrhythmia include evaluation for a precipitating etiology (e.g., mitral stenosis, thyrotoxicosis), control of the ventricular rate and, in cases of atrial fibrillation of recent onset, restoration and maintenance of sinus rhythm.

To decrease the ventricular response, drugs such as beta blockers (esmolol, propranolol), and calcium channel blockers (verapamil, diltiazem) are commonly used. Traditionally, digoxin has been of therapeutic value in further decreasing AV node conduction, although it may be a less desirable drug in the acute setting. Pharmacologic agents that may be of benefit in the medical conversion of atrial fibrillation to sinus rhythm include beta-blocking drugs, class IA (quinidine, procainamide, disopyramide), class IC antiarrhythmic agents (flecainide, propafenone), and class III drugs (amiodarone, sotalol). Ibutilide is effective for the conversion of recent-onset fibrillation or flutter to sinus rhythm. It was the first "pure" class III antiarrhythmic drug to become available. The major toxicity of ibutilide is the development of ventricular dysrhythmias (2–5% of patients).

8. What important factors should be considered in the management of patients with atrial fibrillation?

The choice of therapy in patients with atrial fibrillation is influenced by the clinical state of the patient, ventricular function (normal or impaired), and whether Wolff-Parkinson-White (pre-excitation) syndrome is present. The duration of atrial fibrillation (less or more than 48 hours) is an important factor in the selection of strategies to convert atrial fibrillation to sinus rhythm. Cardioversion (electrical or chemical) in patients with atrial fibrillation of unknown duration or beyond 48 hours of onset may be associated with embolization of atrial thrombi in patients with inadequate anticoagulation.

9. Describe the major electrophysiologic effects of cardiac glycosides and explain their role in the management of symptomatic supraventricular dysrhythmias.

Digitalis glycosides have been used for many years as first-line pharmacologic agents in the management of certain dysrhythmias. The electrophysiologic properties of these drugs are the result of direct effects on cardiac tissues (through inhibition of the sarcolemmic sodium pump) and indirect effects via the autonomic nervous system. Digitalis is known to increase the refractory period and decrease the conduction velocity of the specialized cardiac conduction system, slow the sinus rate (primarily by enhancing vagal discharge), and shorten the refractory period in atrial and ventricular muscle.

In view of the fact that the onset of the digitalis effect may be delayed (up to 5 hrs), this drug may be less than ideal in the treatment of acute symptomatic tachycardias. Despite this fact, digitalis glycosides remain useful in controlling the ventricular response in atrial tachyarrhythmias, particularly during atrial flutter or fibrillation.

10. Describe the adverse effects of digitalis therapy.

Toxic manifestations of digitalis therapy may be classified as cardiac and noncardiac. Cardiac toxicity includes sinus bradycardia, AV block, junctional escape rhythms, ectopic beats, and atrial or ventricular dysrhythmias. Noncardiac manifestations of digitalis toxicity include gastrointestinal (nausea, vomiting, anorexia) and neurologic symptoms (headache, lethargy, weakness, confusion, seizure), and visual disturbances. Although nonspecific, noncardiac symptoms are the earliest manifestations of digitalis toxicity.

11. How are ventricular tachyarrhythmias clinically classified?

Ventricular tachycardia is a dysrhythmia characterized by a series of at least three repetitive excitations that arise distal to the bifurcation of the bundle of His, in the specialized cardiac conduction system, or in the ventricular myocardium. These tachyarrhythmias may be classified for practical purposes as monomorphic (same QRS morphology) or polymorphic (variable QRS morphology), nonsustained or sustained. Ventricular dysrhythmias are most commonly encountered in the clinical settings of coronary artery disease and cardiomyopathy. They are also seen in association with hypoxia, metabolic disturbances (hypokalemia, hypomagnesemia), and digitalis toxicity.

12. Describe the treatment of ventricular tachycardia.
Aggressive treatment of acute ventricular tachycardia is indicated in view of frequently associated hemodynamic instability and potential deterioration of the rhythm into ventricular fibrillation. In many cases, cardioversion is the treatment of choice. In other acute situations, antiarrhythmic drug interventions may also play an important role. Agents that may be useful include lidocaine, procainamide, amiodarone, or sotalol. The intravenous administration of beta-blockers and magnesium may also be of benefit. It is important to treat underlying ischemia or electrolyte abnormalities.

13. Describe the treatment of torsade de pointes.
Torsade de pointes is a specific form of ventricular dysrhythmia characterized by QRS complexes of changing amplitude that appear to twist on its axis. The ventricular rates are often variable and typically very rapid. This polymorphic tachycardia is frequently seen in the setting of a prolonged QT interval and may lead to ventricular fibrillation. Treatment consists of discontinuation of any potentially offending agents and correction of electrolyte abnormalities. Other acute management options include either atrial or ventricular pacing, isoproterenol infusion, or beta blockade. Intravenous magnesium therapy has been used successfully even in the absence of documented serum magnesium abnormalities. Overdrive pacing also may be of benefit.

14. Describe the pharmacology of drugs used in the acute therapy of ventricular dysrhythmias.
Lidocaine is one of the antiarrhythmic drugs most frequently used in the intensive care environment. This drug is a short acting, intravenous type IB antiarrhythmic agent used primarily in patients with acute myocardial infarction or recurrent ventricular tachyarrhythmias. This is the drug of choice for suppression of frequent ventricular ectopy, warning dysrhythmias, and for prevention of recurrence of ventricular tachycardia/fibrillation. Lidocaine is rapidly metabolized in the liver and therefore drugs (e.g., cimetidine) or conditions (e.g., severe congestive heart failure) associated with reductions in hepatic blood flow may result in decreased metabolism of lidocaine. The recommended dosage includes an initial bolus of 1–2 mg/kg intravenously and if ineffective, additional boluses of 1 mg/kg may be repeated. The maintenance infusion rate ranges from 1–4 mg/min.

Procainamide is a type IA antiarrhythmic agent useful in the management of both atrial and ventricular dysrhythmias. This drug is more effective than lidocaine in acutely terminating sustained ventricular tachycardia. Procainamide may be administered via the oral, intravenous, or intramuscular routes. The drug is eliminated by the kidneys (50–60%) and via hepatic metabolism (10–30%). For the treatment of acute rhythm disturbances, intravenous loading (doses of 10–15 mg/kg) is usually required, and a continuous infusion may be initiated (at 1–4 mg/min).

Amiodarone has a wide spectrum of actions with multiple and complex electrophysiologic effects that encompass all four antiarrhythmic drug classes. It binds extensively to most tissues, accounting for its extremely prolonged elimination. Several drug administration schemes are available. For wide-complex tachycardia, recommended therapy consists of a rapid infusion (150 mg IV over 10 min), followed by a slow infusion (360 mg IV over 6 hours). For maintenance therapy, an infusion of 540 mg over 18 hours is suggested.

Sotalol nonselectively blocks beta-adrenergic receptors in a competitive fashion. It also prolongs action potential duration and increases the refractory period of most cardiac tissues. Sotalol is available in oral form in the U.S. and is given intravenously in countries where approved as a 1–1.5 mg/kg load followed by infusion at a rate of 10 mg/min.

15. List factors leading to hemodynamic deterioration during a tachycardia.

Supraventricular and ventricular tachyarrhythmias may produce symptoms and hemo-dynamic disturbances ranging from mild to severe in nature. Major factors that contribute to hemodynamic decompensation during tachycardia include: increases in myocardial oxygen consumption, shortening of the diastolic period, loss of synchronous left ventricular activation, and atrioventricular asynchrony.

16. Discuss the role of nonpharmacologic therapy of cardiac tachyarrhythmias.

Interventions such as vagal maneuvers, rapid atrial pacing, and cardioversion may play a diagnostic and/or therapeutic role in the treatment of supraventricular tachycardias. Direct current electrical cardioversion/defibrillation should be considered for any rhythm that produces rapidly deteriorating hemodynamic stability such as hypotension, congestive heart failure, or angina, and does not respond promptly to medical management.

BIBLIOGRAPHY

1. Atlee JL: Perioperative cardiac dysrhythmias: Diagnosis and management. Anesthesiology 86:1397–1424, 1997.
2. Grant AO: On the mechanism of action of antiarrhythmic agents. Am Heart J 123:1130–1136, 1992.
3. Hastillo A, Hess ML: Diagnosis and treatment of cardiac arrhythmias. In Shoemaker WC, Ayres SM, Greuviik A, Holbrook P (eds): Textbook of Critical Care. Philadelphia, W.B. Saunders, 1995, pp 502–513.
4. Lazzaro R: From first class to third class: Recent upheaval in antiarrhythmic therapy: Lessions from clinical trials. Am J Cardiol 78(Suppl 4A):28–33, 1996.
5. Mason JW: A comparison of seven antiarrhythmic drugs in patients with ventricular tachyarrhythmias. N Engl J Med 329:452–458, 1993.
6. Murray KT: Ibutilide. Circulation 97:493–497, 1998.
7. Prystowsky EN: Supraventricular arrhythmias. In Messerli FH (ed): Cardiovascular Drug Therapy. Philadelphia, W.B. Saunders, 1996, pp 1207–1228.
8. Prystowsky EN, Klein GJ: Pharmacologic therapy. In Prystowsky EN, Klein GJ (eds): Cardiac Arrhythmias: An Integrated Approach for the Clinician. New York, McGraw-Hill, 1994, pp 359–390.
9. Santoro IH, Soble JS, Bump TE: Rhythm disturbances. In Hall JB, Schmidt GA, Wood LDH (eds): Principles of Critical Care. New York, McGraw-Hill, 1992, pp 1503–1524.
10. Surawicz B: Arrythmias. In Messerli FH (ed): Cardiovascular Drug Therapy. Philadelphia, W.B. Saunders, 1996, pp 13–16.
11. Vaughan Williams EM: A classification of antiarrhythmic actions reassessed after a decade of new drugs. J Clin Pharmacol 24:129–147, 1984.

XIII. Surgery and Trauma

76. BURNS

James Jeng, M.D., and Mark W. Bowyer, M.D.

1. Describe the epidemiology of burns in the United States.

The most recent data demonstrate an annual incidence of 1.25 million burns (1992) with 51,000 acute hospital admissions (1991 to 1993 average) and 5500 deaths from fire and burns (1991). Most burns are cared for on an outpatient basis, and more than 80% of all burns affect less than 20% of the body. Scalds are the most common cause of burn admissions. Although they account for a small fraction of burn admissions (4%), house fires cause at least 70% of all burn-related deaths, 75% of which are directly attributable to inhalation injury. The age distribution of burns is bimodal with a peak incidence of burns in patients less than 5 years of age. A second smaller peak occurs in the 30- to 35-year-old range. Besides age, factors influencing the likelihood of thermal injury include sex, occupation, and economic status.

2. What amount of thermal energy is required to cause injury?

The severity of a thermal injury is related to temperature and duration of contact. A heat source less than 45°C (113°F) will result in no injury, regardless of duration of exposure. As the heat intensity increases, the duration of exposure necessary to cause a significant burn decreases. Exposure to water at 54° C (129.2° F) for 30 seconds causes a partial-thickness burn.

3. What are the priorities in the initial management of burns?

The initial priority in the field is to stop the burning process by extinguishing the flames, washing away any offending chemicals, or removing the patient from contact with the electric current. Next, the ABCs (airway, breathing, circulation) of standard cardiopulmonary resuscitation are followed. Carbon monoxide poisoning should be assumed for any patient burned in a closed space, and 100% oxygen by a nonrebreathing mask should be administered. Some evidence suggests that cold water soaks or icepacks applied to burns within 15 minutes of the injury can reduce the amount of tissue destruction. Larger burns should not be treated in this fashion because of the risk of potentially life-threatening hypothermia. All patients should be covered with a blanket to conserve body heat. Prompt transport to a hospital is the next step. If transport can be accomplished in 45 minutes or less and the patient's only injury is burns, intravenous fluids need not be started in the field. Emergency department care is an extension of prehospital care. Tesuscitation is begun with crystalloid, and urine output followed closely after placement of a urethral catheter. Other life-threatening injuries are attended to. Finally, the extent and depth of burns are estimated and resuscitation fluid needs are calculated.

4. How is the depth of a burn categorized?

Traditionally, the depth of burns has been classified as first-, second-, or third-degree. The depth of a burn determines the type of medical care required, the healing time or need for grafting, and the ultimate cosmetic result. **First-degree burns** are the most superficial type and involve only the epidermis. The skin is pink or red and dry with no or only small blisters. This is exemplified by a sunburn. Healing occurs in less than 1 week. **Second-degree burns** or partial-thickness burns are subcategorized into superficial and deep. Superficial dermal injuries are produced by brief exposures to hot liquids or flames. The skin is bright red and moist with blisters and is extremely hypersensitive. Healing occurs in 10–21 days. Deep dermal injuries, caused by more prolonged exposure to the above, are characterized by dark red or yellow-white skin with large bullae. Healing is very slow, taking longer than 3 weeks, and often results in marked hypertrophic scar formation. **Third-degree or full-thickness burns** are caused by prolonged exposure to hot objects or flames or by high-voltage electricity or concentrated chemicals. The entire dermis is destroyed, and the burn has a pearly white, charred, or parchmentlike appearance. The burn is dry and leathery with thrombosed vessels visible through the eschar. It is hypalgesic because the cutaneous nerves are destroyed. Reepithelialization will never occur, and grafting is required.

5. How is the extent of burn injury estimated?

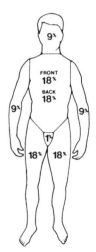

In determining the extent of burns, first- degree burns are ignored. For adults, the portion of the body involved with second- and third-degree burns can be estimated using the rule of nines. This rule divides the body into segments, each of which represents roughly 9% of the total body surface area: 9% for the head and neck and each upper extremity, 18% for each lower extremity, the anterior trunk, and the posterior trunk, and 1% for the genitalia and perineum. In pediatric patients, however, the distribution of total body surface area is different, as the head and neck comprise a greater percentage and the lower extremities a lesser. Therefore, for an accurate estimate, a burn chart is needed. Furthermore, small burns, and irregularly disposed burns can be estimated using the surface of a patient's hand as representative of 1% of the total body surface.

6. What are the indications for referral to a burn center?

Various criteria have been itemized as indications for transfer to a burn center and vary from source to source. Furthermore, the need to transfer a patient to a burn unit is mostly influenced by local capabilities. The following are some general guidelines:
- Full-thickness burns > 5% total body surface area (TBSA)
- Burns > 20% TBSA in patients 10–50 years of age
- Burns > 10% TBSA in patients less than 10 or greater than 50 years of age
- Significant burns involving the face, hands, feet, genitalia, or major joints
- Significant electrical, chemical, or inhalation injury
- Preexisting illness or concomitant trauma which could complicate management and increase mortality.

7. How are burn patients resuscitated?

Several formulas have been proposed for estimating the burn patient's fluid requirements. The two most common formulas are the Parkland formula and the modified Brooke formula. Both estimate the patient's fluid requirements for the first 24 hours after a burn. One-half of the estimate is given over the first 8 hours, and the second half is administered over the next 16 hours. The Parkland formula estimates the fluid needs as 4 ml/kg body weight/% TBSA burns (given as lactated Ringer's solution), whereas the modified Brooke formula estimates the fluid requirement as 2 ml/kg/% (also given as lactated Ringer's solution). In an environment in which hourly urine outputs can be monitored, these formulas serve only to determine an initial fluid rate, which is then continuously adjusted to achieve an hourly urine output between 30 and 50 ml in 70-kg adult. It is important to emphasize that the fluids to be given in the first 8 hours are for the **first 8 hours after burn injury**, not for the first 8 hours after admission. Furthermore, in patients in whom there is a significant delay (more than 2 hours) in the initiation of resuscitation, more resuscitation fluid is frequently needed. Both formulas withhold colloid-containing fluids until the second 24 hours after burn injury. In the first 24 hours there is a significant capillary leak so that colloids can cross into the interstitium, making subsequent fluid management more difficult.

8. What factors determine a burn patient's prognosis?

The three major factors influencing a burn patient's survival are the extent of the burn, age, and the presence or absence of inhalation injury. Larger burns, extremes of age, and patients with inhalation injury fare worse. The standard statistic for assessing the patient's mortality is the LA_{50}, the extent of the burn associated with death in 50% of patients having burns of that extent. With the advent of fluid resuscitation, topical antimicrobial therapy, early excision and grafting, and nutritional support, the LA_{50} has improved significantly. For young adults (15–40 years of age), the LA_{50} is approximately 70%. Infectious complications remain the principal cause of death; pneumonia has surpassed invasive burn wound infections as the most common infectious complication.

9. What are the principles of burn wound care?

Care of the burn wound is divided into three stages: (1) the presurgical stage, during which the primary goal is to decrease the incidence of burn wound infection with topical antibacterial agents; (2) the surgical phase, during which the wounds are excised of all necrotic material and covered either with autologous skin grafts or with a temporary biologic dressing or biosynthetic skin substitute; and (3) the period after the wound is covered when the primay goals are to minimize graft loss, prevent wound contracture, and maximize physical and occupational function/rehabilitation.

10. What antimicrobial agents are used in burn wound care?

After an airway is ensured, resuscitation begun, and associated injuries addressed, attention can be given to the burn wound itself. The burn is gently bathed, and all loose necrotic tissue, including intact bullae, are debrided. After thorough debridement, an accurate mapping of the burn on an injury diagram can be accomplished. The primary initial goal of burn wound care then becomes control of infection until spontaneous healing or surgical closure occurs. The injured and nonviable tissue predisposes the burn wound to colonization and subsequent invasion of organisms into viable tissue. The avascular nature of the wound prevents delivery of blood-borne host defenses as well as systemically administered antibiotics. Therefore, topical antimicrobials are used.

In the United States, two topical agents are most commonly used: mafenide acetate (Sulfamylon) and silver sulfadiazine (Silvadene). Sulfamylon cream has the advantages of excellent gram-negative coverage and good eschar penetration. Its disadvantages are pain when it is applied to partial-thickness burns and metabolic acidosis secondary to inhibition of carbonic anhydrase. Silvadene cream has enhanced yeast coverage and is painless on application; however, it has decreased eschar penetration and decreased gram-negative coverage. Furthermore, it may cause myeloid toxicity manifest by granulocytopenia. Several other topical agents are used on a less frequent basis (e.g., silver nitrate solution) or are just beginning to become more widely accepted (e.g., Acticoat, a silver-impregnated fabric).

11. How are burn wound infections diagnosed?

Fever, tachycardia, glucose intolerance, and leukocytosis are of little assistance in diagnosing infection in the burn patient because these changes are common components of the normal response to burn injury in the absence of infection. However, trends in their patterns can be helpful in arriving at the clinical conclusion of burn wound infection.

Therefore, given the unreliability of systemic indicators of infection, a daily inspection of the entire burn is compulsory to detect early evidence of invasive infection. Wound changes associated with invasive infection include a focal brown or black discoloration of the eschar, sudden conversion of a partial-thickness injury to full-thickness wound, and rapid separation of the eschar. All of these signs, however, are nonspecific. Surface culture techniques are also unreliable. The definitive technique for assessing burn wound infection is histologic examination of a burn wound biopsy (500 mg). Identification of microorganisms in viable tissue confirms the diagnosis of an invasive burn wound infection (to be distinguished from simple colonization of the eschar).

12. How are burn wound infections treated?

Once invasive burn wound infection is confirmed histologically, rapid and aggressive therapy is mandated, as the mortality of burn wound invasion, particularly with systemic dissemination, is extremely high. If another topical agent is being used, it is stopped and Sulfamylon is applied twice daily. Empirical systemic therapy is inititaed, guided by the burn unit's microbial surveillance program. Above all else, as soon as the patient can tolerate general anesthesia, all infected tissue is excised.

13. What factors raise the suspicion of an inhalation injury?

Inhalation injury is common in patients with an impaired mental status (alcohol or drugs), in trauma patients, and in patients who have been burned in a closed space. However, in reports on patients who have inhalation injuries, up to 30% of the patients sustained their burns in an open area. Thus, the occurrence of a burn in an open area does not preclude airway injury. The most sensitive physical finding indicative of inhalation injury is facial burns. Ninety percent of patients who have inhalation injury have facial burns. This finding, however, is not highly specific, as only 50% of patients with facial burns have inhalation injury. Other physical findings suggestive of inhalation injury are inflammation of the oropharyngeal mucosa, singed nasal hair, hoarseness, stridor, wheezing, and rales. Carbonaceous sputum, while pathognomonic for inhalation injury, is present less than half of the time. Definitive diagnosis is made by bronchoscopic confirmation of soot or erythema in the trachea.

14. How are inhalation injuries diagnosed and managed?

Inhalation injury can be divided into upper and lower airway injuries, although the two can occur concurrently. A normal chest roentgenogram and arterial blood gas on admission are typical for patients with inhalation injury and are thus of little use in diagnosing airway injury. The flexible fiberoptic bronchoscope is used for diagnosing and managing airway injury. The patient can be examined with an endotracheal tube threaded over the bronchoscope. Significant supraglottic edema mandates intubation. Lesser degrees of airway edema are managed with humidified air and possibly racemic epinephrine. The lower airways should also be examined for evidence of erythema, edema, mucosal sloughing, or carbonaceous material. Xenon[133] ventilation scans, when performed in the first 24 hours, can also help diagnose lower airway injury. Management of lower airway injury is entirely supportive and involves treating pulmonary edema and pneumonia, the two major consequences of lower airway injury. Prophylactic antibiotics and steroids have not been shown to be beneficial.

15. How is carbon monoxide poisoning diagnosed and managed?

Carbon monoxide avidly binds to hemoglobin with an affinity 200 times greater than that of oxygen. This reduces the oxygen-delivering capacity of blood and causes tissue hypoxia. The clinical manifestations of carbon monoxide poisoning relate to the central nervous system and to the heart. Confusion, agitation, loss of consciousness, and myocardial depression can be seen. The classic cherry-red lips are seen infrequently. Diagnosis is confirmed by directly measuring carboxyhemoglobin levels. Optimal therapy for carbon monoxide poisoning is 100% oxygen by face mask or endotracheal tube. This thereapy should be begun in the field for all patients burned in a closed space, involved in a combustion incident, or with an altered sensorium. Hyperbaric oxygen clearly accelerates carbon monoxide elimination. However, its superiority to normobaric 100% oxygen in increasing survival or decreasing long-term neurologic sequelae remains unproven. Furthermore, it carries the risks of inducing seizures, causing pulmonary injury, and impairing immunity. Pulse oximetry is misleading in carbon monoxide poisoning and demonstrates falsely elevated saturation levels.

16. When should escharotomy be done?

As edema forms below the inelastic eschar of a circumferential full-thickness burn, tissue pressure increases to the point that venous pressure is exceeded and tissue perfusion is impaired. Cyanosis, delayed capillary refilling, and neurologic changes all suggest poor perfusion. Using Doppler ultrasound, demonstration of absent or progressively diminishing pulsatile flow in the palmar arch or in the posterior tibial artery is an indication for escharotomy. Escharotomies can be performed at the bedside without anesthesia because the incisions are made through insensate full-thickness burns. The incision is carried from the proximal to the distal margin of the encircling burn on the midlateral and/or midmedial aspect of the limb. The incision should cross the joints and be deep enough to allow the cut edges of the eschar to separate. Circumferential torso burns may impair ventilation by restricting chest wall motion, in which case bilateral anterior axillary line escharotomies are performed. Electrocautery is an expedient technique for performing escharotomies but should not be used on hands and feet. Be prepared to control several sites of cutaneous bleeding with any technique.

17. What biologic dressings and skin substitutes are available?

When burns are so extensive that available donor sites are limited, biologic dressings must be used. The gold standard for biologic dressings remains living, cutaneous allografts (homografts, cadaver skin), which become vascularized by the host and act for all intents and purposes like the patient's native skin. Availability, processing and storage requirements and the theoretical risk for disease transmission, however, must be factored into the decision to use cutaneous allografts. Alternatives are cutaneous xenografts (porcine) or amniotic membranes (very rare in the U.S.). Neither is vascularized by the host or protects as well against microbes. The limitations of biologic dressings have led to the development of skin substitutes. Two commonly used skin substitutes for third-degree burns (TransCyte and Integra) employ collagen-based dermal analogs with a silicone epidermal analog. The silicone layers are ultimately removed, and the wound is grafted with epithelial tissue. TransCyte is also useful for temporary coverage of partial-thickness burns and may enhance their healing. Keratinocytes can be harvested from a small skin biopsy and used to create cultured epidermal autografts (CEAs). The take of CEAs has not been outstanding (because of the lack of a dermis) and in some studies has been inversely proportional to the extent of the burn. Thus, the amount of burn definitively closed by CEAs is small. The shortcomings of CEAs have served as a stimulus for the development of culture-derived composite tissue with a dermal analog and an adherent cultured epidermis. Appligraft, the first commercial example of such a composite culture-derived skin substitute, is beginning to gain some acceptance in closing full-thickness wounds of limited size. This continues to be an area of major research in burn care.

18. How are chemical burns managed?

Chemical injury is caused by the thermal energy produced when strong acids and strong alkalis react with tissue. Chemical burns are managed by irrigating away the offending agent. Powders should be brushed away before skin lavage. Acids can usually be removed by 30–60 minutes of water irrigation. Alkalis, because of their greater tissue avidity, cause more severe damage and may require hours of lavage. Neutralizing agents are avoided because the heat that they generate can cause further damage. White phosphorus burns can be hazardous because the retained phosphorus particles ignite on exposure to air. These burns can be bathed with copper sulfate, which forms a cupric phosphide coating over the particles and impedes ignition. However, the absorbed copper may cause hemolysis and renal failure. Therefore, the safer approach is the continuous application of water-soaked dressings until the particles are removed. They can be identified under ultraviolet light in the operating room.

19. How are electrical burns managed?

Electric current damages tissue by the conversion of electric energy into heat. The effects of electricity depend on voltage, type of current (alternating or direct), pathway, and duration of contact. Alternating current is more dangerous because of its tetanic effect as well as its potential to cause cardiac or pulmonary arrest. Cutaneous injury occurs at the entrance and exit sites, as well as at sites of arcing across flexor surfaces. After cessation of current flow, the body acts as a radiator, and deeper tissues that cool more slowly suffer greater injury. Patients with electrical injury frequently have considerably less cutaneous damage than deeper injury, which may lead to an underestimation of their fluid needs. Underresuscitation coupled with rhabdomyolysis leads to renal failure. It is therefore important to maintain a brisk hourly urine output (~ 70–100 ml/hr in a full-sized adult) in electrically injured patients and to consider alkalinizing the urine to prevent myoglobin precipitation in the renal tubules. Deep muscle injury and the resultant edema commonly cause a compartment syndrome, necessitating fasciotomy. At operation, the viability of the deep muscles must be assessed because nonviable perosseous muscle may underlie more superficial viable muscle. Spinal compression fractures may occur due to tetanic muscle contractions and cataracts may develop, particularly in patients with a contact point on the head.

20. What are the systemic consequences of burn injury?

The systemic response to burn injury involves all organ systems; a biphasic pattern of early hypofunction and later hyperfunction characterizes the multisystem response to any injury. As with any major injury, the body increases secretion of catecholamines, cortisol, glucagon, renin-angiotensin, antidiuretic hormone, and aldosterone. The consequence is a tendency toward retention of sodium and water and excretion of potassium by the kidney. Profound hypermetabolism occurs following the burn, with an increase in metabolic rate and oxygen consumption, which remain elevated until the wound is covered. The evaporative water loss from the wound may reach 300 ml/m²/hr, which markedly increases heat loss. In addition, immunologic abnormalities in burn patients may predispose them to infection.

21. What are the nutritional requirements of the burn patient?

Burn patients demonstrate marked hypermetabolism and increased catabolism of lean body mass. Nutritional management is aimed at supplying total caloric and nitrogen needs to spare the body tissue mass as much as possible. Total caloric requirements can be calculated with the formula: 25 kcal × body weight (kg) + 40 kcal × % TBSA burn. Of the total calories, 20–25% should be protein. Vitamins and minerals are supplied at 2–3 times the recommended daily allowance. The preferred route is via the intestinal tract, with parenteral nutrition reserved only for patients unable to tolerate enteral nutrition.

22. What are the major complications associated with burns?

Infection remains the most frequent cause of morbidity and mortality in burn patients. With the advent of topical antimicrobials and early excision and grafting, pneumonia has emerged as the most common cause of life-threatening sepsis. Gastrointestinal complications include Curling's ulcers (stress ulceration of the stomach and duodenum in burn patients) and acalculous cholecystitis.

BIBLIOGRAPHY

1. Arturson G: Forty years in burns research—the postburn inflammatory response. Burns 26:599–604, 2000.
2. Brigham PA, McLoughlin E: Burn incidence and medical care use in the United States: Estimate, trends, and data sources. J Burn Care Rehab 17:95–107, 1996.
3 Cioffi WG: What's new in burns and metabolism. J Am Coll Surg 192:241–254, 2001.
4. Demling RH, Seigne P: Metabolic management of patients with severe burns. World J Surg 24:673–680, 2000.
5. Innes ME, Umraw N, Fish JS, et al: The use of silver-coated dressings on donor site wounds: A prospective, controlled, matched pair study. Burns 27:621–627, 2001.
6. Periti P, Donati L: Survival and therapy of burn patients at the threshold of the twenty-first century: a review. J Chemother 7:475–502, 1995.
7. Pruitt BA, Goodwin CW, Cioffi WG Jr: Thermal injuries. In Davis JH (ed): Surgery: A Problem-Solving Approach, 2nd ed. St. Louis, Mosby, 1995, pp 643–720.
8. Shakespeare P: Burn wound healing and skin substitutes. Burns 27:517–522, 2001.
9. Sheridan RL: Comprehensive treatment of burns. Curr Probl Surg 38:657–756, 2001.
10. Yowler CJ, Fratianne RB: Current status of burn resuscitation. Clin Plast Surg 27:1–10, 2000.

77. THE ACUTE ABDOMEN

Kim F.Rhoads, M.D., and Madhulika G. Varma, M.D.

1. What is an acute abdomen?

The term *acute abdomen* refers to the extreme end of a spectrum of abdominal pain. It is characterized by sudden or gradual onset of moderate-to-severe abdominal pain that persists over several hours. The presentation can vary from localized abdominal pain and tenderness to diffuse pain associated with sepsis, circulatory collapse, and obtundation. It is important to recognize that not all cases of acute abdominal pain require surgery.

2. What types of stimulation cause abdominal pain?

Visceral sensation is mediated by autonomic afferents found in the walls of hollow viscera and in the capsule of solid organs. Direct injury such as cutting, crushing, or burning causes very little pain. Spasm, distention, inflammation, and ischemia are the primary causes of pain in these organs. In contrast, the parietal peritoneum, abdominal wall, and diaphragm receive somatic sensory innervation. Therefore, direct injury to these structures by cutting, crushing, or chemical irritation produces significant abdominal pain.

3. Define referred pain. To what sites do various abdominal organs refer pain?

The term *referred pain* denotes a noxious sensation perceived at a site distant from the primary stimulus. Referred pain occurs because afferent nerves from abdominal viscera enter the spinal cord at levels often remote from the site of injury or irritation. In some cases, the initial pain symptoms may be located at a referred site. This commonly happens in appendicitis, in which the onset of pain is experienced in the periumbilical region (appendiceal afferents enter the spinal cord at T10) before migrating to the right lower quadrant. Other organs have different sites of referred pain: inflammation of the gallbladder may be perceived as scapular or shoulder pain, obstruction of the ureter as testicular pain, and an incarcerated obturator hernia as medial thigh pain.

4. What are the initial maneuvers in the treatment of the acute abdomen?

The initial assessment of the patient, regardless of the primary complaint, should begin with the ABCs (airway, breathing, and circulation). The patient should avoid oral ingestion (NPO), and intravenous fluid resuscitation should be undertaken with the guidance of serum electrolytes. If physical exam or radiographic studies suggest evidence of obstruction, a nasogastric tube should be placed for palliation of emesis and decompression of gastrointestinal air. Surgical consultation should be obtained early in the course of illness, particularly in patients with evidence of intestinal obstruction, perforation, or ischemia. Prompt surgical evaluation should also be obtained when signs of peritoneal or visceral inflammation are present.

5. How do you evaluate any complaint of abdominal pain?

Whether the patient presents with abdominal pain or develops symptoms of abdominal pain after being admitted for another condition, the initial evaluation should always be the same. A thorough history is essential and includes location and time of onset of pain, any change in location or severity of pain, and description of quality of the pain (i.e., sharp, stabbing, dull aching, or burning). Associated symptoms such as vomiting, anorexia, change in bowel habits, urinary complaints, or gynecologic symptoms should be elicited but are nonspecific and therefore nondiagnostic. Blood in vomit or stool or a history of melena is useful. Physical examination should begin with a careful observation of the patient's position in bed and voluntary mobility during the course of the examination. The writhing of a patient with visceral pain (e.g., intestinal or ureteral colic) contrasts sharply with the motionless appearance of the patient with parietal pain (e.g., appendicitis or peritonitis). The shape and contour of the abdomen (scaphoid vs. distended) should also be noted. Auscultation of all quadrants for presence of bowel sounds, and abdominal bruits should be performed before manual palpation. Palpation begins in the least tender area of the abdomen and progresses to the most tender. Peritoneal signs, when present, can be elicited by gentle percussion of the abdomen or by asking the patient to cough. Deep palpation to produce rebound is unnecessary and creates discomfort. The examination of the acute abdomen is incomplete without a digital rectal exam. The digital exam may reveal the presence of tumor or gastrointestinal bleeding and can provide an assessment of pelvic peritoneal irritation or inflammation.

6. Which tests are helpful in diagnosing the cause of abdominal pain?

The most important tools in the investigation of abdominal pain are the history and physical exam. Laboratory investigations conducted on admission are also very helpful. A complete blood count can be informative in cases of infection and gastrointestinal bleeding. Serum electrolytes, blood urea nitrogen (BUN), and creatinine give some indication of chronicity of illness and help guide resuscitation efforts. Arterial blood gases can be useful to evaluate metabolic acidosis. Serum amylase, although used primarily as an indicator of acute pancreatitis, can also be abnormally elevated in patients with strangulated or ischemic bowel and perforated ulcer. Urinalysis should be included in any work-up of abdominal pain and may suggest nephrolithiasis, urinary tract infection, or other renal pathology as the cause. If the history and physical examination leave little doubt about the diagnosis, radiographic examination is often unnecessary and may lead to delay in resuscitation and therapy. However, selective use of abdominal imaging techniques can be valuable. Plain radiographs of the chest should be part of a complete series of plain films of the abdomen. These films help rule out nonsurgical, thoracic causes of abdominal pain and also may detect free air from a perforated viscus below the diaphragm. Plain films of the abdomen can reveal dilation of the small or large intestine, air-fluid levels, calcified rim around an abdominal aortic aneurysm, or free air within the abdominal cavity. Ultrasound accurately identifies gallstones, can evaluate the size of the biliary ducts, and is gaining wide acceptance in the evaluation of acute appendicitis. Ultrasound is also useful in evaluating the size of an abdominal aortic aneurysm (AAA) but does not detect aneurysmal leaks. Computed tomography (CT) scan with intravenous and oral contrast is quite useful in evaluating the patient with a long history of previous abdominal operations and can clearly identify AAA and its attendant complications. Angiography is rarely used except when mesenteric arterial occlusion is suspected and the patient is hemodynamically stable enough to undergo a somewhat lengthy procedure.

7. Is the differential diagnosis of abdominal pain in the ICU different from that in the emergency department (ED)?

The specific illnesses that cause abdominal pain in the ED are also seen in the ICU. However, many of the nonabdominal conditions that cause a patient to become critically ill can cause abdominal pain. Malnutrition, sepsis, acute respiratory distress syndrome, myocardial infarction, pulmonary embolus, and multiple-organ trauma may promote the development of acute abdominal processes. Common sources of abdominal pain in the ICU include peptic ulcer disease with bleeding or perforation, mesenteric ischemia, acalculous cholecystitis, and acute pancreatitis. These conditions can be exacerbated by malnutrition and ICU-related physiologic stress.

8. Does the differential diagnosis of abdominal pain vary by age?

Yes. In infants and children, the most common diagnoses are intussusception, intestinal volvulus, and incarcerated inguinal hernias. In adolescents, the most common causes of acute abdominal pain are trauma, appendicitis, and mesenteric adenitis. In young adults, appendicitis, inflammatory bowel disease, and gynecologic conditions lead the differential diagnosis. In adults and elderly patients, the differential diagnosis reflects age and underlying comorbidities. Malignancy, diverticulosis, gallbladder disease, and peptic ulcer disease are frequent diagnoses. Given its bimodal distribution by age, appendicitis also must be considered early in the evaluation of elderly patients, because the consequences of rupture in elderly patients can be catastrophic.

9. How does immunocompetence affect the diagnosis and treatment of abdominal pain?

Immunocompromised patients are at risk for unusual as well as common causes of abdominal pain. Given the central role of neutrophils in the inflammatory pathway of the peritoneum, immunocompromised patients, such as patients with HIV and patients taking steroids or on chronic immunosuppression therapy, have a blunted response to the disease process. For this reason, they often present later in the course of illness with more advanced disease. Furthermore, suggestive symptoms and signs, such as fever or elevation of the white blood cell count, may or may not be present, making the diagnosis of intrabdominal pathology difficult. In assessing abdominal pain in immunocompromised patients, it is also important to consider causes related to the underlying immunosuppressive condition. Examples include infection with opportunistic organisms, neoplasm (particularly intestinal lymphomas), neutropenic enterocolitis, side effects of medication, and unusual forms of biliary tract disease. A heightened awareness of these possibilities is necessary to diagnose and intervene early in these potentially treatable conditions.

10. Name some vascular causes of acute abdominal pain. How and in whom do they present?

Ruptured AAA presents with sudden onset of intense back pain due to dissection of tissue in the retroperitoneum with the spread of blood. Patients may be diaphoretic and hypotensive with palpable, pulsatile, expansile mid-epigastric mass. CT scan may aid in diagnosis in hemodynamically stable patients. If the diagnosis is strongly suspected in a patient with history of AAA, surgical intervention should not be delayed by imaging studies.

Visceral artery aneurysms present with acute abdominal pain and possible rupture. Some patients may present with a sentinel GI bleed. Visceral aneurysms should be considered in young, pregnant women with abdominal pain and patients with fibromuscular disease, vasculitis, or history of ongoing pancreatitis. Sixty percent are splenic, 20% hepatic. Superior mesenteric and celiac artery aneurysms occur in fewer than 5% of vascular-related abdominal pain cases.

Acute aortic dissection usually presents with sudden onset of tearing pain localized to the area between the scapula; however, abdominal pain can occur when the false lumen occludes renal or mesenteric arteries (5–17% of dissections). Because the pathophysiology is based on medial degeneration, this condition occurs in patients generally younger than those with advanced atherosclerotic disease.

Acute mesenteric ischemia presents with pain out of proportion to the physical exam. The cause can be embolic, thrombotic, or nonocclusive. Therefore, it should be suspected in patients with a history of atrial fibrillation or hypercoaguable states and patients with congestive heart failure or low-flow hemodynamic states.

11. What is Ogilvie's syndrome?

Ogilvie's syndrome, or pseudo-obstruction of the colon, is marked by massive dilation of the colon without mechanical obstruction. It is seen most commonly in elderly, debilitated patients and patients immobilized by orthopedic procedures or neurologic disorders such as Parkinson's disease. It is also seen in the presence of electrolyte derangements. If dilation of the cecum exceeds 9–12 cm (as estimated on plain films of the abdomen), the risk of perforation is significant. Treatment begins with colonoscopic or rectal tube decompression of the colon. Medical therapy includes administration of neostigmine (2.5mg IV over 3 minutes). Treatment should be undertaken in a monitored setting because of the risk of bradycardia with systemic infusions. If these maneuvers fail, surgical decompression with cecotomy may be required.

12. Compare the clinical features and differential diagnosis of small bowel vs. large bowel obstruction.

Although the pathophysiologic endpoints are similar in small and large bowel obstruction, it is important to differentiate the two because of their underlying causes and significant variation in surgical therapy. **Small bowel obstruction** (SBO) generally begins with the sudden onset of sharp, colicky, diffuse abdominal pain. Between episodes of cramping, the patient may be pain-free. Nausea and emesis can follow the onset of pain and may relieve it in some cases. Emesis in SBO tends to be frequent and bilious, gradually becoming more feculent as the process continues. Bowel sounds may be high-pitched with audible rushes as cramping intensifies. Tachycardia is common, and hypotension and dehydration develop as fluid loss from vomiting continues. Fever may or may not be present. Laboratory data reveal an increase in hematocrit caused by dehydration. The white blood cell count may be elevated if the duration of obstruction has been several hours or more. Plain films of the abdomen characteristically show bowel dilatation, air–fluid levels, and a nonobstructed colon with air and feces. If the obstruction in proximal, the plain films may be unremarkable. CT scan is highly sensitive for diagnosing SBO. The scan may show a clear transition point from dilated to decompressed small intestine. The top differential diagnoses for SBO (in order of decreasing frequency) are adhesions, incarcerated hernia, and neoplastic disease.

In contrast, **large bowel obstruction** (LBO) occurs in older patients and tends to have a gradual onset, presenting with constipation and abdominal distention. Nausea and vomiting are late findings. The patient may give a history of pencil-thin or blood-streaked stools. Vital signs may be within normal range, depending on the duration of the obstruction. The abdomen is tympanitic to percussion, and pain is minimal, unless peritonitis is present. Laboratory data reveal normal hematocrit and white blood cell count, unless there is ongoing infection or ischemia. Plain films of the abdomen show marked dilation of the colon proximal to the point of obstruction. Colonoscopic decompression is frequently successful in cases of sigmoid volvulus. Barium enema can be diagnostic for other conditions. CT scan with rectal contrast may show evidence of diverticulitis or malignancy as the source of obstruction. The most frequent causes of LBO in the United States are cancer, volvulus, and diverticular disease.

13. Name some nonsurgical causes of acute abdominal pain.

Numerous medical conditions can cause abdominal pain and even mimic an acute abdomen, obscuring the abilitiy to diagnose truly surgical conditions. These commonly include myocardial infarction, pneumonia, sickle cell pain crisis, spontaneous bacterial peritonitis, infectious gastroenteritis, typhlitis, leukemia, poisoning, pancreatitis, inflammatory bowel disease without perforation, hepatitis, and pelvic inflammatory disease.

BIBLIOGRAPHY

1. Boey JH: The acute abdomen. In Way LW (ed): Current Surgical Diagnosis and Treatment, 10th ed. Appleton & Lange, Norwalk 1994.
2. Cameron JL: Current Surgical Therapy, 4th ed. St. Louis, Mosby, 1992.
3. Greenfield L, et al: Essentials of Surgery—Scientific Principles and Practice, 2nd ed. Philadelphia, J.B. Lippincott, 1997.
4. Holder WD: Intestinal obstruction. Gastroenterol Clin North Am 17:317–323; 1988.
5. Jorgensen J, Hawkins R: Abdominal vascular catastrophes. Surg Clin North Am 77:1305–1321, 1997.
6. Martin RF, Flynn P: The acute abdomen in the critically ill patient. Surg Clin North Am 77:1455–1464, 1997.
7. Murr M, Sarr M: The surgeon's role in the treatment of chronic intestinal pseudo-obstruction. Am J Gastroenterol 90:2147–2151, 1995.
8. Neblett WW, Pietsch JB: Acute abdominal conditions in children and adolescents. Surg Clin North Am. Vol 68:415–429, 1988.
9. Sabiston DC: Textbook of Surgery: The Biological Basis of Modern Surgical Practice, 15th ed. Philadelphia, W.B. Saunders, 1997.
10. Silen W: Cope's Early Diagnosis of the Acute Abdomen, 17th ed. New York, Oxford University Press, 1987.
11. Zenilman M: Surgery in the nursing home patient. Surg Clin North Am 74:63–77, 1994.

78. DIAGNOSTIC PERITONEAL LAVAGE

Walter L. Biffl, M.D., and Ernest E. Moore, M.D.

1. What is diagnostic peritoneal lavage (DPL)?

DPL is a procedure that was developed by H. D. Root and associates in 1965 for the evaluation of patients with acute blunt abdominal trauma. DPL replaced the four-quadrant peritoneal tap that was popular at that time. The unique feature of DPL, in addition to aspirating the peritoneal cavity, is the introduction of fluid that is recovered and analyzed for cellular, enzyme, and particulate content.

2. What are the clinical situations in which DPL may be valuable?

DPL became the gold standard for evaluation of blunt abdominal trauma in the early 1970s. In the late 1970s, studies from Brooklyn, Dallas, and Denver expanded the role of DPL to penetrating wounds, particularly stab wounds to the anterior abdomen and lower chest. More recently DPL has been applied in the diagnosis of acute peritonitis and staging of acute pancreatitis, with generally favorable results.

3. What techniques are available to introduce the DPL catheter into the peritoneum?

Conceptually there are three approaches: open, semi-open, and closed. The **open** technique consists of an incision through the abdominal wall, placing the catheter into the peritoneal cavity under direct vision. The **semi-open** technique limits the incision to the skin with a small nick in the fascia; the catheter, with trocar in place, is advanced across the peritoneum. The **closed** technique is placement of the catheter with trocar in place through the abdominal wall. Variants of this procedure use a Veress needle to penetrate the peritoneal cavity or a guidewire to facilitate more controlled tunneling of the catheter.

4. What are the advantages and disadvantages of these techniques?

The open technique has been considered the standard because it is the most secure route into the peritoneal cavity and is safest procedure in patients with previous abdominal surgery, pelvic fracture, or pregnancy. The disadvantages of the open approach include its additional time and risk of wound infection. The closed technique of DPL is the quickest and perhaps easiest to perform. The major disadvantage is the blind nature with its inherent risk of injuring underlying abdominal viscera. This risk, however, can be minimized by using a Seldinger (guidewire) technique or Veress needle.

5. Must DPL be performed in the operating room?

No. DPL can be performed readily in the emergency department, intensive care unit, or hospital ward. However, it must be performed in a sterile fashion and, optimally, under conscious sedation.

6. What are the complications of DPL?

In the non-obese patient who has not had a previous abdominal operation or infection, the technical complications are less than 0.5%, with an additional 1% risk of infection. The mechanical constraints of obesity or intestinal adhesions increase these risks. Furthermore, patients with underlying portal hypertension have a substantial risk of bleeding.

7. Can DPL be performed in patients with previous abdominal surgery?

Even with preexistent laparotomy, DPL can be performed with either open or closed technique. If done carefully, both approaches are safe, but extensive adhesions may compartmentalize the peritoneal cavity and thus render the lavage falsely negative.

8. Can DPL be performed in pregnant patients?

The open technique is mandatory in gravid patients. The catheter entrance site chosen is at the top of the fundus of the uterus, and, accordingly, in later pregnancy the catheter entrance site is in the supraumbilical region. Although a theoretical concern, DPL has not been associated with induction of labor.

9. What is the sensitivity for intraperitoneal bleeding?

The false-negative rate is less than 1%. The test is extremely useful in blunt trauma because the predominant intraperitoneal injuries are to the spleen and liver. The major limitations of DPL are in the identification of diaphragmatic rupture or perforation of hollow viscera, including the gastrointestinal tract and bladder. The incidence of false-negative studies based on red blood cell analysis with isolated small perforations to these structures is considerable because such lesions tend to bleed minimally.

10. What criteria of bleeding are considered significant after blunt abdominal trauma?

Aspiration of greater than 10 ml of free blood (a "grossly positive" result) is considered an indication for laparotomy. If the aspirate is not grosslypositive, the lavage is done with 1 liter (15 ml/kg in children) of warm saline, and the effluent is analyzed in the laboratory. A red blood cell (RBC) count exceeding $100,000/ml^3$ is considered positive. The inability to read newsprint through the effluent is *not* a reliable indicator of positive lavage. It is important to collect at least 600 ml of effluent to avoid misleading results.

11. What additional indices are considered significant for DPL in blunt abdominal trauma?

Initial aspiration of enteric contents warrants prompt laparotomy. A white blood cell (WBC) count exceeding $500/mm^3$ has been considered significant, but several recent series have shown that this leukocytosis frequently occurs without associated visceral injury. Alternative criteria have been proposed, but the current standard is to repeat the DPL in 4 hours and operate if the WBC count remains elevated. The utility of biochemical markers in the lavage effluent is controversial. A bilirubin level greater than serum level is highly suggestive of gallbladder perforation. Amylase and alkaline phosphatase levels appear useful, but the threshold for laparotomy is time-dependent.

12. Has contrast-enhanced CT scanning or ultrasonography eliminated the need for DPL in the evaluation of blunt abdominal trauma?

Abdominal CT scanning has clearly reduced the need for DPL (see Controversy). Ultrasound has proved to be a rapid and reliable test for intraabdominal hemorrhage following blunt abdominal trauma. In addition, it offers the opportunity to assess the heart and pericardial space. It is easily repeated, portable, and noninvasive, making it ideal for serial examinations. However, it cannot provide information about hollow viscus injuries beyond the presence of fluid. Thus, DPL still has a place in the evaluation of bluntly injured patients.

13. Is DPL useful in the evaluation of penetrating abdominal wounds?

In many centers DPL has become the mainstay for evaluating stab wounds to the anterior abdomen. These patients are generally difficult to assess because of intoxication and pain emanating from the abdominal wall stab wound. Stab wounds to the anterior abdomen penetrate the peritoneum in approximately two-thirds of patients, of whom about half incur significant visceral injury. Thus, only one of three patients with a stab wound to the anterior abdomen requires laparotomy. Local wound exploration and DPL provide a safe, quick, and cost effective means of triaging these patients. The DPL criteria for abdominal exploration in stab wounds are similar to those for blunt abdominal trauma. There is a much higher rate of isolated hollow visceral injury following a stab wound (2–5% of patients with a negative DPL have perforation of the small bowel, stomach, or, in rare cases, the colon. For that reason, all patients undergoing DPL for stab wounds must be observed in the hospital for at least 24 hours, and laparotomy should be performed promptly for any signs of peritoneal irritation.

14. Are the criteria for operation different when DPL is used to evaluate the possibility of abdominal injury via a lower chest wound?

Because small injuries to the diaphragm may bleed minimally, the threshold for laparotomy is reduced in the evaluation of lower chest stab wounds. An RBC count exceeding 10,000/mm^3 (i.e., exceeding the value that could be ascribed to the DPL technique) is considered positive. However, diaphragmatic injury may yield < 10,000 RBC/mm^3. Thoracoscopy and laparoscopy are used in the evaluation of RBC counts 1000–10,000/mm^3 in this setting.

15. Is DPL useful in the evaluation of abdominal gunshot wounds?

Abdominal gunshot wounds pose a much greater threat for visceral injury than stab wounds. The incidence of significant visceral damage when the missile penetrates the peritoneum approximates 95%. Therefore, it is routine policy to perform laparotomy when the missile appears to have entered the peritoneal cavity. However, in a select group of patients in whom a low-energy missile appears to remain extraperitoneal, DPL may be used as an adjunctive test to avoid laparotomy. In such cases, the RBC threshold is 10,000/mm^3; the rationale is similar to that applied to penetrating wounds to the lower chest.

16. Does DPL have any value in the evaluation of the patient with potential intraabdominal infection?

Several groups have advocated the use of DPL in the evaluation of critically ill patients in the ICU with potential intraperitoneal sepsis. The most useful lavage marker appears to be the leukocyte count; i.e., a WBC count exceeding 500/mm^3 is specific for intraperitoneal inflammation. Nonperforated inflammatory lesions of the peritoneal cavity may not manifest changes in the lavage fluid. To enhance the sensitivity for abdominal infection, other groups have suggested measurement of endotoxin, lactate, or a variety of enzymes. These reports are promising but inconclusive. Several authors have advocated DPL for the staging of acute pancreatitis, but precise markers remain to be established. Some groups suggest the relative levels of amylase and lipase compared with serum are prognostic; others suggest that blood-tinged lavage or ascitic fluid implies pancreatic necrosis.

CONTROVERSY

17. What is the best test for the evaluation of blunt abdominal trauma?

For DPL: DPL is a rapid, safe, and highly sensitive test for intraperitoneal blood. The procedure can be performed during the initial evaluation of the injured patient while other resuscitative maneuvers are ongoing. Thus, DPL is an extremely valuable triage tool in the multisystem-injured patient who remains in shock.

Against DPL: Paradoxically, the major downfall of DPL is that it is too sensitive for intraperitoneal blood and does not indicate the source of bleeding. In the past several years, there has been growing enthusiasm for nonoperative management of solid organ injuries, particularly the spleen. Furthermore, DPL may be falsely positive in as many as 15% of patients with major pelvic fracture because of RBC diapedesis. DPL does not sample the retroperitoneum; therefore, injuries to the pancreas, duodenum, urinary tract, and major vascular structures may be missed.

For CT scanning: CT scanning affords the opportunity to manage solid organ injuries nonoperatively and can identify many hollow visceral injuries.

Against CT scanning: The logistics of removing a critically injured patient from the ED is less than optimal. In addition, there are risks associated with oral contrast material (aspiration) as well as with intravenous contrast material.

For ultrasound: Ultrasound is rapid, noninvasive, and accurate for the detection of intraabdominal hemorrhage, making it the test of choice in the initial evaluation of the multisystem-injured patient. It is portable and easily repeated, allowing its use for serial examination in any locale. Proficiency is gained rapidly and thus does not require additional personnel present. Additional information can be obtained regarding the heart and pericardial space.

Against ultrasound: Ultrasound cannot evaluate the retroperitoneum, does not identify the precise site of hemorrhage, and offers no information about hollow viscus injuries other than free fluid.

BIBLIOGRAPHY

1. Branney SW, Moore EE, Cantrill SV, et al: Ultrasound based key clinical pathway reduces the use of hospital resources for the evaluation of blunt abdominal trauma. J Trauma 42:1086–1090, 1997.
2. De Maria EJ,. Dalton JM, Gore DC, et al: Complementary roles of laparoscopic abdominal exploration and diagnostic peritoneal lavage for evaluating tabe wounds: A propsective study. J Laparoendosc Adv Surg Tech A 10:131–136, 2000.
3. Feliciano V, Bitondo-Dyer CG: Vagaries of the lavage white blood cell count in evaluating abdominal stab wounds. Am J Surg 168:680–684, 1994.
4. Gonzalez RP, Ickler J, Gachassin P: Complementary roles of diagnostic peritoneal lavage and computed tomography in the evaluation of blunt abdominal trauma. J Trauma 51:1128–1136, 2001.
5. Hodgson NF, Stewart TC, Girotti MJ: Open or closed diagnostic peritoneal lavage for abdominal trauma? Ameta-analysis. J Trauma 48:1091–1095, 2000.
6. Kelemen JJ III, Martin RR, Obney JA, et al: Evaluation of diagnostic peritoneal lavage in stable patients with gunshot wounds in the abdomen. Arch Surg 132:909–913, 1997.
7. McAnena OJ, Max JA, Moore EE: Peritoneal lavage enzyme determinations following blunt and penetrating abdominal trauma. J Trauma 31:1161–1164, 1991.
8. Moore JB, Alden AW, Rodman GH: Is closed diagnostic peritoneal lavage contraindicated in patients with previous abdominal surgery? Acad Emerg Med 4:287–290, 1997.
9. Saunders CJ, Battistella FD, Whetzel TP, Stokes RB: Percutaneous diagnostic peritoneal lavage using a Veress needle versus an open technique: A prospective randomized trial. J Trauma 44:883–888, 1998.
10. Sullivan KR, Nelson MJ, Tandberg D: Incremental analysis of diagnostic peritoneal lavage fluid in adult abdominal trauma. Am J Emerg Med 15:277–279, 1997.
11. Walsh RM, Popovich MJ, Hoadley J: Bedside diagnostic laparoscopy and peritoneal lavage in the intensive care unit. Surg Endosc 12:1408–1409, 1998.

79. WOUND INFECTION AND DEHISCENCE

Thomas F. Rehring, M.D.

1. Define the scope of the problem of surgical wound infection.

Wound infections, now more appropriately termed surgical site infections (SSIs), are the second most common nosocomial infection in the United States, accounting for 3.7 million excess hospital days and over 1.6 billion dollars in hospital charges annually.

2. What are the classic signs and symptoms that herald wound infection?

Local signs include warmth, erythema, pain, and swelling (classically described as calor, rubor, dolor, and tumor). Systemic signs are less common (15% of cases) but may include elevation in temperature or rigors.

3. Which wounds are likely to become infected?

Traditionally, operations were divided into clean, clean-contaminated, and contaminated cases, thus implying a proportionate risk of infection. This scheme of stratification fails to account for intrinsic patient- and operation-specific risk factors for the development of an SSI. Subsequently, an index was developed in concert with the Centers for Disease Control and Prevention to predict SSI rates more accurately and and to compare rates between institutions and surgeons (National Nosocomial Infections Surveillance System Basic SSI Risk Index). This index includes the patient's American Society of Anesthesiologists (ASA) preoperative score, the type of operation, and the duration of the operation. The overall rate of SSIs is approximately

3%. Acceptable rates of infection are 1–3% for clean wounds (e.g., herniorrhaphy), 3–7% for for clean-contaminated (e.g., biliary), and 6–15% for contaminated (e.g., colorectal), and 7–40% for dirty-infected (e.g., abscess drainage). This degree of overlap encompasses the variability due to the factors listed in question 5.

4. What are the common infecting organisms?
Gram-positive bacteria are isolated in over 46% of SSIs from clean cases. Generally, they are skin contaminants from the patient's flora. In clean-contaminated and dirty cases, the organisms also may be from the source of the contamination (e.g., colon, stomach).

5. What are the risk factors for wound infection?
• Patient factors: extremes of age, malnutrition, obesity, diabetes, immunosuppression, cancer, smoking, corticosteroids, irradiation.
• Preoperative factors: hospitalization, early shaving vs. clipping, prior antibiotic therapy.
• Intraoperative factors: normothermia, contamination, duration of operation.
• Local factors: blood supply, local hypoxia, dead space, foreign body, hematoma.

6. When are prophylactic antibiotics indicated?
For clean-contaminated cases, prophylactic antibiotics have been shown to decrease the incidence of postoperative wound infection. By definition, antibiotic administration in contaminated and dirty-infected wounds is therapeutic, not prophylactic. The routine administration of antibiotics for prophylaxis in clean cases continues to be controversial; however, a large, prospective randomized trial has demonstrated a 48% decrease in wound infection in breast biopsy and herniorrhaphy with antibiotic prophylaxis. Current consensus opinion recommends prophylaxis in high-risk clean operations in which foreign bodies are implanted (e.g., vascular graft, cardiac valve, total joint replacement).

7. Besides antibiotics, what other therapeutic interventions may limit the chance of a postoperative wound infection?
1. Keep the patient warm during surgery. Maintenance of normothermia during colonic surgery has been shown to decrease wound infection rates threefold (6% vs. 19%) in a recent prospective, randomized trial.
2. Provide supplemental oxygen perioperatively. In a recent prospective, randomized study of patients undergoing colorectal procedures, the perioperative administration of 80% oxygen decreased SSIs by 50% (5.2% vs. 11.2%).

8. When do SSIs typically manifest?
Generally, 3–7 days postoperatively.

9. What should be done with a red, indurated abdominal incision?
Individual surgeons vary as to whether they take all of the skin suture and subcutaneous sutures out and open the entire wound or remove a limited portion of the skin sutures (and subcutaneous sutures, if present). Anaerobic and aerobic cultures should be obtained, followed by local wound care. Most superficial infections do not require systemic antibiotics; however, extensive infections or those with significant cellulitis may benefit.

10. Describe the routine care for a wound allowed to close secondarily.
Necrotic tissue is an ideal bacterial growth medium. Bacterial overgrowth inhibits epithelialization and wound healing. Local wound care, therefore, is critical. Routine care involves sterile wet-to-dry normal saline dressings changed 2 or 3 times/day to aid in debridement of necrotic tissue. Provision of a moist environment and removal of devitalized tissue are the critical points; however, novel commerical topical agents to assist in healing are continually marketed, and wound care specialists abound.

11. What is delayed primary closure?

In an effort to reduce the risk of wound infection in contaminated or dirty cases to rates similar to clean cases, wounds can be closed in a delayed fashion. At the time of surgery, sutures are placed loosely in the skin and left untied. For the first 4 or 5 days postoperatively, the wound is packed with gauze and changed two or three times a day. The wound is then inspected. If it appears clean, the sutures are tied, bringing the wound edges together. This allows more rapid healing and a smaller scar, and avoids the potential for early wound infection.

12. What is the most worrisome diagnosis in a patient 12 hours postoperatively with a temperature of 39°C, a very painful wound with erythema, bullae, and a thin, serosanguinous discharge?

Clostridial myonecrosis.

13. In the same patient, what is the diagnosis if the wound is very erythematous, no bullae are noted, and a Gram stain of expressed fluid demonstrates many leukocytes and gram-positive cocci?

Group A β-hemolytic streptococcal infection. Treatment includes high-dose IV penicillin and surgical debridement.

14. What is gas gangrene? How is it treated?

Gas gangrene is another term for clostridial myonecrosis. It generally occurs 24–48 hours after trauma or abdominal surgery and presents as pain and edema with minimal erythema that rapidly progresses to hemorrhagic bullae. Also noted is a thin, watery, foul-smelling discharge with Gram stain findings remarkable for few leukocytes but abundant gram-positive rods. Crepitance in the wound is a late finding and corresponds with mortality. Mortality rates approach 60%. Treatment relies on early diagnosis, aggressive surgical debridement, antibiotics, and supportive care.

15. True or false: Most infections with gas in the soft tissue involve _Clostridium_ species.

False. Although gas in the soft tissues generally implies a surgical infection, most cases are necrotizing infections caused by other pathogens.

16. What is necrotizing fasciitis?

This worrisome diagnosis is characterized by widespread fascial necrosis with relative sparing of the skin and underlying muscle. It is uniformaly fatal if left untreated and requires a high index of suspicion for diagnosis. Commonly it presents as a slowly advancing cellulitis that progresses to firm or "woody" induration of the subcutaneous tissues. A thin, brown exudate may be expressed from the wound. A lack of response to nonoperative therapy or signs of systemic toxicity may be the only indications of underlying necrosis.

Necrotizing fasciitis may develp after relatively minor abrasions, insect bites, lacerations, or superficial wound infections in trauma or abdominal surgery. It also is seen in IV drug abusers. Ninety percent of cases are polymicrobial. Treatment relies primarily on early surgical debridement augmented by broad-spectrum antibiotics and supportive care. Antibiotics initially should be chosen to ensure coverage of aerobic gram-positive and gram-negative organisms and anaerobes, then tailored to the specific organisms that are cultured. In a recent series, the mortality rate of necrotizing fasciitis approached 30%.

17. What is Fournier's gangrene? How is it treated?

Necrotizing fasciitis of the perineum. Like other forms of necrotizing fasciitis, if left untreated, it progresses to systemic sepsis, multiple-organ failure, and death. Treatment consists of early diagnosis, early and repeated radical debridement, diversion of the fecal stream (colostomy), and broad-spectrum antibiotics.

18. Explain hyperbaric oxygen treatment.

Patients are placed in a specialized chamber at three times atmospheric pressure. Hyperbaric oxygen inhibits the production of clostridial alpha toxin. In theory, therefore, treatment with hyperbaric oxygen should limit the mortality rate and extent of tissue loss incurred with severe necrotizing soft tissue infections, particularly those caused by Clostridium species. However, despite experimental evidence suggesting a benefit in animals, no controlled prospective clinical trial has demonstrated efficacy above and beyond debridement and antibiotics. Hyperbaric oxygen, therefore, remains a controversial component in the care of profoundly ill patients with necrotizing fasciitis.

19. What are the risk factors for a wound dehiscence?

At risk are elderly, debilitated, malnourished and obese patients. Contributing factors include infection, corticosteroid therapy, ascites, diabetes, radiation, or any process which increases intraabdominal pressure. Of ultimate importance, however, is the technical adequacy of the closure. Appropriate placement and tension of sutures are critical. It is unlikely, however, that interrupted vs. running sutures or choice of incision (vertical vs. transverse) contributes significantly to the incidence of dehiscence. However, a recent meta-analysis suggested a decreased rate of incisional hernia with nonabsorbable suture placed in a running fashion.

20. Which signs herald wound dehiscences?

Serosanguinous discharge from a wound greater than 24 hours postoperatively must *always* be considered a wound dehiscence until proved otherwise.

21. Do retention sutures prevent dehiscence?

No. They reduce the likelihood of evisceration. Classically, retention sutures are heavy, nonabsorbable sutures traversing all layers of the abdominal wall, reinforcing the normal fascial closure.

22. What is the difference between wound dehiscence and evisceration?

Dehiscence means that the abdominal fascia is not intact. It is diagnosed by gently probing the wound with a sterile, gloved finger to document separation of the fascia. Evisceration is protrusion of abdominal contents (usually small bowel) through the wound.

23. How do you manage dehiscence? Evisceration?

If the surgeon is unsure of the diagnosis, the wound may be gently explored at the bedside with a sterile glove, noting the integrity of the fascia and the contents of the wound cavity. In general, **dehiscences** should be closed operatively. In certain difficult extenuating circumstances (chronic intraabdominal sepsis), a small dehiscence may be left open, simply accepting the fact that an incisional hernia will result.

In **evisceration**, the exposed bowels should be wrapped in sterile, saline-soaked towels and the patient returned promptly to the operating room for definitive closure.

BIBLIOGRAPHY

1. Green R, Dafoe D, Raffin T: Necrotizing fasciitis. Chest 110:219–229, 1996.
2. Greif R, Akca O, Horn EP, et al: Supplemental perioperative oxygen to reduce the incidence of surgical-wound infection. Outcomes Research Group. N Engl J Med 342:161–167, 2000.
3. Hodgson NC, Malthaner RA, Ostbye T: The search for an ideal method of abdominal fascial closure: A meta-analysis. Ann Surg 231:436–442, 2000.
4. Horan TC, Gaynes RP, Martone W, et al: CDC definitions of nosocomial surgical site infections, 1992: A modification of CDC definitions of surgical wound infections. Infect Control Hosp Epidemiol 13:606–608, 1992.
5. Kurz A, Sessler DI, Lenhardt R: Perioperative normothermia to reduce the incidence of surgical-wound infection and shorten hospitalization. Study of Wound Infection and Temperature Group. N Engl J Med 334:1209–1215, 1996.
6. National Nosocomial and Infections Surveillance (NNIS) System Report: Data summary from January 1992–June 2001, issued August 2001. Am J Infect Control 29:404–421, 2001.
7. Nichols RL, Florman S: Clinical presentations of soft-tissue infections and surgical site infections. Clin Infect Dis 33(Suppl 2):S84–S93, 2001.

80. PNEUMOTHORAX

Michael E. Hanley, M.D.

1. What are the major etiologic classifications of pneumothoraces?

Pneumothoraces are classified as spontaneous or traumatic. **Spontaneous** pneumothoraces occur without antecedent trauma or other obvious cause. A spontaneous pneumothorax that occurs in an individual without underlying lung disease is termed a primary spontaneous pneumothorax. A secondary spontaneous pneumothorax occurs as a complication of underlying lung disease. **Traumatic** pneumothoraces result from direct or indirect trauma to the chest and are further classified as iatrogenic or noniatrogenic.

2. What are the major causes of spontaneous pneumothoraces?

Primary spontaneous pneumothoraces result from rupture of subpleural emphysematous blebs. Although these blebs may be congenital, they most likely result from airway inflammation. Cigarette smoking in particular is a significant risk factor.

Secondary spontaneous pneumothoraces may occur as a complication of any lung disease. The most common lung disease associated with this type of pneumothorax is chronic obstructive pulmonary disease (COPD), accounting for up to 67% of cases. Other lung diseases more frequently associated with secondary spontaneous pneumothoraces include asthma, cystic fibrosis, Marfan's syndrome, pulmonary alveolar proteinosis, pulmonary infarction, *Pneumocystis carinii* pneumonia, granulomatous diseases such as tuberculosis, sarcoidosis and berylliosis, and interstitial lung diseases including idiopathic pulmonary fibrosis, scleroderma, rheumatoid lung disease, eosinophilic granuloma, lymphangioleiomyomatosis and tuberous sclerosis.

3. What are the common causes of pneumothorax in critically ill patients?

Most pneumothoraces that develop in the intensive care unit are due either to antecedent noniatrogenic chest trauma or to iatrogenic causes. Common causes of iatrogenic pneumothorax include positive-pressure ventilation, central venous catheter placement, thoracentesis, tracheostomy, nasogastric tube placement (due to inadvertent insertion of the nasogastric tube into the tracheobronchial tree), bronchoscopy (especially if transbronchial biopsy is performed), pericardiocentesis, transthoracic needle aspiration, and cardiopulmonary resuscitation. Secondary spontaneous pneumothorax also occasionally develops in critically ill patients, especially those with chronic obstructive pulmonary disease, asthma, interstitial lung disease, necrotizing lung infections, and *P. carinii* pneumonia.

4. What measures reduce the risk of iatrogenic pneumothorax in patients receiving positive pressure ventilation?

End-inspiratory plateau pressure should be kept < 35 cm H_2O, and both peak end-expiratory pressure (PEEP) and auto-PEEP levels should be minimized. Approaches that may help to achieve these goals include using smaller tidal volumes (5–10 ml/kg) in patients with underlying lung disease, utilizing permissive hypercapnea when a high minute ventilation is required, and using high inspiratory flow rates. In addition, thoracentesis and subclavian/internal jugular venous lines insertion should be performed with utmost care in high-risk patients.

5. Describe the clinical manifestations of pneumothoraces.

Dyspnea and chest pain (usually localized to the side of the pneumothorax) are the most common symptoms in primary spontaneous pneumothorax. The most common physical signs are tachycardia and an abnormal chest exam. The latter includes ipsilateral expansion of the chest and decreased or absent tactile fremitus. Chest percussion and auscultation reveal ipsilateral hyperresonance and decreased or absent breath sounds. The trachea may be deviated toward the contralateral side.

The symptoms in secondary spontaneous pneumothoraces are more severe than for primary pneumothoraces because the pulmonary reserve is already compromised by underlying lung pathology. Dyspnea occurs in virtually all patients and commonly appears to be out of proportion to the size of the pneumothorax. Cyanosis and hypotension are more common. Because the chest examination is already abnormal and many of the physical signs associated with the underlying lung disease are similar to those associated with pneumothoraces, side-to-side differences in the examination of the chest may not be as apparent.

6. What subtle signs or symptoms should prompt consideration of pneumothorax in mechanically ventilated patients?

The sudden onset of any of the following should raise the possibility of a pneumothorax in mechanically ventilated patients:
- Decline in oxygen saturation
- Agitation
- Respiratory distress
- "Fighting the ventilator"
- Sudden increase in peak inspiratory and/or static airway pressure
- Hypotension
- Cardiovascular collapse
- Pulseless electrical activity

7. How is the diagnosis of pneumothorax established in critically ill patients?

A pneumothorax should be suspected in any critically ill patient who develops unexplained hypoxemia, dyspnea, or chest pain or who has physical findings consistent with the condition. The diagnosis is established by demonstrating typical chest roentgenographic findings, including a thin pleural line and the absence of lung parenchymal markings between the pleural line and chest wall. However, when the chest roentgenogram is obtained with the patient in the supine position, free pleural air will collect anteriorly and may not be readily apparent. The presence of a pneumothorax in these cases is suggested by evidence of an increase in the size of the ipsilateral hemithorax, including contralateral shift of the mediastinum and heart, as well as depression of the ipsilateral hemidiaphragm. In such cases, chest roentgenograms obtained at expiration, in the lateral decubitus position, or as cross-table lateral view may be useful in confirming the presence of free pleural air. If chest roentgenograms are nondiagnostic and the patient is sufficiently stable for transport, computed tomography (CT) of the chest may be required to prove the diagnosis.

8. Describe the treatment of a pneumothorax.

Most pneumothoraces in the critically ill patient are either secondary spontaneous or traumatic. Tube thoracostomy should be performed in almost all secondary spontaneous or noniatrogenic, traumatic pneumothoraces, especially if mechanical ventilation is required. Proper positioning of the thoracostomy tube is important in obtaining complete evacuation of the free pleural air. The tube should be directed to an anterior/apical position in a patient at bed rest. Tube thoracostomy should also be performed for all iatrogenic pneumothoraces due to positive pressure ventilation. Other forms of iatrogenic pneumothorax require tube thoracostomy only if the pneumothorax (1) is large (greater than 40%), (2) is associated with significant symptoms or arterial blood gas abnormalities, (3) progressively enlarges, (4) does not respond to simple aspiration, or (5) occurs in a patient requiring positive-pressure ventilation.

9. Does the development of a pneumothorax portend a worse prognosis for patients with acute respiratory distress syndrome (ARDS)?

No. The association of pneumothorax and other air leaks (extrusion of of any air outside the tracheobronchial tree) with mortality was recently studied in 725 patients with ARDS involved in an aerosolized synthetic surfactant protocol. The 30-day mortality rate for patients who developed a pneumothorax was 46% compared with 40% in patients without pneumothorax (p = 0.35). Similarly, the 30-day mortality rate for patients with any type of air leak was 45.5% compared with 39.0% for patients without air leaks (p = 0.28).

10. What are the potential physiologic consequences of a bronchopleural fistula in mechanically ventilated patients?

A bronchopleural fistula (BPF) is generally defined as an air leak that persists for longer than 24 hours after evacuation of a pneumothorax. Large BPF in patients receiving positive pressure ventilation may be associated with inability to maintain adequate alveolar ventilation through loss of effective tidal volume, inappropriate cycling of the ventilator, incomplete lung reexpansion, and inability to apply PEEP.

11. Describe the management of a persistent BPF.

Management focuses on minimizing air flow through the fistula while maintaining complete evacuation of the pleural space. This is primarily accomplished in patients breathing spontaneously (negative pressure ventilation) by altering the level of suction applied to the pleural space. The optimal amount of suction must be determined on an individual basis, as the level of suction at which gas flow through the fistula is minimized varies.

Gas flow across a BPF in mechanically ventilated patients is also influenced by peak inspiratory and mean airway pressures. Management of BPFs in this setting includes measures that minimize airway pressures while maintaining adequate ventilation. This is accomplished by minimizing positive end-expiratory pressure, tidal volume, number of mechanically delivered breaths per minute, and inspiratory time. Mechanical ventilation should be discontinued as soon as possible.

If a BPF does not close after 5–7 days of chest tube drainage or if adequate ventilation cannot be maintained because of the size of the air leak, suturing or resection of the fistula with scarification of the pleura by either thoracoscopy or open thoracotomy should be considered. The decision to perform this procedure should include a consideration of the operative risk to the patient. Prolonged chest tube drainage, intrabronchial bronchoscopic instillation of materials (Gelfoam or tissue adhesives such as cyanoacrylate-based or fibrin glues) designed to occlude the fistula, differential lung ventilation, or synchronized chest tube occlusion should be considered in patients whose operative risk is increased by significant underlying lung disease or other medical problems.

12. What is reexpansion pulmonary edema? What is the risk of its occurrence after evacuation of a pneumothorax? How can the risk be minimized?

Reexpansion pulmonary edema involves the development of unilateral pulmonary edema following reexpansion of a collapsed lung. The risk and severity of reexpansion pulmonary edema appear to be related to the duration of the pneumothorax as well as the magnitude of negative pressure applied to the pleural space to reexpand the lung.

The exact incidence of reexpansion pulmonary edema following treatment of pneumothoraces in humans is unknown but it is rare. However, the associated mortality is between 10% and 20%.

The risk can be minimized by withholding pleural suction during the immediate treatment of pneumothoraces of either unknown duration or duration greater than 3 days. If the pneumothorax is not completely evacuated after 24–48 hours of water seal or if significant respiratory compromise requires more rapid evacuation, low levels of negative pressure (less than 20 cm H_2O) may be applied to the pleural space. Nonetheless, reexpansion pulmonary edema has been reported even under these conditions.

13. What is a tension pneumothorax? What are its clinical manifestations?

A tension pneumothorax occurs when the pleural pressure within a pneumothorax is greater than atmospheric pressure throughout expiration and often during inspiration. Tension pneumothoraces generally result from a one-way valve phenomenon and most frequently occur in patients receiving positive-pressure ventilation.

Clinical manifestations include sudden deterioration with rapid, labored breathing, cyanosis, and respiratory distress. The patient is commonly diaphoretic with cardiovascular instability characterized by tachycardia and hypotension. Physical examination demonstrates the findings typically associated with a pneumothorax, but with evidence of a marked increase in the size of the ipsilateral hemithorax, including contralateral shift of the trachea. Arterial blood gases commonly demonstrate severe hypoxemia and occasionally hypercapnia with respiratory acidosis.

14. Describe the treatment for a tension pneumothorax.

Untreated tension pneumothoraces are associated with a high mortality and therefore represent medical emergencies. When the diagnosis is suspected and the patient exhibits significant hemodynamic instability, time should not be wasted pursuing roentgenographic confirmation. High levels (FiO_2 = 100%) of supplemental oxygen should be administered and the free pleural air evacuated. This is best accomplished by emergent placement of a tube thoracostomy. If the diagnosis is in question or a tube thoracostomy is not readily available, an alternative approach includes insertion of a large-bore needle attached to a three-way stopcock with a 50-ml syringe partially filled with sterile saline into the pleural space. The needle is inserted under sterile conditions through the second anterior intercostal space in the midclavicular line while the patient is supine. After the needle has been inserted, the plunger is withdrawn from the syringe. The presence of a tension pneumothorax is confirmed if air bubbles up through the saline. When a tension pneumothorax is present, the needle should be left in place until air ceases to bubble through the saline and a tube thoracostomy is performed. If air does not bubble up into the syringe, a tension pneumothorax is not present and the needle may be removed.

CONTROVERSIES

15. What size chest tube is required to perform a tube thoracostomy for pneumothoraces?

Small:

1. Small catheters may be safely inserted using the trocar method, require little nursing care after insertion, and readily allow ambulation when suction is not required if combined with a Heimlich valve.

2. Small chest tubes successfully evacuated 90% of pneumothoraces in two studies of selected patients. Failures were attributed to kinking, inadvertent removal by the patient, occlusion of tube by pleural fluid, malposition, and presence of a large BPF.

3. Although rare, insertion of large tubes is associated with laceration of the diaphragm, lung, and liver.

Large:

1. Almost 50% of pneumothoraces were not successfully managed by small chest tubes in one series. Occlusion or external kinking of the catheter was implicated as the reason for failure in most of the cases.

2. Patients with large BPF on mechanical ventilation frequently require continuous evacuation of large volumes of pleural air. This cannot be accomplished with small-bore chest tubes.

16. Is high-frequency jet ventilation (HFJV) effective in managing large BPFs?

Yes:

1. In experimental animal models, HFJV decreased gas flow through BPFs and improved gas exchange.

2. In a number of studies a significant number of patients with large BPFs but otherwise normal lungs who had failed conventional ventilation were successfully ventilated with HFJV. However, HFJV also failed to ventilate a number of patients with significant parenchymal lung disease and BPFs.

No:

1. Several studies have reported that although gas flow through BPFs decreased in some patients with HFJV, it increased in other patients. In addition, gas exchange (oxygenation) frequently worsened after HFJV was initiated.

2. HFJV is a rarely performed mode of ventilation that is labor intensive; proper application requires a high level of familiarity by physicians and respiratory therapists.

17. Should a tube thoracostomy be removed immediately in patients receiving positive pressure ventilation once the air leak has resolved and the lung is completely reexpanded?

Yes:

1. The tube thoracostomy is no longer required to evacuate air after the BPF has closed and all air has been evacuated. At this point, the chest tube is only a potential source of infection, both at its insertion site and in the pleural space.

2. Patients can be closely monitored and chest tubes reinserted if a pneumothorax recurs.

3. Routine insertion of a prophylactic tube thoracostomy is not indicated in mechanically ventilated patients.

No:

1. Risk of a recurrent pneumothorax remains high in mechanically ventilated patients, especially if they have acute respiratory distress syndrome (ARDS) or a necrotic lung process.

2. Most pneumothoraces in mechanically ventilated patients present under tension. Tension pneumothoraces are associated with a higher mortality, especially if there is delay in diagnosis or treatment.

BIBLIOGRAPHY

1. Albeda SM, Hansen-Flaschen JH, Taylor E, et al: Evaluation of high-frequency jet ventilation in patients with bronchopleural fistulas by quantification of the air leak. Anesthesiology 63:551–554, 1985.
2. Barton ED: Tension pneumothorax. Curr Opin Pulm Med 5:269–274, 1999.
3. Baumann MH, Sahn SA: Medical management and therapy of bronchopleural fistulas in the mechanically ventilated patient. Chest 97:721–728, 1990.
4. Baumann MH, Sahn SA: Tension pneumothorax: Diagnostic and therapeutic pitfalls. Crit Care Med 21:177–179, 1993.
5. Baumann MH, Strange C, Heffner JF, et al: Management of spontaneous pneumothorax: An American College of Chest Physicians Delphi Consensus Statement. Chest 119:590–602, 2001.
6. Bishop MJ, Benson MS, Sato P, Pierson DJ: Comparison of high-frequency jet ventilation with conventional mechanical ventilation for bronchopleural fistula. Anesth Analg 66:833–838, 1987.
7. Gammon R, Shin M, Buchalter S: Pulmonary barotrauma in mechanical ventilation: Patterns and risk factors. Chest 105:568–572, 1992.
8. Heffner JE, McDonald J, Barbieri C: Recurrent pneumothoraces in ventilated patients despite ipsilateral chest tubes. Chest 108:1053–1058, 1995.
9. Mahfood S, Hix WR, Aaron BL, et al: Re-expansion pulmonary edema. Ann Thorac Surg 45:340–345, 1989.
10. Pavlin DJ, Raghu G, Rogers TR, Cheney FW: Re-expansion hypotension: A complication of rapid evacuation of prolonged pneumothorax. Chest 89:70–74, 1986.
11. Powner DJ, Cline CD, Rodman GH: Effect of chest tube suction on gas flow through a bronchopleural fistula. Crit Care Med 13:99–101, 1985.
12. Rankine JJ, Thomas AN, Fluechter D: Diagnosis of pneumothorax in critically ill adults. Postgrad Med J 76:399–404, 2000.
13. Strange C: Pleural complications in the intensive care unit. Clin Chest Med 20:317–327, 1999.
14. Weg J, Anzueto S, Balk RA, et al: The relationship of pneumothorax and other air leaks to mortality in the acute respiratory distress syndrome. N Engl J Med 338:341–346, 1998.

81. FLAIL CHEST AND PULMONARY CONTUSION

Rosemary A. Kozar, M.D., Ph.D,.James B. Haenel, R.R.T., and Frederick A. Moore, M.D.

1. What is a flail chest? How is it diagnosed?

A radiographic diagnosis of flail chest may be made when three or more consecutive ribs or costal cartilages are fractured in two or more places or six consecutive ribs are fractured. These circumscribed segments, having lost continuity with the rigid thorax, move inward with inspiration and push outward with exhalation, thus moving paradoxically. Presenting symptoms of pain, tachypnea, dyspnea, and thoracic splinting, along with chest wall contusions, tenderness, crepitance, and palpable rib fractures, are suggestive, but **paradoxical chest wall motion** is the diagnostic *sine qua non*. Detection often requires careful inspection of the two hemithoraces throughout the respiratory cycle to appreciate subtle paradoxical movement. Mechanical ventilation eliminates this abnormal motion because of positive pressure throughout the respiratory cycle, and subcutaneous emphysema, obesity, or large breasts may obscure the involved segment. Flail chest is frequently not conspicuous upon emergency department presentation because of secondary muscle splinting. With time, the flail becomes apparent as pain relief is achieved and the underlying pulmonary contusion worsens. The latter causes decreased pulmonary compliance. For effective ventilation, greater transthoracic pressure is required, which accentuates paradoxical motion. Consequently, patients sustaining severe blunt chest trauma must be carefully observed for at least 24 hours to detect a flail segment, which may herald respiratory failure. The chest film is helpful in identifying multiple displaced rib fractures, but will not reveal cartilaginous disruptions. The major value of routine chest x-ray lies in detecting associated chest injuries such as pneumothorax, hemothorax, or early pulmonary contusion.

2. What is a pulmonary contusion? How is it diagnosed?

The spectrum of lung parenchymal injury following a blunt chest impact ranges from simple contusion to frank laceration. Pulmonary contusion, by far the most frequent variant, is merely a bruise of the lung. Direct injury causes pulmonary vascular damage with secondary alveolar hemorrhage. In the early phase, these flooded alveoli are poorly perfused; consequently, little shunt exists. However, tissue inflammation develops rapidly and the resultant surrounding pulmonary edema produces regional alterations in compliance and airway resistance, leading to localized ventilation-perfusion mismatch.

The diagnosis is radiologic. The classic finding is a nonsegmental pulmonary infiltrate that occurs within 12–24 hours of injury. The infiltrate may consist of irregular nodular densities that are discrete or confluent, a homogeneous consolidation, or a diffuse patchy pattern. If seen on early chest x-ray, a more severe contusion is likely. Early pulmonary contusion infiltrates are due to alveolar hemorrhage. On the other hand, aspiration and reexpansion of collapsed right upper lobe (due to right mainstem intubation) are causes of early chest x-ray findings that are misdiagnosed as a pulmonary contusion. In most cases the infiltrates do not become apparent until after fluid resuscitation. Pulmonary contusions tend to worsen over 24–48 hours and then slowly resolve unless complicated by infection, ARDS, or cavitation (see question 16).

3. What causes a pulmonary contusion?

The basic argument is whether shear stress (tearing tissues) or bursting forces (popping the balloons) cause the tissue injury; it is likely that both elements are operational. It has been demonstrated in an animal model that impact velocity and chest wall displacement determine the severity and distribution of parenchymal injury. A high-velocity, low-displacement impact (T-bone motor vehicle accident) causes peripheral alveolar lung injury, whereas a low-velocity, high-displacement impact (crush) produces central parenchymal and major bronchial disruptions.

4. In their severe forms, flail chest and pulmonary contusion often coexist. What is the incidence of other concomitant injuries?

More than 90% of patients have associated intrathoracic injuries, including pulmonary contusion, hemothorax, or both. Three out of four patients require tube thoracostomy for hemopneumothorax. Extrathoracic injuries are common: head injuries occur in 40%, major fractures in 40%, and intraabdominal injuries in 30%.

5. What is the mortality rate and cause of death in combined flail chest/pulmonary contusion injuries?

Despite tremendous advances in trauma and critical care, current mortality is 25%. Improved prehospital care no doubt contributes to this persistently high mortality by delivering more severely injured patients to the reporting trauma centers. Early deaths are due to extrathoracic hemorrhage (e.g., pelvic fracture, liver injuries), and head injury; late mortality relates to sepsis and multiple organ failure. Factors that portend a poor outcome include presence of shock (blood pressure < 90 mmHg), high Injury Severity Score (ISS > 25), associated head injury (Glasgow coma scale < 7), falls from great heights (> 20 feet), preexisting disease (atherosclerotic heart disease, COPD, Laennec's cirrhosis), and advanced age (> 65 yr).

6. Describe the initial priorities in the management of patients with severe blunt chest trauma.

Patient management is prioritized according to the physiologic need for survival. The initial ABCs (airway, breathing, circulation) of advance trauma life support (ATLS) are directed at establishing peripheral oxygen delivery before a specific diagnosis is made. Prophylactic tube thoracostomy for suspected hemopneumothorax, empirical tracheal intubation, and mechanical ventilation are clearly warranted in the unstable, multisystem-injured patient with chest injuries. If time permits, cervical spine fractures should be excluded so that a large-bore orotracheal tube can be placed safely. Volume resuscitation is initiated promptly since hypovolemia is the most likely cause of reversible postinjury shock. The early use of crystalloid versus colloid is an unresolved controversy, and both will leak through damaged capillary endothelium. Most authorities agree that albumin or artificial plasma expanders are no more effective in restoring tissue perfusion than when adequate sodium is provided. Moreover, colloids are costly and may aggravate pulmonary complications in the setting of disrupted capillary membranes. We prefer isotonic saline for emergent resuscitation. When crystalloid infusions exceed 50 cc/kg in the ER, blood is administered to increase oxygen-carrying capacity. The next step is to assess life-threatening sources of hemorrhage as well as the presence of cardiogenic shock. Patients who cannot be resuscitated quickly in the ED must be treated definitively in the OR. Once life-threatening injuries have been treated, all efforts are directed at completing resuscitation. Core hypothermia is reversed, metabolic acidosis corrected, and mechanical ventilation is optimized.

7. What are the basic treatment strategies for flail chest/pulmonary contusions?

The tenets of management center on five principles: close observation of respiratory status if not intubated (see question 8), ample pain control, aggressive lung physiotherapy, early mobilization, and adequate nutrition. Pulmonary care should center on measures to prevent atelectasis, including incentive spirometry in all nonventilated patients and intermittent positive-pressure breathing for patients who fail incentive spirometry. Adequate pain control can seldom be obtained without intravenous narcotics, including patient-controlled analgesia. Important adjuncts to pain control include epidural analgesia and, more recently, continuous intercostal nerve blockade. Early restoration of mobility, including early fixation of lung bone and pelvic fractures when possible, is also beneficial.

8. What are the pitfalls in pain management of nonintubated patients with blunt chest trauma?

Sufficient pain control is the vital adjunct that permits patient mobilization, deep breathing, and secretion clearance. Pain from multiple rib, long bone, and pelvic fractures is surprisingly variable and difficult to evaluate clinically. Intermittent dosing of intravenous naroctics can oversedate if large doses are administered and can depress respiratory efforts and cough reflex, whereas long intervals allow the patients to experience cycles of significant pain and anxiety. Participation in respiratory care is thus limited to both ends of this dosing regimen. Small parenteral dosing at short intervals is preferred. We have found the patient controlled analgesia (PCA) device to be invaluable in achieving this goal. But irrespective of how sophisticated we become in delivering systemic analgesia, the primary limitation is depression in respiratory drive, and therefore regional anesthetic techniques have been aggressively pursued for the spontaneously breathing, chest-injured patient. Intercostal nerve blocks are highly effective for simple rib fractures, but are not suitable for flail chest injuries because of the multiple ribs involved and the repetition that is therapeutically necessary. Although intercostal and intrapleural catheter infusions of anesthetics have been described, the most convincingly successful application of regional anesthesia in chest trauma is continuous epidural infusion of local anesthetics or narcotics or, more recently, continuous intercostal nerve blockade with local anesthetic.

9. Which respiratory therapy procedure(s) should be ordered for patients with significant blunt chest trauma?

Vigorous ambulation remains the best method of restoring normal respiratory physiology; early removal of monitoring lines, chest tubes, and Foley catheters should be considered to achieve this goal.

Loss of lung volume is the major mechanism contributing to postsurgical pulmonary complication, and maximal lung expansion can best be achieved with the **incentive spirometer** (IS), which permits maximal inspiration without resistance while it provides visual quantification of the patient's efforts. This "incentive" encourages the patient to repeat the effort frequently. A major advantage is that IS can be performed with little supervision at frequent enough intervals (10 times per hour) to maintain lung volume. It also provides an effective means of monitoring a patient's progress. An abrupt setback may signal inadequate pain relief, progression of the pulmonary contusion, or onset of a new problem such as lobar collapse or pneumothorax.

Intermittent positive-pressure breathing (IPPB) is labor intensive and is reserved for patients who cannot generate adequate inspiratory lung volume with IS. It is generally performed at 4-hour intervals to promote coughing and improve ventilation as well as deliver bronchodilators.

Chest physiotherapy (CPT) is another frequently employed modality and consists of postural drainage, enhanced coughing maneuvers, chest vibration, and chest percussion. Despite its widespread use, prospective studies have shown no advantage of routine CPT in postsurgical prophylaxis, and it may actually worsen oxygenation. We limit its use to patients with tenacious secretions as well as adjunct to the treatment of lobar collapse. Obviously chest percussion will not be tolerated in the face of multiple rib fractures, but **positional drainage and coughing** can be quite effective.

10. Do all patients with flail chest require mechanical ventilation? Why or why not?

No. Only selected patients with flail chest require mechanical ventilation. Recent studies have shown that patients who are not intubated but are treated with aggressive pulmonary care have significantly shorter ICU stays, less pneumonia, and reduced mortality.

Roughly 20% need short-term ventilation for nonthoracic indications, primarily head injuries or major operative intervention, and another 40% are mechanically ventilated because of respiratory failure. Standard intubation criteria can be used. Inadequate oxygenation is defined as PaO_2/FiO_2 ratio < 250 or alveolar-arterial oxygen gradient > 400 mmHg. Measures of impaired ventilation include respiratory rate > 35 breaths per minute, $PaCO_2$ > 50 mmHg, or respiratory acidosis with a pH < 7.25. Other factors to consider are mental status, physiologic reserve (age, chronic disease), and metabolic stress (shock, associated injuries, ISS).

11. What is the optimal mode of ventilation for patients with flail chest or pulmonary contusion?

The optimal mode of ventilation continues to be debated. The decision depends on the time after injury and degree of pulmonary dysfunction. In the early phase of multisystem resuscitation, CO_2 production may increase abruptly (resuscitation, hypermetabolism, sepsis) or CO_2 elimination may deteriorate suddenly (mucous plug, bronchospasm, ARDS), both sharply increasing minute ventilation demands. The issue here is whether to provide full ventilatory support (with the assist control [AC] mode, high-rate intermittent mandatory ventilation, or pressure control) or partial ventilatory support with pressure support (PS) or bilevel partial airway pressure (BIPAP). As ventilation requirements increase, patients who receive full ventilatory support are prone to develop auto-PEEP. (See question 12.) On the other hand, with partial ventilatory support, the patient is required to supply added work of breathing and consequently must be monitored closely for hypoventilation (respiratory acidosis). The chest-injured patient is particularly vulnerable to fail on partial ventilatory support because the work of breathing is high (decreased compliance, increased airway resistance), plus the ability to contribute added ventilation is limited by chest wall pain and mechanics. PS and airway pressure release ventilation (APRV), which are popular weaning modes, should not be used in the acute setting because as compliance worsens tidal volumes will decrease, and there will be progressive loss of lung volume. Note that when using AC or IMV in patients with severe unilateral pulmonary contusions, tidal volumes are delivered unevenly. This can result in overdistention of the normal lung and underdistention of the injured lung. In this setting, independent lung ventilation via a double lumen endotracheal tube can be life-saving. This, however, is quite labor intensive and cannot be maintained for long periods.

Patients who were intubated for nonthoracic indications and those whose pulmonary dysfunction improves should be extubated as soon as possible to avoid bacterial contamination of the contused lung and receive adequate pain relief as well as aggressive pulmonary care to avoid loss of lung volume and reintubation. Patients who cannot be extubated should receive partial ventilatory support (we prefer IMV/PS or bilevel) with PEEP or CPAP to maintain functional residual capacity. The patients are encouraged to contribute as much ventilation as they can because this will result in less positive airway pressure and better matching of ventilation and perfusion. Patients whose pulmonary function continues to deteriorate (i.e., worsening oxygenation) may be better served by utilizing low tidal volume ventilation (4–7 ml/kg) with permissive hypercapnia. The continued use of large tidal volumes (10–12 ml/kg) and high ventilatory rates to maintain a normal $PaCO_2$ is believed to cause iatrogenic barotrauma. Clinical studies have shown low tidal volume ventilation to be well tolerated and to be associated with better than expected outcomes.

12. What is the role of positive end-expiratory pressure (PEEP) in the management of blunt chest trauma?

For the past two decades PEEP has been an invaluable adjunct to ventilator management of hypoxic postinjury respiratory failure. Improvement in arterial oxygenation results from an increase in alveolar size and recruitment. Presumptive application in multisystem trauma may limit atelectasis, decrease exposure to high inspired oxygen concentration, and even attenuate the natural history of acute lung injury, but indiscriminate use may have profound adverse effects. In the hypovolemic patient, PEEP can embarrass cardiac work. It also produces barotrauma, raises intracranial pressure, promotes accumulation of lung fluid, and increases pulmonary vascular resistance. In flail chest/pulmonary contusion where regional differences in compliance and airway resistance exist, PEEP can accentuate V/Q mismatch. We routinely apply 5 cm H_2O PEEP. If FiO_2 cannot be lowered to at least 0.60 within 12 hours, additional PEEP is used. As acute respiratory failure resolves, PEEP levels are weaned.

13. Are there alternative means to avoid intubation/mechanical ventilation in patients with severe blunt chest trauma?

Mask CPAP is particularly attractive for the patient who initially does not require emergent intubation. CPAP restores functional residual capacity, improves compliance, and stabilizes the flail segment until the underlying pulmonary contusion resolves, thus eliminating the need for intubation/mechanical ventilation. Ideally, mask CPAP should be applied prior to severe hypoxemia and there should be no evidence of CO_2 retention. The patient should be alert with a functioning nasogastric tube to prevent serious aspiration. Patients with maxillofacial injuries may not tolerate the tightly applied mask and are at risk for pneumocephalus if a basilar skull fracture exists.

14. What is the long-term morbidity in flail chest injuries?
Lone-term disability has not been well studied. In a recent review of 32 patients with flail chest with a mean follow-up of 5 years, only 12 (38%) had returned to full-time employment. Most complaints were subjective, such as chest tightness, pain, and decreased activity level. Another study reported on 22 patients with isolated flail chest injuries. Follow-up was 2 months to 2 years. Two-thirds experienced long-term morbidity. Persistent chest wall pain, dyspnea on exertion, and chest wall deformity were the most frequent complaints. Five (22%) remained disabled. Additional studies are clearly needed.

15. Are prophylactic antibiotics indicated in severe chest trauma?
No clear data address this issue in severely injured patients. The best available data are derived from studies of trauma patients requiring chest tubes. Prospective randomized trials offer conflicting results, but a recent meta-analysis suggests that prophylactic antibiotics can reduce empyemas. Given that our empyema rate is quite low, we do not routinely administer prophylactic antibiotics. Pneumonia is the major source of septic morbidity and most occur late. A short early course of antibiotics does not prevent late pneumonias, whereas longer coverage selects out a more virulent host flora. On the other hand, patients with combined flail chest/pulmonary contusion are at increased risk for early pneumonia secondary to aspiration. They typically have evolving chest x-ray infiltrates and hypermetabolism, which makes the diagnosis of early pneumonia difficult. When clinical judgment suggests infection, patients should be presumptively treated. A sputum Gram stain should be obtained to determine the most likely pathogen. The most frequent isolates are *Staphylococcus aureus*, *Haemophilus influenzae*, and normal oral flora.

16. What is posttraumatic pulmonary pseudocyst (PPP)? How is it managed?
PPP describes an air- or fluid-filled intraparenchymal that occurs in the setting of blunt chest trauma. PPP, although unusual, should be considered in all adults sustaining a serious pulmonary contusion. The pseudocyst typically evolves over the first week as a nonspecific air- or fluid-filled loculation seen on plain films. CT scanning of the chest is critical to define air-fluid levels seen on plain films, but its use should be limited to patients with signs of sepsis. In our experience with adult patients, infected pseudocysts are not responsive to antibiotics. Prompt diagnostic aspiration is valuable. Simple infected pseudocysts should be drained percutaneously; complex pseudocysts should be considered for early thoracotomy with the anticipation that formal lobectomy may be necessary.

BIBLIOGRAPHY

1. Acute Respiratory Distress Syndrome Neworks: Ventilation with lower tidal volumes as compared with traditional tidal volumes for acute lung injury and the acute respiratory distress syndrome. N Engl J Med 342:1301–1308, 2000.
2. Bolliger CT, Van Eden SF: Treatment of multiple rib-fractures randomized controlled trial comparing ventilatory with nonventilatory management. Chest 97:943–948, 1990.
3. Ciraulo DL, Elliott D, Mitchell KA, et al: Flail chest as a marker for significant injuries. J Am Coll Surg 178:466–470, 1994.
4. Clark GC, Shecter WP, Trunkey DD: Variables affecting outcome in blunt chest trauma: Flail chest vs. pulmonary contusion. J Trauma 28:298–304, 1988.
5. Haenel JB, Moore FA, Moore EE: Pulmonary consequences of severe chest trauma. Resp Care Clin North Am 2:401–424, 1996.
6. Haenel JB, Moore FA, Moore EE, et al: Continuous intercostal nerve block for amelioration of multiple rib fracture pain. J Trauma 38:22–29, 1995.

7. Hurst JM, Dehaven CB, Branson RD: Comparison of conventional mechanical ventilation and synchronous independent lung ventilation (SILV) in the treatment of unilateral lung injury. J Trauma 25:766–787, 1985.
8. Mackersie RC, Shackford SR, Hoyt DB, et al: Continuous epidural fentanyl analgesia: Ventilatory function improvement with routine use in treatment of blunt chest injury. J Trauma 27:1207–1212, 1987.
9. McIntyre RC, Haenel JB, Moore FA, et al: Cardiovascular effect of permissive hypercapnea in adult respiratory distress syndrome. J Trauma 37:433–439, 1994.
10. Moore FA, Moore EE, Haenel JB, et al: Post-traumatic pulmonary pseudocyst in the adult: Pathophysiology, recognition, and selective management. J Trauma 29:1380–1385, 1989.
11. Shackford SR: Blunt chest trauma in the intensivist's perspective. J Intens Care Med 1:125–136, 1986.
12. Shapiro BA, Cane RD, Harrison RA: Positive end-expiratory pressure therapy in adults with special reference to acute lung injury: A review of the literature and suggested clinical correlations. Crit Care Med 12:127–141, 1984.
13. Tanaka H, Maemura T, Yukioka T, et al: Surgical stabilization or internal pneumatic stabilization? An evaluation study of management of severe flail chest patients. J Trauma 41:200, 1996.
14. Voggenreiter G, Neudeck F, Aufmkolk M, et al: Operative chest wall stabilization in flail chest: Outcomes of patients with or without pulmonary contusion. J Am Coll Surg 187:130–138, 1998.

82. FAT EMBOLISM SYNDROME

Patrick Nana-Sinkam, M.D., and Mark W. Geraci, M.D.

1. Define fat embolism syndrome (FES).

FES is a clinical condition characterized by the classic triad of respiratory insufficiency, global neurologic dysfunction, and petechial rash. It most commonly occurs after fractures of long bones or other instances of bone marrow disruption that result in the appearance of free fat and fatty acids in the blood, lungs, kidneys, and other organs. The classic triad is seen in 0.5–2% of solitary long bone fractures; however, the incidence approaches 5–10% in multiple fractures with pelvic involvement. FES should be distinguished from isolated fat embolism, which may or may not be associated with clinically significant embolization.

2. When was FES first recognized?

The first description of the FES was offered by Zenker in 1862. He described the findings of microscopic fat emboli in the lungs of a patient who had been killed after being crushed between two railroad cars, and proposed that the ensuing respiratory compromise was the cause of death. Although his patient had fractured ribs, Zenker postulated that the embolized fat originated from the contents of a lacerated stomach having entered torn hepatic veins.

3. Describe the pathogenesis of FES.

The pathogenesis is controversial. The most cogent and widely accepted theory holds that embolic marrow fat derived from the fracture site is the central inciting agent. The fat is concentrated in the pulmonary bed and serves to activate the clotting cascade, increase platelet function and fibrinolytic activity, and induce catecholamine-mediated mobilization of free fatty acids. These free fatty acids directly increase capillary permeability. Along with the release of inflammatory mediators, the final common pathway results in critical impairment of gas exchange, and a form of adult respiratory distress syndrome. A more recent theory argues that fat embolism may be derived in part from chylomicrons and very-low-density lipoproteins agglutinated in the plasma. Acute-phase reactant proteins, particularly C-reactive protein (CRP), have been involved in the process of causing agglutination of intravenous fat emulsions in trauma victims and other critically ill patients.

4. Who is at risk for FES?

Fat embolism to the lungs and peripheral microcirculation occurs in over 90% of long bone fractures; however, only some 2–5% of patients develop the clinical syndrome. FES most commonly occurs after femoral and pelvic fractures but also has been reported after fractures of the humerus. The incidence in children is 100 times less frequent than in adults with comparable injuries. This finding is secondary to differences in either the content or composition of marrow fat. Certain clinical conditions cause increased liquid marrow fat content and medullary cavity enlargement, which can predispose to the FES.

Causes of Fat Embolism Syndrome

Fractures (>90% of all cases)	Steroid therapy
Nontraumatic orthopedic procedures, mainly joint reconstruction	Decompression sickness and high altitude flights
Burns	Parenteral infusion of lipids
Osteomyelitis	Bone marrow harvesting and transplant
Myelodysplastic syndromes	Liposuction
Collagen vascular diseases	Alcoholic liver disease
Sickle cell disease	Epilepsy
Pancreatitis	Cardiopulmonary bypass
Diabetes mellitus	Use of propofol in the intensive care unit
After extracorporeal circulation	

5. Describe the clinical presentation of FES.

The clinical presentation is usually marked by a latency period of 12–72 hours. Respiratory impairment leads to hypoxemia in up to 30% of patients and, on rare occasions, to respiratory failure requiring mechanical ventilation. The chest x-ray often shows diffuse pulmonary infiltrates. Cerebral symptoms may occur in 60% of patients and tend to follow the pulmonary symptoms. Central nervous system impairment may range from restlessness, confusion, and focal deficits to seizures and coma and may occur without evidence of respiratory insufficiency. A petechial rash appears in 50% of patients and is usually found on the neck, axilla, trunk or conjunctivae. The rash is short-lived, usually lasting for only 6 hours.

6. How is FES diagnosed?

The diagnosis is made on clinical grounds and diagnostic criteria are varied. The two most widely accepted criteria are presented. Gurd's (1970) criteria are grouped into major and minor features. Schonfeld (1983) advocates a fat embolism index score.

Diagnosis of FES According to Gurd's (1970) Criteria*

Major features	Minor features	Laboratory features
• Respiratory insufficiency	• Fever	• Anemia
• Cerebral involvement	• Tachycardia	• Thrombocytopenia
• Petechial rash	• Retinal changes	• Elevated erythrocyte sedimentation rate
	• Jaundice	• Fat macroglobulinemia
	• Renal changes	

* A positive diagnosis requires one major feature plus four minor features and fat macroglobulinemia.

Diagnosis of FES According to Schonfeld's (1983) Criteria*

SYMPTOM	SCORE
Petechiae	5
Diffuse alveolar infiltrates	4
Hypoxemia (PaO$_2$, 70 torr)	3
Confusion	1
Fever (≥ 38° C)	1
Heart rate ≥ 120/min	1
Respiratory rate ≥ 30/min	1

* A positive diagnosis has a cumulative score ≥ 5.

7. Are there specific tests to aid in the diagnosis of FES?

There is no single test to diagnose FES, but a pattern of biochemical abnormalities may be seen. Hematologic studies may reveal decreased hematocrit and platelets, whereas fibrin degradation products, prothrombin time, erythrocyte sedimentation rate, and C5a levels are often all elevated. Biochemical abnormalities include lowered calcium and the presence of fat microaggregates in samples of clotted blood. In a large series studied prospectively, the commonly held tenet of fat globules presenting in the urine was not found in any patient with FES. Recently, both bronchoalveolar lavage (looking for fat droplets in alveolar macrophages) and pulmonary artery catheter blood sampling for cytology have been proposed as methods of early diagnosis of FES. Unfortunately, both lack specificity. Radiographic studies are particularly useful in cases of suspected cerebral involvement. Although computed tomography of the brain may be normal, magnetic resonance imaging characteristically reveals multiple high-density lesions on T2-weighted imaged and low-density lesions on T1-weighted images. Common areas of involvement include basal ganglia, corpus callosum, cerebral deep white matter, and cerebellar hemispheres. Findings on imaging tend to resolve with clinical improvement.

8. How is FES treated?

A number of treatment modalities have been studied. The use of ethanol, heparin, low-molecular-weight dextran, and hypertonic glucose has shown inconsistent results and none is currently advocated. The first successful treatment of FES with corticosteroids was reported by Ashbaugh and Petty in 1966. In a well-designed, prospective, randomized, double-blind study of patients at high risk for FES, Schonfeld et al. demonstrated that prophylactic use of methylprednisolone, 7.5 mg/kg intravenously every 6 hours for 12 doses, significantly reduced the incidence of the FES. Lindeque et al. found similar results even with less stringent diagnostic criteria, using a dose of methylprednisolone of 30 mg/kg IV on admission and a single repeat dose after 4 hours. In both studies, the use of steroids had no adverse effects on fracture healing. The mechanism of steroid effectiveness likely involves membrane stabilization, limitation in the rise of plasma free fatty acids, and inhibition of the complement-mediated leukocyte aggregation. The effectiveness of steroids other than for prophylaxis remains to be tested. In short, the treatment includes aggressive supportive care, early ventilatory support, and early steroid use.

9. Does early operative intervention change outcome?

Retrospective studies seem to confirm that early operative stabilization of fractures within the first 24 hours reduces the incidence of acute respiratory distress syndrome (ARDS) from 75% for delayed surgery to 17% for early surgery. Obviating the development of ARDS provides a survival advantage and decreases morbidity as well as hospital stay.

10. What is the prognosis for patients with FES?

Mortality often depends on the underlying extent of injury. For uncomplicated FES, though, the mortality is often much less than for other types of ARDS, and is most often quoted as 10%. FES is self-limited, and, provided oxygenation is maintained, pulmonary function can be expected to return to normal. Most of the long-term morbidity is associated with cerebral complications, particularly focal neurologic deficits.

BIBLIOGRAPHY

1. Ashbaugh DG, Petty TL: The use of corticosteroids in the treatment of respiratory failure associated with massive fat embolism. Surg Gynecol Obstet 123:493–500, 1966.
2. Chastre J, Fagon JY, Soler P, et al: Bronchoalveolar lavage for rapid diagnosis of the fat embolism syndrome in trauma patients. Ann Intern Med 113:583–588, 1990.
3. Gosling HR, Pellegrini VD: Fat embolism syndrome: A review of the pathophysiology and physiological basis of treatment. Clin Orthop 165:68–82, 1982.
4. Gurd AR: Fat embolism: An aid to diagnosis. J Bone Joint Surg 52:732–737, 1970.
5. Hulman G: The pathogenesis of fat embolism. J Pathol 76:3–9, 1995.

6. Johnson KD, Cadambi A, Seibert GB: Incidence of adult respiratory distress syndrome in patients with multiple musculoskeletal injuries: Effects of early operative stabilization of fractures. J Trauma 25:375–384, 1985.
7. Johnson MJ, Lucas GL: Fat embolism syndrome. Orthopedics 19:41–48, 1996.
8. Lindeque BGP, Schoeman HS, Dommisse GF, et al: Fat embolism and the fat embolism syndrome: A double-blind therapeutic study. J Bone Joint Surg 69B:128–131, 1987.
9. Mellor A, Soni N: Fat embolism. Anaesthesia 56:145–154, 2001.
10. Parizel PM, Demey HE, Veeckmans G, et al: Early diagnosis of cerebral fat embolism syndrome by diffusion-weighted MRI (starfield pattern). Stroke 32:2942–2944, 2001.
11. Peltier LE: Fat embolism: A perspective. Clin Orthop 232:263–270, 1988.
12. Roger N, Xambet A, Agusti C, et al: Role of bronchoalveolar lavage in the diagnosis of fat embolism syndrome. Eur Respir J 8:1275–1280, 1995.
13. Schonfeld SA, Ploysongsang Y, DiLisio R, et al: Fat embolism prophylaxis with corticosteroids: A prospective study in high-risk patients. Ann Intern Med 99:438–443, 1983.
14. ten Duis HJ: The fat embolism syndrome. Injury 28:77–85, 1997.
15. Van Besouw JP, Hinds CJ: Fat embolism syndrome. Br J Hosp Med 42:304–311, 1989.
16. Vedrinne JM, Guillaume C, Gagnieu MC, et al: Bronchoalveolar lavage in trauma patients for the diagnosis of fat embolism. Chest 102:1323–1327, 1992.
17. Zenker FA: Beitrage zur normalen und pathologischen Anatomie der Lunge. Dresden, J Braunsdorf, 1862.

83. MYOCARDIAL CONTUSION

John C. Messenger, M.D., and Eugene E. Wolfel, M.D.

1. What causes cardiac injury in blunt chest trauma?

Nonpenetrating cardiac trauma is most often associated with motor vehicle accidents, often due to steering wheel trauma or blunt chest trauma experienced by unrestrained passengers. Chest injuries account for 25% of the 50,000–60,000 deaths per year due to auto accidents and contribute significantly to another 25% of deaths. The incidence of myocardial contusion varies depending on the diagnostic modality and criteria used, but ranges in the literature from 8–71%. Other causes include direct blows to the chest, falls from heights, crush injuries and, rarely, a kick from a large animal. Myocardial contusion is part of a spectrum of injuries now called blunt cardiac injury (BCI).

2. What is myocardial contusion?

Myocardial contusion results from direct damage to the myocardium without traumatic involvement of the coronary arteries. Pathologically, there is evidence of myocyte injury with cell necrosis, edema, and interstitial hemorrhage. Often, injury is limited to the subepicardial or subendocardial tissue without evidence of transmural injury. Clinically, the diagnosis depends on the noninvasive test used to define it, as there is no accepted "gold standard" other than autopsy findings. In general, it refers to transient myocardial dysfunction associated with or without laboratory evidence of myocardial necrosis. The majority of myocardial contusions diagnosed by radionuclide study or echocardiogram resolve during follow-up, revealing the transient nature of this injury. Due to the anterior location of the right ventricle, it is not surprising it is the most common site of contusion. One echo study detected myocardial contusion (defined as a wall motion abnormality) in 31 of 105 patients with blunt chest trauma. Right ventricular (RV) and left ventricular (LV) contusions were present in 17 (55%), RV contusion alone in 12 (39%), and LV contusion alone in 2 (6%).

3. What other myocardial injuries may be associated with blunt chest trauma?

Most other injuries of the myocardium associated with blunt chest trauma have accompanying myocardial contusion. These complications include laceration and/or rupture of the atria or ventricles (atrial rupture is much more common), perforation of the interventricular septum, and development of ventricular aneurysm or pseudoaneurysm. Direct injury to the coronary arteries, with resultant thrombosis or dissection can result in myocardial damage similar to atherosclerotic myocardial infarction.

4. Are there associated chest injuries that make myocardial contusion more likely after blunt chest trauma?

Severe cardiac injury can occur with minimal or absent external signs of chest injury. However, in general, patients with more severe chest trauma, particularly those requiring care in the ICU, tend to have a higher incidence of myocardial contusion. Associated chest injuries in one large series included rib and clavicle fracture (50%), pulmonary contusion (44%), pneumothorax (33%), hemothorax (30%), flail chest (18.5%), sternal fracture (7%), and great vessel injury (7%). With any blunt trauma to the chest, the level of suspicion should be high for possible cardiac injury, particularly if faced with arrhythmias or refractory hypotension.

5. What clinical features associated with blunt chest trauma suggest myocardial contusion?

Myocardial contusion is usually clinically silent. Chest pain is very common in patients with suspected myocardial contusion and is usually related to other thoracic injuries. The pain of classic angina is unusual. Patients who present with unexplained sinus tachycardia or hemodynamic instability may have the first manifestations of myocardial dysfunction, but the possibility of pericardial tamponade should always be entertained. The presence of ventricular ectopy in the absence of significant hypoxemia or electrolyte abnormalities may indicate myocardial contusion, especially if seen early in the clinical course. Shock is rare, and if related to a cardiac cause, it usually represents tamponade, cardiac rupture or aortic dissection. The finding of a pericardial rub or the presence of an S3 on cardiac exam and rales on auscultation of the lungs suggest myocardial dysfunction and should raise suspicion for contusion.

6. What is the role of electrocardiography (EKG) in the diagnosis of myocardial contusion?

The EKG continues to play an important role in identifying patients with suspected myocardial contusion who require more aggressive diagnostic testing and monitoring. According to recent guidelines, an admission EKG should be performed for all patients in whom BCI is suspected. EKG findings that are considered abnormal include atrial or ventricular arrhythmias, ST-segment depression or elevation, marked T-wave inversions, interventricular conduction delay, or bundle-branch block. When EKG findings are compared with results of gated blood pool scan, thallium SPECT scans, or echocardiography, which detected wall motion abnormalities suggestive of myocardial contusion, it is clear that EKG is neither sensitive nor specific in the diagnosis of myocardial contusions. Nonetheless, multiple studies have demonstrated that the presence of a normal EKG in a hemodynamically stable patient identifies a group who are at low risk for complications. Ventricular arrhythmias, if present, can be a reasonable indicator of myocardial contusion, if they occur in the absence of other known arrhythmogenic factors.

7. What is the role of cardiac enzyme determinations in the diagnosis of myocardial contusion?

CK-MB. The MB fraction of creatine kinase is believed to be a highly sensitive routine test in the diagnosis of myocardial necrosis. Its efficacy is well established in myocardial infarction. Because myocardial contusion requires myocyte necrosis, one would think that measuring CK-MB would be useful. However, it is clear that CK-MB is neither sensitive nor specific in the diagnosis of myocardial contusion based on positive echocardiographic and radionuclide imaging studies. This may be due to a very small release of CK-MB with right ventricular contusions, or to the size and depth of myocardial damage from blunt trauma. In addition, it does not predict cardiac complications in patients with suspected myocardial contusion. Several recent studies have shown no utility to the test, and it currently should not be used routinely in patients suspected of having myocardial contusion.

Cardiac troponin T and I. Cardiac troponin T (cTnT) and cardiac troponin I (cTnI) are regulatory proteins found exclusively in cardiac tissue. Recent studies have shown that it has a high sensitivity for detecting myocardial injury and an improved specificity over CK-MB. One study in patients with blunt chest trauma revealed a very high sensitivity and specificity for cTnI when echocardiography was used to detect wall motion abnormalities suggestive of myocardial contusion. Its superior specificity over CK-MB is most likely related to its exclusive presence in the myocardium. Nonetheless, several recent studies assessing the utility of troponins in BCI have revealed that, despite increased specificity compared with CK-MB, they have low sensitivity and low predictive value in diagnosing myocardial contusion and do not affect management of patients.

8. How is echocardiography used in the diagnosis and management of myocardial contusion?

Transthoracic echocardiogram (TTE). The use of two-dimensional echocardiography along with Doppler ultrasound is a very useful diagnostic tool in the assessment of myocardial contusion. It is portable, allowing rapid bedside diagnosis. The presence of segmental wall motion abnormalities suggest contusion, and many investigators are using echo as the gold standard currently. It is also useful for assessing the pericardial space as well as valve structure and integrity. Potential complications of myocardial contusion, such as right or left ventricular mural thrombus, aneurysm or pseudoaneurysm, can also be recognized. In several studies, however, failure to achieve adequate images occurred in 15–62% of patients studied, limiting the usefulness of this test. Of greater importance, echocardiography does not allow prediction of a subgroup of patients with cardiac complications.

Transesophageal echocardiogram (TEE). Several recent studies have examined the usefulness of TEE in patients with blunt chest trauma. It is a more "invasive" test than transthoracic echo, but has a very high success rate and very few complications. In one recent study, cardiac contusion was diagnosed by TEE in 34% of patients with injuries from blunt chest trauma. In addition, it is a very useful tool for the diagnosis of traumatic aortic rupture, and is comparable to CT scan or aortography. However, TEE does not appear superior to TTE in predicting a subgroup of patients at increased risk for cardiac complications and adds to cost.

9. Does imaging of the heart with radioisotopes help in the diagnosis of myocardial contusion?

Imaging techniques such as technetium pyrophosphate (infarct scanning), thallium scintigraphy, or radionuclide ventriculography have been studied extensively in the past but have fallen out of favor. In general, these studies are expensive and have failed to predict patients at risk of cardiac complications from cardiac cntusionis. In particular, they add little if echocardiography is performed.

10. What are the indications for invasive cardiac diagnostic studies in myocardial contusion?

Invasive studies are generally not used to make the diagnosis. If there is strong suspicion of coronary involvement with the development of new pathologic Q waves, significant ST elevation in 2 adjacent leads on the EKG, or the presence of a continuous cardiac murmur suggesting a possible coronary artery fistula, then coronary arteriography is indicated. Right heart catheterization with a balloon flotation pulmonary artery catheter may be useful in patients with hemodynamic instability. The equilibration of intracardiac pressures, particularly with elevated right atrial and pulmonary capillary wedge pressure, is highly suggestive of pericardial tamponade. In addition, right ventricular injury, left ventricular dysfunction, and pulmonary artery hypertension can be diagnosed in this manner. By sampling blood for oxygen saturation in the various right heart chambers, a diagnosis of traumatic intracardiac left-to-right shunt can be made. All of these conditions are relatively uncommon and can be made noninvasively now with echo-Doppler study.

11. Based on the above information, what is the optimal approach to the diagnosis of myocardial contusion?

It is clear in looking at the literature that the problem with this diagnosis is the lack of an easily obtainable gold standard. More recently, investigators have moved away from trying to make the diagnosis of myocardial contusion and have tried to focus on the risk factors that predict cardiac complications in patients who have blunt chest trauma. A high index of suspicion for the diagnosis is essential. Upon arrival in the emergency department, a brief physical exam to assess for JVD, pulmonary rales, or the presence of a third heart sound or rub should be performed. An initial EKG should be obtained to assess for significant abnormalities (conduction block, atrial or ventricular arrhythmias or significant ST elevation or depression). Finally, a chest x-ray should be performed. There is no need to draw cardiac enzymes unless the EKG reveals changes suggestive of ischemia or infarction, and serial enzymes should not be drawn routinely. In the setting of an anbormal EKG, cardiac troponin I or T appears to be superior to CK-MB and should be used, if available. Patients with a prior cardiac history may benefit from early evaluation with echocardiography. In patients with suspected myocardial contusion and significant arrhythmias or hemodyamic instability, TTE should be performeded. If necessary, TEE may be performed if the TTE is nondiagnostic.

12. Describe the standard treatment of myocardial contusion.

The overwhelming majority of patients with myocardial contusion have no significant hemodynamic or electrical instability. The mere presence of myocardial contusion does not allow accurate prediction of patients who will develop cardiac complications. Therefore, the hospital course should be dictated by the extent of associated injuries. Asymptomatic patients with no associated injuries may be discharged from the emergency department after short observation if the EKG does not reveal significant abnormalities. Patients who have a prior history of coronary artery disease may be monitored on telemetry for 24 hours and have serial EKGs; however, serial cardiac enzymes should not be ordered routinely. The overwhelming majority of patients with cardiac contusions that go on to develop cardiac complications (arrhythmias, heart failure) will do so while being monitored in the ICU, as they tend to have more associated injuries that require treatment in an intensive care setting. In several large studies, there have not been any cardiac-related deaths in patients triaged to telemetry or regular ward beds.

Unlike anesthetic risks associated with recent myocardial infarction, patients with myocardial contusion appear to have a very low risk associated with anesthesia, and operative treatment should not be delayed in this patient population. If necessary, invasive hemodynamic monitoring may be performed in patients with suspected LV dysfunction. If there is an associated mural thrombus, the embolic risks must be weighed against the risk of bleeding related to anticoagulation in patients suffering blunt chest trauma. Usually patients with myocardial contusion require no specific follow-up, unless they have a complicated cardiac clinical course. In patients with severe wall motion abnormalities noted on echo, a follow-up echo should be performed at 4–6 weeks to exclude the rare late complications of aneurysm or pseudoaneurysm. Wall motion abnormalities resolve in between 80 and 90% of patients with initial abnormal findings.

CONTROVERSIES

13. Is routine hospitalization with EKG monitoring required in all cases of blunt chest trauma with suspected myocardial contusion?

For:

1. Some patients will have unrecognized significant myocardial injury that may result in serious ventricular arrhythmias or other cardiac complications.

2. Because myocardial dysfunction has been evident on echocardiograms even in the presence of a normal 12-lead EKG and normal cardiac enzymes, all patients should be observed for possible adverse cardiac events.

Against:

1. The prognosis in these patients is excellent and their clinical course is dictated by noncardiac injuries. Therefore, in patients with no significant injuries, a short period of monitoring in the emergency department is sufficient.

2. Several clinical factors may be used to identify a higher risk group for further observation: the elderly, presence of arrhythmias or conduction defects on initial EKG, hemodynamic

abnormalities or abnormalities on chest x-ray, or prior cardiac history. These are the patients who should be admitted for further cardiac monitoring and possible diagnostic work-up.

14. Should echocardiograms be used in the standard evaluation of patients with blunt chest trauma for possible myocardial contusion?

For: These studies are the most sensitive means of determining injury to the myocardium and are useful in detecting possible serious cardiac complications from this injury. They will affect the subsequent length of hospitalization and further treatment of patients with blunt chest trauma.

Against: These studies are expensive and do not accurately predict which patients will go on to develop cardiac complications that will require intervention. The prognosis in uncomplicated patients with blunt chest trauma is excellent, and these studies only add to the cost of the hospitalization. Even if wall motion abnormalities are found, they resolve in 80–90% of cases on follow-up. The clinical outcome of these patients is determined by the extent of the noncardiac injuries. Only cardiac rupture has a profound effect on survival, and most of these patients expire before arrival at the emergency department.

15. Should all patients with sternal fractures be considered to have myocardial contusions and admitted for monitoring?

For: Sternal fractures are often an indication of serious intrathoracic injury, usually involving motor vehicle crashes, and are believed to be associated with a high rate of cardiac contusion.

Against: Isolated sternal fractures are common and increasing in frequency. Hemodynamically stable patients with a normal chest x-ray and a normal EKG have a very low rate of complications. Such patients can be safely discharged with oral pain medication and outpatient clinical follow-up.

BIBLIOGRAPHY

1. Adams JE, Davila-Roman VG, Bessey PQ, et al: Improved detection of cardiac contusion with cardiac troponin I. Am Heart J 131:308–312, 1996.
2. Bertinchant JP, Polge A, Mohty D, et al: Evaluation of incidence, clinical significance, and prognostic value of circulating cardiac troponin I and T elevation in hemodynamically stable patients with suspected myocardial contusion after blunt chest trauma. J Trauma 48:924–931, 2000.
3. Biffl WL, Moore FA, Moore EE, et al: Cardiac enzymes are irrelevant in the patient with suspected myocardial contusion. Am J Surg 169:523–528, 1994.
4. Chirillo F, Totis O, Cavarzerani A, et al: Usefulness of transthoracic and transoesophageal echocardiography in recognition and management of cardiovascular injuries after blunt chest trauma. Heart 75:301–306, 1996.
5. Collins JN, Cole FJ, Weireter LJ, et al: The usefulness of serum troponin levels in evaluating cardiac injury. Am Surg 67:821–826, 2001.
6. Feghali NT, Prisant LM: Blunt myocardial injury. Chest 108:1673–1677, 1995.
7. Hossack KF, Moreno CA, Vanway CW, Burdick DC: Frequency of cardiac contusion in nonpenetrating chest injury. Am J Cardiol 61:392–394, 1988.
8. Karalis DG, Victor MF, Davis GA, et al: The role of echocardiography in blunt chest trauma: A transthoracic and transesophageal echocardiographic study. J Trauma 36:53–58, 1994.
9. Nagy KK, Krosner SM, Roberts RR, et al: Determining which patients require evaluation for blunt cardiac injury following blunt chest trauma. World J Surg 25:108–111, 2001.
10. Pasuale M, Fabian TC: Practice management guidelines for trauma for the Eastern Association for the Surgery of Trauma. J Trauma 44:941–945, 1998.
11. Pretre R, Chilcott M: Blunt trauma to the heart and great vessels. N Engl J Med 336:626–632, 1997.
12. Ross P, Degutis L, Baker CC: Cardiac contusion: The effect on operative management of the patient with trauma injuries. Arch Surg 124:506–507, 1989.
13. Sadaba JR, Oswal D, Munsch CM: Management of isolated sternal fractures: Determining the risk of blunt cardiac injury. Ann R Coll Surg Engl 82:162–166, 2000.
14. Tenzer ML: The spectrum of myocardial contusion: A review. J Trauma 25:620–627, 1985.
15. Weiss RL, Brier JA, O'Connor W, et al: The usefulness of transesophageal echocardiography in diagnosing cardiac contusions. Chest 109:73–77, 1996.
16. Wisner DH, Reed WH, Riddick RS: Suspected myocardial contusion: Triage and indications for monitoring. Ann Surg 212:82–86, 1990.

84. LIVER AND HEART TRANSPLANTATION

Claus U. Niemann, M.D.

LIVER TRANSPLANTATION

1. How many liver transplantations are performed in the U.S. annually?

In 2000, 4954 liver transplantations were performed in the U.S, including increasing numbers from living liver donors. As of Janaury 2002, 18,710 patients are on the waiting list for liver transplantation. Approximately 1750 patients die annually while awaiting liver transplantation. Nationwide, the 3-year survival rate is 76%.

2. What are the indications for liver transplantation?

The list of diseases treatable by liver transplantation has increased steadily. The most common causes of end-stage liver disease leading to transplantation are chronic viral hepatitis B or C and alcoholic liver disease. The causes of chronic liver disease can be classified as follows:

Noncholestatic cirrhosis: alcohol, hepatitis A, B, C, and D, cryptogenic autoimmune disease, drug-induced cirrhosis.

Cholestatic cirrhosis: primary biliary cirrhosis, secondary biliary cirrhosis, primary sclerosing cholangitis.

Acute hepatic necrosis: of unknown cause, drug-induced disease, acute hepatitis, environmental exposure (e.g., mushrooms).

Metabolic disease: Wilson's disease, hemochromatosis, primary oxalosis, glycogen storage disease, alpha-1-antitrypsin deficiency, tyrosinemia, homozygous hyperlipidemia.

Malignant neoplasm: hepatocellular carcinoma, hepatoma and cirrhosis, bile duct carcinoma, hepatoblastoma, hemangiosarcoma.

Miscellaneous: biliary atresia (most common indication in children), cystic fibrosis, polycystic liver disease, Budd-Chiari syndrome, neonatal hepatitis

The Child-Turcotte-Pugh (CTP) classification has been used widely as an index of disease severity for patients with end-stage liver disease and until recently was used for the organ allocation algorithm. Because of the shortcomings of CTP scores and subsequent limitation in organ allocation, however, the model for end-stage liver disease (MELD) has been introduced. The MELD risk score is a mathematical formula that includes creatinine, bilirubin, and international normalized ratio (INR). It does not include the cause of liver disease.

3. Why is a patient rejected for liver transplantation?

Reasons to deny transplant may vary from center to center. Liver transplantation is an extremely stressful procedure for patients. Significant coronary artery disease, cardiac dysfunction, and pulmonary hypertension are considered contraindications for liver transplantation. Uncontrolled infection or sepsis also excludes a patient from transplantation. A positive HIV test without evidence of AIDS, however, is *not* a contraindication. In general, advanced malignant hepatic disease and metastatic disease are considered contraindications, as is uncontrolled and markedly elevated intracerebral pressure (ICP) in the case of fulminant hepatic failure. Psychosocial factors such as active alcohol abuse or lack of a good social support system may lead to exclusion. Hence, it is important to evaluate patients adequately in the preoperative phase and to order necessary diagnostic tests. Old age per se is not a reason to deny liver transplantation; patients older than 65 years now receive transplants with increasing frequency.

4. Describe the clinical problems of the typical patient before transplantation.

Virtually every organ system can be altered by end-stage liver failure. Consequently, global assessment and consideration of all organ systems are of paramount importance.

Central nervous system: hepatic encephalopathy and increased ICP in acute hepatic failure.

Cardiovascular system: hyperdynamic circulation, cirrhotic cardiomyopathy.

Respiratory system: hepatopulmonary syndrome ($PaO_2 < 70$ mmHg or AaO_2 gradient > 20 mmHg, intrapulmonary vascular dilation), portopulmonary hypertension (precapillary/arteriolar pulmonary hypertension, mPAP > 25 mmHg at rest, primary pulmonary hypertension ruled out).

Gastrointestinal (GI) system: portal hypertension with possible upper GI bleed, ascites.

Hematologic system: anemia, thrombocytopenia (sequestration into spleen), prolonged prothrombin time/partial thromboplastin time, decreased fibrinogen, and low-grade DIC.

Renal system: hepatorenal syndrome, acute tubular necrosis.

Miscellaneous: electrolyte disturbances of virtually any kind, immunosuppression, malnutrition with ascites.

5. What are the common perioperative complications of liver transplantations?

Perioperative complications depend on the medical condition of the recipient (see question 4). Hemodynamic instability due to blood loss and massive fluid shifts, severe coagulopathy, electrolyte/glucose abnormalities, renal dysfunction, and respiratory compromise are frequently seen. Ultrasound is warranted if patency of the hepatic artery and portal vein is in doubt. Thrombosis of the hepatic artery also requires retransplantation. Biliary leakage or bleeding is also seen postoperatively. In addition, complications may be due to poor organ quality. Organ quality depends on multiple factors, including donor age, organ ischemia time, and mechanism of death. Primary nonfunction of the donor organ, often manifesting immediately after transplantation, requires immediate retransplantation.

6. What are the indicators of good graft function in the immediate perioperative period?

Bile production (intraoperatively), correction of negative base excess, improvement in prothrombin time, and decreasing requirements for fresh frozen plasma.

7. Does every liver transplant patient need to stay intubated and be admitted to the ICU postoperatively?

Postoperative intubation is not required as long as significant respiratory compromise or concern about airway protection is absent. Patients are extubated in the operating room with increasing frequency. Fluid shifts or blood loss per se should be considered an indication for postoperative intubation. Most centers admit patients to the ICU for monitoring purposes. Certain centers, however, admit uncomplicated cases to the post-anesthesia care unit and then discharge them to the floor.

8. Describe patient management in the immediate postoperative period.

The perioperative course of patients undergoing liver transplantation is unpredictable and may range from uncomplicated to extremely complex. Frequent assessment of cardiac and pulmonary function, serum glucose/electrolytes, renal and liver function, and coagulation and blood count is of great importance. In most cases, therapy is supportive and follows guidelines established for all intensive care patients. However, certain aspects require special attention.

Coagulopathy/bleeding. Occasionally patients require postoperative fresh frozen plasma (FFP) to offset an initially sluggish liver function. FFP requirements are considered an indirect measurement of postoperative liver function. In general, FFP infusion can be weaned over the first few postoperative hours. Aprotinin and aminocaproic acid are used in cases of severe coagulopathies, which are not thought to be well controlled by FFP alone. Of note, some centers use these agents routinely in the perioperative phase to minimize blood loss. The need to administer platelets or cyroprecipitate is relatively low and reserved for selected cases. Lastly, one should have a low threshold for re-exploration. Leakage from vascular anastomosis sites, "bleeders," and diminished flow in the hepatic artery or portal vein should always be kept in mind.

Renal function. Renal dysfunction is common preoperatively and often worsens during the immediate postoperative period because of temporary renal outflow obstruction during surgery when the inferior vena cava is clamped for insertion of the donor liver. Intraoperatively venovenous bypass ameliorates the outflow obstruction but is not used at many centers. Close postoperative monitoring of renal function and supportive therapy with adequate fluid status, Lasix, and dopamine often suffice. In some cases, continuous renal replacement therapy (continuous venovenous hemofiltration [CVVH]) through the immediate postoperative period assists recovery of renal function.

Glucose/electrolytes. With adequate postoperative liver function and steriod administration, patients tend to be hyperglycemic, which may warrant an insulin drip. Depending on renal function and diuretic therapy, potassium can be either high or low. Calcium homeostasis is usually not a problem in the postoperative period.

Immunosuppression. Allograft rejection can occur at any point after surgery and is classified as hyperacute, acute, or chronic. Patients usually are started on immunosuppressive therapy immediately after surgery. Common drugs, often used in combination, include cyclosporine, tacrolimus, sirolimus, mycophenolate mofetil, and steroids. These agents can cauase various side effects, including undesired drug interactions, hypertension, hyperlipidemia, osteoporosis, thrombocytopenia, and atherosclerotic disease.

HEART TRANSPLANTATION

9. How many heart transplantations are performed in the U.S. annually?

In 2000, 2198 heart transplantatinos were performed in the U.S. As of January 2002, 4139 patients are on the waiting list for heart transplantation. Nationwide the 3-year survival rate is 77%.

10. What are the indications for heart transplantation?

Cardiac transplantation has become an accepted treatment for selected patients with end-stage heart failure. As for liver transplantation, the number of candidates and the waiting time have increased over the past years. The most common causes of end-stage heart disease leading to heart transplantation are cardiomyopathy and coronary artery disease. The causes of end-stage heart disease can be classified as follows:

Dilated cardiomyopathy: viral, idiopathic, postpartum, familial, adriamycin-induced, and ischemic cardiomyopathy; myocarditis.

Restricted cardiomyopathy: sarcoidosis, amyloidosis, endocardial fibrosis, idiopathic disease, radiation- or chemotherapy-induced disease.

Retransplantation/graft failure: primary failure; hyperacute, acute, or chronic rejection; nonspecific cause; restrictive/constrictive disease; coronary artery disease.

Other: congenital disease, valvular disease, hypertrophic cardiomyopathy.

Medical treatment of patients with end-stage heart disease continuously improves, and selected patients can be managed medically with symptomatic and survival outcomes similar to those of heart transplantation. Hence, heart transplantation should be offered to patients who experience severe disability due to cardiac disease despite optimal medical treatment and have no major contraindications to heart transplantation.

11. Why is a patient rejected for heart transplantation?

Similar criteria are applied as for patients with end-stage liver disease but vary somewhat from center to center. Significant irreversible pulmonary hypertension; renal, hepatic, or cerebrovascular disease; and chronic obstructive pulmonary disease are contraindications. In addition, lack of compliance, psychological instability, lack of supportive social environment, and active drug abuse may exclude a patient from heart transplantation. Old age per se is not a reason to deny heart transplantation; patients older than 65 years receive transplants with increasing frequency.

12. Describe the pathophysiology of the typical patient before heart transplantation.

In most cases, the pathophysiology is determined primarily by end-stage cardiomyopathy. Systolic and diastolic dysfunction is common. Subsequently, increased left ventricular pressures may lead to pulmonary congestion and edema. Increased autonomic sympathetic tone results in vasoconstriction and, in combination with ventricular dilatation, increased myocardial wall tension. Therapy (diuretics, vasodilators) aimed at symptom amelioration may result in hypokalemia, hypomagnesemia, and hypovolemia. As for all transplant patients, careful screening and monitoring for coexistent medical problems such as renal dysfunction are prudent.

13. Describe the typical pathophysiology after heart transplantation.

Cardiac denervation is a usual consequence of heart transplantation, and reinnervation is absent or rare. Although baseline cardiac function is maintained, cardiac response to demand is altered significantly. Heart rate can be increased only gradually by circulating catecholamines. Consequently, patients depend mainly on elevated stroke volumes—and hence on preload—to increase cardiac output. Maintenance of adequate preload is crucial. Denervation also affects pharmacologic therapy. Drugs that act on the heart indirectly (mediated through either the sympathetic or parasympathetic nervous system) are generally ineffective. Drugs that act directly on the heart are thus the agents of choice to modify cardiac physiology. In addition, denervation of the heart prevents the recipient from experiencing chest pain during myocardial ischemia.

14. What are the common complications of heart transplantation?

Although long-term survival has improved significantly, a number of complications may occur after transplantation. Examples include right ventricular failure/pulmonary hypertension, systemic hypertension, cardiac dysrhythmias, bleeding, early graft failure, allograft rejection, accelerated allograft coronary artery disease, renal dysfunction, and malignancy. Immunosuppressive agents can cause similar complications as outlined under liver transplantation. The postoperative stability of the patient is also affected by donor characteristis and operative technique. The bicaval technique is used most frequently.

15. Describe the management of the heart transplant recipient in the immediate postoperative period.

Postoperative care is similar to that of other cardiac surgical patients. However, based on the unique pathophysiology after heart transplantation (see question 13), close cardiac monitoring via EKG, arterial blood pressure, central venous pressure, and pulmonary artery pressure is important. The transplanted heart and its hemodynamic performance are highly dependent on preload, particularly in the early postoperative phase when myocardial dysfunction, relative bradycardia, and atrioventricular valve incompetence are present. Patients require continuous beta-adrenergic infusion (isoproterenol) for chronotropy or inotropy; in most cases, therapy can be weaned within a few days. However, certain aspects require special attention:

Increased pulmonary vascular resistance (PVR)/right ventricular failure. Because fixed pulmonary hypertension was excluded preoperatively, postoperative increases in PVR are usually transient and treatable. If untreated, however, they can lead to right ventricular failure. Vasodilators (e.g., prostaglandin E1, nitrates, hydralazine, inhaled nitric oxide) and occasionally a ventricular assist device can be used to control elevated PVR. Therapy may result in systemic hypotension, which requires an infusion of alpha agonists.

Cardiac dysrhythmias. Bradycardia, which is common postoperatively, can be treated with isoproterenol. In addition, isoproterenol also acts as a pulmonary vasodilator. Atrial and ventricular tachyarrhythmias are quite common after heart transplantation. Graft rejection may be responsible for such arrhythmias and needs to be ruled out before initiation of pharmacologic treatment.

Immunosuppression. Allograft rejection can occur at any time after surgery and is classified as hyperacute, acute, or chronic. Patients usually are started on immunosuppressive therapy immediately after surgery. Common drugs, often used in combination, are cyclosporine, tacrolimus, sirolimus, mycophenolate mofetil, azathioprine, and steroids. These agents can cause various side effects, including undesired drug interactions, hypertension, hyperlipidemia, osteoporosis, thrombocytopenia, and atherosclerotic disease.

Hyperacute rejection/early graft failure. Diagnosis of rejection of the transplanted heart is difficult and relies mainly on endomyocardial biopsy, particularly in view of vague clinical symptoms and no reliable serologic markers. Serial biopsies are performed postoperatively to detect any sign of rejection.

16. What pharmacologic agents are effective or ineffective in persons with heart transplants?
Atropine: no effect.
Beta blockers: decrease heart rate and blood pressure; also decrease exercise capacity.
Calcium channel blockers: decrease blood pressure and heart rate (especially in sinoatrial node dysfunction).
Digitalis: no effect on sinoatrial and atrioventricular function; increases cardiac output.
Dobutamine: increases cardiac output.
Dopamine: increases cardiac output; mild increase in heart rate.
Epinephrine: increases cardiac output and heart rate.
Norepinephrine: increases cardiac output and heart rate; increases systolic blood pressure.
Isoproterenol: increases heart rate and cardiac output; decreases pulmonary and arterial pressure.
Nitrates: cause venous and arterial dilation.
Phosphodiesterase inhibitors: increase cardiac output, cause vasodilation.
Quinidine: decreases conduction throught the atrioventricular node.

BIBLIOGRAPHY

1. Baker K, Nasraway SA: Multiple organ failure during critical illness: How organ failure influences outcome in liver disease and liver transplantation. 6:S5–S9, 2000.
2. Blanche C, Blanche DA, Kearney B, et al: Heart transplantation in patients seventy years of age and older: A comparative analysis of outcome. 121:532–541, 2001.
3. Brann WM, Bennett LE, Keck BM, Hosenpud JD: Morbidity, functional status, and immunosuppressive therapy after heart transplantation: An analysis of the joint International Society for Heart and Lung Transplantation/United Network for Organ Sharing. Thorac Reg 17:374–382, 1998.
4. Cardenas A, Uriz J, Gines P, Arroyo V: Heptorenal syndrome. 6:S63–S71, 2000.
5. Carithers RL Jr: Liver transplantation. Am Assoc Study Liver Dis 6:122–135, 2000.
6. Carton EG, Plevak DJ, Kranner PW, et al: Perioperative care of the liver transplant patient: Part 2. 78:382–399, 1994.
7. Carton EG, Rettke SR, Plevak DJ, et al: Perioperative care of the liver transplant patient: Part 1. 78:120–123, 1994.
8. Fazel S, Everson SA, Stitt LW, et al: Predictors of general surgical complications after heart transplantation. 93:52–59, 2001.
9. Gridelli B, Remuzzi G: Strategies for making more organs available for transplantation. 343:404–410, 2000.
10. Hunt SA: Who and when to consider for heart transplantation. 9:18–20, 2001.
11. Kang Y: Coagulapathies in hepatic disease. 6:S72–S75, 2000.
12. Krowka MJ: Hepatopulmonary syndrome: Recent literature (1997 to 1999) and implications for liver transplantation. 6:S31–S35, 2000.
13. Mandell MS: Critical care issues: Portopulmonary hypertension. 6:S36–S43, 2000.
14. Miniati DN, Robbins RC: Heart transplantation: A thirty-year perspective. 53:189–205, 2002.
15. Quinlan JJ, Firestone S, Firestone LL: Anesthesia for heart, lung, and heart-lung transplantation. In Kaplan JA (ed): Cardiac Anesthesia, 4th ed. Philadelphia, W.B. Saunders, 1999.
16. United Network for Organ Sharing (UNOS): www.unos.org (accessed February 2002).

XIV. Perioperative Care

85. POSTOPERATIVE CARE OF CARDIOTHORACIC SURGERY PATIENTS

Jason Widrich, M.D., and Mark T. Grabovac, M.D.

1. What issues need to be addressed immediately after cardiothoracic surgery?

The first hours after cardiac surgery are an unstable and critical period. The most immediate concerns are to ensure adequate oxygenation and ventilation and to maintain hemodynamic stability. Patients are initially mechanically ventilated on 100% oxygen while a chest x-ray is obtained. Physiologic monitoring, including pulse oximetry, arterial pressure, electrocardiography, central venous pressure, pulmonary artery pressure (if available), chest tube output, and urine output should be established as soon as possible after arrival in the intensive care unit (ICU). During this period attention is given to rewarming the patient and correcting acid–base, electrolyte, and coagulation abnormalities. Blood pressure and contractility are supported with vasoactive medications as needed. If necessary, adequate cardiac rhythm can be achieved via a temporary cardiac pacemaker or antiarrhythmic drugs. Assessment of coagulation and bleeding is guided by measurement of chest tube output, reports of prior or ongoing transfusions by the intraoperative personnel, and objective laboratory testing.

2. Describe the Fick equation and the most commonly used method for measuring cardiac output after cardiac surgery.

The Fick equation is a mass balance equation: the quantity of a compound consumed by an organ in a closed system is equal to the product of the flow to that organ and the change in concentration of the compound as it is consumed. For oxygen, if consumption is designated as VO_2 and the change in oxygen content as $(a-v)DO_2$, flow from the heart (Q or cardiac output) can be expressed as follows:

$$VO_2 = Q \times (a\text{-}v)\, DO_2$$

VO_2 is the measured or estimated oxygen consumption (approximately 3 ml/kg/min), and $(a\text{-}v)$ DO_2 is the change in oxygen content from mixed venous blood (obtained from the pulmonary artery) to arterial blood (obtained peripherally).

The most commonly used method of determining cardiac output (CO) after cardiac surgery is the thermodilution technique, using a pulmonary artery (PA) catheter. The thermodilution technique involves injecting a known volume of saline at a specific temperature from the proximal port of the PA catheter and measuring the temperature change at the distal tip. The time integral of the change in temperature yields a measurement of CO. Note that valvular regurgitation or intracardiac shunting can cause significant inaccuracy in the measurement of CO by thermodilution.

3. How are systemic vascular resistance (SVR) and peripheral vascular resistance (PVR) calculated? What is cardiac index?

SVR is a derived quantity that reflects the arterial tone against which the left side of heart must work (afterload). A normal range for SVR is 800–1000 dynes·sec/cm^5. SVR is calculated by the following equation, in which MAP = mean arterial pressure and CVP = central venous pressure:

$$SVR = \frac{(MAP - CVP) \times 80}{CO} \left[dynes \cdot sec \Big/ _{cm^5} \right]$$

PVR reflects the resistance against which the right heart must work. A normal range is 150–250 dynes·sec/cm^5. PVR is calculated by the following equation, in which PAmean = mean pulmonary artery pressure and PCWP = pulmonary capillary wedge pressure:

$$PVR = \frac{(PAmean - PCWP) \times 80}{CO} \left[dynes \cdot sec \Big/ _{cm^5} \right]$$

Cardiac index is defined as CO (L/min) divided by the body surface area (m^2) and thus normalizes CO for body size. A cardiac index > 2.2 L/min/m^2 is considered adequate; < 2.0 L/min/m^2 is considered the threshold for intervention.

4. Is a PA catheter indicated for all patients after cardiac surgery?

Certain centers use PA catheters in most of their patients. However, with the advent of routine intraoperative transesophageal echocardiography (TEE), the use of PA catheters has decreased. For unstable patients with significant myocardial dysfunction or with underlying pulmonary hypertension, measurement of CO and PA pressure may be help to guide therapy. Results from various studies of the risks and benefits of a PA catheter are sufficiently conflicting that the decision to use it should not be automatic.

5. How is low CO diagnosed and managed in the postoperative period? What is the significance of postoperative hypertension? How is it managed?

Findings associated with low CO include hypotension, oliguria, tachycardia, cold extremities, and arrhythmias. Ventricular function reaches its nadir by 5 hours after cardiopulmonary bypass and normally recovers within 24–48 hours. The approach to diagnosis and management should address the factors that determine CO: preload, afterload, heart rate/rhythm, and contractility.

Decreased preload can be due to hypovolemia, hemorrhage, vasodilation from rewarming, and/or tamponade. Management consists of proper resuscitation with IV fluids, correction of anemia with blood products, pharmacologic support of blood pressure, and surgical intervention to stop bleeding or relieve tamponade. A pulmonary artery occlusion pressure (PAOP) or wedge pressure of 15–18 mmHg is often adequate for the compliant ventricle, whereas the noncompliant ventricle may require a PAOP > 20 mmHg. Echocardiography also can be used to assess for hypovolemia or tamponade.

Postoperative hypertension is the most frequent manifestation of increased afterload. Hypertension most often occurs in response to hypothermia, pain, or anxiety with an associated increase in catecholamine levels. It can cause hemorrhage at suture lines, aortic dissection, or cerebrovascular accident. Hypertension also increases the likelihood of ventricular dysfunction and myocardial ischemia. Therapy includes deepening of sedation, alleviation of pain, correction of hypothermia, and use of vasodilators to decrease blood pressure.

Maintenance of sinus rhythm in the range of 80–100 beats/min is generally optimal in the postoperative period. This rate gives the heart adequate time for coronary perfusion and generation of an adequate stroke volume. The maintenance of sinus rhythm provides atrial kick and lowers the risk for embolic events. Pharmacologic treatment of arrhythmia or use of a pacemaker is often necessary.

Myocardial dysfunction is common after cardiac surgery. Aside from visualizing left ventricular function on TEE, depressed contractility should be considered as the cause of low CO when preload, afterload, and heart rate have already been optimized. Various inotropic drugs can be selected for these purposes.

6. What does an intra-aortic balloon pump (IABP) do? What other devices perform similar functions?

The IABP is a mechanical assist device used to improve CO in patients not responsive to pharmacologic therapy by decreasing afterload and increasing coronary artery perfusion. A balloon is placed percutaneously via the femoral circulation and positioned in the descending aorta above the renal arteries. The balloon is triggered to inflate during diastole (at the incisura of the a-line tracing or ECG T-wave), thus augmenting coronary blood flow. The balloon pump is timed most frequently to inflate once with every beat (1:1) or with every other beat (1:2). A mistimed balloon can significantly compromise coronary perfusion and ventricular function. Complications include embolization in patients with severe atherosclerotic or calcific disease of the aorta, thrombosis, thrombocytopenia, aortic occlusion, infection, leg ischemia, renal ischemia, and hemolysis. Contraindications to the IABP include aortic insufficiency and aneurysmal disease of the aorta.

The left ventricular assist device (LVAD) is a pump that connects the left atrium or ventricle to the aorta and augments blood flow. Patients supported by an LVAD need to remain anticoagulated until they can be weaned from the additional support. Twenty to 30% of patients requiring LVADs in the postoperative period are successfully weaned and survive to discharge. These devices were previously in operation exclusively outside the body, but technologic improvements have created smaller devices that are almost totally implantable. Now some patients are considered for LVADs for long-term use.

7. What is cardiac tamponade? How is it diagnosed and managed?

Cardiac tamponade is a mechanical restriction in cardiac filling resulting from blood clots or fluid in the mediastinum. The incidence of tamponade requiring drainage after cardiac surgery is less than 1%. Signs include a progressive decrease in pulse pressure, abrupt decrease in chest tube drainage, equalization of right- and left-sided pressures measured with a PA catheter, an exaggerated x descent on a CVP tracing, or a widened mediastinum on chest x-ray. Definitive diagnosis is made by echocardiographic detection of clot or fluid compressing the heart. Initial therapy includes optimization of preload with IV fluids, maintenance of heart rate, and inotropic support. If possible, the patient should be kept spontaneously ventilating because increased intrathoracic pressure from positive-pressure ventilation can further compromise ventricular filling. The definitive management of tamponade is surgical evacuation of blood and clot.

8. What are the most common arrhythmias after cardiac surgery? How are they treated?

The most common arrhythmias are sinus bradycardia and tachycardia, followed by atrial arrhythmias. Sinus bradycardia and slow junctional rhythms occur frequently during the recovery of the myocardium from hypothermia. Temporary pacing of atria and/or ventricles is the therapy of choice and is accomplished via epicardial pacing wires placed intraoperatively. Drugs that augment both heart rate and contractility (dopamine, epinephrine, norepinephrine) can be used in patients with both low CO and sinus bradycardia.

Sinus tachycardia after cardiac surgery often can be attributed to pain, low CO, hypovolemia, infection, ischemia, tamponade, or drug withdrawal (beta blockers). These underlying causes need to be considered and ruled out before therapy is initiated because the management of each is different.

Atrial fibrillation (AF) usually occurs within 1–5 days after cardiac surgery, with an incidence of 40% after coronary artery bypass grafting and 60% after valvular surgery. Risk factors include advanced age, pericarditis, increased atrial size, long bypass time, chronic obstructive pulmonary disease, renal failure, and valvular surgery. Most cases of AF resolve in 6–8 weeks without further cardiovascular morbidity, but AF does carry an increased risk of stroke. Rapid atrial (overdrive) pacing or cardioversion may be necessary in unstable patients. Inability to convert AF requires use of anticoagulants to prevent thrombosis and embolization. New data about pretreatment with amiodarone, beta blockers, and/or magnesium have focused attention on prophylaxis of AF and other arrhythmias. Although amiodarone has gained popularity for prophylaxis and treatment of arrhythmias in most patient groups, it slightly increases the risk of acute respiratory distress syndrome (ARDS) after cardiac surgery.

Ventricular arrhythmias also can occur in the postoperative period as a result of electrolyte imbalance, ischemia, hypoxia, or increased sympathetic tone. Treatment should include stabilization with correction of the underlying cause, appropriate drug therapy, and/or electrical cardioversion.

9. How is perioperative myocardial infarction (MI) diagnosed?

The diagnosis of MI after cardiac surgery is a complex problem. Suspicion should be elevated in patients who require prolonged or excessive inotropic support for lower CO and patients who have ventricular arrhythmias or other physical signs and symptoms consistent with MI. After surgery, a 12-lead ECG is ordered to establish a new baseline for comparison. The pre- and postoperative ECGs generally are not identical, and new intraventricular conduction delays such as left bundle-branch block can make interpretation of ST segments difficult. Despite these changes, substantial ST-segment elevations or depressions need to be addressed, and the leads in which the changes occur may indicate the anatomic location of the suspected ischemia.

TEE has been shown to display wall motion abnormalities associated with ischemia earlier and with greater sensitivity than ST-segment changes on ECG. TEE also can be used to distinguish hypovolemia from contractile dysfunction.

The enzymes creatine kinase (CK-MB) or cardiac troponin I (cTnI) often are used to diagnose Q-wave and non–Q-wave MI. After cardiac surgery, elevations in both enzymes are expected, and the levels required for diagnosis of MI are controversial. Recent studies indicate that cTnI is more sensitive and specific for MI than CK-MB. A cTnI value 24 hours after cardiac surgery that is higher than the cTnI value at the 12-hour mark is cause for concern. Larger studies are needed to determine the efficacy of using cTnI and the threshold values required to diagnose an infarction after bypass surgery.

10. What pulmonary complications should be considered in the postoperative period?

After cardiovascular complications, pulmonary complications are the leading cause of morbidity after cardiac surgery. Many patients undergoing cardiac surgery have a history of smoking and frequently have underlying chronic obstructive pulmonary disease (COPD) that may require perioperative treatment. Both lung and chest wall compliance are reduced for approximately 1 week after surgery, and overall lung function remains abnormal for 6 weeks or more. Patients in severe pain from sternotomy and thoracotomy incisions or with phrenic nerve injury are not able to cooperate with deep breathing exercises. The resulting drop in vital capacity, forced expiratory volume in 1 second, and functional residual capacity sets the stage for atelectasis, ventilation–perfusion mismatch, and pneumonia. In addition, massive resuscitation, low CO, sepsis, and gastric aspiration can lead to acute lung injury and ARDS. The primary management of these problems includes supportive measures, pulmonary suctioning, incentive spirometry, positive end-expiratory pressure (PEEP), bronchodilator therapy, antibiotics (if indicated), and IV or neuraxial medications for pain.

Inhaled nitric oxide (NO) after cardiopulmonary bypass (CPB) has received attention for patients with hypoxia and increased pulmonary vascular resistance. Its ability to vasodilate the pulmonary circulation without significant effect on SVR can improve CO in this group of patients. Studies of the efficacy and safety of NO in cardiac surgery patients are pending.

11. Describe the approach to the bleeding patient after cardiac surgery.

Patients returning from cardiac surgery may already have had significant blood loss and received blood products intraoperatively to correct the associated coagulopathy. A residual effect from heparin administered intraoperatively also may contribute to postoperative coagulopathy. Heparin-associated coagulopathy can result from heparin that has not been completely reversed or from reinfusion of blood, collected from the bypass machine, that contains residual heparin. Coagulopathy from the effect of heparin can be corrected with additional doses of protamine.

Delayed capillary refill, pale conjunctiva, falling blood pressure, hypoxemia, and/or tachycardia are signs of the bleeding or anemic patient. Excessive saturation of the surgical dressings and high output from the chest tubes are also indicators of bleeding. Output from the chest tube should be less than 200 ml in the first hour and should decrease substantially over the next several hours. In patients with a high chest tube input, a precipitous decrease may be an early sign of tamponade.

Transfusion triggers for patients after cardiac surgery are frequently different from those in other critically ill patients. The goal for transfusion of packed red blood cells and whole blood is to maintain a hematocrit value of 30%. This level of hemoglobin optimizes the balance between blood viscosity and oxygen-carrying capacity.

The treatment of bleeding secondary to coagulopathy involves a multilevel approach. Frequently ordered laboratory tests include prothrombin time (PT), partial thromboplastin time (PTT), fibrinogen, and platelets. Isolated elevation of PTT implies inadequate reversal of heparin effect that can be corrected with protamine. Elevation of PT alone or both PT and PTT often points to a need for fresh frozen plasma. Decreased platelet count (< 100) requires platelet transfusion, whereas decreased fibrinogen (< 150) may require cryoprecipitate. For patients whose coagulopathy or bleeding does not correct with appropriate management, other causes need to be considered (disseminated intravascular coagulation, sepsis, GI bleed, shock liver). Bleeding despite normal coagulation studies often requires re-exploration to treat a surgical cause.

12. Describe the neurologic complications that may occur after cardiac surgery and CPB.
The neurologic complications of cardiac surgery can be categorized as vascular, encephalopathic, cognitive, and neuropathic. The incidence of postoperative stroke resulting in death or disability is 3–5%. The prevalence of stroke increases with the presence of atherosclerotic disease in the ascending aorta, advanced age, atrial fibrillation, or ventricular thrombi. In addition, the combination of coronary artery bypass grafting (CABG) and carotid endarterectomy carries a higher risk of cerebrovascular accident than either procedure performed on separate admissions.

Postoperative encephalopathy is evidenced by disorientation, somnolence, agitation, and delirium. Advanced age, long CPB times, and sleep deprivation are risk factors for ICU psychosis. Other disorders that can cause delirium should be considered, including sepsis, hypoxia, renal failure, withdrawal, metabolic causes, and medications (nitroprusside). Acute agitation can be treated with haloperidol or other antipsychotic medications. The condition is often self-limited and improves once the patient can be moved out of the ICU to less stimulating surroundings.

Neurocognitive and neuropsychological testing reveals that many patients develop subtle cognitive deficits that can be detected at 6 months after CPB. Fine motor skills, recall, and memory have been shown to be impaired to some degree.

Neuropathic injury can result from malpositioned extremities, brachial plexus injury from sternal retraction, and direct injury to nerves from thoracotomy incisions.

13. What complications may affect renal function after cardiac surgery?
The overall frequency of renal failure requiring dialysis is 2–3% after cardiac surgery. Oliguric renal failure carries a much higher mortality and morbidity than nonoliguric renal failure in the postoperative period. A transient rise in creatinine occurs in many patients in the first 48 hours after cardiac surgery. For persistent elevation after 48 hours, prerenal (hypovolemia and low CO), renal (drugs, sepsis), and postrenal (obstruction) causes should be considered. Management consists of maintaining urine output and optimizing renal perfusion. Although diuretics or low-dose (renal-dose) dopamine often is administered in clinical practice, little evidence solidly supports their efficacy in improving outcomes.

14. Discuss the gastrointestinal complications after cardiac surgery.
Postoperative nausea, constipation, and ileus often result from narcotic effects and/or postoperative bowel edema and normally resolve within 24–48 hours. Shock liver can result from hepatic hypoperfusion and is evidenced by low CO in conjunction with elevated liver function tests and bilirubin. Critically ill patients also are at increased risk of GI bleeding and should receive prophylactic therapy with a proton pump inhibitor and/or an H_2 blocker.

15. How may cardiac surgery affect insulin requirements?
Insulin requirements increase after CPB, especially in diabetic patients. Glucose levels should be expected to remain elevated in diabetic patients for the first 24 hours after surgery. Treatment consists of insulin infusion as needed. It also has been shown that hyperglycemia in diabetic patients in the first 2 days after surgery is an independent (and possibly the leading) risk

factor for development of deep sternal wound infection. Use of a continuous IV insulin infusion with a goal glucose level of 150–200 mg/dl significantly reduces the incidence of deep sternal wound infection in diabetic patients.

16. How can cardiac surgery induce an autoimmune response?
Repeated exposure to heparin can induce an antibody-mediated thrombocytopenia known as heparin-induced thrombocytopenia (HIT). Postpericardiotomy syndrome is characterized by unexplained fever, chest pain, and effusions after cardiac surgery. Severe immune reactions to the bypass circuit, protamine (anaphylactoid), or transfused blood products (anaphylaxis or hemolytic reaction) also may occur.

17. What infectious complications may be associated with cardiac surgery?
Pneumonia and sternal wound infections have a significant impact on length of ICU stay. Sternal wound infection can result in sternum malunion. Risk factors include obesity, bilateral grafting of internal mammary arteries in a diabetic patient, emergency operation, re-exploration, and use of a tracheostomy.

18. When is profound hypothermia used? What complications may result?
Profound hypothermia (18°C) with circulatory arrest (total cessation of circulatory flow) is used most often for cerebral protection during repair of the aortic arch and some pediatric procedures. Longer periods of hypothermia are associated with increased bleeding and a higher incidence of neurologic complications.

19. What risks are associated with repeat CABG?
Patients who have had multiple cardiac procedures are at higher risk for low CO syndromes, ischemia, arrhythmias, bleeding, and lung injury due to massive transfusions.

20. Define off-pump coronary artery bypass (OPCAB). What are its advantages?
Surgery is done on the beating heart with the use of stabilizers to keep certain sections of the myocardium relatively immobile. OPCAB avoids many of the problems associated with CPB and has been associated with quicker extubation, recovery, and discharge. Some centers have even performed OPCAB under epidural anesthesia with conscious sedation. OPCAB procedures have allowed some centers to bypass the ICU altogether with the use of step-down units and telemetry beds. Larger studies are pending, but initial reports have cited a lower incidence of cardiac, pulmonary, and neurologic complications with OPCAB.

21. What complications are associated with valvular disease?
Mitral stenosis. Arrhythmias, particularly atrial fibrillation, are common both pre- and postoperatively as a result of left atrial enlargement. Pulmonary hypertension may complicate management. Most of the valvular disorders require postoperative anticoagulation therapy, especially if an artificial valve is placed.

Mitral regurgitation. Reports of a normal ejection fraction preoperatively may be misleading because the ventricle has been pumping a fraction of its stroke volume into the systemic circulation and frequently a larger fraction of stroke volume into the low-resistance left atrium. Mitral valve repair or replacement may lead to acute failure because the ventricle cannot accommodate the increased afterload.

Aortic stenosis. Maintenance of sinus rhythm and after load are critical to the management of patients with uncorrected aortic stenosis. Patients who are asymptomatic preoperatively are at at significantly higher risk of mortality after aortic valve replacement. The hypertrophied left ventricle is at high risk for ischemia in the postoperative period, even after aortic valve replacement.

22. What issues are crucial in adult congenital heart disease?
This exhaustive topic has many variations, but it has become increasingly important because of the number of children with congenital disorders who survive to adulthood. Vital issues

include the presence or absence of cyanosis, the prior and corrected anatomy, pulmonary hypertension, polycythemia, and the dependence of the patient on the balance between systemic and pulmonary resistance/circulation. These issues guide oxygenation, hemodynamic, acid–base, transfusion, and ventilatory goals.

23. Describe some of the approaches to pain management after cardiac surgery. How has the approach changed in the past decade?

In the 1970s and 1980s the mainstays of anesthetic management were high-dose narcotics (fentanyl, 20 µg/kg), high-dose benzodiazepines (chlordiazepoxide or midazolam), and long-acting muscle relaxants (pancuronium). The intraoperative and postoperative management of pain were linked because patients remained intubated and sedated in the ICU overnight as they recovered from the anesthetic.

Patients who can be awakened earlier and extubated have no additional morbidity or mortality. The idea of "fast-track" management (rapid extubation and recovery) has led to significantly shorter ICU and hospital lengths of stay. Techniques using newer intravenous and inhaled anesthetics that allow smaller doses of long-acting narcotics and benzodiazepines have had a significant impact on recovery times.

The most recent technique, which has both supporters and critics, is the use of neuraxial medications for intraoperative and postoperative pain control. Many centers have significantly reduced the amount of IV narcotics and the systemic side effects of respiratory depression, nausea, and ileus with the use of long-acting morphine preparations given intrathecally (< 8 µg/kg).

Recent reports of OPCAB in awake patients using an epidural catheter as the primary source of anesthesia have shown that the epidural can be a safe and effective technique. The long-term benefit obtained from attenuation of the stress response as a result of epidural anesthesia is a topic of much interest and controversy. This benefit must be weighed against the higher risk of an epidural hematoma in the fully heparinized patient. If blood is aspirated from what is believed to be the epidural space during needle placement, most centers delay the procedure rather than risk an epidural hematoma.

24. Discuss the role of process- or protocol-driven care for cardiac patients.

Many medical centers have improved their outcomes by adopting specific procedures and algorithms. Cardiac surgical care is a process involving unique decisions made by cardiologists, surgeons, anesthesiologists, and ICU personnel from the preoperative assessment until discharge. Review of the literature and the experience of other medical centers with the most successful practices (benchmarking) can lead to the discovery of areas that can be improved. Examples of common problems that can be address in this manner include bleeding, infection, neurologic outcome, pulmonary morbidity (ARDS, fast-track extubation), and cardiovascular morbidity (arrhythmia, low-output syndrome, use of monitors).

The Northern New England Cardiovascular Disease Group is an example of a network of hospitals from six states that have applied this technique to the cardiovascular surgery process. As a result of their efforts, they have been able to decrease significantly the time to extubation, rate of sternal wound infection, number of transfusions of non–red blood cell products, rate of surgical re-exploration, and length of stay. Another group recently reported that "standardization" of anesthetic, surgical, and ICU techniques for uncomplicated CABG with CPB has decreased the time to discharge to 4 days in 80% of patients. Many centers are attempting to find ways to bypass the ICU altogether for uncomplicated patients with aggressive weaning of support and use of step-down (lower level of activity) units.

BIBLIOGRAPHY

1. Bharucha DB, Kowey PR: Management and prevention of atrial fibrillation after cardiovascular surgery. Am J Cardiol 85:20D–24D, 2000.
2. Chaney MA: Intrathecal morphine for coronary artery bypass grafting and early extubation. Analges Anesthes 84:241–248, 1997.

3. Cleveland JC Jr: Off-pump coronary artery bypass grafting decreases risk adjusted mortality and morbidity. Ann Thorac Surg 72:1282–1288, 2001.
4. Hogue CW Jr: Cardiac and neurologic complications identify risks for mortality for both men and women undergoing coronary artery bypass graft surgery. Anesthesiology 95:1074–1078, 2001.
5. Kumon K: Nitric oxide inhalation as chemical assist for circulation in patients after cardiovascular surgery. Artif Organs 23:169–174, 1999.
6. Marie-Odile B: Cardiac troponin I: Contribution to the diagnosis of perioperative myocardial infarction and various complications of cardiac surgery. Crit Care Med 29:1880-1886, 2001.
7. Meade MO: Trials comparing early vs. late extubation following cardiovascular surgery. Chest 120:445S–453S, 2001.
8. Morris DC, St. Claire D: Management of patients after cardiac surgery. Curr Probl Cardiol Apr:167–228, 1999.
9. Nuttall GA: Efficacy of a simple intraoperative transfusion algorithm for nonerythrocyte component utilization after cardiopulmonary bypass. Anesthesiology 94:771–778, 2001.
10. Ovrum E: Rapid recovery protocol applied to 5,658 consecutive "on-pump" coronary bypass patients. Ann Thorac Surg 70:2008–2012, 2000.
11. Paiste J: Minimally invasive coronary artery bypass surgery under high thoracic epidural Analges Anesthes 2001.
12. Reyes A, Gema V: Early vs. conventional extubation after cardiac surgery with cardiopulmonary bypass. Chest 112:193–201, 1997.
13. Roach GW: Adverse cerebral outcomes after coronary artery bypass surgery. N Engl J Med 335:1857–1863, 1996.

86. UPPER AIRWAY OBSTRUCTION

Jean-François Pittet, M.D.

1. Define upper airway obstruction.

Upper airway obstruction is the blockage of air between the nose and the mouth and the tracheal bifurcation. It may be complete or incomplete and is often life-threatening when it occurs below the hypopharynx, where the cross-sectional diameter of the airway is the smallest.

2. What is the clinical presentation of upper airway obstruction?

Three phases of physiologic change occur in acute airway obstruction before death:

1. The first phase (1–3 min duration) is characterized by a marked sympathetic response with an increase in blood pressure, pulse, and respiratory rate, and an increase in the work of breathing. Then, PaO decreases and $PaCO_2$ increases, causing a fall in pH. The patient is still conscious and choking, making paradoxic respirations that do not result in air movement. The patient rapidly becomes cyanotic.

2. During the second phase (2–5 min duration), blood pressure and heart rate fall rapidly, respiratory movements diminish, and the patient loses consciousness.

3. The third and final phase (5–8 min after beginning the airway obstruction) is characterized by asystole; the cardiac rhythm degenerates from sinus to nodal bradycardia, then to idioventricular rhythms, and terminates in asystole or ventricular fibrillation.

The same physiologic changes occur in partial upper airway obstruction but more slowly and to lesser degrees. However, when symptoms are present, the obstruction should be considered as substantial because mild obstruction is generally asymptomatic.

3. Do the signs of upper airway obstruction depend on its location?

Yes. Airway obstruction produces different anatomic and physiologic changes depending on whether it is fixed or variable, extrathoracic or intrathoracic. An extrathoracic obstruction with a mobile airway wall produces more symptoms during inspiration because the airway lumen is normally more narrow during inspiration in its extrathoracic portion. A mobile intrathoracic obstruction causes more symptoms during expiration. However, if the airway obstruction is fixed, both inspiratory and expiratory flow will be limited equally, because changes in transmural pressure cannot modify the diameter of the airway.

4. What should be included in the physical examination of a patient presenting with an upper airway obstruction?

The oral cavity is inspected, avoiding instrumentation in patients with suspected epiglottitis and severe airway obstruction. Auscultation over the larynx, trachea, and both lungs is done to exclude tension pneumothorax. Flail chest, which may mimic airway obstruction, also should be excluded. The physician should listen for stridor, which may be inspiratory (supraglottic obstruction), expiratory (intraglottic obstruction), or both. Its presence signifies an airway diameter of 5 mm or less in adults.

5. Can airway obstruction be precisely located?

Yes. Neck and chest x-rays (anteroposterior and lateral views), airway tomography, CT scan, pulmonary function testing, and, if necessary, bronchoscopy can localize the airway obstruction.

6. What causes upper airway obstruction?

The site of an upper airway obstruction may be extrathoracic or intrathoracic, and localized within the lumen, in the wall, or extrinsic to the wall of an anatomic or artificial airway. The following clinical conditions may be associated with upper airway obstruction:

- Infection: acute epiglottitis, tonsillitis, peritonsillar and retropharyngeal abscess, diphtheria, Ludwig's angina, and laryngitis
- Mass lesions: benign and malignant tumors, traumatic hematomas, and hematomas secondary to anticoagulants
- Head and neck trauma
- Foreign body aspiration (café coronary)
- Inflammation: angioneurotic edema, anaphylaxis, inhalation of corrosives and toxins, thermal burns
- Vocal cord pathology: laryngospasm, bilateral vocal cord paralysis
- Cricoarytenoid arthritis
- Sleep apnea syndrome

7. What is the clinical presentation of upper airway infection?

Acute infectious epiglottis is unusual but not rare in adults. Adults have a longer prodromal state than children, as more inflammatory edema is needed to produce symptoms at the larger glottic opening. As in children, *Hemophilus influenzae* is the most common organism, but pneumococcus, Staphylococcus, and Streptococcus have been incriminated. The initial symptoms are a muffled voice, signs and symptoms out of proportion to the degree of oropharyngeal obstruction, and some early signs of upper airway obstruction. Although indirect laryngoscopy has been considered to be dangerous in patients with severe airway obstruction, this procedure should be performed in patients with milder symptoms in order to establish the diagnosis. **Acute and chronic tonsillitis** can cause an upper airway obstruction and lead to the development of a sleep apnea syndrome associated with snoring, restless sleep, chronic mouth-breathing, daytime hypersomnolence, and morning headache. **Peritonsillar abscess** may threaten the upper airway as an obstruction mass lesion and may also threaten the airway by rupturing and causing pulmonary aspiration. **Ludwig's angina** is an infection of the floor of the mouth, usually due to the spread of infection from the lower molar teeth. It is characterized by rock-hard swelling of the area, with elevation of the base of the tongue and with both paralaryngeal and glottic edema.

8. What is café coronary? Which patients are at risk?

Café coronary, or aspiration of partially chewed food, usually occurs in elderly persons with altered consciousness, decreased gag reflexes, or dentures. Individuals who are taking drugs with anticholinergic effects are at risk for swallowing a large bolus of food and having it obstruct the glottis. Although food appears to be the most common obstructing foreign body, dentures, loose teeth, or other objects should be considered.

9. Which patients are at greatest risk for nonpenetrating trauma to the upper airway?

Young adult men with sport injuries and patients who suffer blunt trauma from motor vehicle accidents are at the greatest risk. The presence of a cervical spine injury should be considered when the initial mechanism of upper airway injury is associated with dissipation of high energy to the tissues of the neck. These lesions are often characterized by the presence of a large hematoma, subcutaneous emphysema, and the development of stridor.

10. What is the clinical presentation of laryngeal edema?

Laryngeal edema occurs within minutes during an allergic response or as part of anaphylaxis. There is usually angioneurotic edema of the tongue, the lips, or the supraglottic tissues as well as the subglottic tissues. This edema can result in complete airway obstruction. Some patients may also have a cardiovascular collapse, severe bronchoconstriction, urticaria, and diarrhea. The most frequent etiologies are hymenoptera bites, shellfish allergies, and drug allergies. Laryngeal edema may also occur in patients with extrinsic asthma as part of an acute attack or in patients with C1 esterase inhibitor deficiency (hereditary angioneurotic edema).

11. What is the treatment of foreign body aspiration?

For obstruction of the supraglottic area, the Heimlich maneuver (abdominal thrust) is indicated. If it is not successful, laryngoscopy and extraction of the foreign body by suction and/or by forceps is mandatory. A cricothyroidotomy may be life-saving if the foreign body is impacted in a subglottic site. In the presence of viscous particulate matter, endotracheal intubation (with a long endotracheal tube) may be helpful.

Extraction of foreign bodies from the trachea requires judgment because aggressive treatment may be more detrimental than helpful. If air movement is present, supplemental oxygen should be provided. A rigid bronchoscopy should be considered quickly. A mixture of helium and oxygen (80:20) may be administered in certain patients for a short interval to reduce the work of breathing. This gas mixture is given by endotracheal tube or by a tightly fitting, nonrebreathing mask. Such treatment has been reported to decrease airway resistance in normal volunteers by 23% during quiet breathing and to decrease airway resistance by 49% during panting. This decrease in airway resistance may be explained by a reduction in gas density (the density of helium is roughly one-third that of oxygen or air), by elimination of turbulence downstream from the obstruction, and by a reduction in the tendency for the airways to collapse downstream from the obstruction.

12. What is the treatment of trauma to the upper airway?

In complete airway obstruction, transtracheal jet ventilation is probably the best procedure. Various devices have been developed to facilitate this procedure. Basically, a catheter attached to a syringe is inserted into the trachea across the crycothyroid membrane. The transtracheal ventilation system is then attached to the intratracheal catheter. Surgical cricothyroidotomy (opening the cricothyroid membrane with a scalpel and inserting a small endotracheal tube) is an alternative treatment. A classic tracheotomy requires more skill and training and is not the standard technique for managing acute upper airway obstruction. Indeed, the presence of a severe contusion of the neck soft tissues may make tracheotomy particularly difficult. With less severe injuries, endotracheal intubation may exacerbate injuries.

Even in patients with minimal symptoms of airway obstruction, prophylactic intubation may need to be considered, particularly in patients who have suffered thermal burns. In such cases, endotracheal intubation has to be atraumatic, so the use of a fibroscope may be helpful.

13. What is the treatment of epiglottitis in adult patients?

Endotracheal intubation should be performed early, once the diagnosis becomes clear. Inhalation anesthesia with 100% oxygen is preferable to the use of intravenous hypnotics and muscle relaxants in order for the patient to maintain spontaneous breathing during the whole procedure. Monitoring of oxyhemoglobin saturation with pulse oximetry is highly desirable. After intubation, secure fixation of the endotracheal tube is mandatory. There is no need for mechanical ventilation if the lungs are not involved. Patients should receive antibiotics effective against *Hemophilus influenzae* and may usually be extubated within 2 or 3 days when air leak exists around the endotracheal tube with a deflated cuff.

14. What is the treatment for laryngeal edema secondary to anaphylaxis?
The management of acute anaphylaxis reactions is described elsewhere in this book and will not be repeated here. Briefly, the management of severe cases includes endotracheal intubation, or cricothyroidotomy if necessary, and intravenous epinephrine (0.2–0.5 mg). In milder cases, 0.3 mg of epinephrine subcutaneously may be sufficient. The use of corticosteroids and antihistamines is of secondary importance in the acute care of these patients.

15. Describe the management of patients with known upper airway obstrution at extubation.
Patients with known upper airway obstruction are also at risk at the time of extubation. Before extubation it is important to determine the possible presence of an obstruction above the vocal cords by direct visualization of both the pharynx and and the larynx (direct laryngoscopy, visualization with the aid of an a flexible bronchoscope). To determine whether there is still an obstruction below the vocal cords, it is useful to deflate the cuff of the endotracheal tube before extubation and to measure the pressure that induces an air leak around the endotracheal tube (leak test). A low pressure (5–10 cmH$_2$O) indicates sufficient space between the endotracheal tube and the wall of the trachea.

BIBLIOGRAPHY

1. Curtis JL, Mahlmeister M, Fink JB, et al: Helium-oxygen gas therapy: Use and availability for the emergency treatment of inoperable airway obstruction. Chest 90:455–457, 1986.
2. DeWeese EL, Sullivan TY, Yu PL: Ventilatory and occlusion pressure responses to helium breathing. J Appl Physiol 54:1525–1531, 1983.
3. Jacobson S: Upper airway obstruction. Emerg Med Clin North Am 7:205–217, 1989.
4. Jorden RC: Airway management. Emerg Med Clin North Am 6:671–686, 1988.
5. Jorden RC: Percutaneous transtracheal ventilation. Emerg Med Clin North Am 6:745–752, 1988.
6. Walls RM: Cricothyroidotomy. Emerg Med Clin North Am 6:725–736, 1988.

87. COMPLICATIONS OF GENERAL ANESTHESIA

Jean-François Pittet, M.D.

1. What is the incidence of complications due to general anesthesia?
In a review of 112,000 anesthetic procedures, Cohen et al. reported an 8–10% rate of complications during and after general anesthesia; the incidence of life-threatening complications was less than 1%. Many postoperative problems described as complications of anesthesia are a combination of preexisting disease and extent of surgery, regardless of the anesthetic technique.

2. What causes central nervous system (CNS) dysfunction after general anesthesia?
CNS dysfunction may be due to decreased oxygen availability, increased oxygen consumption, or a specific drug effect. Decreased oxygen availability is the most common cause and results generally from problems with anesthesia equipment. The increased use of monitors to measure oxygenation (such as pulse oximeters) should reduce the incidence of this tragic complication.

3. What measures should be taken if the patient suffers cerebral insult during general anesthesia?

First, attempt to keep the patient hemodynamically stable. The following techniques specific to resuscitation of the brain may be used:

1. Improve cerebral perfusion pressure by maintaining an adequate systemic arterial pressure.

2. Lower intracranial pressure by decreasing cerebral blood flow through increases in respiratory rate (thereby decreasing arterial PCO_2) and decreasing free brain water with diuretics (mannitol, furosemide).

3. Improve venous return by keeping the head elevated to 30° or greater and by avoiding positive end-expiratory pressure if oxygenation is not compromised.

4. Administer drugs to decrease the cerebral metabolic rate (barbiturates, phenytoin).

4. What causes changes in heart rate during general anesthesia?

Abnormalities in heart rate are defined as a sinus rhythm less than 50 beats/min (bradycardia) or more than 100 beats/min (tachycardia). In general, tachycardia is more deleterious because of the reduction of diastolic filling time of the coronary circulation. The cause of sinus tachycardia is usually increased sympathetic activity secondary to inadequate anesthesia. Preoperative conditions such as anxiety, cardiac disease, fever, burns, or hyperthyroidism may also cause tachycardia. Intraoperatively, drug effect (atropine, pancuronium, isoflurane), hyperthermia, thyroid storm, and pheochromocytoma should be considered in the differential diagnosis.

Bradycardia is important when the decrease in cardiac output leads to impairment of organ perfusion. The most common causes are increased vagal tone from traction or pressure on body tissues with vagal innervation (i.e., mesenteric traction), and drug effects (i.e., suxamethonium, halothane, high-dose opioids). Treatment includes stopping vagal stimulus, administering IV atropine (0.5–1 mg), and reducing the inspired concentration of the halogenated agent.

5. Which arrhythmias should be treated?

Cardiac dysrhythmias may occur in 60% or more patients undergoing anesthesia when continuous methods are used for surveillance. All arrhythmias produce some decrease in cardiac output and should be treated if there is a significant decrease in cardiac output. Treatment should be instituted for arrhythmias causing hypotension and those resulting in myocardial ischemia, or when ventricular fibrillation or asystole is present.

6. Describe the treatment of supraventricular tachyarrhythmias observed during general anesthesia.

Treatment depends on the rate and rhythm and the degree of decrease in cardiac output. Adequate oxygenation and ventilation and sufficient anesthetic depth are of paramount importance. If the arrhythmia persists, IV adenosine (6–12 mg) may be the drug of choice. Verapamil (5 mg infused over 1–2 min) and propranolol (0.5–1 mg IV) may also be used to slow the ventricular response.

7. Can general anesthesia make preexisting cardiac conduction block worse?

Yes. In such cases, the risk of asystole and sudden death must be weighed against the morbidity of placing a temporary or permanent pacemaker. Pacing is not indicated in asymptomatic type II AV block or congenital heart block. Patients with asymptomatic type II AV block as well as those with symptomatic bradycardia require a pacemaker.

8. Are ventricular arrhythmias common during general anesthesia?

Yes. The most frequent cause is sympathetic overactivity of endogenous or exogenous origin. Endogenous causes are anxiety, primary hypertension, pheochromocytoma, and surgical stimulation. Exogenous causes are hypoxia, hypercapnia, and drug interactions (i.e., epinephrine and volatile anesthetics). Lidocaine (IV bolus of 50–100 mg) is the drug of choice for emergent acute ventricular arrhythmias.

9. Do electrolyte disturbances induce ventricular arrhythmias?
Yes—specifically, acute hypokalemia. Hyperventilation lowers serum potassium by 0.5 mmol/L for every 9.7 mmHg reduction in $PaCO_2$. The safe level of serum potassium is around 3.3 mmol/L and may be higher in patients taking digitalis or with ischemic myocardial disease. Transport of potassium in cells is facilitated by concomitant administration of 10% glucose with insulin (0.5 unit/2 gm of glucose). ECG monitoring is essential during this treatment.

10. Does cardiac arrest occur without preceding signs during general anesthesia?
Generally, there are warning signs. Cardiac arrest is normally preceded by a progressive bradycardia. The incidence of cardiac arrest during general anesthesia is estimated to be 6–10 per 10,000 anesthesia. The most important causes include overdose of anesthetics, inadequate ventilation, long periods of hypotension, or anaphylactoid reaction to anesthetic agents or other drugs.

11. What is the risk of myocardial infarction (MI) during anesthesia?
The risk of MI is low (0.1%) in patients without preoperative cardiac disease. In patients with a previous MI, the risk decreases as the time interval to surgery increases. During the first 3 months after an MI, the risk of reinfarction during anesthesia is 5–6%, with an overall mortality of 35% for a patient optimally monitored and treated. The risk decreases to 2% after 6 months. Elderly patients (> 70 years old) undergoing noncardiac surgery who have chronic stable angina, previous MI, or ECG signs of myocardial ischemia are at increased risk for perioperative MI or cardiac death. In patients with coronary artery disease, early postoperative myocardial ischemia is an important correlate of adverse cardiac outcome. Perioperative beta blockade has been shown to decrease perioperative myocardial ischemia and to improve mortality rates in high-risk patients; perioperatife beta blockade should be offered to patients at risk. In patients with contraindications to beta blockade (e.g., asthma, bradycardia), consider perioperative alpha agonist therap, which also has been shown to improve ischemia and patient outcomes.

12. Does anesthetic technique play a significant role in the development of perioperative MI?
No. No study has demonstrated a difference in the risk of perioperative MI between patients undergoing general or regional anesthesia with sufficient intravenous sedation. The general aim with either technique is to maintain a slightly depressed mean arterial pressure and avoid tachycardia, hypertension, and severe hypotension.

13. What are the most important causes of changes in systemic arterial pressure during anesthesia?
The causes of arterial hypotension during anesthesia include a change in cardiac rate, rhythm or contractility, a decrease in systemic vascular resistance, or a decrease in circulating blood volume. The causes of arterial hypertension during general anesthesia include increased cardiac contractility or increased systemic vascular resistance. The latter is the result of increased sympathetic tone, either endogenous (anxiety, pain) or exogenous (inadequate anesthesia, ketamine).

14. What are the most important respiratory complications observed during general anesthesia?
Laryngospasm, bronchospasm, obstruction of the endotracheal tube, and pneumothorax.

15. Discuss the causes and treatments of laryngospasm.
Laryngospasm may result from edema of the airway, a reflex response to local irritation (i.e., presence of secretions), or inadequate anesthesia. Laryngospasm may be partial or complete. Partial spasm is audible if the airway has narrowed to 5 mm or less (in adults). Treatment includes ventilation with 100% oxygen and a low level PEEP (5 cmH$_2$O), correction of the cause, and deepening of anesthesia. A short-acting neuromuscular blocking agent may be used to relieve the spasm.

16. Discuss the causes and treatment of bronchospasm.

Factors predisposing to bronchospasm include preoperative wheezing, endotracheal intubation of an inadequately anesthetized patient, placement of the endotracheal tube near or at the carina, surgical stimulus, or aspiration of gastric contents. Treatment includes ventilation with 100% oxygen and aerosol of a beta agonist through the endotracheal tube to relieve the spasm. Increasing the concentration of volatile anesthetics is helpful, although halothane has the potential of causing cardiac arrhythmias in a hypoxic, hypercapnic patient. Isoflurane is probably the volatile agent least likely to trigger such arrhythmias.

17. When is a pneumothorax a problem intraoperatively?

A small pleural leak rapidly increased the effect of positive-pressure ventilation and the influx of nitrous oxide into the pleural space. Pneumothoraces frequently accompany central line placements, nephrectomies, thoracotomies, median sternotomies, and abdominal procedures adjacent to the diaphragm.

18. How does anesthesia contribute to postoperative abnormalities in gas exchange?

Postoperative abnormalities in gas exchange present two temporal patterns:

1. Transient postoperative hypoxemia is mostly due to the reduction of the postoperative hypoxic and hypercapnic drive induced by narcotics used for induction and maintenance of anesthesia (particularly in elderly patients), a residual effect of muscle relaxants used intraoperatively, the loss of pulmonary hypoxic vasoconstrictive reflexes following the administration of volatile anesthetic agents, and increased oxygen consumption due to hypertonic muscles and shivering.

2. A second pattern lasts several hours to days because of the effect of anesthesia and surgery on the chest-wall system, and this pattern appears to be an important factor contributing to the postoperative morbidity of anesthesia and surgery.

19. Describe the effect of general anesthesia on the lung-chest-wall system.

Induction of anesthesia, within 5 minutes, causes the development of compression atelectasis in the dependent part of the lung in 90% of supine subjects without preexisting lung diseases. Application of 10 cm H_2O of PEEP eliminates the atelectasis, which then reappears within 1 minute after discontinuation of PEEP. Compression atelectasis is due to a reduction in functional residual capacity, probably secondary to the relaxation of the chest wall muscles (rib cage and diaphragm) caused by the induction of anesthesia.

20. Does the extent of atelectasis correlate with impairment of gas exchange during anesthesia?

Yes. In patients with healthy lungs, a strong correlation was found during anesthesia between the amount of atelectasis and the percentage of shunt. In patients who did not develop atelectasis, there was no increase in shunt and no impairment of gas exchange during general anesthesia.

21. What causes postoperative hypothermia?

Postoperative hypothermia results from the combined effects of radiation and convective heat loss during anesthesia. Additional causes include the use of dry inspired gases and muscle relaxants that prevent shivering. Postoperative hypothermia is associated with hypoperfusion of peripheral tissues, resulting in tissue hypoxia and metabolic acidosis, coagulopathy, hypertension, and tachycardia. Therefore, patients admitted to the PACU with a core temperature < 35°C should be actively rewarmed with warmed blankets, radiant heating, or reflective coverings. In addition, such patients should receive supplemental oxygen.

22. What is the most frequent cause of postoperative nausea?

The presence of nitrous oxide in the stomach is one of the major causes of postoperative nausea. At an alveolar nitrous oxide concentration of 75%, bowel volume increases by 0.5 L/hr. Another important cause of postoperative nausea is the administration of narcotics for postoperative analgesia.

23. Does the anesthetic technique influence the liver blood supply?

Yes. Both regional and general anesthesia produce a decrease in hepatic blood flow in a dose-dependent fashion. If volatile anesthetic agents are used, isoflurane is the drug of choice to ensure maintenance of hepatic oxygenation. As hypocapnia also decreases hepatic blood flow, arterial PCO_2 should also be carefully controlled.

24. Does anesthesia influence the immune response of the patient?

Yes. Anesthesia may produce underactivity or overactivity of the immune response. All anesthetic agents produce a short-term and reversible decrease in chemotactic migration, phagocytic activity, and bactericidal function of neutrophils. However, antibody production remains unchanged. The drug most frequently implicated is nitrous oxide, which inactivates the methionine synthetase, leading to oxidation of vitamin B12, an important compound in DNA synthesis.

Overactivity of the immune system during general anesthesia is characterized by anaphylactoid reactions to intravenous anesthetic agents. Specific mechanisms by which the majority of anaphylactoid reactions occur are anaphylaxis (type 1 hypersensitivity), activation of complement system (classic or alternate pathway activation), and direct histamine liberation. Irrespective of the initial mechanism, the final pathway of an anaphylactoid response is the deregulation of mast cells with release of mediator substances. Mediator release is triggered by calcium transport through specific channels into the mast cells. Mediators are preformed or membrane-derived. Preformed granule substances include histamine, eosinophil chemotactic factors of anaphylaxis (ECF-A), and neutrophil chemotactic factor. Membrane-derived factors are leukotrienes and prostaglandins, both formed from arachidonic acid as part of the process that triggers calcium influx. More than 90% of reactions occur within 5 minutes after drug administration. Delayed hypersensitivity (type 4) reactions are rare.

25. What are the target organs of anaphylactoid reactions during general anesthesia?

Principal target organs are the skin, and the cardiovascular, respiratory, and gastrointestinal systems. Skin is involved in 75% of major hypersensitivity reactions (erythema with or without urticaria or angioedema). Hypotension occurs in 80% of patients because of H1- and H2-receptor activation and intravascular volume depletion secondary to translocation of fluid by capillary leakage. Cardiac arrhythmias are reported in 10–15% of patients as a result of effect of histamine on cardiac conduction system, endogenous release and exogenous administration of catecholamines, concurrent administration of volatile anesthetic agents, and presence of hypoxia, hypercarbia, and acidosis. Bronchospasm occurs in 30% of patients. It is mediated by the effect of histamine on H1 bronchial smooth muscle receptors, prostaglandins D_2 and F_2-alpha, and leukotrienes C_4 and D_4. Pulmonary edema occurs rarely. Abdominal pain, diarrhea, and vomiting are frequent during the recovery period, possibly because of a histamine-enhanced peristaltic activity.

26. Which drugs are implicated anesthetic anaphylactoid reaction?

Although all agents given during general anesthesia may induce the release of mediators from mast cells, the following agents are most frequently implicated in major anaphylactoid reactions: neuromuscular blocking agents (suxamethonium, alcuronium, gallamine, and tubocurarine), barbiturates (thiopental and methohexital), colloid solutions (gelatin, dextran, hetastarch), local anesthetics (procaine), and a polyoxylated castor oil (Cremophor EL) used to solubilize many anesthetic agents.

BIBLIOGRAPHY

1. Altee JL, Bosnjack ZJ: Mechanisms for cardiac dysrhythmias during anesthesia. Anesthesiology 72:347–374, 1990.
2. Cohen MM, Duncan PG, Pope WDB, Wolkenstein C: A surgery of 11,000 anesthetics at one teaching hospital (1975–1983). Can Anaesth Soc J 33:22, 1986.
3. Davies JM: Complications of general anesthesia. In Nimmo G (eds): Anesthesia. London, Blackwell Scientific Publications, 1989, pp 502–521.

4. Frost AM: Management of head injury. Can Anaesth Soc J 32:S32, 1985.
5. Grief R, Akca O, Horn EP, et al: Supplemental perioperative oxygen to reduce the incidence of surgical-wound infection. Outcomes Research Group. N Engl J Med 342:161–167, 2000.
6. Haagensen R, Steen PA: Perioperative myocardial infarction. Br J Anaesth 61:24, 1988.
7. Jakobsen CJ, Billie S, Ahlburg P, et al: Perioperative metoprolol reduces the frequency of atrial fibrillation after thoracotomy for lung resection. J Cardiothorac Vasc Anesth 11:746–751, 1997.
8. Lee TH, Marcantonia ER, Mangione CM, et al: Derivation and prospective validation of a simple index for prediction of cardiac risk of major noncardiac surgery. Circulation 100:1043–1049, 1999.
9. Magnusson L, Zemgulis V, Wicky S, et al: Atelectasis is a major cause of hypoxemia and shunt after cardiopulmonary bypass: An experimental study. Anesthesiology 87:1153–1163, 1997.
10. Mangano DT, Browner WS, Hollenberg M, et al: Association of perioperative myocardial ischemia with cardiac morbidity and mortality in men undergoing noncardiac surgery. N Engl J Med 323:1781, 1990.
11. Mangano DT, Layug EL, Wallace A, Tateo I: Effect of atenolol on mortality and cardiovascular morbidity after noncardiac surgery. N Engl J Med 335:1713–1720, 1996.
12. McGovern B: Hypokalemia and cardiac arrhythmias. Anesthesiology 63:127, 1985.
13. Mellin-Olsen J, Fasting S, Gisvold SE: Routine preoperative gastric emptying is seldom indicated. A study of 85,594 anaesthetics with special focus on aspiration pneumonia. Acta Anaesthesiol Scand 40:1184–1188, 1996.
14. Mitchel CK, Smoger SH, Pfeifer MP, et al: Multivariate analysis of factors associated with postoperative pulmonary complications following general elective surgery. Arch Surg 133:194–198, 1998.
15. Palazzo MGA, Strunin L: Anesthesia and emesis. I. Etiology. Can Anaesth Soc J 31:178, 1984.
16. Poldermans D, Boersma E, Bax J, et al: The effect of bisoprolol on perioperative mortality and myocardial infarction in high-risk patients undergoing vascular surgery. N Engl J Med 341:1789–1794, 1999.
17. Rao TLK, JAcobs KH, El-Etr AA: Reinfarction following anesthesia in patients with myocardial infarction. Anesthesiology 59:449, 1983.
18. Shah KB, Kleinman BS, Rao TLK, et al: Angina and other risk factors in patients with cardiac diseases undergoing noncardiac operations. Anesth Analg 70:240, 1990.

XV. Sedation and Pain Management

88. USE OF PARALYTIC AGENTS IN THE INTENSIVE CARE UNIT

William B. Cammarano, M.D., and Jean-François Pittet, M.D.

1. What are the two major types of muscle relaxants?

Depolarizing (e.g., succinylcholine). These act by binding to acetylcholine receptor sites and depolarizing the postjunctional membrane, preventing further muscle action potentials. This results in the relaxation of skeletal muscle. These drugs act very quickly but the effect is brief.

Nondepolarizing (e.g., pancuronium, atracurium, vecuronium). These act by competing with acetycholine for binding to the nerve endplate, but they prevent depolarization of the nerve. These agents tend to be intermediate- to long-acting relative to the depolarizing agents.

2. When should succinylcholine be used?

Critically ill patients frequently require emergent intubation. Because some patients will have full stomachs (e.g., newly admitted patients) or delayed gastric emptying (abdominal trauma, ileus, sepsis, etc.), it is imperative that intubation be done quickly in a well-controlled setting. Succinylcholine causes muscle relaxation within 30 seconds, which, in general lasts 10–15 minutes, making it useful in these situations.

3. What are the contraindications to the use of succinylcholine?

Succinylcholine causes serum potassium to increase, so it should not be used in patients with hyperkalemia. Other patients at risk for an exaggerated increase in serum potassium levels include those with renal failure, burns, crush injury, upper motor neuron injury, and lower motor neuron injury.

4. What are the indications for nondepolarizing muscle relaxants in the ICU?

Improved forms of mechanical ventilation and optimal administration of sedatives and analgesics have decreased the need for muscle relaxants. The major indications include:

- Control of shivering after cardiopulmonary bypass surgery
- Temporary control of agitated, sedated, ventilated patients
- Facilitation of mechanical ventilation in patients with severely impaired lung mechanics
- Patients in status asthmaticus who fail to respond to conventional therapy
- Control of intracranial pressure in ventilated neurosurgical or neurologic patients
- Control of painful cramps in patients with tetanus
- Decrease in oxygen consumption with improvement in visceral organ perfusion in patients with respiratory failure

5. How can we monitor the level of neuromuscular blockade in the ICU?

When a muscle relaxant is used, its effects should be monitored. Boluses or infusion rate can be adjusted to optimize the level of neuromuscular blockade. The most commonly used technique is the detection of supramaximal train-of-four stimuli delivered by a nerve stimulator usually attached over the ulnar or orbicularis nerve. The movements of the thumb or the contractions of the orbicularis muscle are observed visually. The general goal is to maintain the infusion rate of muscle relaxant at a level that produces the first twitch of the train of four. In some cases, subcutaneous edema, which is common in ICU patients, may interfere with the stimulus applied to the ulnar or orbicularis nerve. It is possible to decrease the importance of this problem by exerting a gentle pressure on the electrode for a few minutes before applying the electrical stimulus.

6. What are the risks related to use of nondepolarizing muscle relaxants in the ICU?

Prolonged use is associated with (1) inability to clear pulmonary secretions secondary to the suppression of cough, (2) atrophy of skeletal muscles, (3) venous thrombosis and pulmonary embolism, (4) osteoporosis with impairment of calcium-phosphorus balance, (5) psychic trauma if the patient is not adequately sedated while paralyzed, (6) skin breakdown, and (7) injuries to nerves and limbs secondary to poor positioning.

The patient's safety rests entirely with the medical staff and the available hemodynamic monitors, so all alarms should be activated and quickly heeded. Close attention should be paid to any changes in vital signs, as they may provide subtle clues to significant changes in clinical status.

7. Is it true that patients paralyzed with muscle relaxants are "unconscious"?

No. These patients are awake and can feel pain, so it is imperative that they receive adequate sedation and analgesia.

8. What are the most useful nondepolarizing muscle relaxants for ICU patients?

Pancuronium (Pavulon), atracurium (Tracrium), vecuronium (Norcuron), rocuronium (Zemuron), and cisatracurium (Nimbex).

9. How do you decide which agent to use?

Atracurium is spontaneously degraded in plasma rather than eliminated by the kidneys or liver, so it may be the drug of choice for patients with renal or hepatic failure. One potential serious side effect is substantial histamine release; thus it may be relatively contraindicated in patients with significant cardiovascular disease, asthma, or anaphylactoid reactions.

Vecuronium does not produce histamine release or cardiovascular instability, so it is potentially useful in patients with bronchospasm or cardiopulmonary disease. The drug is primarily metabolized by the liver and excreted in bile, and thus is useful for patients with renal failure. Prolonged neuromuscular blockade may occur in patients with hepatic failure.

Rocuronium is a newer nondepolarizing neuromuscular blocking agent with an intermediate duration and very rapid onset of action. When given as a bolus of 0.6–1.0 mg/kg, blockade is almost always achieved within 2 minutes. Its main metabolite, 17-deacetylrocuronium, has only 5–10% activity compared with the parent drug.

Pancuronium does not produce histamine release and prevents vagally mediated bradycardia, so it may be useful in patients with cardiovascular disease, however, tachycardia develops occasionally, which must be considered. Because 90% of the drug is renally excreted and 10% is metabolized by the liver, renal and hepatic function need to be monitored closely. Pancuronium is significantly less expensive than either vecuronium or atracurium.

Cisatracurium, one of the isomers of atracurium, is four times more potent than the parent drug. It seems to release less histamine than atraciurum, although its cardiovascular stability is comparable to that of atracurium. Clinical experience with cisatracurium in the ICU is limited.

10. What are the recommended dosages for nondepolarizing agents?

	Pancuronium	Vecuronium	Rocuronium	Atracurium	Cisatracurium
IV bolus	0.06–0.1 mg/kg	0.1 mg/kg	0.6–1.0 mg/kg	0.3–0.6 mg/kg	0.15 mg/kg
Infusion rate	0.03 mg/kg/hr	0.08 mg/kg/hr	0.01 mg/kg/hr	0.25 mg/kg/hr	0.1 mg/kg/hr

11. Discuss the clinically significant interactions between muscle relaxants and other drugs used in the ICU.

The following drugs have been shown to potentiate neuromuscular blockage: furosemide, type 1 antidysrhythmics, calcium channel blockers, magnesium, aminoglycosides, clindamycin, lithium, and nitroglycerin. Other drugs such as theophylline, azathioprine, and possibly steroids have been shown to decrease the level and duration of neuromuscular blockage.

12. Is prolonged neuromuscular weakness a significant problem in the ICU?
Yes. Prolonged weakness (lasting up to 84 days) has been reported with the use of nondepolarizing muscle relaxants in the ICU. Most cases have implicated vecuronium and pancuronium. There appear to be two distinct types of prolonged neuromuscular blockade related to these drugs in the ICU. The first type is a pharmacokinetic problem related to alterations in drug clearance and the formation of active metabolites; the second is a functional neuromuscular junction problem **not** related to abnormal pharmacokinetics.

13. When should an active metabolite be suspected as the cause for prolonged neuromuscular blockade in the ICU?
An active metabolite of vecuronium, 3-desacetylvecuronium, having a prolonged half-life, has caused prolonged weakness in ICU patients receiving vecuronium for greater than 48 hours. Patients at high risk appear to be those with (1) renal failure, (2) hypermagnesemia, (3) metabolic acidosis, or (4) those of female gender.

14. When should a functional neuromuscular abnormality be suspected as a cause of prolonged weakness?
As stated above, a number of drugs can cause weakness. Other factors, including poor nutrition, infections, atrophy, and demyelination (e.g. chronic inflammatory demyelinating polyneuropathy), may also contribute to prolonged weakness, with or without the use of neuromuscular blocking agents. However, it is becoming increasingly clear that the combination of steroidal neuromuscular blocking agents (vecuronium and pancuronium) with high-dose corticosteroids may result in an increased incidence of prolonged weakness in ICU patients. Severe asthmatics appear to be at high risk, and vecuronium or pancuronium should be used with caution in these patients.

15. Can prolonged neuromuscular blockade be prevented in the ICU?
Further studies are needed to determine the safety of neuromuscular blockers in the ICU and whether complications may be avoided by monitoring depth of blockade. Common sense recommendations seem prudent. First, one should use neuromuscular blocking agents only when indicated, in the lowest effective dose, and for the shortest duration as clinical circumstances allow. Second, one should consider avoiding the use of vecuronium or pancuronium in patients with renal failure. Third, one should consider the avoidance of steroidal muscle relaxants (vecuronium or pancuronium) in patients receiving corticosteroids. Fourth, one should monitor depth of blockade with a nerve stimulator in order to maintain at least one twitch on a train of four.

16. What is the best way to terminate the actions of muscular relaxants?
The best way is to ventilate the patients and wait until these drugs are metabolized or excreted. Assessment of the level of neuromuscular blockage by nerve stimulator may be useful in some circumstances.

17. Which drugs can be used to terminate the action of muscle relaxants?
Nondepolarizing muscle relaxants may be antagonized by anticholinesterase drugs, which block the hydrolysis of acetylcholine. As a result, acetylcholine accumulates at the neuromuscular junction and antagonizes the blockage.

18. What is the usual dosage of anticholinesterase drugs?
The following drugs may be administered in an IV bolus: neostigmine, 0.03–0.06 mg/kg; pyridostigmine, 0.1–0.2 mg/kg; edrophonium, 0.5–1.0 mg/kg.

19. What is the most common side effect of anticholinesterase drugs?
The most common side effect is excessive stimulation of cholinergic receptors in the peripheral nervous system, which elicits bradycardia, vasodilation, contraction of ureter and bronchioles,

increased gastrointestinal motility and secretion of hydrogen chloride from gastric parietal cells, increased secretory gland activity, and miosis. To counteract these effects, it is customary to administer anticholinesterase drugs in combination with atropine (0.01–0.02 mg/kg IV) or glycopyrrolate (0.01 mg/kg IV).

BIBLIOGRAPHY

1. Gilston A: Paralysis or sedation for controlled ventilation. Lancet 1:480, 1980.
2. Green D: Paralysis or sedation for controlled ventilation. Lancet 1:715, 1980.
3. Lumb PD: Sedatives and muscle relaxants in the intensive care unit. In Fuhrman BP, Shoemaker WC (eds): Critical Care: State of the Art, Vol. 10. Fullerton, CA, Society for Critical Care Medicine, 1989, p 145.
4. Marik PE, Kaufman D: The effects of neuromuscular paralysis on systemic and splanchnic oxygen utilization in mechanically ventilated patients. Chest 109:1038–1042, 1996.
5. Miller-Jones CMH: Paralysis or sedation for controlled ventilation. Lancet 1:312, 1980.
6. Partridge BL: Clinical use of muscle relaxants: Avoiding the complications. Prog Anesthesiol 4:314–323, 1990.
7. Rudis MI, Sikora CA, Angus E, et al: A prospective, randomized, controlled evaluation of peripheral nerve stimulation versus standard clinical dosing of neuromuscular blocking agents in critically ill patients. Crit Care Med 25:575–583, 1997.
8. Schapera A: The use of neuromuscular blocking agents in the intensive care unit. Pulmonary and Critical Care Update 5:1–7, 1990.
9. Segredo V, Caldwell JE, Matthay MA, et al: Persistent paralysis in critically ill patients after long-term administration of vecuronium. N Engl J Med 327:524–528, 1992.
10. Watling SM, Dastra JF: Prolonged paralysis in intensive care unit patients after the use of neuromuscular blocking agents: A review of the literature. Crit Care Med 22:884–893, 1994.

89. PAIN MANAGEMENT IN THE INTENSIVE CARE UNIT

William B. Cammarano, M.D., Daniel Burkhardt, M.D., and Jean-François Pittet, M.D.

1. Is the relief of pain generally adequate in ICU patients?

Probably not. Many studies have reported that inadequate pain relief is common after surgery. The potential for inadequate analgesia is probably greater in ICU patients, who are often confused, paralyzed, or unable to communicate.

2. Why do ICU patients often receive inadequate analgesia?

Physicians frequently underestimate the amount of pain patients are experiencing and are overly concerned about side effects of treatment.

3. Why is it important to provide adequate pain relief?

Aside from humanitarian reasons, adequate analgesia has a number of benefits:

- Prevention of deep venous thrombosis and lung embolism by earlier patient mobilization.
- Attenuation of the stress response and more rapid normalization of the overactivity of the nervous system (tachycardia, hypertension, increased systemic vascular resistance and oxygen consumption), which is poorly tolerated by critically ill or geriatric patients.
- Provision of analgesia with epidural local anesthetics and/or opioids may prevent pulmonary complications in patients having blunt chest trauma.
- Some data suggest that the combination of intraoperative epidural anesthesia followed by postoperative epidural analgesia may improve outcome in certain vascular surgery patients.

4. Are pain-stimulating factors present in the ICU environment?

Yes. Admission to an ICU provokes anxiety, which leads to sleep deprivation and discomfort and increases the perception of pain. Noise, a common problem in the ICU, interferes with sleep and has been found to increase analgesic requirements. Restraints and forced immobility due to numerous tubes and catheters also exacerbate pain.

5. What methods can be used for relieving pain in the ICU?

Opioid or nonopioid analgesics and regional nerve blocks are the classic methods. Other methods such as electroanalgesia, psychotherapy, or hypnosis should also be considered.

6. What are the opioids currently recommended for routine parenteral administration in ICU patients?

Currently morphine, fentanyl and hydromorphone (Dilaudid) are recommended for routine parenteral analgesia in ICU patients.

Morphine: a naturally occurring opioid with a long clinical history and therefore excellent physician familiarity with its use. It is relatively hydrophilic compared to fentanyl and hydromorphone, and therefore is less potent and has a slower onset. Because of its greater water solubility, it does have a longer duration of action than the other two agents. The time to peak onset for morphine (by bolus) is approximately 20–30 minutes, and duration of action is 2–4 hours.

Fentanyl: a synthetic, highly potent and lipid soluble opioid. It has a potency 80–100 fold greater than morphine, and because of its great lipid solubility, it also has a much more rapid onset time and shorter duration of action. The time to peak onset for fentanyl (by bolus) is 1–3 minutes, and duration of action is 30–45 minutes. Because of its short duration of action, fentanyl is an excellent drug administered by infusion. After long-term use (3–4 days), one can expect a significant increase in the duration of action of fentanyl.

Hydromorphone: a semisynthetic opioid which is highly lipid soluble and more potent than morphine (5–10 fold greater). Its time to peak effect (by bolus) is 10–20 minutes, and duration of action is 1–3 hours.

7. When should fentanyl or hydromorphone be used instead of morphine?

Morphine has a more potent effect in reducing preload (and therefore blood pressure) than either fentanyl or hydromorphone, and therefore should not be used in the acutely hemodynamically unstable patient, especially if hypovolemia is suspected or confirmed. Glucuronide metabolites with analgesic properties and very long half-lives exist for morphine and may accumulate in patients with renal failure; therefore, fentanyl or hydromorphone may be preferable in such patients. Finally, histamine release may occur with morphine administration, and if this is a clinical problem, fentanyl or hydromorphone may also be preferable in this setting.

8. What are reasonable starting doses for opioids in adult ICU patients?

Suggested Doses of Opioids for Adult ICU Patients

	BOLUS	INFUSION	PCA BOLUS
Morphine	2–5 mg	2–10 mg/hr	0.5–1.0 mg
Fentanyl	25–100 µg	25–100 µg/hr	10–25 µg
Hydromorphone	0.5–1 mg	0.5–2 mg/hr	0.2–0.3 mg

9. Which opioids should be avoided in the ICU for routine analgesia?

Meperidine and the mixed agonist/antagonist opioids should be avoided. Meperidine, a low- potency opioid, is metabolized to a potentially proconvulsant compound (normeperidine), which can be especially troublesome in patients with renal failure. Mixed agonist/antagonist agents may precipitate withdrawal syndrome in patients who have developed tolerance or dependence to opioids.

10. Which opioid is most effective at terminating postoperative shivering?

Postoperative shivering can increase oxygen consumption three- to four-fold in postoperative patients and may be especially detrimental if it occurs in patients with ischemic heart disease or reduced cardiovascular reserve. Meperidine is useful in the treatment of postoperative shivering and has been demonstrated to be superior to morphine and fentanyl for this indication. An intravenous dose of 10–25 mg (which is usually subanalgesic) is usually adequate.

11. What are the indications for opioid analgesics in the ICU?

Opioids are administered most often for pain relief. They are used for their beneficial side effects, including sedation, depression of respiratory drive, and attenuation of psychologic discomfort.

12. How can opioid analgesics be administered to ICU patients?

Opioids are administered orally, rectally, sublingually/transbucally, intramuscularly, or intravenously as repeated boluses or as continuous infusions, in the epidural space or spinal space, or transmdermally. Intravenously administered opioids can be given by the nurse or by the patient through patient-controlled analgesia (PCA). The intramuscular route should not be used for administration of opioids to ICU patients, because the serum drug levels are extremely variable.

13. Does the achievement of pain relief correlate with the blood level of opioid analgesics?

Yes. It is generally accepted that analgesia occurs when a definite blood level of opioids has been achieved (analgesia threshold). This blood level is not the same for all patients. Therefore, the concept of a minimum effect analgesic concentration (MEAC) has been proposed and corresponds to the minimum blood level of opioid that provides effective analgesia for an individual patient. Each patient has a different MEAC, which changes as the intensity of pain changes. As physical tolerance develops, a progressively higher serum level is required to achieve the same degree of analgesia.

14. What are the advantages and disadvantages of intermittent IV bolus and continuous IV infusion of opioid analgesics?

Intermittent IV boluses of opioids can relieve pain effectively if the patient is observed closely to determine when the blood level of opioid is below the MEAC. This method prevents drug accumulation and allows rapid drug elimination when the drug is stopped. In practice, close evaluation of a patient's pain is seldom possible because ICU nurses are busy. In addition, an accurate assessment of the level of analgesia in intubated, mechanically ventilated patients is understandably difficult. Even so, efforts should be made to quantify objectively the patient's level of pain (the visual analog scale [VAS] is an excellent method to achieve this goal).

Continuous IV infusions of opioids easily maintain a blood drug level above the MEAC. This technique needs minimal nursing care and often provides good analgesia. However, excessive drug accumulation may occur, particularly in patients with hepatic or renal failure. The use of newer opioids, such as fentanyl, which have more rapid onsets and shorter half-lives may be advantageous. The difficult problem when using continuous IV infusion of narcotics is determining the proper dose. An objective clinical assessment of analgesia is difficult, and the patient should therefore be consulted about his or her pain relief (see above).

15. Does ketamine have a role as an anaglesic/sedative agent in the ICU?

Recent national guidelines do not recommend the use of ketamine, a phencyclidine derivative, in the ICU because of its many unwanted side effects. The most important are elevations in blood pressure, heart rate, and intracranial as well as increased airway secretions. Morever, vivid dreams and hallucinations may be a problem in 30% of patients on discontinuation of the drug. However, because of its potent analgesic effect and rapid onset and short duration of action, IV boluses of ketamine (0.5–1.0 mg/kg) have been used in ICU patients to enhance tolerance of limited but painful procedures, such as dressing changes for burns. The guideline emphasizes that ketamine should not be the primary analgesic/sedative agent for ICU patients. It is a popular drug for dressing changes because it leads to less respiratory depression than equianalgesic doses of opioids. If ketamine is used, a hypnotic/anxioilytic agent should be administered to avoid vivid dreams and hallucinations.

16. What is patient-controlled analgesia (PCA)?

PCA is a system that allows the patient to monitor his or her own blood level of opioid analgesia by its effect on pain, and to self-administer the drug to achieve pain relief. This system was developed about 25 years ago but recently became more popular with the wide availability of commercial devices.

17. What is the goal of PCA?

The goal of PCA is to produce a relatively stable and effective level of opioids by allowing the patient to receive multiple small boluses following an initial loading dose. This allows the patient to maintain his or her opioid blood level above the MEAC. PCA may also be used with continuous IV infusion of opioids.

18. Is there an advantage to continuous opioid infusions delivered by PCA?

Probably not. The advantages of a continuous opioid infusion delivered by PCA are questionable for several reasons. First, PCA continuous infusions bypass the intrinsic safety feature of standard, bolus-only PCA by allowing opioids to be continuously delivered even if sedation is excessive. Second, studies have demonstrated that postoperative patients treated with PCA plus continuous infusion have no improvement in analgesia, but have a significantly greater number of side effects compared to postoperative patients receiving standard PCA.

19. What are the characteristics of PCA devices?

PCA devices are microprocessor-based pumps that can deliver opioids on demand. The following parameters can be set on the pump: the dose administered when the patient pushes the button, the lock-out interval or length of time between doses, the maximal dose to be given, the initial loading dose, and a bolus dose that can be used for extreme pain.

20. Do patients receive more opioids when using PCA than they do with other traditional techniques?

No. Studies have shown that PCA patients used more opioids on the first day but less on subsequent days. The risk of addiction is minimal. Patients prefer this pain-relief technique because they control analgesia administration.

21. What are the undesirable side effects of intravenous opioids?

Examples include respiratory depression; euphoria and development of addiction; a withdrawal syndrome when narcotics are administered over a long period (0.1 mg IV clonidine, twice daily, may be helpful in this situation); increased gastric, pancreatic, and biliary secretions; increased tone in anal, biliary, and ileocolic sphincters; release of histamine (morphine, meperidine); and development of seizures (fentanyl, sulfentanil), particularly in patients with chronic renal failure.

22. What is the rationale for using epidural opioid analgesia in the ICU?

Administration of opioids into the epidural space produces safe and effective analgesia equal or superior to that produced by conventional analgesic techniques. However, epidural opioid analgesia has been associated with less sedation, greater improvement in postoperative pulmonary function, earlier ambulation, decreased morbidity, and shorter hospital stay compared with other analgesic techniques.

23. How can opioids be administered in the epidural space?

Techniques of epidural opioid administration include intermittent boluses, continuous infusion, or epidural PCA. Although adequate analgesia may be obtained with all of these techniques, continuous epidural infusion of narcotics allows a more selective titration of analgesia, and the use of more lipophilic opioids with short duration of action and less intrinsic risk of respiratory depression. The concomitant use of local anesthetics is performed more safely (stable sympathetic blockage) with this technique than with repeated boluses.

24. What are the undesirable side effects of epidural opioids? How are they managed?

Respiratory depression, particularly in elderly patients, is the most serious side effect. Respiratory depression following epidural morphine has been reported to be biphasic: an early phase resulting from absorption in epidural veins and circulatory redistribution to the brain, and a late phase resulting from the cephalic movement of the morphine in the cerebrospinal fluid. Avoidance of large doses of epidural opioids, careful titration of analgesia, and use of lipophilic narcotics may significantly increase the margin of safety with this technique.

Side effects of epidural opioids include itching, nausea and vomiting, urine retention, and decreased gastrointestinal motility. Itching, nausea and vomiting may be treated by very small IV doses of naloxone (0.04–0.08 mg), which do not completely antagonize the epidural analgesia and do not produce the undesirable side effects (hypertension, cardiac arrhythmias, lung edema, and sudden death) observed after greater doses (0.4 mg).

25. What is the rationale for using nonopioid analgesics in the ICU?

Nonopioid analgesics (prostaglandin inhibitors) are particularly effective in reducing muscular and skeletal pain and may decrease the need for opioids. They are often more effective than opioids in reducing pain from pleural or pericardial rubs, a pain that responds poorly to opioids. They are also useful in providing analgesia for neurosurgical patients who are not ventilated, because opioids may reduce respiratory drive and lead to CO_2 retention and increased intracranial pressure in patients with poor cerebral compliance.

At present, only one nonopioid analgesic (ketorolac) is widely available in a parenteral preparation. Most of these compounds decrease platelet function and therefore may interfere with hemostasis. Prostaglandins are involved in the regulation of the renal function. Their inhibition by nonopioid analgesia may lead to sodium and water retention, hyperkalemia, increased blood pressure, and impaired response to diuretics. Gastrointestinal bleeding is not uncommon with the use of nonopioid analgesics and may be especially poorly tolerated in critically ill patients. Acetaminophen is often used as a nonopioid anaglesic; high doses, however, cause liver toxicity and should not be given to patients with liver disease or patients who consume large quantities of alcohol.

26. What are the advantages of regional blocks for ICU patients?

The greatest advantage of regional anesthesia is the production of pain relief superior both in quality and duration to that obtained by IV opioids. In particular, regional blocks provide sufficient analgesia for movement and physiotherapy, whereas opioids only eliminate pain at rest. Other advantages include a greater improvement in respiratory function by inhibition of muscle spasms, the provision of analgesia with a minimum of sedation which may facilitate neurologic assessment, less constipation, and a possible reduction in the incidence of thromboembolic phenomena.

27. What are the limitations to regional anesthesia in the ICU?

Regional blocks are time-consuming, difficult to perform, and contraindicated in patients who have a coagulopathy or receive anticoagulants. Epidural or other catheters used to administer local anesthetics continuously may become infected. Local anesthetics have a low therapeutic/toxic ratio and may accumulate easily, particularly in patients with renal or hepatic failure.

28. Is regional analgesia safe in the setting of deep vein thrombosis (DVT) prophylaxis with unfractionated or low molecular weight heparin (LMWH)?

Regional analgesia is not contraindicated in the setting of minidose (i.e., 5000 units subcutaneous injection every 12 hours) unfractionated heparin administration for DVT prophylaxis, although practitioners must be vigilant for the development of epidural hematoma in this setting.

Although not contraindicated, the use of epidural analgesia in the setting of LMWH requires greater care as a number of epidural/spinal hematomas have been reported in this setting. Recommendations are available regarding the placement and removal of epidural catheters in the setting of concomitant LMWH use.

29. Are hypnosis and relaxation-associated strategies useful for treating acute pain in the ICU?
Yes. Hypnotic strategies have been used successfully for treating acute pain in the ICU, particularly for patients suffering extensive burns. Hypnosis has been hypothesized to reduce pain through mechanisms such as control of attention or dissociation. During hypnosis, suggestions are combined with imagery to enhance the feeling of comfort.

30. Does hypnosis decrease acute pain in every ICU patient?
No. The reduction of pain depends on the suggestibility of the patient. Moreover, it appears that effective pain reduction is consistently achieved when patients have had sufficient practice with such techniques.

BIBLIOGRAPHY

1. Austin KL, Stapleton JV, Mather LE: Multiple intramuscular injections: A major source of variability in analgesic response to meperidine. Pain 8:46–62, 1980.
2. Bion JF, Logan BK, Newman PM, et al: Sedation in intensive care: Morphine and renal function. Intens Care Med 12:359, 1986.
3. Cicala RS, Voeller GR, Fox T, et al: Epidural analgesia in thoracic trauma: Effects of lumbar morphine and thoracic bupivicaine on pulmonary function. Crit Care Med 18:229–231, 1990.
4. Donovan M, Dillon P, McGuire L: Incidence and characteristics of pain in a sample of medical-surgical inpatients. Pain 30:69, 1987.
5. Ferrante FM, Orav EJ, Rocco AG, et al: A statistical model for pain in patient-controlled analgesia and conventional intramuscular opioid regimens. Anesth Analg 67:457, 1988.
6. Forrest WH, Smethurst PWR, Kienitz ME: Self-administration of intravenous analgesics. Anesthesiology 33:363, 1970.
7. Hansell NH: The behavioral effect of noise on man: The patient with "intensive care unit psychosis." Heart Lung 13:59, 1984.
8. Horlocker T: Low molecular weight heparin and central neuraxial anesthesia. Am Soc of Reg Anesth News (February); 5–6, 1996.
9. Jones J, Hoggart B, Withey J, et al: What the patient says: A study of reactions to an intensive care unit. Intensive Care Med 5:89, 1979.
10. Pansard JL, Mankikian B, Bertrand M, et al: Effects of thoracic extradural block on diaphragmatic electrical activity and contractility after upper abdominal surgery. Anesthesiology 78:63–71, 1993.
11. Parker RK, Holtmann B, White PF: Effects of a nighttime opioid infusion with PCA therapy on patient comfort and analgesic requirements after abdominal hysterectomy. Anesthesiology 76:362–367, 1992.
12. Pauca AL, Savage RT, Simpson S, et al: Effect of pethidine, fentanyl and morphine on postoperative shivering in man. Acta Anaesthesiol Scand 28:138-143, 1984.
13. Peck CL: Psychological factors in acute pain management. In Cousins MJ, Phillips GD (eds): Acute Pain Management. New York, Churchill Livingstone, 1985, pp 251.
14. Pflug AE, Murphy TM, Butler SH, et al: The effects of postoperative peridural analgesia on pulmonary therapy and pulmonary complications. Anesthesiology 41:8, 1974.
15. Rowbotham DJ: Cisapride and anesthesia. Br J Anaesth 62:121, 1989.
16. Shapiro B, Warren J, Egol A, et al: Practice parameters for intravenous analgesia and sedation for adult patients in the intensive care unit: an executive summary. Crit Care Med 23:1596–1600, 1995.
17. Yeager MP, Glass DD, Neff RK, et al: Epidural anesthesia in high-risk patients. Anesthesiology 66:729, 1987.

90. SEDATION

Jill A. Rebuck, Pharm. D., B.C.P.S.

1. What is the goal of sedation in most critically ill patients?

To decrease the level of anxiety and agitation and to produce a calm but communicative state while minimizing patient discomfort.

2. What is the prefered analgesic for mechanically ventilated patients in the ICU?

Morphine sulfate, although fentanyl should be considered if the patient has a morphine allergy, symptoms of histamine release, or hemodynamic instability during morphine infusion. Both agents undergo hepatic elimination. Morphine, however, possesses a potent active metabolite, morphine-6-glucoronide, which is renally excreted and may accumulate in patients with significant renal failure. Fentanyl is extremely lipophilic compared with morphine and has a more rapid onset and shorter duration of action; in addition, it is 100 times more potent than morphine. Typical bolus doses of morphine include 2–10 mg every 2–4 hours or infusions of 1–5 mg/hr compared with 1–2 μg/kg every hour or infusion of 50–150 μg/hr for fentanyl.

3. Describe the therapeutic effects of benzodiazepines.

The therapeutic effects of benzodiazepines are caused by alterations primarily on binding to the gamma-aminobutyric acid (GABA) neurotransimtter. Benzodiazepines have antianxiety, sedative, anticonvulsant, hypnotic, and muscle-relaxant properties. Because they have no analgesic activity, an analgesic agent such as morphine should be prescribed.

4. What is the benzodiazepine of choice for sedation in the ICU?

Midazolam is preferred for short-term (< 24-hour) therapy, whereas lorazepam is indicated for prolonged treatment (> 24 hours) of anxiety. Midazolam is a short-acting agent that rapidly penetrates the central nervous system (CNS) and produces onset of sedation within 2–2.5 minutes and possesses an active metabolite, 1-hydroxymidazolam. Lorazepam is an intermediate-acting benzodiazepine that is less lipophilic than midazolam and thus has a slightly delayed onset of action. Lorazepam has less potential for peripheral accumulation and no active metabolites; it also has been shown to produce more rapid awakening with prolonged administration.

5. What sedative should be chosen for patients who require neurologic monitoring?

Propofol is preferred for intubated patients who require rapid titration to multiple levels of sedation for neurologic monitoring. Subanesthetic doses produce effects of anxiolysis and amnesia. Propofol has a rapid onset of action and brief effect due to rapid CNS penetration and redistribution. Elimination is reduced in elderly patients but not in patients with renal or hepatic disease. Long-term infusions result in accumulation in lipid stores, although on discontinuation a rapid 50% decrease in serum concentration occurs in most patients.

6. Which medication is useful for the treatment of ICU delirium?

Haloperidol is the preferred agent for treatment of delirium in adult ICU patients. It is a neuroleptic that binds to postsynaptic dopamine receptors and has strong central antidopaminergic activity. All patients should be monitored closely for extrapyramidal side effects, presence of neuroleptic malignant syndrome, and QT prolongation, which may lead to torsades de pointes. Necessary dosages vary, although many patients are controlled with the administration of 2–5 mg intravenously every 4–6 hours. On rare occasions, ICU patients may require a continuous infusion to control agitation, with dosages of 3–25 mg/hr reported in a limited number of patients.

7. How does daily assessment of an ICU patient receiving continuous sedation improve outcome?

Interrupting continuous sedation (e.g., with midazolam or propofol) until the patient awakens each day shortens the duration of mechanical ventilation as well as length of stay in the ICU. Thus, it is important to assess each patient daily by performing wake-up examinations and decreasing the infusion rate appropriately, as tolerated by the patient, to eliminate prolonged recovery.

8. How do you best control the specific level of sedation for each patient?

Several scales are available to improve control of the individual level of sedation for each patient, including the Ramsay, Sedation-Agitation, and Motor Activity Assessment Scales. For example, if the Ramsay Scale is used, patients are maintained at a specific Ramsay level, noted as a number from 1 to 6. Most patients require a Ramsay level of 3 (responding to commands) or 4 (brisk response to stimulus such as light glabellar tap or loud auditory stimulus). Sedation scales are powerful tools because they allow the ICU practitioner to indicate a specific level of sedation to the nursing staff and also decrease the possibility of oversedation.

9. Name various complications that may be seen in agitated adult patients in the ICU.

Agitation, a definite problem in critically ill patients, may be due to pain, anxiety, or disorientation. Complications in agitated patients may include self-extubation, removal of arterial lines and venous catheters, increased oxygen requirements, and the negative effect incurred when the patient cannot participate in improving his or her own care. Efforts must be made to identify the cause of agitation (e.g., hypoxia, alcohol withdrawal, pain, sleep disturbances) before pharmacologic agents are administered.

10. What reversal agent is available for oversedation due to benzodiazepines?

Flumazenil antagonizes the actions of benzodiazepines on the CNS by competitively inhibiting activity at the benzodiazepine recognition site on the GABA/benzodiazepine receptor complex. Of importance, flumazenil does not antagonize effects of opioids or other nonbenzodiazepine sedatives. Flumazenil is administered at a dose of 0.2 mg intravenously over 15 seconds; the dose can be repeated as necessary to a maximal total dose of 1 mg. Onset of reversal occurs within 1–2 minutes after injection. Flumazenil may lower the seizure threshold in patients with a predisposition to seizure activity and thus is not recommended in patients with a seizure disorder, patients receiving sedation for intracranial pressure control, and patients presenting with cyclic antidepressant overdose.

11. What is the most effective way to decrease the time required to achieve adequate sedation when lorazepam is prescribed for prolonged therapy?

Lorazepam is an intermediate-acting benzodiazepine with a slightly delayed onset of action. When it is used as a continuous infusion for prolonged sedation (> 24 hours), dosing during administration influences time to adequate sedation. Patients should receive a bolus dose (typically 2 mg) before the continuous infusion is initiated. Further increases in infusion rate should be accompanied by an additional bolus of medication. Otherwise, once the drip is initiated, patients require longer periods to reach steady state and thus may risk oversedation later because of unnecessary increases in infusion rates secondary to inadequate initial sedation.

12. Which agent—midazolam or profofol—is preferred for short-term sedation in the ICU?

Either is acceptable. The two agents are equally effective in providing adequate short-term sedation to critically ill patients. Patients who receive propofol infusions tend to have a shorter time to extubation, although this does not necessarily correlate with decreased length of stay in the ICU. Midazolam may provide less expensive sedation for most patients and is typically preferred in patients who do not require frequent neurologic monitoring.

13. What anxiety-related issue must be considered in patients who have an inadequate response to appropriate sedation therapy?

It is important to assess the level of pain control, because most sedatives do not have analgesic properties. In addition, ICU delirium, which may further complicate the clinical picture, should be considered in the differential diagnosis.

14. Do all patients paralyzed in the ICU require concurrent sedation?

Yes. All paralyzed patients must receive concurrent analgesia and sedation, because neuromuscular blocking agents do not reduce either pain or anxiety.

15. What is the potential role of dexmedetomidine (Precedex) in the postoperative surgical ICU patient?

Dexmedetomidine, which has unique alpha$_2$-adrenergic properties, recently became available as an intravenous sedative agent for use in patients undergoing initital mechanical ventilation. Potential advantages related to its use include ease of patient awakening on stimulation during sedative infusion, decreased requirements for pain medication, increased ability of patients to communicate with caregivers, and lack of respiratory depression, which may allow faster ventilator weaning either in the immediate postoperative period or in long-term patients having difficulty with weaning from the ventilator because of agitation when the current sedative is discontinued. The loading dose of 1 μg/kg over 10 minutes may result in significant hypotension; thus, the dose should be either decreased (0.5 μg/kg) or prolonged (20- to 30-minute infusion). The loading dose is followed by a continuous infusion of 0.2–7 μg/kg/hr. Bradycardia and hypotension, especially in hypovolemic patients, are the most prominent adverse effects.

BIBLIOGRAPHY

1. Chamorro C, et al: Comparative study of propofol versus midazolam in the sedation of critically ill patients: Results of a prospective, randomized, multicenter trial. Crit Care Med 24:932–939, 1996.
2. Durbin CG: Sedation in the critically ill patient. New Horizons 2:64–74, 1994.
3. Jacobi J, et al: Clinical practice guidelines for the sustained use of sedatives and analgesics in the critically ill adult. Crit Care Med 30:119–141, 2002.
4. Kress JP, et al: Daily interruption of sedative infusions in critically ill patients undergoing mechanical ventilation. N Engl J Med 342:1471–1477, 2000.
5. Ostermann ME, et al: Sedation in the intensive care unit. JAMA 283:1451–1459, 2000.
6. Pohlman AS, et al: Continuous intravenous infusions of lorazepam versus midazolam for sedation during mechanical ventilatory support: A prospective, randomized study. Crit Care Med 22:1241–1247, 1994.
7. Riker RR, et al: Continuous infusion of haloperidol controls agitation in critically ill patients. Crit Care Med 22:433–440, 1995.
8. Shapiro BA, et al: Practice parameters for intravenous analgesia and sedation for adult patients in the intensive care unit: An executive summary. Crit Care Med 23:1596–1600, 1995.
9. Young C, et al: Sedation in the intensive care unit. Crit Care Med 28:854–866, 2000.

XVI. Radiology

91. CT SCANNING OF THE CHEST AND ABDOMEN IN THE ICU SETTING

Suzanne Z. Barkin, M.D., and Randall M. Patten, M.D.

1. Is computed tomography (CT) scanning of the chest useful in the ICU patient, especially considering such problems as patient transport and monitoring?

Yes. In select groups of patients, CT scanning has contributed additional information and altered management in up to 70% of those scanned.

2. What are indications for CT scanning of the chest in the ICU patient?

- To explore differential considerations when the clinical course is not explained by plain chest and abdominal x-ray findings.
- To distinguish pleural from parenchymal disease; to distinguish lung abscess versus empyema.
- To determine the presence or position of a pneumothorax, particularly a loculated one, and document position of chest tube(s).
- To further define equivocal findings on plain x-ray studies: for example, cavity or pneumatocele vs. uninvolved lung, pulmonary nodules, or mediastinal abnormalities.
- To diagnose pulmonary thromboembolism.

3. How does CT scanning of the chest add information not readily detectable by portable radiography?

The combination of contrast resolution over a wide range of densities and thin (usually 1 cm or less) axial sectioning provides greater anatomic detail of the mediastinum, lungs, and pleura. Confusing and overlapping shadows are eliminated, allowing clarification of anatomic relationships in a two-dimensional (and potentially three-dimensional) perspective.

4. What are some findings on chest CT scans that may be unsuspected on portable chest radiographs, and that may significantly affect patient management?

Pneumothorax, pleural effusion, pericardial effusion, lung abscess, cavity, lung laceration, empyema, mediastinal abnormalities (hematoma, adenopathy, abscess), and atelectasis (especially left upper lobe, which may be difficult to evaluate on a plain AP portable film). An abnormal chest tube position may be clarified. Occasionally, diffuse edema or focal pneumonia may be more readily detected by CT.

5. When is CT scanning of the abdomen indicated in the critically ill patient?

Indications include suspected abscess, abdominal symptoms not explained by physical examination, and persistent and unexplained acidosis following surgery or trauma. CT also can be used to differentiate ileus from mechanical small bowel obstruction, with occasional determination of cause.

6. What findings on abdominal CT scan may not be apparent on plain films?

Abscess, organomegaly, pancreatic pseudocyst or phlegmon, small bowel obstruction (especially with fluid filled bowel), bowel wall edema or pneumatosis, free intraperitoneal air, air in portal veins or biliary tree, ascites, abdominal aortic aneurysm, and retroperitoneal processes may be detected. Chest processes such as pneumothorax, pleural effusion, or lower lobe pneumonia may also be identified on the upper slices.

7. What is helical (spiral) CT? What are its advantages?

Helical CT permits simultaneous patient translation and data acquisition through a continuously rotating x-ray source and detector array combined with a high-heat-capacity x-ray tube. Advantages are significantly shorter scanning time and markedly decreased artifact from respiratory motion. Reformation of images in coronal, sagittal, or three-dimensional planes is possible. Helical CT can quickly image opacified blood vessels, making CT angiography an alternative to catheter angiography in patients with emergent vascular problems.

8. When is iodinated intravenous contrast indicated in CT of the chest or abdomen?

Chest: delineates mediastinal abnormalities, vascular vs. nonvascular masses, evaluation of hilar adenopathy vs. enlarged pulmonary arteries, thoracic aortic dissection, or aneurysm. Contrast is *not* needed for evaluation of pleural vs. parenchymal disease, lung nodules, abscesses, etc.

Abdomen: contrast is generally helpful in evaluating liver, spleen, pancreas, kidneys, and bladder for focal abnormalities. It is generally used in patients with multiple injuries. Abdominal aortic aneurysm and possible leak are well evaluated with contrast-enhanced CT. However, abdominal CT without intravenous contrast may still be quite valuable if contrast is contraindicated.

9. What are the risks of intravenously administered iodinated contrast? What are the contraindications?

Risks: (1) Allergic reaction is usually mild. Mild reactions are even less frequent with nonionic contrast agents. Severe reactions occur in about 1/3,000–1/14,000 cases, and death as a result of contrast material has been reported in about 1/14,000–1/117,000 cases. The number of mild and moderate reactions has decreased with the more common administration of nonionic agents. (2) Renal failure may occur, but this risk in the normal patient is small. Risk is increased in patients with dehydration, previously existing renal disease, and diabetes with abnormal creatinine. (3) Extravasation of contrast into soft tissues may produce tissue necrosis.

Contraindications: Previous severe reaction or preexisting nephropathy, particularly in a diabetic.

10. How may the risks of intravenous contrast be minimized?

Renal failure. Adequate hydration is extremely important. In patients with mild preexisting nephropathy, mannitol may be administered immediately prior to and following the procedure. Creatinine should be measured in patients at risk; with significant elevation of creatinine, alternative diagnostic methods should be sought. CT with only oral contrast may still be an extremely useful diagnostic procedure.

Allergic reaction. Pretreatment with corticosteroids (e.g., 32 mg of methylprednisolone orally 12 and 2 hours prior to administration) has been reported to decrease the incidence of allergic reactions but remains controversial. Low-osmolality nonionic contrast materials appear to be associated with a significantly decreased incidence of allergic reaction.

11. What is the value of oral contrast in CT scanning of the abdomen? Which oral contrast agent is used?

Oral contrast is essential to distinguish fluid-filled loops of bowel from abnormal collections, such as abscess or tumor, which are both soft-tissue density by CT. Very dilute (1–2% w/v) barium or water-soluble contrast (diatrizoate or ioxaglate at about 2% iodine) is used. Meticulous attention to administration (orally or nasogastrically) is necessary for good GI contrast. Ideally, 1000 cc should be administered in 3–4 doses every 20–30 minutes to opacify the entire bowel. If pelvic or paracolic gutter pathology is of particular interest, dilute barium or water-soluble enema may be given just prior to the CT scan.

12. What previous studies interfere with CT scanning of the body?

Barium in the GI tract from a prior study will cause marked degradation of the CT image. Barium is so dense that extensive streak artifact is created, in the same manner that a piece of metal creates streak artifact. This artifact may also degrade images of the lung bases on a chest CT scan. CT scanning should be delayed until barium is cleared from the GI tract. Certain procedures performed prior to CT scanning may create iatrogenic abnormalities. For example, diagnostic peritoneal lavage prior to abdominal CT scanning may introduce pneumoperitoneum and free intraperitoneal fluid, which are indistinguishable from findings secondary to bowel perforation.

13. How may subsequent studies be affected by prior CT with intravenous and/or oral contrast?
Intravenous contrast administers a large (about 30 gm) load of iodine to the body. A significant amount is taken up by the thyroid, and the thyroid becomes saturated with iodine. Iodine-uptake studies or thyroid scanning with radioactive iodine may be affected for up to 2 years.

Closely administered doses of intravenous contrast (e.g., for CT and angiography) will increase the incidence of renal failure, especially in patients with underlying nephropathy. It is best to try to schedule contrast studies several days apart, ensuring adequate hydration between examinations.

The oral contrast for CT, although it is very faint on plain films, will affect visibility of mucosal detail on subsequent GI examinations. GI examinations should be scheduled after oral contrast has cleared the GI tract. Occasionally the density of contrast in the GI tract may interfere with angiographic or interventional procedures as well.

CONTROVERSIES

14. What is the best imaging technique for diagnosis of an abdominal abscess?
a. **CT scanning**
Advantages: Overall, the most accurate; sensitive for fluid collections; can be used to guide percutaneous drainage.
Disadvantages: Patient must be transported; diffuse process may be difficult to detect; uninfected fluid collections may not always be distinguishable from abscess; adequate bowel opacification with oral contrast is needed.
b. **Ultrasound**
Advantages: May be done portably; no ionizing radiation; fairly sensitive for evaluating liver, gallbladder, kidneys, and female pelvis.
Disadvantages: Least sensitive (particularly in left upper quadrant and mid abdomen); very dependent on operator skill; infected and uninfected fluid not distinguishable.
c. **Gallium scanning**
Advantages: Very sensitive; can detect diffuse inflammation; whole body imaging.
Disadvantages: Imaging after 24–72 hours; extensive overlapping physiologic uptake; less anatomic resolution; less specific (e.g., uptake in neoplasms, uninfected inflammatory processes); best in chronic infection.
d. **Indium-labeled leukocyte imaging**
Advantages: Very sensitive; more specific for infection than gallium; best in acute infectious processes.
Disadvantages: Images at 24 hours; less anatomic resolution; less specific than CT; overlapping physiologic uptake limits diagnosis.
In most cases, CT should be the imaging technique of choice. If the patient cannot be transported, ultrasound may be helpful. Nuclear medicine studies may add information when clinical suspicion is high and other images are negative.

15. What is the procedure of choice for diagnosing thoracic aortic dissection?
a. **Dynamic, contrast-enhanced helical CT**
Advantages: Noninvasive (arterial puncture not required); more sensitive than angiography; demonstrates accompanying pathology (e.g., periaortic hematoma from rupture or pericardial effusion); multiplanar reconstruction can clarify anatomy; helical scanning is very rapid.

Disadvantages: Intimal flap may be obscured by motion; involvement of coronary and brachiocephalic arteries may not be accurately assessed; does not demonstrate aortic insufficiency.

b. **Aortography**

Advantages: Rapid film sequence demonstrates the timing of filling of true and false lumens; intimal flap may be better demonstrated; anatomy of coronary arteries and great vessels better delineated; demonstrates aortic insufficiency.

Disadvantages: Invasive; higher risk; less sensitive for intramural hematoma than CT or MRI.

c. **Magnetic resonance imaging**

Advantages: Contrast not required; imaging in any plane; no ionizing radiation; equal sensitivity to CT.

Disadvantages: Limitations on emergency availability; limits on life-support equipment; long imaging times requiring the patient to lie very still; small bore size; cannot image intimal calcifications; not as accurate as CT for branch vessel involvement.

CT scanning is useful in excluding dissection when the index of suspicion is low, the chest x-ray abnormal, and the patient is debilitated. Aortography may be the initial study in surgical candidates when there is a high suspicion of dissection. When there is a strong suspicion of dissection but the initial study is normal or nondiagnostic, both CT and angiography may be necessary to make a definitive diagnosis.

d. **Transesophageal echocardiography (TEE)**

Advantages: Portable; high sensitivity for dissection of descending aorta.

Disadvantages: Highly operator-dependent; difficulty in visualization of ascending aorta and branch vessels; less accurate than CT or MRI for location of intimal flap or intramural hematoma.

CT, MRI, or TEE may be used in the initial evaluation of a patient with suspected aortic dissection. CT is the most specific, and is rapid and readily available. Aortography may be needed preoperatively to evaluate great vessel involvement and aortic regurgitation. MRI is an excellent modality for follow-up of postoperative patients or patients with chronic dissection.

BIBLIOGRAPHY

1. Cochran St, Bomyea K, Sayre JW: Trends in adverse events after IV administration of contrast media. Am J Roentgen 176:1385–1388, 2001.
2. Cohan RH, Dunnick NR: Intravascular contrast media: Adverse reactions. AJR 149:665, 1987.
3. Goodman LR: Congestive heart failure and adult respiratory distress syndrome. New insights using computed tomography. Radiol Clin North Am 34:33–46, 1996.
4. Jacobs JE, Birnbaum BA: Abdominal computed tomography of intensive care unit patients. Semin Roentgenol 32:128–141, 1997.
5. Katayama H, Yamaguchi K, Kozuka T, et al: Adverse reactions to ionic and nonionic contrast media. Radiology 175:621, 1990.
6. Laissy JP, Blanc F, Soyer P, et al: Thoracic aortic dissection: Diagnosis with transesophageal echocardiography versus MR imaging. Radiology 194:331–336, 1995.
7. McDowell RK, Dawson SL: Evaluation of the abdomen in sepsis of unknown origin. Radiol Clin North Am 34:177–190, 1996.
8. McLean TR, Thornby J, Svensson LG: Predicting the results and outcome of patients who undergo abdominal CT scanning while in the surgical intensive care unit. Am Surg 59:610–614, 1993.
9. Miller WT: Thoracic computed tomography in the intensive care unit. Semin Roentgenol 32:117–121, 1997.
10. Novelline RA, Rhea JT, Rao PM, Stuk JL: Helical CT in emergency radiology. Radiology 213:321–339, 1999.
11. Paulin S: Imaging of suspected aortic dissection. Am J Roentgen 161:494–495, 1993.
12. Sebastia C, Pallisa E, Quiroga S, et al: Aortic dissection: Diagnosis and follow-up with helical CT. Radiographics 19:45–60, 1999.
13. Sommer T, Feshke W, Holzknecht N, et al: Aortic dissection: A comparative study of diagnosis with spiral CT, multiplanar transesophageal echocardiography and MR imaging. Radiology 199:347–352, 1996.
14. Soulen RL, Duman RJ, Hoeffner E: Magnetic resonance imaging in the critical care setting. Crit Care Clin 10:401–416, 1994.
15. Wiener MD, Garay SM, Leitman BS, et al: Imaging of the intensive care unit patient. Clin Chest Med 12:169–198, 1991.

92. ULTRASONOGRAPHY

Suzanne Z. Barkin, M.D., and Julia A. Drose, B.A., R.D.M.S., R.D.C.S., R.V.T.

GENERAL CONCEPTS

1. Which abdominal structures are best evaluated by ultrasound?
Ultrasound can evaluate any solid, soft-tissue organ. In the abdomen, this includes liver, spleen, and kidneys. It is also useful to evaluate fluid-filled structures such as the gallbladder, bile ducts, and abdominal vasculature (e.g., aorta, inferior vena cava). Ultrasound is not useful in evaluating air-filled structures such as bowel, lung, or bone.

2. Which structures in the pelvis are best evaluated by ultrasound?
Ultrasound is useful in evaluating the uterus and ovaries for the presence of solid masses or fluid-filled structures such as ovarian cysts. Because of the large amount of bowel located in the pelvis, the patient must have a full urinary bladder in order to permit evaluation of the uterus and ovaries when scanning transabdominally. An endovaginal ultrasound may be performed, obviating the need for a full urinary bladder. This entails using an endovaginal transducer, which is placed inside the vagina next to the cervix. A closer evaluation of the uterus, ovaries, and fallopian tubes can be achieved with this method in some cases. Some structures such as early gestational sacs or hydrosalpinx, which may not be evident by transabdominal sonography, may be seen using an endovaginal probe. Conversely, masses arising from the fundus of the uterus or ovarian masses located high in the pelvis may be missed by endovaginal ultrasound alone.

3. When is ultrasound useful in evaluation of the chest?
Although ultrasound is not able to evaluate lungs, it can identify pleural fluid and guide a needle for thoracentesis. Some chest masses such as mediastinal lymph nodes may be evaluated, although CT is the modality of choice. Ultrasound is an excellent tool for evaluating structure and function of the heart.

4. Which vascular structures can be evaluated by ultrasound?
Almost any vascular structure that is not surrounded by air or bowel can be evaluated using diagnostic ultrasound. In the abdomen this includes evaluating the aorta for aneurysm, the inferior vena cava and renal veins for clot, and the renal arteries for stenosis. Peripheral vasculature that can be evaluated by ultrasound includes the carotid arteries and jugular veins in the neck, subclavian and axillary veins of the upper torso, the deep venous and arterial system of the upper extremities, and the iliac and femoral arteries and deep venous system of the lower extremities.

5. When is Doppler ultrasound useful?
Doppler ultrasound can be used to evaluate any vascular structure for presence, direction, and velocity of flow, and to differentiate type of flow, i.e., arterial vs. venous.

6. When is ultrasound valuable intraoperatively?
Intraoperative ultrasound is useful in the brain to help identify the location of a tumor and to assist in ventricular shunt placement. It may also be useful in locating tumors of the spinal cord or abdomen, in evaluating the carotid artery following arthrectomy, or in evaluating function after cardiac valve replacement to assure that appropriate blood flow has been established. It also has been used successfully in transplant surgery to establish the immediate presence of blood flow.

453

7. How good is portable ultrasound compared with studies done in the radiology department?

All real-time ultrasound units are portable, but there are still drawbacks to doing a portable examination. Ultrasound equipment may not fit in small spaces such as ICU rooms. In addition, patient rooms may not block out enough light, therefore hindering the ability to see the ultrasound monitor well enough to perform the exam. Other problems include monitors that the patient has on, which can interfere with the sound transmission of the ultrasound transducer. Also, many intensive care patients have tubes, lines, or bandages that limit access of the ultrasound transducer.

VASCULAR APPLICATIONS

8. What noninvasive modalities can be used to evaluate a patient with deep venous thrombosis (DVT)?

Ultrasound is currently the modality of choice. The veins and thrombi can be directly visualized with real-time ultrasound. Pulsed and color Doppler can help confirm the presence or absence of blood flow and evidence of clot.

9. Can the veins distal to the popliteal vein in patients with suspected DVT be visualized using ultrasound?

The calf veins can be visualized with ultrasound; however, because of the multiple branching of these vessels, they are not routinely studied. The proximal segment of the anterior tibial and posterior tibial-peroneal trunks are frequently included on the exam.

10. Can ultrasound be used as a primary modality to evaluate the carotid arteries for stenosis and plaque identification and characterization?

Yes. Sonographic imaging using pulsed and color Doppler is currently the method of choice for evaluating the carotid arteries. Plaque morphology and flow characteristics can be assessed.

ABDOMINAL APPLICATIONS

11. When is ultrasound better than CT scanning in the abdomen?

Ultrasound is inherently better than CT scanning when looking for gallstones or deciding when the consistency of a mass is cystic vs. solid. It is also the method of choice for evaluating hydronephrosis and vascular flow patterns. Both ultrasound and CT are equally good when evaluating abdominal aortic aneurysms; however, ultrasound is less expensive and does not use ionizing radiation. When evaluating the pancreas or looking for an abscess or bowel lesions, CT is the method of choice because of the inability of ultrasound to penetrate bowel.

12. What is the role of ultrasound in the diagnosis of appendicitis?

Historically, appendicitis has been a clinical diagnosis. However, ultrasound with graded compression may be useful in confirming the diagnosis. An inflamed appendix on ultrasound is differentiated from normal bowel by size, shape, location, and absence of peristalsis. It is also difficult to compress and is relatively rigid. Wall-thickening and fluid around the appendix are other signs. The McBurney sign, producing moderate tenderness with the ultrasound transducer, is frequently seen. Increased vascularity secondary to hyperemia may be appreciated with color Doppler. However, CT still has increased sensitivity over ultrasound in making a definitive diagnosis of appendicitis; therefore, it may be the imaging method of choice in most cases.

13. What is the most sensitive exam to diagnose appendicitis?

CT and MR imaging have been shown to be more sensitive than ultrasonography; however, ultrasound is relatively quick and accurate in diagnosing or excluding uncomplicated appendicitis. Ultrasound is lower in cost and should be used for initial imaging. Laparoscopic exploration is definitive, and in certain settings clinical observation is warranted.

14. Which modality is best for evaluating hepatic pathology?
Ultrasonography is probably the best method of screening patients for suspected hepatic pathology. It is noninvasive, can be performed rapidly, provides excellent results, and is the least expensive of available imaging tests. It is also usually better in characterizing lesions that have been detected, in distinguishing simple cysts from noncystic lesions, and in diagnosing anatomic variants. CT may be needed as a secondary imaging modality once an abnormality has been identified.

15. What is the differential diagnosis of a solid hepatic lesion?
A single, solid lesion in the liver statistically represents a cavernous hemangioma. These are usually small and found in patients who are asymptomatic. A large solid lesion may be more indicative of neoplasm, with hepatocellular carcinoma being the most common primary malignant tumor of the liver. Multiple solid lesions may also represent cavernous hemangiomas or, more likely, metastatic disease. Other possibilities include hepatic adenomas or focal nodular hyperplasia.

16. When is ultrasound useful in evaluating the biliary system?
Ultrasound is the procedure of choice for evaluating the biliary system because of its high sensitivity and accuracy in detecting gallstones and for detecting biliary dilatation.

17. What other gallbladder abnormalities can be detected by ultrasound?
Sonography can be used to detect diffuse wall thickening, which is diagnosed when the wall is more than 3 mm thick. Polyps or masses of the gallbladder may also be identified as foci that do not move or shadow. Other conditions seen by ultrasound include echogenic bile or sludge, or pericholecystic fluid, most often due to acute cholecystitis.

18. When should ultrasound be used to evaluate the pancreas?
Ultrasound is valuable in examining the size and echotexture of the pancreas and accompanying lesions and the presence of a dilated pancreatic duct. However, adequate visualization of the pancreas is often obscured by the ribs, stomach, and colon. Therefore, a CT scan may be the modality of choice.

GENITOURINARY APPLICATIONS

19. When is ultrasound useful in evaluating urinary tract abnormalities?
Ultrasound is usually the modality of choice when evaluating the kidneys. Renal anatomy can be well delineated with the superior resolution provided by currently available ultrasound units. The internal architecture of the kidney is now routinely displayed with a clarity approaching that of the cut surface of a gross anatomic specimen. Not only can the kidney be evaluated for anatomic abnormalities, but with the use of Doppler and color flow imaging, renal blood flow alterations can be identified and studied. Furthermore, with ultrasound guidance, biopsy of renal masses or renal parenchyma can be performed and fluids aspirated. Ultrasound is very useful in identifying and following dilatation of the renal pelvis and dilated ureters. The urinary bladder may also be evaluated for the presence of masses. Nephrolithiasis is best evaluated by nonenhanced CT.

20. When a patient presents with an acutely painful scrotum, which imaging studies are most helpful in making the diagnosis?
It is important to differentiate torsion of the testis from epididymitis and/or orchitis when there is no history of trauma, because torsion requires immediate surgical intervention. (A nuclear medicine scan in the acute setting should be performed first with technetium 99m sodium pertechnetate. This study is 95% accurate in the first 6 hours in distinguishing torsion from epididymitis. Ultrasound can be done following the nuclear medicine study.)
Clinically, torsion and epididymitis/orchitis may be difficult to differentiate; however, ultrasonographically they can usually be differentiated based on the morphologic, color flow, and pulsed Doppler waveform findings. State-of-the-art ultasound equipment in conjunction with

operator experience is sensitive enough to make the diagnosis of testicular torsion, based on the absence of color and pulsed Doppler flow within the testis.

When an intratesticular lesion is considered with a palpable scrotal mass, ultrasonography is excellent and is the first imaging study that should be ordered. However, there is no way to delineate malignant from benign lesions, except with surgery. Any intratesticular lesion should be considered malignant until proved otherwise.

GYNECOLOGIC APPLICATIONS

21. What are the advantages of transabdominal versus endovaginal sonography?

Transabdominal and endovaginal ultrasound are best used in an additive fashion. Endovaginal ultrasound may be able to detect an intrauterine pregnancy earlier than transabdominal. It also enables visualization of structures sometimes missed by transabdominal ultrasound such as an ectopic pregnancy, tubal ovarian abscess, and small fibroids. However, large ovarian masses or fibroids, especially those located high in the pelvis, may be missed by endovaginal ultrasound because they are too far from the endovaginal probe to be visualized. Bowel may also obscure normal ovaries and ovarian masses when using an endovaginal probe, whereas a full bladder and a transabdominal probe may facilitate their visualization.

22. What are the ultrasound findings in pelvic inflammatory disease?

They are usually nonspecific and therefore cannot definitively make the diagnosis, but a constellation of sonographic findings may be present. Because the infection affects the endometrium, early findings may include a prominent and hyperechoic endometrium surrounded by a hypoechoic ring, or a definitive fluid collection may be seen within the endometrium. A subtle hypoechogenicity of the uterus may signal early uterine infection. Indistinct borders of pelvic structures and posterior cul-de-sac fluid may also be present. As the infection ascends, acute salpingitis results. When this occurs, dilated cystic or complex structures may be seen, representing a hydrosalpinx or pyosalpinx. Pyosalpinx is usually a unilateral process but may be seen bilaterally. Severe pelvic inflammatory disease may appear as an indistinct complex mass.

23. When should you see a gestational sac, fetal pole, and fetal heartbeat by transabdominal ultrasound versus transvaginal ultrasound?

By transabdominal ultrasound, a gestational sac may often be seen as early as 5 weeks' gestational age. The secondary yolk sac becomes visible at approximately 5–5.5 weeks, and shortly thereafter (by 6.5 weeks) a small fetal pole containing a flickering fetal heart can be seen adjacent or near the yolk sac. The use of transvaginal transducers permits these structures to be seen approximately 1 week earlier.

24. What are the ultrasound criteria for an ectopic pregnancy?

The only conclusive criteria for excluding an ectopic pregnancy by ultrasound is to demonstrate a viable intrauterine pregnancy occupying a high fundal position in the endometrium. The coexistence of intrauterine and extrauterine gestations occurs 1 in 6000 cases and is considered a rare phenomenon. The appearance of a sac-like structure within the endometrium itself is not diagnostic of an intrauterine pregnancy because a similar structure termed "pseudogestational sac" can accompany an ectopic pregnancy. Ultrasound may provide a definitive diagnosis of an ectopic pregnancy only if an ectopic gestational sac is visualized outside of the uterus and fetal heart movements are demonstrable within it.

25. What is the sonographic appearance of hydatidiform mole?

A variable appearance is possible by ultrasound. Some first-trimester moles may simulate anembryonic gestation, missed abortion, degenerating fibroid, or hydropic placenta. Others may appear as an echogenic mass filling the entire uterine cavity. The more advanced hydatidiform mole, which contains numerous hydropic villi, can be well visualized by sonography. It appears as a large, soft-tissue mass containing cystic spaces of various sizes. Large multiseptated ovarian cysts (theca lutein cysts) may be present. Whenever these criteria are seen, careful clinical correlation is important in differentiating the possible causes.

BIBLIOGRAPHY

1. Berland LL, Lawson TL, Folley WD: Porta hepatis: Sonographic discrimination of bile ducts from arteries with pulsed Doppler with new anatomic criteria. AJR 138:833, 1982.
2. Bernardino NE, Thomas JL, Maklad N: Hepatic sonography: Technical considerations, present applications, and possible future. Radiology 142:249, 1982.
3. Brown J, Hammers L, Barton J, et al: Quantitative Doppler assessment of acute scrotal inflammation. Radiology 197:427–431, 1995.
4. Carroll BA, Gross DM: High frequency scrotal sonography. AJR 140:511–515, 1983.
5. Cronan JJ, Dorfman GS, Scola FH, et al: Deep venous thrombosis: US assessment using vein compression. Radiology 162:191–194, 1987.
6. Goldstein SR, Snyder JR, Watson C, e al: Very early pregnancy detection with endovaginal ultrasound. Obstet Gynecol 72:200–204, 1988.
7. Graif M, Mannor A, Itzchak Y: Sonographic differentiation of extra- and intrahepatic masses. AJR 141:553, 1983.
8. Grant EG: Duplex ultrasonography: Its expanding role in noninvasive vascular diagnosis. Radiol Clin North Am 23:563–582, 1985.
9. Grant EG, Raqavendra N, McNamara RO: Color Doppler depicts flow patterns in legs. Diagn Imaging 11:140–146, 1990.
10. Groseman H, Rosenberg ER, Bowey JD, et al: Sonographic diagnosis of renal cystic diseases. AJR 140:81, 1983.
11. Hessler PC, Hill DS, Detorie FM, Rocco AF: High accuracy sonographic recognition of gallstones. AJR 136:157, 1981.
12. Hill MC: Pancreatic sonography: An update. In Saunders RC (ed): Ultrasound Annual. New York, Raven Press, 1982.
13. Incesu L, Coskun A, Selcuk MB, et al: Acute appendicitis: MR imaging and sonographic correlation. Am J Radiol 168:669–674, 1997.
14. Kane RA: Sonographic anatomy of the liver. In Raymond HW, Zwiebel WJ (eds): Seminars in Ultrasound, Vol. 2. New York, Grune & Stratton, 1981.
15. Mendelson EB, Bohm-Velez M, Neiman HL, et al: Transvaginal sonography in imaging. Semin Ultrasound CT MR 9:102–121, 1988.
16. Mittlestaedt CA: Abdominal Ultrasound. New York, Churchill Livingstone, 1987.
17. Renz J, Merritt CRM, Bluth EI: Sonographic evaluation of carotid plaque. Appl Radiol 8:29–32, 1990.
18. Rifkin MD, Kurtz AB, Goldberg BB: Epididymis examined by ultrasound. Radiology 151:187–190, 1984.
19. Rosenfield AT: Ultrasound evaluation of renal parenchymal disease and hydronephrosis. Urol Radiol 4:125, 1982.
20. Rumack CM, Wilson SR, Charboneau JM: Diagnostic Ultrasound, 2nd ed. St. Louis, Mosby, 1998.
21. Sarti D: Diagnostic Ultrasound: Text and Cases, 2nd ed. Chicago, Year Book Medical Publishers, 1987.
22. Sexton CC, Zeman RK: Correlation of computed tomography, sonography and gross anatomy of liver. AJR 141:711, 1983.

93. INTERVENTIONAL RADIOLOGY

Douglas M. Coldwell, Ph.D., M.D.

1. What are the indications for a transjugular intrahepatic portosystemic shunt (TIPS)?
With better techniques, the rate of failed sclerotherapy in a patient who is actively bleeding from esophageal or gastric varices has improved dramatically so that the most common indication for TIPS is in patients with intractable ascites who are refractory to medical therapy and require frequent paracenteses or patients with hydrothorax due to ascites, which usually results from a rent in the diaphragm. Hemorrhage that cannot be stopped with sclerotherapy, usually in gastric varices, is a less common indication.

2. How is the liver disease of cirrohotic patients graded?

Child-Pugh System (Modified)

POINTS	1	2	3
Albumin	>3.5	2.8–3.5	< 2.8
Bilirubin	< 2.5	2.5–4	> 4
Prothrombin time	< 4	4–6	> 6
Ascites	None	Mild	Moderate
Encephalopathy	None	Mild	Moderate

Grade A: total is 5–6 points   **Grade B:** total is 7–9 points   **Grade C:** total is 9–15 points
In order to be placed on a transplant list, the total must be at least 9.

3. What are the results of TIPS?
Cessation of variceal hemorrhage occurs in approximately 90% of cases, and ascites is diminished or resolved in 70%. Encephalopathy that is either increased or of new onset occurs in 10–15% of cases. The lower the portal-systemic pressure gradient, the greater the likelihood of development of worsened encephalopathy. The complications of intra-abdominal hemorrhage, hepatic failure, or renal failure occur in less than 2% of cases. The 30-day mortality rate is approximately 20% in Child's C cases, which is about half of cases seen in elective portacaval shunts.

4. How long do the shunts last?
Two-thirds of all shunts are patent without intervention for a year. The remaining third have about one intervention and stay patent. With proper follow-up (monthly Duplex ultrasounds) and the necessary intervention, angioplasty, and additional stent placement, virtually all TIPS shunts remain patent for at least a year.

5. Practically speaking, who should get a TIPS?
Any patient who has bled from varices and is a transplantation candidate, who has bled from varices after they have been sclerosed or banded, or who has ascites that requires frequent paracenteses. Child's A patients usually undergo a surgically placed shunt; Child's C patients, a TIPS; and Child's B patients, either, depending on the expertise of the individual institution. Clinical trials are under way to determine the efficacy of TIPS versus sclerotherapy.

6. Embolization is a viable therapy for which patients?
Any patient with a localized source of bleeding (such as a gastric ulcer, Mallory-Weiss gastroesophageal tear, colonic diverticulum, lung tumor, or traumatic injury) or a malignant tumor

that can be isolated from normal tissue (such as a renal cell carcinoma, hepatic primary or metastatic tumor, recurrent renal cell carcinoma in the renal bed with the attendant bleeding and pain, metastatic or primary lung cancer, painful bony metastases). In addition, if the normal tissue in which the tumor is located can be sacrificed, the patient can be embolized. Care must be taken *not* to embolize a hollow viscus (e.g., the stomach or bowel) with fine particulates or tissue adhesives.

7. What are the results of embolization of tumors?
Practically all embolizations of renal or hepatic tumors result in palliation, but a lengthening of survival is not assured. In primary hepatocellular carcinoma, embolization with Lipiodol and doxorubicin has shown impressive survival gains with palliation and a 1-year survival rate of over 70% as opposed to treatment with intravenous chemotherapeutic regimens (survival rate < 20% in a similar set of unresectable patients). New radioactive emoblization agents containing yttrium-90 show promise for dealing with unresectable hepatic tumors.

8. What are the side effects and complications of embolization?
When hepatic or renal tumors are embolized, the postembolization syndrome of nausea, vomiting, fever, pain, leukocytosis, and an increase in liver function tests is expected and lasts for 3–5 days. The fever is nocturnal and spiking and may last for up to 3 weeks without evidence of infection. Patients should be treated symptomatically. If the patient does not improve in a week, the possibility of nontarget embolization with tissue necrosis should be considered. This is unlikely with modern fluoroscopic equipment and the wide availability of microcatheters, which easily allow superselective catheterization. Other complications include tumor lysis syndrome with the shutdown of the kidneys due to tumor degradation products. This complication is preventable, especially when large tumors are involved, by pretreatment with allopurinol.

9. Can interventional radiology help with access problems?
Absolutely yes. Gastrostomy and gastrojejunostomy catheters are more easily, accurately, and inexpensively placed under fluoroscopic guidance than with endoscopy. In addition, the percutaneous placement allows a more directed approach to be performed since the catheter is angled toward the pylorus, permitting ready exchange of a gastrostomy for a gastrojejunostomy catheter. Only a nasogastric tube or feeding tube is necessary prior to placement. Central venous access, particularly the long-term tunnelled variety, is another area that is better addressed with fluoroscopic placement. Since most interventional radiology suites are equipped with more sterile equipment than previously and there are many catheters specially designed for percutaneous placement available, the long-term central venous access placement should be performed with radiologic guidance.

10. What is the role of angiography in lower gastrointestinal hemorrhage (LGIB)?
Its role is both diagnostic and therapeutic. If a patient has LGIB, a nuclear medicine technetium-99m–labeled red blood cell scan should be obtained. If this examination reveals a site of hemorrhage, the patient should be taken immediately (as soon as the scan is positive) to the angiography suite so that a confirmatory arteriogram and embolization of the bleeding site may be performed. Under no circumstances should the patient be taken back to the ICU or placed on the ward between the nuclear medicine scan and the performance of the arteriogram. Becaues of the intermittent nature of the bleeding, close communication among the interventional radiology, nuclear medicine, and admitting services personnel needs to take place so that the arteriogram is not delayed. In essence, the decision for an arteriogram **must** be made prior to the performance of the nuclear medicine scan if the scan is positive.

11. What are the results and complications of embolization of LGIB?
Because the bowel is usually embolized with a nonabsorbable material such as polyvinyl alcohol foam particles, there is approximately a 10% chance that the bowel may infarct. This is acceptable risk in light of the facts that the infarction will occur over a period of several days while the patient is stabilized and that the surgery will be an elective rather than an emergent procedure.

The likelihood of finding the source of the LGIB is very high given a positive nuclear medicine scan and the rapid performance of the arteriogram. If the arteriogram is not positive, 1–4 mg of tissue plasminogen activator, 5000 units of heparin, or vasodilators such as Priscoline or papaverine may be administered intra-arterially in the region where the nuclear medicine scan was positive to incite a LGIB. The only caveat in the performance of these enhancing maneuvers is that the interventional radiologist must be able to embolize the bleeding site.

BIBLIOGRAPHY

1. Coldwell DM (ed): Radiologic Interventions: Embolotherapy. Baltimore, Williams & Wilkins, 1997.
2. Coldwell DM, Ring E, Rees C, et al: Multicenter investigation of the transjugular intrahepatic portosystemic shunt (TIPS): Role in the management of portal hypertension. Radiology 196:335–340, 1995.
3. Heyman MB, LaBerge JM: Role of transjugular intrahepatic portosystemic shunt in the treatment of portal hypertension in pediatric patients. J Pediatr Gastroenterol Nutr 29:240–249, 1999.
4. LaBerge JM, Somberg DA, Lake JR, et al: Two-year outcome following transjugular intrahepatic portosystemic shunt for variceal bleeding: Results in 90 patients. Gastroenterology 108:1143–1151, 1995.
5. Mauro MA, Jacques PF: Insertion of long-term hemodialysis catheters by interventional radiologists: Trend continues. Radiology 198:316, 1996.

XVII. Emergency Medicine

94. TETANUS

Peter T. Pons, M.D.

1. What is tetanus?

Tetanus is acute infection with *Clostridium tetani* (gram-positive anaerobic rod), which produces a neurotoxin (exotoxin) whose primary action is to cause profound skeletal muscle hypertonicity. In the most severe form, the muscle spasms can cause respiratory failure and death. *C. tetani* can be introduced into any wound or open tissue; it proliferates in necrotic or compromised tissue, then elaborates the exotoxin.

2. How does the exotoxin/neurotoxin cause the disease?

C. tetani manufactures three exotoxins: tetanospasmin, tetanolysin, and nonconvulsive neurotoxin. Most clinical manifestations appear to be produced by tetanospasmin. This exotoxin becomes concentrated in the anterior horn of the spinal cord and blocks neurotransmitter release at presynaptic sites of inhibitory neurons, thus causing increased muscle tone, hypertonicity, and muscle spasms. Tetanolysin is a hemolytic toxin that may cause hemolysis and myocardial injury and dysfunction. The role of the third toxin, nonconvulsive neurotoxin, has not been well defined. The toxins spread via lymphatics, blood vessels, and neural pathways to the target organ, alpha motor neurons.

3. Summarize the epidemiology of tetanus.

Incidence and geographic distribution. In the United States, there are approximately 80 cases of tetanus each year; worldwide, there are between 250,000 and 500,000 cases. In the U.S., the disease occurs most commonly in the Southeast; however, the organism is ubiquitous in dirt and dust and is found worldwide. It is less common in cold climates.

Incubation period: varies between 2 and 14 days with a median of 7 days.

Prognosis. The mortality rate is 30% in the U.S. and 40–60% worldwide. The mortality is 100% if the disease becomes manifest within 2 days of injury and infection. Worldwide, 90% of deaths occur in infants.

4. Who is prone to developing tetanus?

General. Most at risk are people who have never been or are inadequately immunized against tetanus. It is estimated that 50–90% of patients in the U.S. are inadequately protected (in most cases, immigrants or adults over the age of 50–60 years who never completed the immunization series). A significant percentage (up to 75%) of elderly patients have inadequate serum levels of antibody against tetanus in numerous studies that measured actual levels.

Neonates. Newborns can acquire tetanus following nonsterile transection of the umbilical cord. In many countries, local remedies such as cow dung, garlic, coffee, and ashes are applied to the umbilical stump to facilitate healing, only to produce tetanus.

Drug abusers. Parenteral drug abusers who administer their drugs by "skin popping" are prone to acquiring tetanus by developing subcutaneous abscesses that support the growth of *C. tetani*.

Septic abortion. Women who have undergone septic abortion are prone to the development of tetanus.

Acne. Cephalic tetanus has been reported as a complication of acne.

5. What sort of wound is prone to infection with *C. tetani*?

Most cases result from accidental soft-tissue injury, such as lacerations, puncture wounds, or burns, which may occur indoors or outdoors. The Centers for Disease Control reported that almost 50% of wounds resulting in tetanus occurred indoors. Many wounds appear quite minor and sometimes cannot be found at the time of presentation of clinical tetanus. Some unusual sources include frostbitten parts, poor dentition, gum ulcers from a denture, and skin infections. *C. tetani* is a strict anaerobe and proliferates only in tissue with low oxygen tension. Necrotic tissue, foreign bodies, and associated infection are predisposing factors. Tetanus has been reported after elective surgery and chronic skin ulceration. The organism itself is not invasive; thus the infection is localized. Once the exotoxin is produced, however, the toxin is transported systemically.

6. What are the clinical manifestations of tetanus?

The most dramatic and obvious findings in tetanus are in the musculoskeletal system. Initial findings are characterized by increased muscle tone, which is usually first noticed in the face and jaw. Trismus, difficulty swallowing, and facial distortion from the muscle spasms (risus sardonicus) develop. Over the next 24–48 hours, generalized muscle hypertonicity develops and muscle spasms may occur. Spasms of neck and back muscles result in opisthotonic posturing. Other findings are low-grade elevation in temperature and pulse, increased or decreased blood pressure, pain associated with the muscle spasms, rigid abdominal wall (also due to muscle spasms but mimicking an acute abdomen), and clear mentation during these episodes. The disease remains "stable" for the next 5–7 days, followed by recovery over the next 7–10 days. Muscle stiffness may remain for up to 2 months. In neonates, the disease is characterized by irritability, difficulty nursing and swallowing, and hypertonicity of the muscles. If the patient survives, recovery occurs without permanent sequelae. The disease does not confer immunity; therefore survivors must be immunized to prevent recurrence.

7. What are the four types of tetanus?

1. **Generalized**. This is the most common form and is manifested by the full constellation of symptoms and signs. The overall mortality rate is approximately 50%.

2. **Neonatal**. Newborns may acquire tetanus from contamination of the umbilical stump. Immunization of the mother can prevent the disease in neonates. The mortality in infants is 50–60%.

3. **Local**. This form is characterized by increased muscle tone near the inoculation site that usually resolves over time. Progression to the generalized form is uncommon but possible.

4. **Cephalic**. This rare form presents with trismus and cranial nerve paralysis (VII most commonly, also III, IV, VI, and XII). Generalized tetanus follows in approximately two-thirds of cases.

8. Are any laboratory studies diagnostic of tetanus?

Virtually all laboratory studies yield nonspecific, nondiagnostic results. Approximately one-third of patients have mild-to-moderate granulocytosis. Decreased hematocrit may be noted, probably secondary to the hemolysin exotoxin. Electrolyte and calcium levels should be normal. As the disease progresses, however, 7% of patients develop the electrolyte picture of inappropriate antidiuretic hormone secretion (SIADH), including decreased sodium and serum osmolality. Arterial blood gases should be monitored to assess pulmonary function. Of note, cultures for *C. tetani* were positive in only one-third of patients diagnosed with tetanus clinically.

9. Which diseases are included in the differential diagnosis?

Hypocalcemia. Decreased serum calcium can produce tetany. Laboratory evaluation is usually diagnostic.

Oral infection or abscess. Infection or abscess in and about the oral cavity (e.g., peritonsillar or dental abscess) can result in trismus or difficulty opening the mouth. Physical examination usually reveals localized swelling and tenderness.

Phenothiazine reaction. Dystonic reactions secondary to phenothiazines may cause muscle rigidity or torticollis. The history usually reveals recent drug use; relief of symptoms occurs with intravenous diphenhydramine.

Black widow spider bite. Pain and muscle spasm are usually acute in onset. Careful physical examination may reveal the telltale spider bite. Administration of calcium intravenously usually relieves the symptoms.

Rabies. Rabies involves the respiratory muscles and muscles of glutition without causing trismus. As the disease progresses, there is progressive alteration in the level of consciousness and increasing fever.

Strychnine poisoning. Muscle spasms (usually involving the upper extremities) and opisthotonus occur; however, facial muscle involvement develops later in the course. Suicidal ideation or possible homicide attempt may be evident by history.

Hyperventilation. Physical examination reveals carpopedal spasm. Arterial blood gas evaluation shows respiratory alkalosis.

10. What are the complications of tetanus?

Spasm of laryngeal muscles, the diaphragm, and other muscles of respiration may produce hypoxia or respiratory arrest. The compromise in respiratory function may lead to atelectasis and pneumonia. Other complications include vertebral subluxation or compression fracture as a result of the profound muscle contractions (usually in children), dehydration, pulmonary edema, and SIADH.

11. How is tetanus treated once it becomes manifest?

The four primary goals of treatment are (1) relief of muscle spasms, (2) support of respiratory status and prevention of complications, (3) treatment of the infection (remove toxin production), and (4) neutralization of any unbound toxin.

1. **Relief of muscle spasms**. The patient should be placed in a darkened room with minimal external stimulation. Diazepam, administered intravenously, is useful for relieving muscle spasms. Oral muscle relaxants such as meprobamate can be used in mild cases or during convalescence. In severe cases not responding to diazepam, chemical paralysis (with intubation and mechanical ventilation) using pancuronium is indicated. The addition of a sedative is helpful in reducing the effect of external stimulation, but careful monitoring of respiratory status is necessary.

2. **Support of respiratory status and prevention of complications**. Close monitoring of the patient's respiratory function is imperative because spasm of laryngeal muscles, the diaphragm, and muscles of respiration can lead to respiratory failure and suffocation. If necessary, endotracheal intubation and mechanical ventilation should be performed. Formal tracheostomy may be needed if intubation cannot be accomplished. Secretions should be suctioned frequently and the patient positioned to minimize aspiration (and decubiti).

3. **Treatment of the infection (remove toxin production)**. When a wound or site of infection is identifiable, any necrotic tissue or foreign material should be removed and any abscess drained. Antibiotics are administered in the hope of preventing further proliferation of the organism and therefore decreasing toxin production, but here is little evidence that the course of the disease is affected. Penicillin is the drug of choice, and tetracycline may be used in penicillin-allergic patients.

4. **Neutralization of unbound toxin**. Human tetanus immune globulin is the medication of choice for neutralization of free exotoxin. The antiserum will not have any effect on toxin already bound in neurons. Equine antiserum can be used if human antiserum is not available; however, hypersensitivity, anaphylaxis, and serum sickness are serious complications. Following recovery, active immunization is necessary because immunity is not acquired by having the disease.

12. Can tetanus be prevented?

Tetanus is easily prevented by immunization and could be virtually eradicated worldwide by an aggressive immunization campaign. Neonatal tetanus is also preventable if the mother is protected because the antibody can pass through the placental barrier. Part of every routine history should include a review of tetanus immunization. Unimmunized patients or those with unclear histories should undergo active immunization with absorbed tetanus toxoid. The first dose should be given at the time of contact, the second dose 1–2 months later, and the third dose 6–12 months after the second dose.

Tetanus Prophylaxis after Injury

		ANTITOXIN	
IMMUNIZATION HISTORY	TOXOID[1]	NON-TETANUS PRONE	TETANUS PRONE
None	Yes	No	Yes
Uncertain or < 3 doses	Yes	No	Yes
3 or more doses	No[2]	No	No

[1] If patient age is less than 7 years, administer toxoid as diphtheria-tetanus-pertussis (DPT). If patient age is greater than 7 years, administer toxoid as tetanus-diphtheria (Td).

[2] Yes, if last prior immunization was greater than 5 years and tetanus-prone wound or 10 years and non–tetanus-prone wound.

When both toxoid and antitoxin are indicated, they may be given at the same time without concern that one will interfere with the action of the other, but separate injection sites should be used.

BIBLIOGRAPHY

1. Alagappan K, Rennie W, Kwiatkowski T, et al: Seroprevalence of tetanus antibodies among adults older than 65 years. Ann Emerg Med 28:18–21, 1996.
2. Alagappan K, Rennie W, Narang V, et al: Immunologic response to tetanus toxoid in geriatric patients. Ann Emerg Med 30:459–462, 1997.
3. American College of Emergency Physicians: Tetanus immunization recommendations for persons seven years of age and older. Ann Emerg Med 15:1111–1112, 1986.
4. American College of Emergency Physicians: Tetanus immunization recommendations for persons less than seven years old. Ann Emerg Med 16:1181–1183, 1987.
5. Centers for Disease Control: Tetanus—United States, 1985–1986. MMWR 36:477–481, 1987.
6. Centers for Disease Control and Prevention: Neonatal tetanus—Montana, 1998. MMWR 47:928–930, 1998.
7. Gergen PJ, McQuillan GM, Kiely M, et al: A population-based serologic survey of immunity to tetanus in the United States. N Engl J Med 332:761–766, 1995.
8. Harding-Goldson HE, Hanna WJ: Tetanus: A recurring intensive care problem. J Trop Med Hyg 98:179–184, 1995.
9. Jagoda A, Riggio SY, Burguieres T: Cephalic tetanus: A case report and review of the literature. Am J Emerg Med 6:128–130, 1988.
10. Luisto M: Unusual and iatrogenic sources of tetanus. Ann Chir Gynaecol 82:25–29, 1993.
11. Peetermans WE, Schepens D: Tetanus—Still a topic of present interest: A report of 27 cases from a Belgian referral hospital. J Intern Med 239:249–252, 1996.
12. Richardson JP, Knight AL: The management and prevention of tetanus. J Emerg Med 11:737–742, 1993.
13. Sangalli M, Chierchini P, Aylward RB, et al: Tetanus: A rare but preventable cause of mortality among drug users and the elderly. Eur J Epidemiol 12:539–540, 1996.
14. Sohat T, Marva E, Sivan Y, et al: Immunologic response to a single dose of tetanus toxoid in older people. J Am Geriatr Soc 48:949–951, 2000.

95. ANAPHYLAXIS

Vincent J. Markovchick, M.D.

1. Define anaphylaxis.

Anaphylaxis is a systemic immediate hypersensitivity reaction of multiple organ systems to an antigen-induced, IgE-mediated immunologic mediator release in previously sensitized individuals.

2. Define anaphylactoid reaction.

This is a potentially fatal syndrome, which is clinically similar to anaphylaxis but is not an IgE-mediated response. It may occur following a single first-time exposure to certain agents, such as radiopaque contrast media.

3. What are the most common causes?
Ingestion, inhalation or parenteral injection of antigens that sensitize predisposed individuals. Common antigens include drugs (e.g., penicillin), foods (shellfish, nuts, egg whites), insect stings (hymenoptera) and bites (snakes), diagnostic agents (ionic contrast media), and physical and environmental agents (latex, exercise and cold). Idiopathic anaphylaxis is a diagnosis of exclusion that is made when no identifiable cause can be determined.

4. What are the most common "target" organs?
The most common organ systems involved are the skin (urticaria, angioedema), mucous membranes (edema), upper respiratory tract (edema and hypersecretions), lower respiratory tract (bronchoconstriction), and cardiovascular system (vasodilatation and cardiovascular collapse).

5. What are the most common signs and symptoms?
The clinical presentation ranges from mild to life-threatening. Mild manifestations, which occur in most people, include urticaria and angioedema. Life-threatening manifestations involve the respiratory and cardiovascular systems. Respiratory signs and symptoms include acute upper airway obstruction presenting with stridor or lower airway manifestations of bronchospasm with diffuse wheezing. Cardiovascular collapse presents in the form of syncope, hypotension, tachycardia, and arrhythmias.

6. What is the role of diagnostic studies?
There is no role for diagnostic studies in anaphylaxis because diagnosis and treatment are based solely on clinical signs and symptoms. There is a role for skin testing either prior to administration of an antigen or in follow-up referral to determine exact allergens involved.

7. What is the differential diagnosis?
Anaphylaxis may be confused with septic and cardiogenic shock, asthma, croup and epiglottitis, vasovagal syncope, and myocardial infarction or any acute cardiovascular or respiratory collapse of unclear etiology.

8. What is the most common form of anaphylaxis? How is it treated?
Urticaria, either simple or confluent, is the most benign and, fortunately, the most common clinical manifestation. This is thought to be due to a capillary leak mediated by histamine release. It may be treated by the administration of antihistamines (orally, intramuscularly, or intravenously) or epinephrine (subcutaneously).

9. Describe the initial treatment for life-threatening forms of anaphylaxis.
1. Upper airway obstruction with stridor and edema should be treated with high-flow nebulized oxygen, racemic epinephrine, and IV epinephrine. If airway obstruction is severe or increases, endotracheal intubation or cricothyroidotomy should be performed.
2. Acute bronchospasm should be treated with epinephrine. Mild to moderate wheezing in patients with a normal blood pressure may be treated with .01 mg/kg of 1:1000 epinephrine administered subcutaneously or IM. If the patient is in severe respiratory distress or has a "quiet" chest, IV epinephrine should be administered via a drip infusion: 1 mg epinephrine in 250 cc D5W at an initial rate of 1 μg/min with titration to desired effect. Bronchospasm refractory to epinephrine may respond to a nebulized beta agonist, such as albuterol sulfate or metaproterenol, in recommended doses.
3. Cardiovascular collapse presenting with hypotension should be treated with a constant infusion of epinephrine, titrating the rate to attain a systolic BP of 100 mm Hg or mean arterial pressure of 80 mm Hg.
4. For patients in full cardiac arrest, administer 0.1–0.2 mg/kg of 1:10,000 epinephrine slow IV push or via endotracheal tube. In addition, immediate endotracheal intubation or cricothyroidostomy should be performed.

10. What are the adjuncts to initial epinephrine and airway management?
If intubation is unsuccessful and cricothyroidostomy is contraindicated, percutaneous transtracheal jet ventilation via needle cricothyroidostomy should be considered, especially in small children. Intravenous diphenhydramine (2 mg/kg) should be administered to all patients. Simultaneous administration of H2 blocker such as cimetadine, 300 mg IV, may be helpful. Aerosolized bronchodilators such as metaproterenol are useful if bronchospasm is present. Corticosteroids are usually given but do not have an immediate positive effect. For refractory hypotension, pressors such as norepinephrine or dopamine may be administered. Glucagon, 1 mg IV q 5 min, may be helpful in "epinephrine-resistant" patients who are on long-term beta-adrenergic blocking agents such as propranolol. Corticosteroids have limited benefit because of the delayed onset of action, but they may be beneficial in patients with prolonged bronchospasm or hypotension.

11. What are the complications of bolus IV epinephrine administration?
When epinephrine 1:10,000 is administered via IV push in patients who have an obtainable blood pressure or pulse, there is significant potential for overtreatment and the potentiation of hypertension, tachycardia, ischemic chest pain, acute myocardial infarction, and ventricular arrhythmias. Extreme care must be exercised in elderly patients and in those with underlying coronary artery disease. It is much safer to administer IV epinephrine by a controlled titratable drip infusion with continuous monitoring of cardiac rhythm and blood pressure.

12. Is there a role for prophylactic treatment in anaphylaxis? How is this performed?
When the potential benefits of treatment or diagnosis outweigh the risks (e.g., administration of antivenom for life- or limb-threatening snake bites), informed consent should be obtained if the patient is competent. Pretreatment with IV Benadryl and corticosteroids should be carried out. An IV epinephrine infusion should be prepared. The patient should be in an ICU setting with continuous monitoring of blood pressure, cardiac rhythm, and oxygen saturation. Full intubation and cricothyroidomy equipment should be at the bedside. Administration of the antigen (e.g., rattlesnake antivenom) should be started very slowly with a physician at the bedside who is capable of immediately administering IV epinephrine and managing the airway. Nonionic contrast medium for diagnostic imaging studies should be administered to patients with a history of anaphylaxis to ionic contrast material.

13. Describe the out-of-hospital treatment of anaphylaxis.
Patients who are known to be at high risk (e.g., previous anaphylactic reaction to hymenoptera) should be prescribed and educated in the self-administration of epinephrine with an autoinjector at the first sign of anaphylactic symptoms. In addition, self-administration of oral dephenhydramine is indicated for the treatment of mild reactions such as urticaria or concomitant with the administration of epinephrine.

BIBLIOGRAPHY

1. Horach A, et al: Severe myocardial ischemia induced by intravenous adrenaline. Br Med J 286:519, 1983.
2. Kemp SF, et al: Anaphylalxis: A review of 266 cases. Arch Intern Med 155:1749–1754, 1995.
3. Lee ML: Glucagon in anaphylaxis [letter]. J Allergy Clin Immunol 69:331, 1981.
4. Lucke WC, Thomas H: Anaphylaxis: Pathophysiology, clinical presentations and treatment. J Emerg Med 1:83–95, 1983.
5. Muellman RL, Tran PT: Allergy, hypersensitivity and anaphylaxis. In Rosen P (ed): Emergency Medicine: Concepts and Clinical Practice, 5th ed. St. Louis, Mosby, 2002, pp 1619–1634.
6. Runge JW, Martinez JC, Cavavuti EM: Histamine antagonists in the treatment of acute allergic reactions. Ann Emerg Med 21:237–242, 1992.
7. Silverman JH, Van Hook C, Haponik EF: Hemodynamic changes in human anaphylaxis. Am J Med 77:341–344, 1984.
8. Volcheck GW, Li JT: Exercise-induced uticaria and anaphylaxis. Mayo Clin Proc 72:140–147, 1997.
9. Weiszer I: Allergic emergencies. In Patterson R (ed): Allergic Diseases: Diagnosis and Management. Philadelphia, J.B. Lippincott, 1980, pp 374–394.

96. HYPOTHERMIA

John A. Marx, M.D.

1. How is hypothermia defined?

Specifically, hypothermia is a core temperature of < 35°C or 95°F. Moderate to severe hypothermia occurs at temperatures below 32.2°C. Physiologically, it is a clinical state of subnormal temperature in which the body is unable to generate sufficient heat to function efficiently. When hypothermia is suspected, it is imperative that thermometers be capable of measuring core temperatures accurately. Many thermometers have a lower limit of 35°C. The rectal temperature is the most practical, although it can lag behind core changes. Ideally the probe should be inserted to 15 cm and not placed in cold feces.

2. What is the function of shivering? When does it occur?

Shivering is modulated by the posterior hypothalamus and spinal cord and is limited by fatigue and glycogen depletion. Shivering is an early response to cold stress and is able to increase the basal metabolic rate 2- to 5-fold. It is operative between 32 and 37°C. Below 32°C, shivering thermogenesis ceasess. There is a progressive depression of the basal metabolic rate down to 24°C. Below 24°C, autonomic and endocrinologic mechanisms for heat conservation are no longer operative.

3. What is the J-wave?

First described in 1938, this electrocardiographic feature is known as the Osborn wave or hypothermic hump. It is seen at the junction of the QRS and ST segments and may appear at temperatures below 32°. It is most often seen in leads II and V6, but in more severe hypothermia may be seen in V3 or V4. Its size is not prognostic but increases with temperature depression. J-waves are typically upright in aV_L, aV_F, and the left precordial leads. The J-wave is not specific for hypothermia and can be seen in cardiac ischemia, sepsis, certain CNS lesions (particularly of the hypothalamus), and occasionally young normothermic patients.

4. What are the five causes of heat loss?

Radiation, conduction, convection, respiration, and evaporation. Approximately 55–65% of heat loss occurs through radiation. Conduction usually is responsible for only 2–3%, but loss by conduction can increase 5-fold in wet clothing and up to 25-fold in cold water. Convection accounts for 10–15% of heat loss and increases markedly with shivering. The heating of inspired air accounts for up to 2–9% of heat loss, and 20–27% is lost via evaporation from the skin and lungs.

5. What are the indications to initiate cardiopulmonary resuscitation (CPR) in the field in a patient with suspected hypothermia?

Apparent rigor mortis and lividity are not necessarily reliable indicators in severe hypothermia. Pupils can be fixed and unreactive at temperatures below 22°C. Peripheral pulses are difficult to palpate in patients with profound bradycardia and vasoconstriction. At least 45–60 seconds should be spent in determining whether spontaneous pulse is present because even extreme bradydysrhythmias may be sufficient to meet the very depressed metabolic needs of the hypothermic patient. Moreover, unnecessary handling, including closed chest compressions, is a purported cause of arrhythmias, although definitive evidence for this is lacking. If no evidence of perfusion can be discerned, an arrest rhythm should be presumed and CPR initiated. Respiratory minute volume is also significantly depressed and careful scrutiny is required to distinguish apnea. A patent airway should always be established, and if the patient is in respiratory arrest, ventilation should be instituted. Endotracheal intubation does not cause dysrhythmias.

CPR in hypothermia is contraindicated under the following circumstances: any signs of life are present, lethal (non–hypothermia-related) injuries are obvious, chest wall compression is impossible due to loss of elasticity, "do not resuscitate" status is verified, or lives of rescuers are endangered by environmental conditions. It may be difficult to distinguish primary from secondary hypothermia (e.g., the patient who dies of cardiac arrest in a cold environment). The oft-quoted maxim that a patient is not dead until warm and dead provides an appropriate caution. Physician judgment is needed, however, to help determine when to begin or cease CRP.

6. What are the current recommendations for rate and technique in CPR?

With regard to duration, it is clear that prolonged closed chest compressions have resuscitated many severely hypothermic patients to normal neurologic status. It is generally recommended that resuscitative measures continue until a core temperature of 35° has been reached before a patient is declared dead. The lowest recorded temperature in a hypothermia survivor is 9°C.

Optimal guidelines for rate and techniques are evolving. In an animal model of hypothermic cardiac arrest, cardiac output and cerebral and myocardial blood flows of 50%, 55%, and 31%, respectively, of those produced during normothermic closed chest compression were achieved. These compare well with the reduced metabolic demands of the hypothermic patient. Because chest wall elasticity and pulmonary compliance are decreased, more force is needed for chest wall compressions in order for adequate intrathoracic pressure gradients to be generated.

7. What is the preferred mode of therapy for ventricular fibrillation in the setting of hypothermia?

Most dysrhythmias of any type will convert spontaneously during rewarming. Ventricular fibrillation occurs at temperatures below 32°C and is most likely to occur at 28°C. The recommended approach to ventricular fibrillation begins with a maximum of 3 shocks (200 joules, then 200–300 joules, then 360 joules). It is unlikely that this will be successful until the core temperature reaches 28–30°C. Bretylium tosylate is the pharmacologic defibrillator of choice for ventricular fibrillation. Magnesium sulfate has also been used successfully in this setting. Lidocaine and propranolol, although not harmful, have little to no efficacy. Procainamide has been reported to increase the incidence of ventricular fibrillation in hypothermia and should not be used. In hypothermia, the fraction of drug bound to protein increases and liver metabolism is decreased. Thus, toxic levels of antiarrhythmics may develop with rewarming. Optimal dosages in this setting are not well established. Recent recommendations suggest that intravenous medications should be administered with increased, albeit unspecified, intervals between doses.

8. What are the basic types of rewarming?

Rewarming Methods

EXTERNAL	INTERNAL	
Passive external rewarming	**Active core rewarming**	
	Airway	Mediastinal
Active external rewarming	Heated intravenous fluid	Diathermy
Truncal	Heated irrigation	Extracorporeal
Arteriovenous anatomoses	Esophageal	Cardiopulmonary bypass
	Gastric	Arteriovenous
	Colonic	Venovenous
	Chest	Dialysis

Passive external rewarming (PER). PER minimizes the normal process of heat loss while it allows the body to rewarm spontaneously via shivering thermogenesis. It is indicated for patients with all levels of hypothermia and is sufficient by itself for mild illness. The technique is to cover the patient with an insulating material in an ambient temperature that exceeds 21°C. In order to be effective, the patient should have a core temperature of 30–32° (i.e., shivering thermogenesis intact), sufficient glycogen stores, and operative metabolic homeostasis. Advantages of the technique include its noninvasivness, simplicity, and maintenance of peripheral vasoconstriction.

Active rewarming. Active rewarming includes techniques that directly transfer heat and is divided into **external (AER)** or **internal core (ACR)** methods. Active rewarming is indicated for patients with moderate or severe hypothermia (< 32°C), cardiovascular instability, endocrine failure, impaired thermoregulation, mild hypothermia with failure to rewarm with PER, and peripheral vasodilatation (traumatic, toxicologic).

AER. In AER, exogenous heat is transferred to the skin via heating pads, heating blankets, radiant light sources, warm water immersion, hot water bottles, and forced air warming systems, in which hot forced air is circulated through a blanket (e.g., Bair Hugger). Forced air warming systems are effective without causing rewarming shock or core temperature afterdrop. Arteriovenous anastomoses techniques have been described, but no data establish their clinical efficacy and safety. AER is not recommended as the sole method of rewarming for patients with moderate to severe hypothermia, but may be successful when combined with ACR methods. The heat source should be applied only to the thorax because heat application to the extremities often produces thermal injury to vasoconstricted and hypoperfused skin and increases the metabolic requirements of the periphery, thus increasing cardiovascular demands. The preferred scenario for AER is acute immersion hypothermia in an otherwise healthy patient.

ACR. These techniques minimize pathophysiologic consequences of rewarming. ACR methods include airway rewarming, intravenous infusion of heated fluid, heated irrigation (esophageal, gastric, colonic, chest, mediastinal), diathermy, and extracorporeal rewarming (cardiopulmonary bypass, arteriovenous rewarming, venovenous rewarming, and hemodialysis).

9. What are the preferred methods of ACR?

A widely used algorithm for ACR in hypothermia is as follows:

Airway rewarming and heated intravenous fluids can be administered safely and effectively in virtually all patients. Those *in extremis* should, in addition, be submitted to extracorporeal rewarming (ECR). Other ACR modalities have less efficacy (heated irrigation), significant complication rates (peritoneal dialysis), or limited experience in humans (diathermy).

A rewarming rate of 1–2.5°C/hour can be achieved with heated (42–46°), humidified oxygen delivery. Heat exchange is augmented depending on technique (endotracheal superior to mask) and volume of minute ventilation. Advantages include technical ease, avoidance of temperature afterdrop, assured oxygen delivery, decreased viscosity of pulmonary secretions, decreased cold-induced bronchorrhea, and modification of the amplitude of shivering, which in severe cases decreases the metabolic demands of the periphery. An additional method of heat inhalation via face mask is continuous positive airway pressure (CPAP). Intravenous fluids can be warmed to 43°C (109°F).

ECR, when available, should be instituted in patients with minimal or absent mechanical cardiac activity. ECR can increase core temperature 1–2°C every 5 minutes with a bypass flow rate of 2–3 L/min. Arteriovenous rewarming is appropriate if systolic blood pressure is 60 mmHg or greater. It is accomplished via the connection of percutaneously placed femoral arterial and venous catheters to a fluid warmer. In venovenous rewarming, blood is routed from a central venous pressure catheter through a warmer and returned through a second central line or a peripheral venous catheter. Hemodialysis, although less rapid and effective, will become more practical with the development of two-way flow catheters.

10. What stabilizing measures should prehospital care providers undertake?

The patient should be handled as gently and carefully as possible because ventricular fibrillation has been ascribed to excessive mechanical stimulation. In cases of immersion, wet clothing should be removed. Further heat loss should be limited by provision of a dry and insulated environment. Blankets, sleeping bags, or aluminum-coated foils can be used for this purpose. Ethanol should not be given because it suppresses shivering thermogenesis, promotes peripheral vasodilatation and can prompt hypoglycemia in these typically glycogen-depleted patients. Massage of the extremities provides unnecessary physical stimulation and, like ethanol, can mitigate both shivering and appropriate peripheral vasoconstriction. If venous access can be acquired, 50 cc of 50% dextrose, 2 mg of naloxone, and 100 mg of thiamine are appropriate. A fluid challenge of D5 0.9% normal saline, 250–500 cc (preferably heated to 43°C), is indicated, as the majority of patients with moderate to severe hypothermia have sustained cold-induced diuresis. Lactated Ringer's solution is a less preferred crystalloid because the hypothermic liver is less able to metabolize lactate.

AER measures are safe in the minimally hypothermic patient but unnecessary. In the patient with moderate to profound hypothermia, only truncal AER should be considered. The only method of ACR appropriate in the field is heated, humidified oxygen. Several portable devices are available for this purpose.

11. What procedures are hazardous in the management of the hypothermic patient?

In patients with moderate and severe hypothermia, cardiac monitoring is indicated and harmless. Central venous pressure catheters can provide useful information and will not precipitate cardiac arrhythmias unless they are inserted into the heart. The placement of pulmonary artery catheters can be quite hazardous in this regard. Transcutaneous pacing is safe. Nasogastric tubes and Foley catheters are frequently required and can be inserted without risk.

Endotracheal intubation was thought to create a higher risk of arrhythmias. However, these reported sequelae were likely coincidental to, rather than caused by, this procedure. Numerous reports have failed to elicit a single case of arrhythmia provoked by endotracheal intubation. Factors that may be responsible for arrhythmias in the immediate post-intubation period include physical stimulation of the patient, acid-base or electrolyte disturbances, and failure to preoxygenate the patient adequately.

12. Are prophylactic antibiotics indicated for hypothermic patients?

Infection, including septicemia (e.g., gram-negative sepsis in adults), may be the cause of, coincident with, or a sequel to hypothermia. Even in the recovery phase of hypothermia, fever as well as other signs of infection are typically absent. Shaking chills caused by sepsis may unwittingly be ascribed to the shivering of hypothermia. Leukocytosis is often absent due to compromised bone marrow release and circulation of neutrophils.

The incidence of infection in hypothermic neonates is quite high and ranges from 41–53% in two series. Pulmonary infections are most commonly found and bacteriology is likely to reveal Enterobacteriaceae, Hemophilus, Staphylococcus or Streptococcus species. In adults, soft-tissue and pulmonary infections are most likely. Occult CNS bacteremia appears to be rare. Gram-negative bacteria, gram-positive cocci, Enterobacteriaceae, and oral anaerobes are likely to be found. The elderly patient with thermoregulatory failure should be considered to have sepsis until proved otherwise.

The key to management is repeated physical examination during and following rewarming. Culture specimens should be secured early in the emergency department course. Lumbar puncture is indicated in adults with persistent altered mental status following rewarming and should be employed more liberally in neonates and the elderly. Antibiotic prophylaxis is recommended for neonates and the elderly. Routine prophylaxis does not appear warranted in hypothermic adults who have no obvious manifestations of infection.

13. What is the relationship of alcohol to hypothermia?

Ethanol has social and pathophysiologic consequences. It is the most frequent associated cause of heat loss in urban hypothermia. Alcoholics are more vulnerable to the hazards of climate because of altered perception due to acute intoxication, inadequate clothing, and insufficient shelter. Heat loss is promoted by peripheral vasodilatation, impaired shivering thermogenesis, and decreased subcutaneous fat caused by malnutrition. There is a strong association between alcohol-induced hypoglycemia and ethanol. An unusual clinical presentation of Wernicke-Korsakoff syndrome is profound hypothermia. This is due to thiamine-depletion-induced hemorrhage in the hypothalamus. The clinical presentation is heralded by hypothermia, bradycardia, hypotension, miosis, and depressed deep tendon reflexes. Therefore, thiamine, 100 mg intravenously, is indicated in hypothermic patients. Magnesium, a necessary co-factor for thiamine, is often depleted in the alcoholic and repletion is required in order for thiamine administration to be effective.

CONTROVERSY

14. Active external rewarming is an effective and safe means of therapy in hypothermia.

For: Certain series report excellent success with the use of AER. The preponderance of data, however, indicate that AER, as an isolated measure of rewarming, is associated with high morbidity and mortality in patients with severe hypothermia. Candidates for AER are previously healthy patients who develop acute hypothermia (e.g., immersion), in whom minimal pathophysiologic changes have occurred. AER in the patient with minimal hypothermia is probably not harmful. The combination of truncal AER (e.g., using forced air warming systems) with core rewarming has been successful in patients who have more serious hypothermic conditions.

Against: Pathophysiologic consequences of AER in moderate and severe hypothermia include sudden peripheral vasodilatation accompanied by shock, afterdrop in core temperature, suppressed shivering thermogenesis with decreased overall rate of core rewarming, increased peripheral metabolic demands, and decreased threshold for ventricular fibrillation due to myocardial thermal gradients. AER should not be used alone in the patient with moderate to severe hypothermia. If AER is used, it should be restricted to the torso to prevent core temperature afterdrop and thermal injury to the extremities.

BIBLIOGRAPHY

1. Danzl DF: Accidental hypothermia. In Marx JA (ed): Rosen's Emergency Medicine: Concepts and Clinical Practice, 5th ed. St. Louis, Mosby, 2002, p 1979.
2. Danzl DF, Pozos RS: Accidental hypothermia. N Engl J Med 331:1756, 1994.
3. Danzl DF, et al: Multicenter hypothermia survey. Ann Emerg Med 16:1042, 1987.
4. Dixon RG, et al: Transcutaneous pacing in a hypothermia dog model. Ann Emerg Med 29:602. 1997.
5. Goheen MSL, et al: Efficacy of forced-air and inhalation rewarming using a human model for severe thyothermia. J Appl Physiol 83:1635, 1997.
6. Gregory JS, et al: Comparison of three methods of rewarming from hypothermia: Advantages of extracorporeal blood warming. J Trauma 31:1247, 1991.
7. Handrigan MT, et al: Factors and methodology in acheiving ideal delivery temperatures for intravenous and lavage fluid in hypothermia. Am J Emerg Med 15:330, 1997.
8. Hypothermia: Guidelines 2000 for CPR and ECC. 102:I-229, 2000.
9. Lazar HL: The treatment of hypothermia. N Engl J Med 337:1545, 1997.
10. Murphy K, Nowak RM, Tomlanovich MC: Use of bretylium tosylate as prophylaxis and treatment in hypothermic ventricular fibrillation in the canine model. Ann Emerg Med 15:1160, 1986.
11. Reuler JB, Girard DE, Conney TG: Wernicke's encephalopathy. N Engl J Med 312:1035, 1985.
12. Silbergleit R, et al: Hypothermia from realistic fluid resuscitation in a model of hemorrhagic shock. Ann Emerg Med 31:339, 1998.
13. Solomon A, Barish RA, Browne B, et al: The electrocardiographic features of hypothermia. J Emerg Med 7:169, 1989.
14. Weinberg AD: The role of inhalation rewarming in the early management of hypothermia. Resusciation 36:101, 1998.

97. HEAT STROKE

Stephen V. Cantrill, M.D.

1. What is heat stroke?
Heat stroke is a rectal temperature of approximately 40.5°C (105°F) or greater in a person with a history of exposure to exercise or increased temperature and humidity with accompanying neurologic disturbance, usually in the form of altered mental status. Anhidrosis (lack of sweating) is not a criterion; sweating may or may not be present.

2. Why is a rectal temperature of 40.5°C selected as the threshold?
A rectal temperature of this magnitude or greater implies that the body's mechanisms for dealing with an increased heat load have been overwhelmed and that the pathologic effects of increased temperature may occur.

3. What are the two types of heat stroke? How do they present?
Classic heat stroke is not associated with exercise, but rather with exposure to high heat and humidity over time. This form of heat stroke has a slow onset, often developing over days. It is common in the elderly and the chronically ill, who may present with anorexia, nausea, vomiting, headache, dizziness, confusion, and hypotension. Anhidrosis is common. **Exertional heat stroke** usually affects young people in good health who are exercising in a hot, humid environment. It is rapid in onset. Nausea, dizziness, and confusion are common. Fatigue, ataxia, coma, and nuchal rigidity or posturing may also occur. Patients often are sweating at the time of presentation.

4. Which populations are at greater risk for heat stroke?
• Extremes of age—due to relatively poor temperature regulation in the young and old
• Chronically ill—especially those on drugs that predispose to heat illness
• Military recruits—especially unacclimated northerners training in the South
• Athletes—most commonly football players and runners
• Laborers—especially if water losses have not been replaced
• Obese individuals—heat dissipation is compromised
• Persons dressed inappropriately for environment or activity level

5. Which drugs predispose a person to heat stroke?
Drugs increasing heat production through increased activity: cocaine, amphetamines, phencyclidine, lysergic acid diethylamide
Drugs decreasing thirst: haloperidol
Drugs decreasing sweating: antihistamines, anticholinergics, phenothiazines, beta blockers

6. What is the most effective measure of the effect of environmental heat in humans?
The commonly measured ambient air temperature is a poor gauge because it does not measure the effect of humidity, wind velocity, and radiational heating. Research has shown that an entity known as the wet bulb globe temperature (WBGT) is a much more accurate measure. The WBGT combines the wet bulb temperature (measuring the effect of humidity and wind velocity), the black globe temperature (measuring radiational heating), and the dry bulb temperature (measuring ambient air temperature). Although rarely used in the civilian world, the WBGT is commonly used by the military as a guide to determine the allowable level of activity.

7. What is the Mean Heat Index? How is it useful?
The Mean Heat Index is a recently devised measure developed by the National Weather Service of how hot the environment actually feels to a person over the course of a day. This value

is computed from a multiregression analysis equation based on ambient temperature and humidity extremes encountered during a 24-hour period. Values > 85°F (29.5°C) are believed to be dangerous to the population at large. The National Weather Service has developed methods to create a forecast giving the probability that a specific locale will exceed a certain Mean Heat Index for up to 7 days in the future. These forecasts can be used by local health and emergency officials to prepare the public for times of increased risk from heat and heat stroke.

8. What is the mortality rate of heat stroke?
Mortality rates vary from zero to 76% in different reports. This high variability is due to the differences in the populations studied. Young, healthy individuals with exertional heat stroke usually do quite well, whereas the elderly, chronically ill suffering classic heat stroke fare quite poorly.

9. What differential diagnoses should be considered in patients presenting with a rectal temperature greater than 40.5°C?

Meningitis	Neuroleptic malignant syndrome
Typhus	Malignant hyperthermia
Falciparum malaria	Thyroid storm
Rocky Mountain spotted fever	Delirium tremens
Hypothalamic lesion	Anticholinergic overdose

10. What are some of the low-level effects of heat stroke?
Cellular hypoxia
Enzyme denaturation and inactivation
Cellular membrane disruption

11. Name some end-organ effects in heat stroke.

Skeletal muscle:	rhabdomyolysis
Cardiac:	hemorrhage, necrosis
Respiratory:	adult respiratory distress syndrome
Renal:	acute tubular necrosis
Hepatic:	centrolobular hepatocellular degeneration
Coagulation:	thrombocytopenia, disseminated intravascular coagulation
Central nervous system:	edema, petechial hemorrhages

12. What is the most important aspect in the treatment of heat stroke?
Rapid cooling. Heat stroke is a true medical emergency in which minutes count. Poor patient outcome is related more to the length of time the temperature remains elevated than to the absolute degree of hyperpyrexia.

13. What treatment modalities are effective for rapid cooling?
Immersion in ice water is effective, although many believe that this must be accompanied by vigorous skin massage to counteract the cutaneous vasoconstriction that may actually impede heat loss. This modality may not be appropriate in the comatose or combative patient. Aggressive evaporative cooling, consisting of treatment with water spray and a forced air stream from a fan, has proved successful. Ice packs and massage may be used. Techniques such as iced gastric lavage and peritoneal lavage have also been reported. Cooling efforts should be ceased when the patient's temperature falls to 38.5°C (101.3°F) to avoid temperature undershoot and shivering.

14. What additional steps should be taken in dealing with heat stroke?
Continuous monitoring of rectal temperature
Supplemental oxygen
Active airway management as indicated

Cardiac monitor and electrocardiogram
Central line or Swan-Ganz catheter placement with CVP/wedge pressure monitoring in the
hypotensive patient
Cautious fluid replacement with normal saline or Ringer's lactate solution
Foley catheter and nasogastric tube placement
Restraints as needed

15. Which laboratory studies are appropriate in the severely ill heat stroke patient?

Arterial blood gases

Serum electrolytes, blood urea nitrogen,
creatinine, glucose

Complete blood count with platelet count

PT/PTT, fibrin degradation products

Liver function tests, creatine kinase

Urinalysis

Serum calcium, phosphate, lactate

16. What complications may occur in patients with heat stroke?

Emesis—especially in the comatose patient
Electrolyte disorders—hypokalemia, hyperkalemia, hyponatremia
Shivering—treat with diazepam, 5 mg IV
Seizures
Acidosis—treat with sodium bicarbonate if severe
Cardiogenic shock—treat with isproterenol; avoid alpha agents
Decreased urinary output—treat with mannitol if necessary
Pulmonary edema—from injudicious fluid replacement
Clotting disorders—may require fresh frozen plasma, heparin, or platelets
Combative, psychotic behavior—IV sedation may be necessary

17. What prognostic signs help to indicate outcome?

The longer the duration of the elevated temperature, the poorer the prognosis. Coma, hypotension, hyperkalemia, and an aspartate aminotransferase level > 1,000 units are associated with a poor prognosis.

18. What steps can be taken to prevent heat stroke?

Adequate fluid intake during periods of high temperature, high humidity, or increased activity
levels
Decreased levels of activity as mandated by the WBGT or Mean Heat Index
Control of ambient temperature and humidity if possible
Appropriate dress for the weather
Prudence during acclimation to a hotter environment
Adjustment of dosages of predisposing drugs, if possible, during hot weather
Awareness of symptoms of impending heat stroke

19. Is dantrolene sodium effective in treating heat stroke?

Dantrolene sodium uncouples the heat-generating mechanism in muscle and is the drug of choice in treating malignant hyperthermia and neuroleptic malignant syndrome, which cause excessive muscular heat production. The potential benefit of this drug in treating heat stroke has been debated. Many investigators are of the opinion that no benefit would accrue, because once treatment has begun, the problem is not heat production but rather heat dissipation. Dog studies have confirmed that administration of dantrolene sodium has no effect on passive cooling rates, pathologic changes, or clinical outcome. Although a human trial demonstrated a significant improvement in cooling rates in patients treated with dantrolene, the trial failed to demonstrate any difference in clinical outcome. In addition, these data have been contradicted by a more recent randomized, double-blind study that showed dantrolene to be ineffective. Routine use of dantrolene sodium in patients with heat stroke is not warranted at this time.

20. What is the most effective means of inducing rapid cooling?

Much discussion has centered on use of immersion, iced gastric lavage, or evaporative cooling of the heat stroke patient, either singly or in combination. Iced peritoneal lavage has also been anecdotally reported. Controlled comparison studies have most commonly used a dog model, which may not adequately represent the human response. At this time, there does not appear to be a "best" method, although many favor evaporative (water spray and forced air) cooling as the best compromise for ease of use, speed of cooling, and patient safety.

BIBLIOGRAPHY

1. American College of Sports Medicine: Heat and cold illnesses during distance running. Med Sci Sports Exerc 28(12):i–x, 1996.
2. Barthel HJ: Exertion-induced heat stroke in a military setting. Milit Med 155:116, 1990.
3. Bourchama A, et al: Activation of coagulation and fibrinolysis in heatstroke. Thromb Haemost 76:909–915, 1996.
3a. Bourchama A, Knochel MD: Heat stroke. N Engl J Med 346:1978–1988, 2002.
4. Channa AB, et al: Is dantrolene effective in heat stroke patients? Crit Care Med 18:290, 1990.
5. Costrini A: Emergency treatment of exertional heatstroke and comparison of whole body cooling techniques. Med Sci Sports Exerc 22:15, 1990.
6. Horowitz BZ: The golden hour in heat stroke: Use of iced peritoneal lavage. Am J Emerg Med 7:616, 1989.
7. Hubbard RW, et al: Novel approaches to the pathophysiology of heatstroke: The energy depletion model. Ann Emerg Med 16:1066–1075, 1987.
8. Hubbard RW: Heatstroke pathophysiology: The energy depletion model. Med Sci Sports Exerc 22:19, 1990.
9. Knochel JP: Environmental heat illness: An eclectic review. Arch Intern Med 133:841–864, 1974.
10. Shibolet S, et al: Heat stroke: A review. Av Space Environ Med 47:280–301, 1976.
11. Sprung CL, et al: The metabolic and respiratory alterations of heat stroke. Arch Intern Med 140:665–669, 1980.
12. Vicario SJ, Okabajue R, Haltom T: Rapid cooling in classic heatstroke. Am J Emerg Med 4:394–398, 1986.
13. White JD, et al: Evaporation versus iced gastric lavage treatment of heatstroke: Comparative efficacy in a canine model. Crit Care Med 15:748–750, 1987.
14. Yarbrough B, Bradham A: Heat illness. In Rosen P, et al (eds): Emergency Medicine, Concepts and Clinical Practice. St. Louis, Mosby, 1998, pp 986–1002.
15. Zuckerman GB, et al: Effects of dantrolene on cooling times and cardiovascular parameters in an immature porcine model of heatstroke. Crit Care Med 25:135–139, 1997.

XVIII. Toxicology

98. GENERAL APPROACH TO POISONINGS
Ken Kulig, M.D.

1. What are the most common causes of death from acute poisoning?

The following drug classes are responsibel for the majority of deaths from both accidental and deliberate self-poisoning:

Analgesics (aspirin, acetaminophen, opiates)	Antispychotics
Antidepressants	Gases and fumes (including carbon
Stimulants	monoxide)
Alcohols	Chemicals (industrial)
Sedatives	Pesticides

These deaths include people found dead in whom the diagnosis of poisoning is made post-mortem and patients who come to medical attention fairly early but receive inadequate treatment.

2. Name the most common causes of death from acute poisoning reported to poison centers.

Category	No.	% of All Exposures in Category
Analgesics	228	0.109
Antidepressants	146	0.241
Stimulants and street drugs	120	0.323
Cardiovascular drugs	102	0.278
Alcohols	89	0.161
Sedative/hypnotics/antipsychotics	83	0.124
Gases and fumes	49	0.105
Chemicals	36	0.066
Anticonvulsants	25	0.136
Insecticides/pesticides (includes rodenticides)	20	0.023
Cleaning substances	17	0.008
Antihistamines	16	0.035
Asthma therapies	15	0.082
Automotive products	14	0.097
Hydrocarbons	10	0.015
Cold and cough preparations	10	0.009

From Litovitz TL, Smilkstein M, Felberg L, et al: 1996 Annual Report of the American Association of Poison Control Centers Toxic Exposure Surveillance System. Am J Emerg Med 14:447–500, 1997, with permission.

3. What is the current role of syrup of ipecac in treating acute poisoning?

Although syrup of ipecac induces vomiting within 20–30 minutes in most persons who are administered a therapeutic dose, very little poison is removed; there are more effective means of decontaminating the gastrointestinal (GI) tract. Ipecac may have a role in treating children at home, who frequently can be administered a dose soon after ingestion. By the time most patients present to a hospital, however, too much time has elapsed for syrup of ipecac to be of benefit. Its use also delays the administration of activated charcoal, which needs to be administered as quickly as possible for maximal benefit. Most toxicologists currently use only activated charcoal without ipecac or lavage as the preferred means of gastrointestinal decontamination.

4. What is the current role of gastric lavage in treating acute poisonings?

Gastric lavage has the advantage over ipecac in that it works faster in emptying stomach contents, and activated charcoal can be administered down the lavage tube before it is pulled. Gastric lavage can be accomplished without prior tracheal intubation in most patients, but it is advised that airway equipment, including suction, be immediately available at the bedside. Placing the patient on his or her left side in mild Trendelenburg position will help to prevent aspiration if vomiting occurs. Nasogastric tubes are too small to remove pills or large pill fragments; whenever gastric lavage is performed, a large-bore (36- or 40-French tube in adults) should be placed through the mouth. A bite block with an oral airway will prevent the patient from biting the tube. Proper location of the lavage tube in the stomach must be verified clinically or radiographically prior to lavage or charcoal administration. Deaths have been reported due to charcoal instillation into the trachea by NG tube.

If gastric lavage is to be at all effective, however, it must be performed soon after ingestion. For this reason, many clinicians do not lavage overdose patients if more than 1 hour has elapsed since ingestion but instead immediately administer activated charcoal either orally or via NG tube. Even then, however, there is a legitimate concern that the procedure may result in major morbidity (e.g., esophageal perforation).

5. Is there a role for cathartics in treating acute poisoning?

The theory behind cathartics is that they will speed up GI transit time, allowing activated charcoal to catch up with pills in the bowel, and also prevent desorption of drug from activated charcoal. A single dose of a cathartic is commonly used, although this practice is of unproven benefit. Multiple-dose cathartics should never be used because life-threatening complications from electrolyte imbalance may result. A single dose of a saline cathartic such as magnesium sulfate or magnesium citrate, or a single dose of sorbitol (approximately 1 gm/kg), is unlikely to be harmful and may be of theoretical benefit.

6. What is the current role of whole-bowel irrigation in the treatment of acute poisoning?

Whole-bowel irrigation uses a polyethylene glycol electrolyte solution such as Golytely or Colyte, which is not adsorbed and will flush drugs or chemicals rapidly through the GI tract. The irrigation fluid is given orally or by NG tube at a dose of 1–2 L/hr. This procedure appears to be most useful when radiopaque tablets or chemicals have been ingested, as their progress through the GI tract can be monitored by radiography. This procedure is also commonly used when packets of street drugs such as heroin or cocaine have been ingested and need to be passed through the GI tract as quickly as possible. The limitations of the procedure are that unless the patient is awake, cooperative, and able to sit on a commode, there is a risk of vomiting and aspiration in addition to the logistical problem of having an unconscious patient in bed with massive diarrhea.

7. What is the role of multiple-dose charcoal in the treatment of acute poisoning?

Multiple-dose charcoal has been shown to enhance the elimination of many drugs that have already been absorbed from the GI tract or that are given intravenously. This process has been called "gastrointestinal dialysis," and has been shown to be quite effective for theophylline and perhaps phenobarbital poisoning. Numerous other drugs have been shown to have their pharmacokinetics altered by multiple-dose charcoal, but is is not clear if this makes a clinical difference. Some of these drugs are listed below; new studies are being currently performed on others. For the majority of acute poisonings in which use of multiple-dose charcoal is being contemplated, the primary reason for giving multiple-dose charcoal is to prevent absorption of drugs from the GI tract, not to enhance their elimination from the blood. In the common case of tricyclic antidepressant overdose, for example, multiple-dose charcoal should be used when large amounts of the antidepressant have been ingested to prevent its absorption (which may be life-threatening) but not to enhance its elimination. Many of these drugs have large volumes of distribution, and increasing elimination of the small amount present in the blood is unlikely to be of benefit.

Drugs with Altered Pharmacokinetics in Response to Multiple-dose Charcoal

Amitriptyline	Dextropropoxyphene	Meprobamate	Piroxicam
Atrazine	Diazepam	Methotrexate	Prophyrins
Carbamazepine	Digitoxin	Nadolol	Proscillaridin
Chlorpropamide	Digoxin	Nortriptyline	Quinine
Cyclosporine	Doxepin	Phenobarbital	Salicylates
Dapsone	Glutethimide	Phenylbutazone	Sotalol
Desmethyldiazepam	Imipramine	Phenytoin	Theophylline

8. Is forced diuresis of benefit in the treatment of acute poisoning?

Very few drugs are excreted unchanged in the urine, so that even increasing urine flow significantly above baseline is unlikely to be of benefit. However, by manipulating the pH of the urine by infusions of bicarbonate solution along with enhanced urine flow, in certain cases drug elimination can be increased. This is most commonly used for salicylates and phenobarbital. By placing 3 ampules of sodium bicarbonate in a liter of D5W along with potassium chloride, and infusing this solution at rates sufficient to produce at least a normal urine flow and a urine pH of 7.5 or greater, the elimination of salicylate and phenobarbital can be increased. Intake and output and urine pH should be monitored hourly with a Foley catheter in place. In the presence of pulmonary or cerebral edema, which can occur in severe salicylate intoxication, alkaline diuresis is dangerous and should not be undertaken.

There is some suggestion that alkaline diuresis workd in a similar manner for chlorophenoxy herbicides, but acute poisonings by these agents are rare. The use of high-volume normal saline to treat lithium intoxication is common, and it is certainly important to maintain adequate urine output and serum sodium in this scenario. It is not clear, however, that forced-saline diuresis for lithium intoxication is of extra benefit over simply ensuring normal renal flow.

9. When are extracorporeal techniques such as hemodialysis or hemoperfusion indicated?

Drugs can be successfully removed by extracorporeal maneuvers only if they have relatively small volumes of distribution and hence are found in significant quantities in the circulation, as opposed to having rapid and thorough tissue distribution. This is the case for only a few drugs. In practice, the drugs most commonly dialyzed after overdose include aspirin, lithium, and perhaps theophylline. Dialysis has the advantage over hemoperfusion in that it is frequently easier and faster to get started and can correct fluid and electrolyte abnormalities as it removes drugs. Charcoal hemoperfusion may be more effective at removing drugs that are highly bound to plasma proteins, as the affinity for charcoal may be higher than the affinity for the protein carrier. The disadvantage of hemoperfusion is that unless frequently performed in skilled hands, the procedure can result in frequent canister clotting. In addition, hypocalcemia and a precipitous drop in platelet count are quite common. Drugs for which charcoal hemoperfusion is frequently employed include theophylline, phenobarbital, and a handful of other less common agents such as paraquat and amatoxin.

10. How can the diagnosis of a drug overdose be made when the patient is unconscious and history is unavailable?

The diagnosis of acute overdose is sometimes difficult to make and requires some detective work on the part of the physician. All unconscious patients should receive dextrose and naloxone (Narcan), and a positive response to either of these is diagnostic. Whenever possible, examination of the pill bottles available to the patient is important, and it is useful to call the pharmacies where the prescriptions were filled to determine if other prescriptions were filled there for different drugs. Discovering which chemical agents were available to the patient, including street drugs, is always important. If track marks are seen, consider street drugs commonly given intravenously such as opiates, cocaine, and amphetamine. The physical examination is extremely useful in narrowing the diagnosis to a class of drug or chemicals. This concept is commonly called toxic syndromes, the most common of which are listed below.

The Most Common Toxic Syndromes

Anticholinergic

Common signs: dementia with mumbling speech, tachycardia, dry flushed skin, dilated pupils, myoclonus, temperature slightly elevated, urinary retention, decreased bowel sounds. Seizures and dysrhythmias may occur in severe cases.

Common causes: antihistamines, antiparkonsonism medication, atropine, scopolamine, amantadine, antipsychotics, antidepressants, antispasmodics, mydriatics, skeletal muscle relaxants, many plants (most notably jimson weed).

Sympathomimetic

Common signs: delusions, paranoia, tachycardia, hypertension, hyperpyrexia, diaphoresis, piloerection, mydriasis, hyperreflexia. Seizures and dysrhythmias may occur in severe cases.

Common causes: cocaine, amphetamine, methamphetamine (and derivatives MDA, MDMA, MDEA, DOB), over-the-counter decongestants (phenylpropanolamine, ephedrine, pseudoephedrine). Caffeine and theophylline overdoses cause similar findings secondary to catecholamine release, except for the organic psychiatric signs.

Opiate/Sedative

Common signs: coma, respiratory depression, miosis, hypotension, bradycardia, hypothermia, pulmonary edema, decreased bowel sounds, hyporeflexia, needle marks.

Common causes: narcotics, barbiturates, benzodiazepines, ethchlorvynol, glutethimide, methyprylon, methaqualone, meprobamate.

Cholinergic

Common signs: confusion/CNS depression, weakness, salivation, lacrimation, urinary and fecal incontinence, GI cramping, emesis, diaphoresis, muscle fasciculations, pulmonary edema, miosis, bradycardia (or tachycardia), seizures.

Common causes: organophosphate and carbamate insecticides, physostigmine, edrophonium, some mushrooms (*Amanita muscaria*, *Amanita pantherina*, Inocybe sp., Clitocybe sp.)

Serotonin

Common signs: fever, tremor, incoordination, agitation, mental status changes, diaphoresis, myoclonus, diarrhea, rigidity.

Common causes: fluoxetine, sertraline, paroxetine, venlafaxine, clomipramine; the preceding drugs in combination with monoamine oxidase inhibitors (MAOs).

---

11. How can a toxicology screen and other ancillary lab tests assist in making the diagnosis of acute poisoning?

Nontoxicologic laboratory tests that are frequently useful include the electrocardiogram, which can help diagnose overdose of tricyclic antidepressants or cardiac medications; chest radiograph, which if demonstrative of noncardiogenic pulmonary edema would make one think of salicylates or opiates; a KUB, looking for radiopaque material, which suggests ingestion of a heavy metal, including iron, phenothiazines, chloral hydrate, or chlorinated hydrocarbon solvents. Liver function tests may help to diagnose ingestion of hepatotoxins such as acetaminophen or carbon tetrachloride. A urinalysis may demonstrate the presence of calcium oxalate crystals, suggesting ethylene glycol poisoning. The acid-base status of the patient is extremely important. Persistent unexplained metabolic acidosis should always prompt the search for other diagnostic clues to aspirin, methanol, or ethylene glycol poisoning. Many other drugs can cause a persistent unexplained metabolic acidosis, including the ingestion of acids themselves, cyanide, carbon monoxide, theophylline, and others. In the work-up of persistent acidosis, a serum osmolality done by freezing point depression can be very useful if it is elevated. A difference between the measured osmolality and the calculated osmolality of greater than 10 is always significant, although a normal osmolol gap does not rule out toxic ingestion.

The toxicology screen, both blood and urine, should be done on any patient who has significant toxicity and when the diagnosis is uncertain. Alternatives to a full toxicology screen include testing discrete serum levels of the toxins in question, doing a urine qualitative test for drugs of abuse, or drawing specimens but holding them until it is determined that a toxicology screen is definitely indicated. More drugs and chemicals are *not* found on typical toxicology screens than *are* found, although the majority of drugs that are commonly ingested are found on comprehensive toxicology screens. It is important to communicate with the laboratory about which drugs are suspected, which drugs the patient takes therapeutically, and the clinical condition of the patient. When there is a discrepancy between clinical suspicion and findings from toxicology screen, it is useful to communicate with the toxicology laboratory and assist them in determining if other tests are likely to be of benefit. Toxicology screens are expensive, frequently inexact, and frequently do not give all the information that is expected by the clinician; thus one must interpret them carefully and know which drugs and chemicals are not screened for.

12. What are some other useful antidotes for common poisonings?

Naloxone and **dextrose** are the most common antidotes and should be given routinely to unconscious overdose patients. Intravenous administration of 2 mg of naloxone that results in awakening of the patient is diagnostic of acute opiate overdose. Lesser doses may be ineffective and should not be used unless it is known that the patient is an opiate addict and that the 2 mg dose of naloxone will precipitate withdrawal. Many drugs and chemicals can cause hypoglycemia, including ethanol, and for this reason dextrose should likewise be given unless it can be very quickly determined that the blood glucose is normal.

Other common antidotes include **physostigmine** for the anticholinergic syndrome. Physostigmine should be used only when the diagnosis of the anticholinergic syndrome is certain, and should seldom if ever be used to treat tricyclic antidepressant poisoning. Seizures and bradydysrhythmias have been reported when used in this setting. A dose of 1–2 mg given slowly intravenously to an adult is usually sufficient.

Digoxin Immune Fab (Digibind or DigiFab) is a safe and effective antidote for digitalis glycoside poisoning and can rapidly reverse coma, dysrhythmias, and hyperkalemia, which can be life threatening. Unlike naloxone, however, Digibind and DigiFab do not work immediately and a full response to therapy may not be seen until approximately 20 minutes after administration. For a life-threatening digitalis overdose when the dose and the serum level are currently unknown, 10 vials of Digibind should be given.

Atropine and **pralidoxime (Protopam)** are antidotes used for cholinesterase inhibitor toxicity. This group of pesticides includes the organophosphates and carbamates, which are commonly found in even household insecticides. Atropine is used to dry up secretions, primarily pulmonary, and pralidoxime is used primarily to reverse the skeletal muscle toxicity of these agents, including weakness and fasciculations.

Flumazenil is a benzodiazepine antagonist that has been shown to be useful in some cases of acute benzodiazepine overdose resulting in significant toxicity. Its use may precipitate benzodiazepine withdrawal, including seizures. It should not be used when tricyclic antidepressants have been co-ingested with benzodiazepines. The usual adult dose is 0.2 mg, followed in 30 seconds by 0.3 mg, followed in 30 seconds by 0.5 mg, repeated up to 3 mg.

Antizol (fomepizole, 4-methyl pyrazole), a recently released blocker of alcohol dehydrogenase, has been used successfully to prevent and treat cases of methanol and ethylene glycol poisoning. In cases of severe, persistent metabolic acidosis, especially in the presence of a significatn osmolal gap thought to represent likely methanol or ethylene glycol intoxication, this antidote should be given slowly at an initial intravenous dose of 15 mg/kg in crystalloid . The next dose of 10 mg/kg is due to be given 12 hours later, allowing enough time for the correct diagnosis to be made before more antidote needs to be given.

BIBLIOGRAPHY

1. ACCT/EAPCCT: Position statement on gastric lavage. J Toxicol Clin Toxicol 35:711–719, 1997.
2. ACCT/EAPCCT: Position statement on single-dose activated charcoal. J Toxicol Clin Toxicol 35: 721–741, 1997.
3. Brent J, McMartin K, Phillips S, et al: Fomepizole for the treatment of methanol poisoning. N Engl J Med 344:424–429, 2001.
4. Kulig K, Bar-Or D, Cantrill SV, et al: Management of acutely poisoned patients without gastric emptying. Ann Emerg Med 14:562–567, 1985.
5. Kulig K: Initial management of toxic ingestions. N Engl J Educ 130:**pages, year.**
6. Merrigan KS, Woodard M, Hedges JR, et al: Prospective evaluation of gastric emptying in the self-poisoned patient. Am J Emerg Med 8:479–483. 1990.
7. Olson KR, Pentel PR, Kelley MT: Physical assessment and differential diagnosis of the poisoned patient. Med Toxicol 2:52–81, 1987.
8. Osterloh JD: Utility and reliability of emergency toxicologic testing. Emerg Med Clin North Am 8:693–723, 1990.
9. Pond SM, Lewis-Driver D, Williams GM, et al: Gastric emptying in acute overdose: A prospective randomized controlled trial. Med J Aust 163:345–349, 1995.
10. Tennenbein M, Cohen S, Sitar DS: Whole bowel irrigation as a decontamination procedure after acute drug overdose. Arch Intern Med 147:905–907, 1987.

99. ASPIRIN INTOXICATION

Ken Kulig, M.D.

1. Is salicylate intoxication a serious problem in adults? Isn't this a pediatric disease?

In a two-year review of salicylate deaths in Ontario published in 1987, 51 cases of salicylate deaths, all in adults, were discovered. Salicylate-caused deaths were more than twice as numerous as any other single drug death during that time. Despite the fact that many of these patients were obviously salicylate toxic in the hospital, unaggressive treatment, including not giving activated charcoal or instituting dialysis, resulted in fatal outcomes.

Aspirin intoxication is a serious adult problem, particularly when chronic toxicity occurs in the elderly, or when the diagnosis is delayed. Physicians get a false sense of security when seeing salicylate levels slowly decline, without recognizing that the reason for the decline may be that the salicylate is moving into tissues (including the brain) and thereby worsening toxicity. Salicylate intoxication resulting in mental status changes, pulmonary edema, or persistent metabolic acidosis should always be taken seriously and treated aggressively in an ICU.

2. What is the cause of death when patients die from salicylate intoxication?

Pulmonary edema and/or cerebral edema are the most common causes of death. Persistent severe metabolic acidosis and hypokalemia may also contribute to the onset of ventricular dysrhythmias. In some patients, precipitous cardiovascular collapse can occur in the absence of obvious pulmonary or cerebral edema. This is generally a late finding seen in the hospital when the patient has been managed unaggressively for many hours.

3. What are the symptoms and signs of aspirin intoxication?

The earliest symptoms are usually nausea, vomiting, tachypnea (which may be perceived by the patient as dyspnea), and tinnitus. These symptoms are self-limited in mild or moderate intoxications. In severe poisonings, persistent vomiting (which may include hematemesis) may occur, and the patient gradually becomes more dyspneic as acidosis and pulmonary problems worsen. Concomitant mental status changes including confusion, bizarre behavior, hallucinations, seizures, and coma, may occur. Hyperpyrexia, sometimes life-threatening, may occur. A mild coagulopathy can be seen with even a single acute ingestion of salicylates. Elevated hepatic enzymes can be seen if the ingestion was chronic.

4. What is the toxic dose of aspirin?

A dose of 150–300 mg/kg (or up to approximately 65 regular-strength tablets in an average-size adult) usually results in mild to moderate toxicity after a single acute ingestion; greater than this amount frequently results in more serious toxicity. Oil of wintergreen is a more dangerous source of salicylate—1 teaspoon contains the equivalent of 21 regular-strength adult aspirin tablets—thus oil of wintergreen intoxications must always be taken seriously. The toxic dose of aspirin during chronic therapy varies from individual to individual. The maximum recommended dose is 8 regular-strength aspirin tablets per day for a normal size adult. Under certain conditions, doses exceeding this may result in drug accumulation and can be life-threatening, especially in the elderly.

5. When should salicylate levels be drawn?

It is common practice to wait 6 hours after an acute overdose to draw an aspirin level, in order to plot the level on the Done nomogram. However, if the patient is symptomatic sooner than this after an acute overdose, it is useful to draw an immediate salicylate level so that therapy can begin prior to 6 hours. If the early level is nondetectable in cases of questionable overdose, then it is relatively certain that salicylate was not ingested. Most hospital laboratories can assess salicylate levels rapidly; in any symptomatic patient, getting a level back as soon as possible after presentation yields useful clinical information.

It is imperative that the correct units be used when interpreting levels. Therapeutic salicylate levels in patients taking aspirin for arthritis are 20–30 mg/dl. Some labs report salicylates in µg/ml. The conversion is mg/dl × 10 = µg/ml. The Done nomogram uses mg/dl.

6. What is the Done nomogram? How should it be used?

The Done nomogram was developed by observing the kinetics of aspirin after overdose in children and in experimental animals. Based on extrapolated half-lives seen, the nomogram was touted to be predictive of degree of toxicity after a single acute aspirin overdose. The Done nomogram is frequently misused and misinterpreted. It should not be used when oil of wintergreen, enteric-coated aspirin tablets, or any of the newer variety of slow-release preparations are ingested. It should never be used in chronic aspirin ingestion. The nomogram should not be used to determine expected toxicity in the patient who is already significantly symptomatic. Finally, in all significant aspirin ingestions, at least two determinations of aspirin level should be done to ensure that it is falling prior to hospital discharge. The clinical status of the patient is always more important than the salicylate level in guiding therapy.

7. What are the indications for alkaline diuresis to treat aspirin intoxication?

An alkaline diuresis is generally safe and quite effective at eliminating aspirin from the body. It should be undertaken in patients who are significantly symptomatic or who have significantly elevated salicylate levels (greater than 40 mg/dl). Adding 3 ampules of sodium bicarbonate to 1 liter of D5W and the appropriate amount of potassium (most aspirin-intoxicated patients are significantly potassium depleted) and running the fluid at a rate fast enough to induce a urine output at least 2 cc/kg/hr will greatly enhance the excretion of salicylate. Contraindications to alkaline diuresis include pulmonary edema, cerebral edema, or oliguric renal failure. Urine output and pH should be closely monitored. Failure to achieve an alkaline urine (pH > 7.5) is often the result of hypokalemia.

8. What are the indications for hemodialysis or hemoperfusion for aspirin poisoning?

Hemodialysis is recommended over hemoperfusion because it can, in addition to rapidly removing aspirin, correct electrolyte and acid-base abnormalities. Indications for hemodialysis include cerebral edema, pulmonary edema, oliguric renal failure, or severe acid-base abnormalities that are not corrected with the usual measures. After acute overdose, dialysis should be considered for serum salicylate levels > 80 mg/dl and probably should be done in most cases with levels > 100 mg/dl.

9. Is there a role for multiple-dose charcoal after aspirin ingestion?

Aspirin tablets can form concretions in the GI tract. Because of their chemical nature, they tend to clump together and slowly release salicylate, which can result in steadily rising levels over long periods of time. For this reason, multiple-dose charcoal may be useful in significant ingestions. Charcoal also slightly enhances the elimination of salicylate that has already been absorbed, and can be used as an adjunct to alkaline diuresis or hemodialysis. Whole-bowel irrigation also may be useful after overdose of enteric-coated tablets.

10. When can patients be safely discharged from the ICU after aspirin poisoning?

In addition to having a return to baseline mental status and pulmonary function, patients should have serial determinations of aspirin level to document that it is going down and that it has at least reached low therapeutic levels (15–20 mg/dl). Vital signs should be normal with no residual tachypnea, and acid-base status should be normal. Even after having charcoal stools, some patients will continue to absorb aspirin from the GI tract, with late intoxication being seen. If the levels are not falling, the patient should be kept in the ICU.

BIBLIOGRAPHY

1. Anderson RJ, Potts DE, Gabow PA, et al: Unrecognized adult salicylate intoxication. Ann Intern Med 85:745–748, 1976.
2. Chapman BJ, Proudfoot AT: Adult salicylate poisoning: Deaths and outcome in patients with high plasma salicylate concentrations. Q J Med 72:699–707, 1989.
3. Done AK: Salicylate intoxication: Significance of measurements of salicylates in blood in cases of acute ingestion. Pediatrics 26:800–807, 1960.
4. Dugandzic RM, Tierney MG, Dickinson GE, et al: Evaluation of the validity of the Done nomogram in the management of acute salicylate intoxication. Ann Emerg Med 18:1186–1190, 1989.
5. Gabow PA, Anderson RJ, Potts DE, et al: Acid-base disturbances in the salicylate-intoxicated adult. Arch Intern Med 138:1481–1484, 1978.
6. Hillman RJ, Prescott LF: Treatment of salicylate poisoning with repeated oral charcoal. Br Med J 291:1492, 1985.
7. Jacobsen D, Wiik-Larsen E, Bredesen JE: Haemodialysis or haemoperfusion in severe salicylate poisoning. Hum Toxicol 7:161–163, 1988.
8. Kulig K: Salicylate intoxication: Is the Done nomogram reliable? AACT Clin-Toxicol Update 3:1, 1990.
9. McGuigan MA: A two-year review of salicylate deaths in Ontario. Arch Intern Med 147:510–512, 1987.
10. Prescott LF, Balali-Mood M, Critchley JA, et al: Diuresis or urinary alkalinization for salicylate poisoning? Br Med J 285:1383–1386, 1982.
11. Vertrees JE, McWilliams BC, Kelly HW: Repeated oral administration of activated charcoal for treating aspirin overdose in young children. Pediatrics 85:594–598, 1990.
12. Walters JS, Woodring JH, Stelling CB, et al: Salicylate-induced pulmonary edema. Radiology 146:289–293, 1983.
13. Wortzman DJ, Grunfeld A: Delayed absorption following enteric-coated aspirin overdose. Ann Emerg Med 16:434–436, 1987.

100. ACETAMINOPHEN OVERDOSE

Ken Kulig, M.D.

1. What are the symptoms and signs after acetaminophen overdose?

Patients are frequently asymptomatic for the first 8–12 hours after even a massive acetaminophen overdose. However, patients who have taken a very large overdose usually develop severe nausea and vomiting at 8–12 hours after ingestion, which can be protracted for the next several days. The skin color can be very pale or pale green, and the patient is frequently diaphoretic during this period of time. As the hepatic enzymes rise, generally beginning between

18 and 24 hours after ingestion, the liver may become enlarged and tender. In severe cases resulting in fulminant hepatic failure, encephalopathy and coma may be seen. Hypoglycemia should always be ruled out in patients with altered mental status after acetaminophen poisoning.

In some cases, significant elevations of blood urea nitrogen and creatinine occur quickly, probably because of some metabolism of acetaminophen to toxic metabolites in the kidney. Frank renal failure is very uncommon, however. Elevations of serum amylase also can occur, usually without clinical findings of pancreatitis.

2. When should an acetaminophen level be obtained after an overdose?
The acetaminophen treatment nomogram can be used only after a single acute overdose when a plasma level is obtained between 4 and 24 hours after ingestion. Levels before 4 hours are difficult to interpret, although if the level is zero, the patient probably has not ingested acetaminophen at all. Levels that are high prior to 4 hours after ingestion may actually fall to below the nomogram line by the time the 4-hour level is obtained. If the time of ingestion is unknown, the acetaminophen level cannot be plotted on the nomogram line. In this case, clinical judgment only must decide whether the antidote is indicated. It is not known how overdoses of sustained relief acetaminophen can be plotted on the nomogram, or if more than one level is required. The regional poison center can be called for advice in these cases. Chronic overdoses, especially in children, are difficult to correlate with acetaminophen levels in regard to need for treatment; the nomogram should not be used.

3. Should activated charcoal be given after an acetaminophen overdose?
Activated charcoal effectively binds acetaminophen in the GI tract and, when given early enough, can help to ensure that the patient does not develop a toxic acetaminophen level and therefore require the antidote. Activated charcoal does not prevent the absorption of N-acetylcysteine (NAC, Mucomyst) to a significant degree unless very large doses of charcoal are given concurrently with the antidote. Even if a dose of activated charcoal has been given, antidotal therapy will probably still be effective. The activated charcoal administered does not have to be removed by lavage tube as previously thought. The dose of Mucomyst does not have to be increased after activated charcoal is given. Instead, the standard doses of 140 mg/kg loading dose followed by 70 mg/kg maintenance doses every 4 hours for 72 hours is sufficient therapy if administered early enough, regardless of the presence of activated charcoal. In selected cases when the acetaminophen level has fallen to zero and hepatic transamines remain normal, less than the full three-day course of oral Mucomyst (sometimes even less than 24 hours) may be sufficient.

4. How does the antidote work?
N-acetylcysteine (NAC, Mucomyst) is thought to work by a variety of mechanisms:
1. By acting as a glutathione surrogate, which detoxifies the toxic metabolite that is formed within liver cells.
2. By being converted to glutathione itself.
3. By blunting the inflammatory response that can contribute to hepatic necrosis.
4. By increasing sulfation of acetaminophen, which also prevents the formation of the toxic metabolite.
If the antidote is given within 8 hours of overdose, it is effective even if the overdose has been massive. If given between 16 and 24 hours after ingestion, it is less effective; and between 16 and 24 hours, it is less effective still. However, Mucomyst may be of some benefit if started at least up to 24 hours, and in some cases appears to be useful even if begun after 24 hours.

5. How should liver function tests be interpreted after an acetaminophen overdose?
It is not uncommon to see hepatic enzymes rise into the tens-of-thousands after an acute acetaminophen overdose without the development of clinically apparent fulminant hepatic failure. When massive hepatic necrosis and hepatic encephalopathy develop, the hepatic enzymes are usually falling 3–5 days after the overdose, whereas the bilirubin and protime continue to rise.

This finding is always of concern, particularly when the bilirubin rises above 5 and the protime rises above 20 seconds. At that time, standard therapy for hepatic failure should be instituted.

6. When can the antidote be stopped?

Sufficient data have been gathered in the United States only for the 72-hour oral NAC protocol and the 48 hour IV NAC protocol. No published studies to date have demonstrated that the antidote can be safely stopped once acetaminophen levels have fallen below the nomogram line, although this practice is becoming more common and appears to be appropriate for patients whose transaminases have remained normal. The 20-hour IV NAC protocol used in Canada and Europe is probably effective for most patients, but is thought not to be as effective as the two longer protocols used in the United States when the overdose has been particularly large and the serum acetaminophen level very high.

7. Should liver transplant be considered after massive acetaminophen overdose?

The majority of patients who develop even major biochemical evidence of liver damage after acetaminophen overdose do well with supportive and antidotal therapy. However, in a subset of patients who have taken a massive overdose and present to the hospital very late, fulminant hepatic necrosis and death from liver failure can occur. Patients who have elevated and rising bilirubin levels and protimes and are becoming encephalopathic should be considered candidates for liver transplantation. The liver transplantation center should be notified as soon as possible about a potential candidate so that a suitable donor can be found if needed.

8. Is there a role for hemodialysis or hemoperfusion after acetaminophen overdose?

N-acetylcysteine works extremely well in preventing hepatic toxicity if given early enough after an overdose. Even when acetaminophen levels are very high, patients treated early enough with the antidote are not candidates for hemodialysis or hemoperfusion. However, patients who present very late (e.g., more than 20 hours after ingestion) who still have high levels of circulating acetaminophen might be candidates for dialysis or hemoperfusion. The procedure will remove only the acetaminophen that is circulating, which may comprise a fraction of the total dose suggested. It is not clear if removing that amount of drug will improve the outcome. These procedures are not generally recommended.

9. Does ethanol ingestion alter the prognosis in acetaminophen-poisoned patients?

The role of ethanol in acetaminophen hepatic toxicity remains somewhat controversial. Chronic ethanol abuse stimulates the P-450 pathway in the liver, which is the pathway responsible for the formation of the toxic metabolite of acetaminophen. However, ethanol itself is partially metabolized by that pathway, and hence competitively inhibits the acetaminophen being metabolized to the toxic metabolite at the same time. It is doubtful that chronic alcoholics who ingest a therapeutic dose of acetaminophen (up to 1 gm/dose and the maximum of 4 gm/day) are at increased risk for hepatic toxicity. The maximum daily dose for acetaminophen should not be exceeded by either alcoholics or nonalcoholics.Chronic alcoholics, who are likely to be malnourished and therefore glutathione-depleted, may be at higher risk for hepatotoxicity when supratherapeutic doses or frank overdoses of aceteminophen have been ingested.

BIBLIOGRAPHY

1. Bernal W, Wendon J, Rela M, et al: Use and outcome of liver transplantation in acetaminophen-induced acute liver failure. Hepatology 27:1050, 1998.
2. Bruno MK Cohen SD, Khairallah EA: Antidotal effectiveness of N-acetylcysteine in reversing acetaminophen-induced hepatotoxicity. Biochem Pharmacol 37:4319, 1998.
3. Curry RW, Robinson JD, Sughurre MJ: Acute renal failure after acetaminophen ingestion. JAMA 247:1012, 1983.
4. Harrison PM, Keays R, Bray GP, et al: Improved outcome of paracetamol-induced fulminant hepatic failure by late administration of acetylcysteine. Lancet 335:1572, 1990.
5. Heubel J: Therapeutic misadventures with acetaminophen: Hepatoxicity after multiple doses in chil-

dren. J Pediatr 132:22, 1998.
6. Prescott LF, Illingworth RN, Critchley JA, et al: Intravenous N-acetylcysteine: The treatment of choice for paracetamol poisoning. Br Med J 2:1097–1100, 1979.
7. Prescott LF: Paracetamol overdosage: Pharmacological considerations and clinical management. Drugs 25:290–314, 1983.
8. Rivera-Panera T, Gugig R, Davis J, et al: Outcome of acetaminophen overdose in pediatric patients and factors contributing to hepatotoxicity. J Pediatr 130:300, 1997.
9. Slattery JT, Wilson JM, Kalhorn TF, Nelson SD: Dose-dependent pharmacokinetics of acetaminophen: Evidence of glutathione depletion in humans. Clin Pharmacol Ther 41:413–418, 1987.
10. Smilkstein MJ, Bronstein AC, Linden CH, et al: Acetaminophen overdose: A 48-hour intravenous N-acetylcysteine protocol. Ann Emerg Med 20:1058–1063, 1991.
11. Smilkstein MJ, Knapp GL, Kulig KW, et al: Efficacy of oral N-acetylcysteine in the treatment of acetaminophen overdose. N Engl J Med 319:1557–1562, 1988.

101. ANTIDEPRESSANT POISONING

Ken Kulig, M.D.

1. Why are antidepressant overdoses so common?

Antidepressants obviously are prescribed to depressed individuals, who constitute the patient population most likely to overdose in a suicide attempt. It is ironic that some of the most dangerous drugs available, the tricyclic antidepressants, are among those prescribed to this high-risk group. The popularity of the selective serotonin reuptake inhibitors (SSRIs), which are much safer than the tricyclics after an overdose, has significantly reduced antidepressant overdose fatalities.

2. What are the symptoms and signs after tricyclic antidepressant overdose?

Very typically, the earliest signs are initial lethargy and perhaps anticholinergic symptoms, including tachycardia and dry mouth. Very rapidly, however, the clinical condition of the patient can deteriorate to include respiratory depression, seizures, myoclonic jerking, hypotension, significant conduction delay, and life-threatening cardiac arrhythmias. This has been termed "catastrophic deterioration," whereby patients can walk into the emergency room with normal vital signs and within 1 hour develop significant life-threatening toxicity.

3. What is the mechanism of death after tricyclic antidepressant overdose?

Up to 80% of fatalities from tricyclic antidepressant overdoses never reach medical attention and victims of overdose are found dead in homes, cars, hotel rooms, etc. Of those who are seen in a hospital, the most common scenario leading to death is a rapid deterioration of vital signs, widening of the QRS on the electrocardiogram, falling blood pressure, and seizures that result in metabolic acidosis, which then makes the cardiac toxicity of the tricyclics worse. Pulseless idioventricular rhythm or asystole then ensues.

4. Are serum levels of tricyclic antidepressants useful?

Serum levels frequently do not correlate well with clinical toxicity, but may be of general academic interest or of forensic interest if the time of the overdose is important. In general, tricyclic antidepressant serum levels greater than 1000 ng/ml usually correspond to life-threatening toxicity. However, levels significantly less than this, even 500 ng/ml, may result in significant CNS and respiratory depression. Many tricyclic antidepressants have active metabolites and the toxicology laboratory will measure these as well. Amitriptyline is metabolized to nortriptyline and imipramine is metabolized to desipramine. Having a higher concentration of the metabolite than the parent compound implies that the overdose occurred many hours previously. In general, serum levels of the SSRIs are not needed after overdose.

5. Of what value is the electrocardiogram in a patient with normal vital signs after an antidepressant overdose?

Cardiac toxicity can be seen on the electrocardiogram even before significant CNS or respiratory depression occurs. The earliest findings consist of a rightward deflection of the terminal 40 msec portion of the QRS complex, followed by widening of the QRS itself due to sodium channel blockers. Widening of the QRS can occur in the absence of other significant toxicity, and means that the patient is more likely subsequently to develop seizures and/or ventricular dysrhythmias. In an unconscious patient in whom the diagnosis is uncertain, seeing a conduction delay on the EKG is useful in diagnosing antidepressant overdose.

6. Which patients need to be admitted after an antidepressant overdose?

Any patient with significant toxicity after tricyclic antidepressant overdose should be admitted to the ICU. Persistent resting tachycardia or persistent lethargy should be construed as indicating significant toxicity. QRS widening on the EKG also mandates ICU admission.

7. When can patients safely be discharged from the ICU?

Patients can leave the ICU when all symptoms and signs of major toxicity have resolved, and the EKG, vital signs, and mental status are back to baseline for at least 12 hours. Late dysrhythmias have been reported. These generally occur in patients who have previously had life-threatening toxicity that has not resolved completely.

8. How should GI decontamination be performed after tricyclic antidepressant overdose?

Syrup of ipecac is always contraindicated after tricyclic antidepressant overdose. Patients can become comatose so quickly that they may be unconscious by the time emesis results. Gastric lavage may be of benefit if performed soon after an overdose, but the lavage fluid may also move tablets through the pylorus and into the small bowel. Activated charcoal should always be administered as quickly as possible, either orally down a nasogastric tube, or down the oral gastric hose prior to gastric lavage being performed.

9. Is there a role for multiple-dose charcoal after antidepressant poisoning?

Although some data suggest that the elimination kinetics of the tricyclics can be altered by multiple-dose charcoal, this is not the primary reason to use multiple-dose charcoal. Tricyclic antidepressants have anticholinergic properties, slow gastric emptying, and decreased intestinal peristalsis. After a large overdose of tricyclic antidepressants, it is imperative to give enough charcoal to adsorb all of the drug found in the GI tract. Hence, multiple doses of charcoal, although they may or may not alter elimination kinetics, may be useful to prevent absorption of drug. Multiple-dose charcoal must always be used with care in the unconscious patient and should not be used if bowel sounds are absent. Multiple-dose cathartics should not be used; however, a single dose of a cathartic with the first dose of charcoal may be useful.

10. How should tricyclic antidepressant seizures be treated?

Initial therapy is identical to the treatment of seizures from other causes. IV diazepam may stop the seizure, but IV phenytoin and/or phenobarbital should also be administered to prevent further seizures. Seizures after antidepressant poisoning are particularly dangerous because they cause acidemia, which makes the cardiac toxicity of the tricyclics worse. Therefore, prevention of seizures is crucial. If the patient has already demonstrated life-threatening toxicity, including conduction disturbances on the EKG, seizure prophylaxis may be indicated. If conservative measures (including diazepam, phenytoin, and phenobarbital) do not stop antidepressant-induced seizures quickly, the patient should be paralyzed or given general anesthesia. Continuous, or at least intermittent, EEG monitoring should be done in these cases.

11. How should the cardiovascular toxicity of antidepressants be treated?

Sinus tachycardia by itself does not require treatment. A conduction disturbance on the EKG may respond to intravenous boluses of sodium bicarbonate or hypertonic saline. Use of phenytoin in this setting is controversial, but there is some evidence that it enhances cardiac conduction and/or prevents seizures in this setting. Slow bicarbonate infusion by putting it in the maintenance IV solution has not been shown to be of benefit. Patients who are intubated should be hyperventilated to keep the arterial pH in the range of 7.45–7.55. Ventricular dysrhythmias can be treated with lidocaine and perhaps bretylium; however, class IA antiarrhythmics (e.g., quinidine) should be avoided.

12. Are the newer antidepressants of different toxicity than the older tricyclics?
Many new antidepressants are on the market and their toxicity does seem to be different. Amoxapine (Asendin) has little or no cardiac toxicity but does seem to cause a higher incidence of seizures and status epilepticus. Trazodone (Desyrel) has little cardiac or CNS toxicity, although a few cases of torsades have been reported. The SSRIs fluoxetine, sertraline, paroxetine, fluvoxamine, citalopram, and venlafaxine usually cause only lethargy after overdose. The serotonin syndrome, characterized by fever, agitation, myoclonus, tremor, incoordination, hyperflexion, diaphoresis, mental status changes, and sometimes rigidity may be seen after overdose.

BIBLIOGRAPHY

1. Boehnert MT, Lovejoy FH: Value of the QRS duration versus the serum drug level in predicting seizures and ventricular arrhythmias after an acute overdose of tricyclic antidepressants. N Engl J Med 313:474–479, 1985.
2. Callahan M, Kassel D: Epidemiology of fatal tricyclic antidepressant ingestion: Implications for management. Ann Emerg Med 14:1–9, 1985.
3. Caravati EM, Bossart PJ: Demographic and electrocardiographic factors associated with severe tricyclic antidepressant toxicity. Clin Toxicol 29:31–43, 1991.
4. Ellison DW, Pentel PR: Clinical features and consequences of seizures due to cyclic antidepressant overdose. Am J Emerg Med 7:5, 1989.
5. Foulke GE, Albertson TE, Walby WF: Tricyclic antidepressant overdose: Emergency department findings as predictors of clinical course. Am J Emerg Med 4:496–500, 1986.
6. Frommer DA, Kulig KW, Marx JA, Rumack B: Tricyclic antidepressant overdose: A review. JAMA 257:521–526, 1987.
7. Lavoie FW, Gansert GG, Weiss RE: Value of initial ECG findings and plasma drug levels in cyclic antidepressant overdose. Ann Emerg Med 19:696–700, 1990.
8. Liebelt EL, Francis PD, Woolf AD: ECG lead aVR versus QRS interval in predicting seizures and arrhythmias in acute tricyclic antidepressant toxicity. Ann Emerg Med 26:195–201, 1995.
9. Niemann JT, Bessen HA, Rothstein RJ, Laks MM: electrocardiographic criteria for tricyclic antidepressant cardiotoxicity. Am J Cardiol 57:1154–1159, 1986.
10. Pentel PR, Benowitz NL: Tricyclic antidepressant poisoning: Management of arrhythmias. Med Toxicol 1:101–121, 1986.
11. Phillips S, Brent J, Kulig K, et al: Fluoxetine versus tricyclic antidepressants: A prospective multicenter study of antidepressant drug overdoses. J Emerg Med 15:439–445, 1997.
12. Wolfe TR, Caravati EM, Rollins DE: Terminal 40-ms frontal plane QRS axis as a marker for tricyclic antidepressant overdose. Ann Emerg Med 18:348–351, 1989.

XIX. Obstetrics

102. CARE OF THE CRITICALLY ILL PREGNANT PATIENT

Stephen E. Lapinsky, M.B., B.Ch., M.Sc., FRCP(C)

1. What conditions may result in admission of pregnant women to the ICU?

A variety of obstetric complications may result in life-threatening illness requiring ICU management. Preeclampsia and its complications (such as acute renal failure, pulmonary edema, seizures [eclampsia], and the HELLP syndrome) are responsible for a large proportion of ICU admissions. Major obstetric hemorrhage and postpartum sepsis are other common obstetric complications resulting in ICU admission. A number of chronic diseases may be exacerbated by pregnancy, such as asthma, systemic lupus erythematosus (SLE), and diabetes. In some geographic areas, trauma is not only a leading cause of ICU admission, but also responsible for the majority of maternal deaths.

2. What are normal arterial blood gas findings in pregnancy?

Pregnancy is associated with an increase in minute ventilation, reaching 20–40% above baseline levels by term. This increase is due to increased carbon dioxide production as well as an increase in respiratory drive mediated largely by progesterone, and results in a low arterial partial pressure of carbon dioxide, at about 30 mmHg. Plasma bicarbonate is decreased to 18–21 mEq/L, maintaining the arterial pH in the range of 7.40–7.45. Alveolar to arterial oxygen tension difference is usually unchanged, and the mean arterial PO_2 is generally about 100 mmHg.

3. How does pregnancy affect pulmonary artery catheter measurements?

Cardiovascular physiology changes significantly during pregnancy, characterized by an increase in blood volume, an elevation in cardiac output, and a small decrease in blood pressure, resulting in a number of changes in the normal hemodynamic values in the third trimester (see table below). Filling pressures (central venous pressure and pulmonary capillary occlusion pressure) are unchanged, while cardiac output is increased by 30–50%. Systemic and pulmonary vascular resistance are reduced by about 20–30%. Oxygen consumption is increased and matched by an increase in oxygen delivery.

Effect of Late Pregnancy on Pulmonary Artery Catheter Measurements

PARAMETER	CHANGE FROM NONPREGNANT VALUE
Central venous pressure	No change
Pulmonary capillary wedge pressure	No change
Cardiac output	30–50% increase
Systemic vascular resistance	20–30% decrease
Pulmonary vascular resistance	20–30% decrease
Oxygen consumption	20–40% increase
Oxygen extraction ratio	No change

4. What factors affect oxygen delivery to the fetus?

Oxygen delivery to the fetus is determined by the maternal arterial oxygen content, uterine blood flow, and placental function. A number of factors may adversely affect blood flow to the uteroplacental vasculature, which is normally maximally vasodilated. A decrease in maternal cardiac output reduces fetal oxygenation. The maternal response to hypotension does not favor the uterus, and catecholamines (endogenous or exogenous) may aggravate fetal hypoxia by producing uterine vasoconstriction. Uterine blood flow may also be reduced by maternal alkalosis and during uterine contractions.

5. Define the supine hypotension syndrome.

In the supine position the gravid uterus may produce significant mechanical obstruction of the inferior vena cava, reducing venous return and resulting in a decrease in cardiac output and hypotension. Maternal syncope or fetal distress may result. Supine hypotension syndrome may be avoided by positioning the patient on her left side, or at least with the right hip slightly elevated. Maternal positioning should be the first response in the management of the hypotensive pregnant patient.

6. What are the principles of management of severe preeclampsia?

The most important aspect of management is the well-timed delivery of the fetus. Supportive treatment involves fluid management, control of hypertension, and prevention of seizures. The preeclamptic patient is usually volume-depleted and requires volume expansion. However, excessive fluid administration may result in pulmonary or cerebral edema due to the markedly reduced plasma colloid osmotic pressure and increased capillary permeability. Pulmonary artery catheterization may be indicated in the persistently oliguric patient or in the presence of pulmonary edema, but most patients can be managed without invasive monitoring. Hypertension is managed to prevent maternal vascular damage, and does not alter the pathologic process of preeclampsia. Commonly used regimens include small boluses of hydralazine (5–10 mg IV), boluses or infusion of labetolol, or oral nifedipine. Seizure prophylaxis should be with magnesium sulfate, using a loading intravenous bolus of 4 g over 20 minutes followed by an infusion of 2–3 g/hr. Toxic levels (usually > 5 mmol/l) can cause respiratory muscle weakness and cardiac conduction defects and are usually seen in the patient with associated renal failure. Hypocalcemia is common and should not be treated unless symptomatic. The effects of magnesium sulfate (toxic as well as therapeutic) can be reversed with intravenous calcium.

7. What are the clinical features of the HELLP syndrome?

The HELLP syndrome is a complication of preeclampsia characterized by multiorgan dysfunction. The diagnostic features are the presence of thrombocytopenia, elevated liver enzymes, and a microangiopathic hemolytic anemia. The patient may present with epigastric or right upper quadrant pain, nausea and vomiting, with or without other features of preeclampsia. Significant hemorrhage may result from the thrombocytopenia. A rare but catastrophic consequence of HELLP syndrome is hepatic hemorrhage, manifesting with sudden shock or acute abdominal pain.

8. What is acute fatty liver of pregnancy?

This is an uncommon complication of pregnancy manifesting with acute fulminant hepatic failure during the third trimester. Increased awareness of this condition has resulted in earlier diagnosis, with milder liver disease and an improved outcome. The clinical presentation is of malaise, anorexia and vomiting, followed by abdominal pain and jaundice. The patient deteriorates rapidly with acute liver failure manifested by coagulopathy, hemorrhage, renal failure, and encephalopathy. Management requires urgent delivery of the fetus and supportive therapy for fulminant hepatic failure.

9. How does amniotic fluid embolism present?

Amniotic fluid embolism is a rare but catastrophic obstetric complication usually associated with labor, delivery, or other uterine manipulations. The typical presentation is a sudden onset of severe dyspnea, hypoxemia, and cardiovascular collapse, which may be accompanied by seizures. The maternal presentation is accompanied or preceded by sudden fetal distress. A significant portion of patients die acutely within the first hour. Survivors commonly develop a disseminated intravascular coagulopathy (DIC), and acute respiratory distress syndrome (ARDS). Management is supportive, and prognosis for mother and fetus is poor.

10. What are the causes of acute respiratory failure in pregnancy?
Respiratory failure may occur as a result of pregnancy-specific complications or other conditions, some of which may be aggravated by the pregnant state (see list, next page). The pregnancy-specific diseases include amniotic fluid embolism, pulmonary edema secondary to the use of tocolytic therapy or related to preeclampsia, or peripartum cardiomyopathy. Although the pregnant patient may have diseases similar to those in the nonpregnant patient, pregnancy may increase the risk of venous thromboembolism, acute asthmatic attacks, and gastric aspiration. Changes in immune function in pregnancy predispose to increased severity of varicella pneumonia as well as Listeria and coccidioidomycosis infections. Of interest is an association between the presence of pyelonephritis and the development of ARDS in pregnancy.

Pregnancy specific: Amniotic fluid embolism
                        Tocolytic pulmonary edema
                        Preeclampsia complicated by pulmonary edema
                        Pulmonary edema due to peripartum cardiomyopathy
                        Obstetric sepsis with ARDS

Risk increased by pregnancy: Venous thromboembolism
                        Asthma
                        Pulmonary edema due to preexisting heart disease
                        Aspiration
                        ARDS associated with pyelonephritis
                        Pneumonia (especially varicella)

11. What are the risks of radiologic procedures in pregnancy?
Despite the potential risk of exposing the fetus to ionizing radiation, radiologic investigations are often necessary for management of critically ill pregnant patients. Estimated fetal radiation exposure varies from less than 0.01 rad (0.0001 Gy) for a chest radiograph to about 2–5 rad (0.02–0.05 Gy) for pelvic computed tomography (CT). Techniques such as shielding the abdomen with lead and using a well-collimated x-ray beam can effectively reduce exposure. The potential adverse effects of uterine exposure to radiation are oncogenicity and teratogenicity. A twofold increased risk of childhood leukemia may occur with relatively low-dose radiation (< 5 rads). Teratogenicity is thought not to occur at low radiation doses; microcephaly and hydrocephaly have been described after exposure of 10–150 rads. Although radiation exposure in pregnancy carries definite risks, the likelihood of any adverse effect is about 0.1% per rad. For exposure less than 5 rads, the risk is far below the spontaneous rate of congenital malformations.

Estimated Fetal Radiation Exposure during Radiographic Studies with Appropriate Shielding

RADIOGRAPHIC STUDY	ESTIMATED FETAL DOSE (RAD)
Chest x-ray	< 0.002
Ventilation-perfusion scan	0.012–0.050
CT scan of head	0.05
CT scan of chest	0.1–1.0
CT scan of abdomen/pelvis	2–5

12. How do the manifestations of severe trauma differ in pregnant patients?
Trauma is a common cause of morbidity and mortality in pregnancy, most commonly due to motor vehicle crashes, falls, and physical abuse. The anatomic and physiologic changes in pregnancy may influence the clinical findings and effects of severe trauma. The increased blood

volume allows the mother to tolerate moderate blood loss initially, but this higher volume of hemorrhage necessitates more rapid intravenous fluid replacement. Occult uterine or retroperitoneal hemorrhage always should be considered. In the third trimester, abdominal trauma usually involves the uterus, whereas the other intra-abdominal organs may be displaced or compressed in the upper abdomen. Physical signs of peritonism may be reduced because of stretching of the peritoneum. The bladder is at increased risk of injury as it extends above the pubis, and it should be remembered that a degree of ureteric dilatation is normal in pregnancy. The fetus is at risk of morbidity because of maternal hypotension, direct injury, fetomaternal hemorrhage, or placental abruption. Fetal or amniotic injury may result in maternal coagulopathy.

13. Is management of cardiac arrest different for the pregnant patient?
   Management of cardiac arrest in pregnancy follows usual protocols with some modifications. CPR in the supine position may cause impaired venous return, so a left lateral tilt position should be used. Alternatively, the uterus may be manually displaced to the left side. Cardiac compression may be technically difficult due to a highly enlarged uterus or engorged breasts. No change in pharmacologic therapy is necessary, and drugs should not be withheld when clinically indicated. Electrical defibrillation may be performed in pregnancy after removal of any fetal monitoring device. When initial attempts at resuscitation have failed, perimortem cesarean section should be considered if the fetus is at a viable gestation. Ideally, this should be initiated within 4 minutes of cardiac arrest for optimal fetal outcome. Cesarean section has been reported to reverse aortocaval compression and allow successful resuscitation of both the mother and infant.

14. How is massive obstetric hemorrhage managed?
   Routine supportive measures as well as specific interventions are used to control bleeding. Supportive measures include adequate venous access, rapid volume replacement, and blood product support. A dilutional coagulopathy should be anticipated. Ultrasound allows assessment of the uterine cavity for retained placental fragments that necessitate uterine curettage. Measures to improve uterine contraction are valuable in the presence of uterine atony. These include uterine massage, intramuscular methylergonovine, and intravenous oxytocin infusion. Methylergonovine should be avoided in the presence of hypertension. Oxytocin is administered in a dose higher than that used for augmentation of labor, e.g., 20–40 units in 1000 ml normal saline is infused at a rate up to a 100 mU/minute. Prostaglandins and their analogues may be beneficial and are replacing ergot preparations. Carboprost tromethamine has been used successfully by intramuscular or intramyometrial injection (0.25 mg).
   If pharmacologic methods fail, invasive approaches may be required. Radiologic embolization of the uterine artery may be used to effectively control hemorrhage. However, in the presence of severe life-threatening bleeding, surgical exploration is necessary to repair lacerations, to reduce blood flow by arterial ligation or, if necessary, to remove the uterus.

15. Which cardiac lesions present problems in pregnancy?
   The marked changes affecting cardiovascular physiology in pregnancy may result in decompensation in the patient with preexisting heart disease. The cardiac output rises during pregnancy, reaching a peak at about 28 weeks, 40–50% above baseline levels. Cardiac lesions limiting cardiac output therefore present the greatest risk. Mitral stenosis is the most common problem-causing valvular lesion. The increased blood volume and cardiac output may precipitate pulmonary edema. The risk of pulmonary edema or hypotension is particularly high during labor due to the poor tolerance of tachycardia and the inability to accommodate the volume shifts of delivery. Aortic stenosis is less common in pregnancy but carries high risks. Pulmonary hypertension is associated with significant morbidity and mortality due to the limitation of cardiac output and the inability to respond to postpartum fluid shifts. Congenital heart abnormalities are generally well tolerated in pregnancy unless complicated by pulmonary hypertension. Pregnancy may predispose to the development of cardiomyopathy.

BIBLIOGRAPHY

1. AMA Division of Drugs and Toxicology: Drug Evaluations Annual 1995. Chicago, American Medical Association, 1995.
2. Briggs GG, Freeman RK, Yaffe SJ: Drugs in Pregnancy and Lactation: A Guide to Fetal and Neonatal Risk, 4th ed. Baltimore, Williams & Wilkins, 1994.
3. Clark SL, Cotton DB, Lee W, et al: Central hemodynamic assessment of normal term pregnancy. Am J Obstet Gynecol 161:1439–1442, 1989.
4. Clark SL, Cotton DB, Hankins GDV, Phelan JP (eds): Critical Care Obstetrics. Boston, Blackwell Scientific Publications, 1991.
5. Hollingsworth HM, Pratter MR, Irwin RS: Acute respiratory failure in pregnancy. J Intensive Care Med 4:11–34, 1989.
6. Lapinsky SE, Kruczynski K, Slutsky AS: Critical care in the pregnant patient. Am J Respir Crit Care Med 152:427–455, 1995.
7. Lapinsky SE: Respiratory care of the critically ill pregnant patient. Current Opin Crit Care 3:1–6, 1996.
8. Pearlman MD, Tintinalli JE: Evaluation and treatment of the gravida and fetus following trauma during pregnancy. Obstet Gynecol Clin North Am 18:371–381, 1991.
9. Rizk N, Kalassian KG, Gilligan T, et al: Obstetric complications in pulmonary and critical care medicine. Chest 110:791–809, 1996.
10. Toppenberg KS, Hill DA, Miller DP: Safety of radiographic imaging during pregnancy. Am Fam Physician 59:1813–1818, 1999.

XX. Psychiatry

103. MANAGEMENT OF THE DANGEROUS PATIENT IN THE ICU

Edmund Casper, M.D., and Elizabeth Cookson, M.D.

1. What kinds of patients raise concerns of dangerousness in the ICU?

Patients can be dangerous to themselves or to others. Patients with the highest potential for danger to others are paranoid patients, who may misperceive care-giving as an attack, and delirious patients, including those who are intoxicated or withdrawing from substance use. Other patients with agitation and cognitive impairment (see Chapter 109) can also strike or kick out. Some patients admitted to the ICU after suicide attempts or self-mutilation (including ingestions and self-inflicted wounds) remain self-destructive and must be monitored closely for further attempts at self-harm.

2. What behavioral signs are red flags for impending violence?

- Increased motor activity
- Prominent startle response
- Heavy/rapid breathing
- Increasingly loud speech, especially if protesting care or expressing anger at caregiver

- Verbal threats or intimidation
- Inability to be calmed or to respond reasonably to verbal assurances or directions
- Increasing physical tension (e.g., rigid body, opening and closing hand into fist)
- Glaring stare

3. What nonpharmacologic approaches can help defuse a potentially violent patient?

Early recognition of the potential for violence can help caregivers exercise caution. A history of becoming combative or aggressive is the best predictor of future outbursts, and multiple scars, old fractures, and missing teeth may indicate a patient who resorts to fighting to resolve conflict. The intoxicated or withdrawing patient is frequently unpredictable.

At the early stages of escalation, verbal reassurance and redirection can be helpful, as can the ongoing presence of a known and trusted relative, friend, or nurse. Explain everything that you need to do before doing it, and ask permission before coming into physical contact with the patient. A dominating, controlling, or confrontational attitude can make the situation worse, as can an attempt to contradict or debate the agitated patient. Some questions can be answered with, "We'll talk about that later," or "Now's not a good time for us to discuss that." If the situation continues to build, inform other staff and ask them to stand by. The presence of additional staff both protects you and communicates to the patient that the situation will stay under control. Many facilities have crisis intervention teams available for such circumstances. If it becomes necessary to subdue the patient forcibly, personnel trained in the institution's protocol should take charge.

4. What medications are available for treatment of agitated, combative, and perhaps paranoid patients?

No medication is approved by the Food and Drug Administration (FDA) for the treatment of agitation or aggression. Nonetheless, at present haloperidol remains the best-studied and most generally accepted agent, although investigations of atypical antipsychotics (e.g., olanzapine, risperidone) are ongoing. Haloperidol is well tolerated in critically ill patients because it has little anticholinergic activity and does not cause hypotension or respiratory depression. Initial doses range from 0.5 to 10 mg, depending on the patient's age, previous exposure to the drug, and degree of agitation. The oral potency is half of the intramuscular (IM) or intravenous (IV) potency (IV use is not FDA-approved). A liquid preparation is also available and rapidly effective. Doses can be adjusted and repeated in 30 minutes. Droperidol also has been used for this indication, but the FDA recently added a "black box" warning because of cases of QT prolongation and/or torsades de pointes at doses at or below the recommended level. Some cases have occurred in patients with no known risk factors for QT prolongation, and some cases have been fatal.

If agitation does not decrease after 2 or 3 doses, 0.5–2 mg of lorazepam can be added IV or IM. Lorazepam is preferred because it is renally excreted and and better absorbed intramuscularly than other benzodiazepines. In alcohol, sedative, or hypnotic withdrawal, benzodiazepines should be used first and haloperidol added if delusions or hallucinations are present.

5. What are the common immediate side effects of haloperidol? How are they treated?

Akathisia ("not to sit," an uncomfortable inner sense of restlessness) can actually increase agitation. Lorazepam is an effective treatment, as is propranolol (in doses ranging from 10 mg 4 times/day to 40 mg 2 times/day).

Dystonias (tonic muscular contractions) generally involve flexors and can be very painful. They usually occur during the first few days of neuroleptic administration; young men are at higher risk. Benztropine, 1–2 mg orally or IM, is quickly effective. Diphenhydramine (50 mg) also may be used IV, IM, or orally. For acute reactions, a repeat dose may be required in 30–60 minutes; the patient is treated with oral doses 2 or 3 times/day thereafter.

If either of these side effects occurs, a lower dose of haloperidol or a different agent should be considered.

6. Under what conditions can a patient be placed on an emergency hold?

State statutes vary considerably. Criteria generally include danger to self or others, based on a probable psychiatric condition, but also may include inability to care for self or need for psychiatric treatment. In some states, a hold lasts up to 72 hours; other states allow up to 3 weeks for evaluation and treatment. One or two parties—usually physicians and/or psychologists—must sign. You must be familiar with local procedures.

7. Under what conditions can a dangerous patient be physically restrained?

A patient who is at imminent risk of hurting self or others can be physically restrained if proper procedures are followed. These procedures are complex and include standards set by the Joint Commission of Accreditation of Healthcare Organizations (JCAHO), federal regulations, and state regulations. Separate standards apply to the care of medical/surgical patients vs. the care of psychiatric patients. Application of restraints to a patient who poses a threat to self or others, based on medical conditions such as delirium, intoxication, withdrawal, traumatic brain injury, or an interictal state, is considered part of the treatment of the medical condition (JCAHO standards TX.7.5–TX.7.5.5). Again, you must be familiar with local procedures. In all cases, careful documentation of the behavior that required restraint and the plan for treating the patient's condition so that restraints can be removed as quickly as possible is critical.

8. What diagnoses are most common among people who attempt suicide?

Approximately 90% of people making serious suicide attempts have a psychiatric diagnosis, and more than half of that group has two or more psychiatric diagnoses. People who attempt suicide have a high risk of mood disorders, nonaffective psychosis, conduct disorder or antisocial personality disorder, and substance use disorders. Other personality disorders (such as narcissistic and borderline) are also common. In some studies, anxiety disorders are overrepresented among successful suicides. Certain medical conditions also increase the risk of suicide, including HIV infection, brain cancers, chronic hemodialysis, and certain neurologic disorders.

9. What factors reflect the severity of a suicide attempt?

Epidemiologically, older white males who are isolated and lack social support are at highest risk of successful suicide. Recent loss of a relationship (by death, separation, or divorce), employment, good health, or housing can be a significant stressor. The depressed and hopeless person may see no option other than suicide. Factors associated with increased risk of successful suicide include psychiatric diagnosis, expectation of death (even more than lethality of means), low likelihood of discovery, lack of relatedness (i.e,. the attempt does not appear to be directed at obtaining a response from another), family history of suicide, history of impulsiveness, past near-lethal suicide attempt, few reasons for living, and ongoing intent and plan.

10. What should be done for the patient who has made a suicide attempt?

People with active suicidal ideation can be very creative, using objects in ways that they were never intended to be used (e.g., tying an EKG lead around the neck). The immediate environment needs to be kept clear of as many potentially dangerous objects as possible (e.g., scissors, needles, bottles of iodine or alcohol, silverware, unnecessary cords). The patient's belongings should be searched so that prescription or other drugs are not easily available for a repeat ingestion. A psychiatric consultation should be initiated as soon as the patient can communicate. Until the patient's lethality is adequately assessed, one-on-one monitoring may be necessary.

11. What is the most therapeutic way to talk to a patient after an apparent suicide attempt?

A direct, honest, and to-the-point discussion is generally most helpful. Suicidality is not a stable trait, but a changing state; it can vary from moment to moment. Almost all suicide attempts involve considerable ambivalence; in other words, patients wish to die at the same time that they wish to live. Most patients with suicidal thoughts or behavior welcome the opportunity to discuss the feelings and events that preceded their suicidal behavior. This kind of discussion can often diminish the suicidal impulse.

12. After an overdose of a number of medications, a patient awakens in the ICU. The patient denies attempting suicide and says, "I got confused and took too many medications by accident." The patient wants to sign out and leave the hospital. How should you respond?

Any patient who needs an ICU level of care for a medication ingestion should be considered dangerous until proved otherwise. The patient should have an immediate psychiatric consultation. If the patient refuses to wait for the consultant, he or she should be placed immediately on an emergency hold. It is generally prudent to request a psychiatric consultation when a patient wants to leave the hospital against medical advice.

13. Discuss common reactions among medical personnel to the patient who has attempted suicide.

Attempted suicide frequently feels like an assault on our professional role. Medical personnel may resent caring for the patient, believing that other patients are more deserving of their attention. Others may become overly solicitous, believing that they can play a unique role in the patient's survival. The stigma against psychiatric disorders still leads many to believe that attempting suicide is a sign of weakness or that the depressed patient's suicidal preoccupations represent a "choice." In addition, by a psychological defense known as projection, the patient may invite rejection. Acknowledgment of such feelings, careful attention to professional standards, and discussions with colleagues are likely to help. If a caregiver finds him- or herself giving a different level of medical attention to the suicidal patient, reassignment of the patient should be considered.

14. What information should be conveyed to the patient in obtaining informed consent for a procedure or treatment?

1. The nature of the procedure
2. The dangers or potential complications of such a procedure
3. The benefits of the procedure
4. Possible side effects of the procedure
5. The potential consequences of not undergoing the procedure
6. Any alternative methods of treatment and their potential risks and benefits

15. Are there conditions when informed consent is not required?

In an emergency situation with immediate need for treatment to preserve life or limb, treatment may be administered without consent.

16. Define competency to consent to treatment. How is it related to the capacity for informed consent?

In all cases, one must clarify the issue by asking, "Competency to do what?" The degree of skill and knowledge needed to manage one's finances, get dressed in the morning, choose a place to live, or consent to medical treatment varies greatly. According to common law, an adult is presumed competent to make medical decisions until he or she is shown to be otherwise through the determination of the court. Strictly speaking, courts determine competency. When we casually refer to "competency" in medical settings, we generally refer to the "capacity for informed consent," which physicians traditionally assess.

17. What are the elements of informed consent?

Four areas are commonly assessed: (1) ability to communicate a choice; (2) appreciation of the situation and its consequences; (3) factual understanding of the issues, including risks, benefits, and alternatives; and (4) rationality of the decision-making process

In practice, the relative risk-to-benefit ratio of the decision or treatment often serves as a guide to how rigorously the capacity for consent needs to be determined. If risk is low and benefit high (e.g., venipuncture for laboratory tests), an affirmative choice (acceptance of the procedure) is taken as presumption of capacity. For higher risk-to-benefit ratios (e.g., surgery), more rigorous assessment of capacity may be indicated.

For example, consider a patient with a subarachnoid hemorrhage requiring evacuation. First, the patient should be able to make a choice and stick to it. The examiner may then test whether the patient is capable of repeating the information given to her—the inability to attend or remember affects the other elements. A combination of written and oral information is ideal. After an explanation of the situation and the proposed procedure, a patient capable of giving informed consent may say, "I have blood inside my skull; you want to take it out. I could have brain damage if you don't do it. The other option is to wait and see if it gets worse, but then it might be too late." With reference to the decision-making process, a very depressed patient may be able to fulfill the other elements of informed consent, but his or her reasoning may demonstrate incompetence. "I know I'll probably die without it, but my life's worthless, so that's OK." Similarly, a paranoid patient may believe that a procedure is dangerous because he or she believes that the physician will insert a tracking device during the operation. Nonetheless, we need to respect the cultural and religious beliefs of our patients and not confuse "rational" with "the decision I would make in the patient's place."

18. How should the patient who refuses all treatment be managed?

The patient's attitude toward treatment and reasons for refusal should be assessed. The patient may be angry about loss of control, afraid of current level of dependence and disability, or unable to accept the condition. Sometimes the patient's refusal comes from rushed or otherwise ineffective communication by the caregiver. An attempt should be made to enlist the patient's participation in the treatment and any decisions that are involved. If the issues underlying refusal are identified and addressed, cooperation and acceptance of treatment often result. If the refusal is not resolved quickly, however, psychiatric consultation and assessment of the patient's capacity for informed decision-making should be obtained.

BIBLIOGRAPHY

1. Beautrais AL, Joyce PR, Mulder RT, et al: Prevalence and comorbidity of mental disorders in persons making serious suicide attempts: A case-control study. Am J Psychiatry 153:1009–1014, 1996.
2. Blanchard JC, Curtis KM: Violence in the emergency department. Emerg Clin North Am 17:717–731, 1999.
3. Comprehensive Accreditation Manual for Hospitals: The Official Handbook. Oakbrook Terrace, TX, Joint Commission Resources, 2001, pp 47–62.

4. Cooper-Patrick I, Crum RM, Ford DE: Identifying suicidal ideation in general medical patients. JAMA 272:1757–1762, 1994.
5. Gutheil TG, Appelbaum PS: Clinical Handbook of Psychiatry and the Law, 3rd ed. Philadelphia, Lippincott Williams & Wilkins, 2000.
6. Harris GT, Rice ME: Risk appraisal and management of violent behavior. Psychiatr Serv 48:1168–1176, 1997.
7. Hughes DH: Management of suicidal and aggressive patients in the medical setting. In Stoudemire A, Fogel BS, Greenberg DB (eds): Psychiatric Care of the Medical Patient, 2nd ed. New York, Oxford University Press, 2000, pp 283–296.
8. Lewis S, Blumenreich P: Defusing the violent patient. RN 56(120:24–29, 1993.
9. Maltsberger JT, Buie DH: Countertransference hate in the treatment of suicidal patient. Arch Gen Psychiatry 30:625–633, 1974.
10. Roth LH, Meisel A, Lidz CW: Tests of competency to consent to treatment. Am J Psychiatry 134:279–284, 1977.

104. DELIRIUM

Marshall R. Thomas, M.D., and Elizabeth Cookson, M.D.

1. What are the organic mental disorders?

Organic mental disorders are neurobehavioral syndromes caused by transient or permanent brain dysfunction. **Delirium**, the most common organic mental disorder, is characterized by widespread cerebral dysfunction, potentially affecting orientation, attention, memory, and higher cognitive functioning, with a fluctuating level of consciousness. The term *organic* is no longer used in the diagnostic nomenclature because it inaccurately implied that mental disorders such as schizophrenia and bipolar disorder did not have organic or neurophysiologic bases. The *Diagnostic and Statistical Manual of Mental Disorders*, 4th ed. (DSM-IV) reassigns the organic mental disorders to the following categories: delirium, dementia, amnestic disorders, mental disorders due to a general medical condition, substance-induced mental disorders, and other cognitive disorders.

2. Define ICU psychosis.

ICU psychosis and **ICU syndrome** are misleading and sometimes dangerous labels describing abnormalities of central nervous system functioning seen in the intensive care unit (ICU). Ot was formerly thought that these syndromes were largely a response to the stress of being in an ICU, with the unfamiliarity of the surroundings, sleep/wake cycle disruptions, and the combined effects of sensory overload and deprivation, can worsen an underlying organic mental disorder. However, most patients so labeled are delirious and require further medical evaluation. A few of the many other terms used and misused to connote delirium include acute organic brain syndrome, metabolic encephalopathy, toxic psychosis, cerebral insufficiency, acute confusional state, and toxic encephalopathy. None of these terms should be thought of as suggesting an etiologic diagnosis.

3. Describe the clinical features of delirium.

The clinical features of delirium are varied, may develop rapidly, and fluctuate over time. Medical patients frequently are delirious either on hospital admission or shortly thereafter; surgical patients are at highest risk on the third postoperative day. The delirious patient exhibits increasing **deficits in attention and concentration** with a **fluctuating level of arousal** that is sometimes interspersed with **lucid intervals**. Memory impairment (especially involving recent events), disorientation, and disorganization of thought and speech may be present. Behaviorally, the patient may display one of three patterns: **hypoactive**, appearing withdrawn, apathetic, or somnolent; **hyperactive**, with physical agitation and restlessness; or (most often) a **mixed picture** with swings between the first two states. The delirious patient may be **emotionally labile**, showing rapid shifts in mood and affect. Perceptual disturbances such as **illusions, delusions,** and **hallucinations** are common; although generally disorganized, they may be paranoid in content. Motor problems such as **myoclonus,** action tremor, myoclonus, asterixis, and muscle tone changes also may occur.

4. How is delirium diagnosed?

Delirium is a clinical diagnosis, made on the basis of history and bedside assessment. The DSM-IV provides the most widely accepted definition (see below). An accurate **history** is necessary to assess whether there has been a change from baseline mental status. Because the delirious patient is often a poor historian, a **thorough chart review** plus histories obtained from past physicians, family, and friends should be part of the data-gathering process. Such detective work may uncover the cause of delirium—for example, a medication error, a previously unsuspected medical disorder, or a covert alcohol or drug problem. The patient's physical status should be further assessed by obtaining **serial physical and neurologic exams,** laboratory studies, and vital signs. The neurologic exam must include a **mental status exam** that assesses level of arousal, attention, concentration, orientation, thought processes, affect, and performance ability (praxis, writing, naming). An exam such as the Folstein Mini-Mental State can be helpful in quantifying such observations. A common error in diagnosing delirium is failure to make serial observations; because the patient's cognitive abilities fluctuate, a single exam showing intact attention and concentration does not necessarily argue against the diagnosis of delirium. The ICU nursing staff can be invaluable in tracking changes over time.

DSM-IV Criteria for Diagnosis of Delirium Due to a General Medical Condition

A. Disturbance of consciousness (i.e., reduced clarity of awareness of the environment) with reduced ability to focus, sustain, or shift attention.

B. A change in cognition (such as memory deficit, disorientation, language disturbance) or the development of a perceptual disturbance that is not better accounted for by a preexisting, established, or evolving dementia.

C. The disturbance develops over a short period of time (usually hours to days) and tends to fluctuate during the course of the day.

D. There is evidence from the history, physical examination, or laboratory findings that the disturbance is caused by the direct physiological consequences of a general medical condition.

From American Psychiatric Association: Diagnostic and Statistical Manual of Mental Disorders, 4th ed. Washington, DC, American Psychiatric Association, 1994.

5. Describe the patient groups at increased risk for delirium.

Approximately one-third of hospitalized medical patients and 60% of elderly patients are delirious at some point in their hospitalization. Nonetheless, one-third to one-half of cases of delirium go unrecognized. Elderly patients, children, postcardiotomy patients, burn patients, patients with drug and alcohol addictions, and patients with preexisting brain disease are at increased risk for developing delirium. Common examples in the latter category include elderly patients with dementia and younger patients with HIV infection. In general, the elderly represent the highest risk category, with the risk of delirium increasing progressively with age. In elderly patients, an altered mental status may be the first indication of a medically significant condition such as a urinary tract infection, dehydration, myocardial infarction, or pneumonia. Specific risk factors for delirium in the elderly include low serum albumin, multiple medications, use of restraints, presence of an indwelling catheter, and iatrogenic complications such as volume overload or hyponatremia. Increasing severity of physiologic stressors, such as more extensive burns or longer operations, also increase the risk of delirium.

6. Why is the diagnosis of delirium so frequently missed?

1. The general physical exam often does not contain an adequate assessment of cognitive functioning. Patients are frequently assumed to be "alert and oriented," and no specific questioning is done.

2. Many clinicians do not realize that delirium is a medical emergency.

3. The fluctuating nature of the syndrome and hence the inconsistency of findings make the recogntion of delirium more difficult.

4. The hypoactive presentation of delirium may go unnoticed; the patient who is shouting or attempting to pull out line and tubes understandably gets more urgent attention than the withdrawn and underactive patient.

The Confusion Assessment Method (CAM) and its adaptation for nonverbal patients, the CAM–ICU, are screening tools for delirium designed to be used by nonpsychiatrically trained interviewers. They can be quite helpful for screening high-risk populations. In lower-risk populations, the CAM's 10% false-positive rate can be troublesome.

7. What are the causes of delirium?

Delirium appears to represent a final common pathway for multiple conditions that interfere with higher cortical functions. Medications are the most common iatrogenic cause of delirium. Sedative-hypnotics, narcotics, and medications with anticholinergic side effects (e.g., prednisolone, cimetidine) are especially problematic. Substance intoxication and withdrawal are also extremely common. Other frequent causes include the following:

• Infections (intacranial and systemic)
• Metabolic derangements (fluid or electrolyte disturbances, acid–base disturbance, hypo- or hyperglycemia, dehydration, liver or renal failure, endocrinopathies [thyroid, parathyroid, pituitary, adrenal glands])
• Trauma (traumatic brain injury, burns, heat or cold exposure)
• Hypoxia or hypercapnia (anemia, cardiac/pulmonary failure, pulmonary embolism)
• Vitamin deficiencies (vitamin B12, folate, thiamine)
• Central nervous system (CNS) disorders (stroke, seizures, space-occupying lesions [tumor, abscess], degenerative disease)
• Vascular disease (hypertensive encephalopathy, lupus cerebritis, subdural or epidural hematoma)

Frequently delirium emerges from multiple factors. Causative factors do not necessarily lead to specific symptom patterns, although atypical presentations(e.g., hypoactivity in a patient withdrawing from alcohol) should prompt further investigation, looking perhaps for pneumonia or subdural hematoma.

8. Which drugs are most likely to be associated with delirium.

Delirium can be associated with any number of drugs. Polypharmacy contributes to delirium in several ways: (1) drugs compete for metabolism, thereby prolonging half-lives; (2) protein displacement changes bioavailability; (3) additive effects occur (e.g., simultaneous use of more than one anticholinergic agent). Drug levels should be monitored, but patients with already compromised brain function may experience CNS toxicity at "therapeutic levels" (e.g., digitalis, lithium). Other acutely ill patients may experience the accumulation of certain drugs (e.g., excessive accumulation of meperidine and its active metabolite normeperidine in patients with renal failure).

Partial List of Drugs That May Cause Delirium in the ICU

Analgesics	**Anti-inflammatory drugs**	**Drug withdrawal**
Meperidine	Adrenocorticotropic hormone	Alcohol
Opiates	Corticosteroids	Barbiturates
Pentazocine	Ibuprofen	Benzodiazepines
Salicylats	Indomethacin	**Sedative-hypnotics**
Antibiotics	Naproxen	Barbiturates
Acyclovir, ganciclovir	Phenylbutane	Benzodiazepines
Aminoglycosides	Steroids	Glutethimide
Amodiaquine	**Antineoplatic drugs**	**Sympathomimetics**
Amphotericin B	Aminoglutethimide	Aminophylline
Cephalexin	Asparaginase	Amphetamines
Cephalosporins	Dacarbazine (DTIC)	Cocaine
Chloramphenicol	5-Fluorouracil	Ephedrine

Table continued on following page

Partial List of Drugs That May Cause Delirium in the ICU (Continued)

Antibiotics *(cont.)*	Antineoplastic drugs *(cont.)*	Sympathomimetics *(cont.)*
Chloroquine	Hexamethylenamine	Epinephrine
Ethambutol	Methotrexate (high doses)	Phenylephrine
Gentamicin	Tamoxifen	Phenylpropanolamine
Interferon	Vinblastine	Theophylline
Sulfonamides	Vincristine	**Miscellaneous drugs**
Tetracycline	**Antiparkinson drugs**	Baclofen
Ticarcillin	Amantadine	Bromides
Vancomycin	Bromocriptine	Chlorpropamide
Anticholinergics	Carbidopa	Cimetidine
Antihistamines (chlorpheniramine)	Levodopa	Disulfiram
Antispasmodics	**Antituberculous drugs**	Ergotamines
Atropine/homatropine	Isoniazid	Lithium
Belladonna alkaloids	Rifampin	Metrizamide
Benztropine	**Cardiac drugs**	Metronidazole
Biperiden	Beta blockers (propranolol)	Phenelzine
Diphenhydramine	Captopril	Podophylline (by absorption)
Phenothiazines (especially thioridazine)	Clonidine	Procarbazine
Promethazine	Digitalis	Propylthiouracil
Scopolamine	Disopyramide	Quinacrine
Tricyclics (especially amitriptyline)	Lidocaine	Ranitidine
Trihexyphenidyl	Methyldopa	Timolol ophthalmic
Anticonvulsants	Mexiletine	
Phenobarbital	Procainamide	
Phenytoin	Quinidine	
Valproic acid	Tocainide	

From Trzepacz PT, Wise MG: Neuropsychiatric aspects of delirium. In Yudofsky SC, Hales RE (eds): The American Psychiatric Press Textbook of Neuropsychiatry, 3rd ed. Washington, DC, American Psychiatric Press, 1997, p 460, with permission.

9. What psychiatric diagnoses may be confused with delirium?

If only one or two symptoms are noted and a fluctuating level of consciousness is missed, delirium may be confused with several psychiatric disorders. A withdrawn, hypoactive patient may appear to be be depressed. Hyperactive and agitated presentations may be mistaken for mania. If hallunincations exist, the patient may be presumed to have schizophrenia. Memory disturbances may raise the diagnostic possibility of dementia; indeed, many patients have both dementia and delirium. However, rapid symptom evolution and fluctuation in level of consciousness are unique to delirium.

10. What laboratory studies are indicated in the work-up of delirium?

The basic studies are complete blood count, comprehensive metabolic panel, urinalysis (and urine culture, when indicated), arterial blood gases, chest x-ray, and electrocardiogram. Serum levels of prescribed medications and toxicology screens (for drugs of abuse) may be quite helpful. Lumbar puncture (LP), electroencephalogram (EEG), magnetic resonance imaging (MRI), or computed tomography (CT) scans also may be indicated. In persistent, unexplained delirium, the laboratory work-up may be extended to include the Venereal Disease Research Laboratory test for syphilis, sedimentation rate, HIV test, antincuclear antibody test, vitamin B12 and folate levels, urinary porphyrins, and a screen for heavy metals.

11. What are the indications for CT scan, MRI, EEG, and LP in the work-up of delirium?

A **CT scan** or **MRI** of the head is performed early in the work-up of delirium in patients with signs of increased intracranial pressure (papilledema or meningeal irritation), focal neurologic findings, significant recent headache or head trauma and in the presence of coma. An **EEG** may be helpful in detecting seizure activity or a focal lesion or in confirming the diagnosis of delirium. Most but not all patients with delirium show generalized diffuse background slowing on EEG that correlates with the severity of the delirium. Although an **LP** may be difficult to perform in the delirious patient, it is indicated if acute bacterial or fungal meningitis is suspected and in the evaluation of mental status changes associated with fever of unknown origin, possible subarachnoid hemorrhage, encephalitis, neurosyphilis, or unexplained seizures.

Although CT scan, MRI, EEG, and LP are not always needed in the work-up of acute delirium, they are usually indicated in the work-up of prolonged delirium of indeterminate etiology.

12. What is the course of delirium?

Delirium is associated with increased complications and longer hospital stay.Although the most common long-term outcome is recovery, morbidity and mortality rates are high. Delirious patients are at risk for seizures, coma, and medical complications related to agitation (e.g., fractures, subdural hematomas, and pulling out of intravenous and intra-arterial lines). Conservatively estimated, 25% of hospitalized delirious patients will die within 3–4 months.

13. How is delirium treated?

The first goal of treatment is to determine the cause(s) of the disorder; then specific treatments can be instituted. The patient with hypertensive encephalopathy can be treated with antihypertensive agents, the patient with alcohol withdrawal can be treated with a benzodiazepine, and the patient with hypoxia and pneumonia can be treated with oxygenation and antibiotics.

In the absence of a specific diagnosis and until the delirium resolves, the patient requires close and frequent supervision. As the diagnostic search continues, nonessential medications are discontinued while vital signs, input and output, laboratory studies, and adequacy of oxygenation are followed. Attempts are made to orient and reassure the patient, provide appropriate levels of environmental stimulation, reestablish a more normal day/night sleep cycle (i.e., dimming the lights at night), minimize immobility, provide assistive devices for sensory deficits, and keep the patient in contact with familiar objects, family, and friends. An estimated 25% reduction in the incidence of delirium can be achieved by decreased use of psychoactive medication, treatment of dehydration, and early mobilization.

14. Describe the pharmacologic management of delirium.

The agitated delirious patient may not respond to verbal or environmental interventions and may require pharmacologic treatment to ensure safety. Although controlled studies are lacking, haloperidol is generally considered the treatment of choice in managing delirium while or until more specific treatment is initiated. Haloperidol is a high-potency neuroleptic agent whose acute side effects may include drug-induced parkinsonism, dystonia, and akathisia. In contrast to other psychotropic agents, haloperidol causes little sedation, respiratory depression, orthostatic hypotension, or cardiac or anticholinergic effects. Haloperidol can be administered orally (in a tablet or liquid concentrate), intramuscularly (IM), or intravenously (IV). IV administration, although used in high doses at some centers, is not approved by the Food and Drug Administration. Cases of QT elongation and torsades de pointes have been reported with high-dose IV administration but are rare with oral administration.

Usually well-tolerated in medically ill patients, haloperidol is prescribed in doses of 2, 5, or 10 mg for younger patients and 0.5, 1, or 2 mg for elderly patients with mild, moderate, or severe agitation, respectively. Intramuscular doses are usually one-half of the oral dose. Doses can be repeated every 30 minutes until the patient is sedated or calm. Once adequate symptomatic control is achieved, a regular dosing schedule can be given, frequently with a larger dose at night. As the patient improves, the dose is usually tapered over several days rather than abruptly discontinued.

The acute dystonia and parkinsonian rigidity associated with neuroleptic agents can be treated with diphenhydramine (25–50 mg PO or IM) or benztropine (1–2 mg PO or IM). Akathisia, a potentially troublesome side effect that may actually worsen agitation, is more likely to respond to low-dose propranolol (20–80 mg/day in divided doses) or lorazepam (1–4 mg/day in divided doses). Atypical antipsychotics such as risperidone (0.25–2 mg twice daily), olanzapine (2.5–20 mg/day), and quietiapine are now used more frequently for delirium because they are less likely to cause extrapyramidal side effects, although research support is scant. Risperidone is available in a liquid form, and olanzapine can be administered in a rapidly dissolving tablet. However, no atypical antipsychotic agent currently availablei in the United States. can be administered in an injectable form.

CONTROVERSY

15. What is the role of benzodiazepines as adjunctive treatment in the agitated, delirious patient?

Excluding alcohol and sedative-hypnotic withdrawal, high-potency neuroleptics are considered the treatment of choice in managing the agitation associated with delirium. Some controversy exists about the adjunctive use of benzodiazepines in this setting.

For: A high-potency neuroleptic such as haloperidol is not particularly sedating; thus, the agitated delirious patient may require high doses to achieve sedation or to become calm. High doses of neuroleptics increase the risk for potentially serious side effects such as neuroleptic malignant syndrome and acute dystonias. Short- or intermediate-acting benzodiazepines can be used adjunctively in this setting for their sedating effects, thereby allowing the use of a relatively lower dose of the antipsychotic agent. Lorazepam may be an especially useful agent because it also treats akathisia

Against: The short-term use of antipsychotic agents in the medically ill population is generally quite safe. In contrast, benzodiazepines can contribute to respiratory depression and in fact may worsen delirium.

BIBLIOGRAPHY

1. American Psychiatric Association: Diagnostic and Statistical Manual of Mental Disorders, 4th ed. Washington, DC, American Psychiatric Association, 1994.
2. American Psychiatric Association: Practice guidelines for the treatment of patients with delirium. Am J Psychiatry 156(Suppl):5, 1999.
3. Casarett D, Inouye SK: Diagnosis and management of delirium near the end of life. Ann Intern Med 135: 32–40, 2001.
4. Ely EW, Margolin R, Francis J, et al: Evaluation of delirium in critically ill patients. Validation of the Confusion Assessment Method for the Intensive Care Unit (CAM–ICU). Crit Care Med 29:1370–1379, 2001.
5. Folstein MF, Folstein SE, McHugh PR: The Folstein Mini-Mental State Examination: A practical method for grading the cognitive state of patients for the clinician. J Psychiatr Res 12:189–198, 1975.
6. Inouye SK, Charpentier PA: Precipitating factors for delirium in hospitalized elderly persons. JAMA 275(11):852–857, 1996.
7. Inouye SK, van Dyck CH, Alessi CA, et al: Clarifying confusion: The Confusion Assessment Method. A new method for detection of delirium. Arch Intern Med 113:941–948, 1990.
8. Koolhoven I, et al: Early diagnosis of delirium after cardiac surgery. Gen Hosp Psychiatry 18:448–451, 1996.
9. Liptzin B: Clinical diagnosis and management of delirium. In Stoudemire A, Fogel BS, Greenberg DB (eds): Psychiatric Care of the Medical Patient, 2nd ed. New York, Oxford University Press, 2000.
10. McGuire BE, Basten CJ, Ryan CJ, Gallagher J: Intensive care unit syndrome: A dangerous misnomer. Arch Intern Med 160:906–909, 2000.
11. Meagher DJ: Delirium: Optimising management. Br Med J 322:144–149, 1996.
12. Sharma ND, Rosman HS, Padhi D, Tisdale JE: Torsades de pointes associated with intravenous haloperidol in critically ill patients. Am J Cardiol 81:238–240, 1998.
13. Trzepacz PT, Wise MG: Neuropsychiatric aspects of delirium. In Yudofsky SC, Hales RE (eds): The American Psychiatric Press Textbook of Neuropsychiatry, 3rd ed. Washington, DC, American Psychiatric Press, 1997, pp 447–470.

105. ANXIETY AND AGITATION IN THE ICU

Marshall R. Thomas, M.D., and Elizabeth Cookson, M.D.

1. Define anxiety and agitation.

Anxiety and agitation are nonspecific signs and symptoms. **Anxiety** can have both psychological (excessive apprehension, fear) and physiologic components (motor tension, autonomic hyperactivity, hypervigilance). **Agitation** is a behavioral sign of excessive motor activity generally associated with discomfort. Both anxiety and agitation can be caused by a broad array of medical and psychiatric conditions, or they may reflect a more purely "psychological reaction" to the circumstances that surround ICU admission. For example, in the ICU agitation is most commonly caused by delirium but also may result from fear, pain, drug withdrawal or toxicity, hypoxia, or akathisia.

2. Which medical conditions are associated with anxiety and agitation?

Medical Conditions Associated with Prominent Symptoms of Anxiety*

Akathisia	Encephalopathy	Parkinson's disease
Angina	Hypercalcemia	Partial complex seizures
Asthma	(hyperparathyroidism)	Pheochromcytoma
Carcionid syndrome	Hypercortisolism	Pneumonia
Cardiac arrhythmias (e.g, PAT)	Hyperkalemia	Pneumothorax
Cardiomyopathies	Hyperthermia	Porphyria
Chronic obstructive pulmonary disease	Hyper- and hypothyroidism	Postconcussive syndrome
Congestive heart failure	Hyperventilation	Poststroke syndrome
Delirium	Hypocalcemia	Pulmonary edema
Dementia	(hypoparathyroidism)	Pulmonary emboli
Drug withdrawal (sedative-hypnotic, opiate, tricyclic antidepressant, alcohol	Hypoglycemia	Respirator dependence
	Hyponatremia	Systemic lupus
	Hypovolemia	erythematosus
Drug toxicities (stimulants, xanthines, sympathomimetics, thyroxine, hallucinogens, anticholinergics	Hypoxia	Tumors in the area of
	Myocardial infarction	the third ventricle
	Pain	Valvular disease

PAT = paroxysmal atrial tachycardia.
* With or without concomitant delirium.

3. Give an expanded list of drugs that are associated with anxiety in the medical setting.

Drugs Associated with Anxiety in the Medical Setting

Dopaminergics	**Anticholinergics**	**Stimulants**	**Sympathomimetics**
Amantadine	Benztropine	Amphetamine	Albuterol
Bromocriptine	Diphenhydramine	Caffeine	Aminophylline
Carbidopa-levodopa	Meperidine	Cocaine	Ephedrine
Metoclopramide	Oxybutynin	Methylphenidate	Epinephrine
Neuroleptics	Pilocarpine (including ocular)	Phenterimine	Isoproterenol
Pergolide	Propantheline	Xanthines	Metaproterenol
	Quinidine		Phenylephrine
	Tricyclic antidepressants		Pseudoephedrine
	Trihexyphenidyl		Theophylline

Table continued on following page

Drugs Associated with Anxiety in the Medical Setting (Continued)

Drug withdrawal	Miscellaneous	Miscellaneous *(cont.)*	Miscellaneous *(cont.)*
Alcohol	Anabolic steroids	Fluoroquinolones	NSAIDs
Antidepressants	Baclofen	Hallucinogens	Procaine derivatives
Barbiturates	Bupropion	Interferon	Progestins
Benzodiazepines	Calcium antagonists	Metrizamide	Selective serotonin
Narcotics	Cycloserine	Metronidazole	reuptake inhibitors
Sedatives	Disopyramide	Mexiletine	Sodium lactate
	Dronabinol	Monosodium glutamate	Sumatriptan
	Estrogens	Nicotinic acid	Thyroxine (in excess)

NSAIDs = nonsteroidal anti-inflammatory drugs.
Adapted from Goldberg RJ, Posner DA: Anxiety in the medically ill. In Stoudemire A, Fogel BS, Greenberg DB (eds): Psychiatric Care of the Medical Patient, 2nd ed. New York, Oxford University Press, 2000, pp 165–180.

4. What is akathisia?

Akathisis (literally, "not to sit") is a side effect of neuroleptics and other dopamine$_2$ receptor blockers (including hydroxyzine, metoclopramide, prochlorperazine, and promethazine). Affected patients become acutely agitated and are unable to stay still. This sensation is frequently difficult to put into words, although some describe it as having "ants in the pants," "skin crawling," or "can't relax." Unfortunately, this syndrome may look just like the original symptoms for which the drug was prescribed. Propranolol (10 mg 4 times/day to 40 mg 3 times/day) is the standard treatment but may not be tolerated by patients in the ICU. Lorazepam (1–2 mg every 1–2 hr until relief is obtained) also can be effective.

5. Describe the symptoms and syndromes associated with alcohol withdrawal.

Thirty to 50% of hospitalized medical patients are thought to have problems with alcohol, and alcohol withdrawal should be considered in any patient who develops extreme anxiety within the first several days of admission to an inpatient service. The every-day drinker may not realize that he or she is at risk for withdrawal symptoms, having had no period without inbibing in many years. Symptoms also may begin in association with a significant decrease in alcohol intake (e.g., the quart-per-day drinker who decreases intake to 1 pint/day). In the ICU, the presence of other medical conditions or the use of concomitant medications (analgesics, beta blockers, and narcotics) may alter the clinical presentation and obscure the diagnosis of acute alcohol withdrawal.

The common and **early signs of alcohol withdrawal** typically occur within 24 hours of cessation or reduction in drinking and include anxiety, irritability, tremulousness, nausea, and vomiting. Other symptoms are malaise, tachycardia, elevated blood pressure, sweating, and orthostatic hypotension, although *characteristic abnormalities in vital signs need not be present.* In milder forms of withdrawal, symptoms peak within 24–48 hours and subside within 5–7 days.

Between 1 and 10% of hospitalized alcoholics develop **alcohol withdrawal delirium** (delirium tremens, DTs) and should be managed in an ICU. Signs and symptoms include confusion, disorientation, fluctuating and clouded consciousness, delusions, paranoia, vivid hallucinations (frequently tactile), marked autonomic arousal, mild fever, agitation, and insomnia. The usual onset is 3–4 days after cessation of drinking, with a peak intensity of symptoms typically occurring on the fourth and fifth days. DTs, however, can occur from 1 to 7 days after alcohol withdrawal. The syndrome is usually self-limited (3–5 days) but in rare cases may extend longer (4–5 weeks). With more modern medical interventions, the previously reported high rate of fatality (20%) is now less than 1%.

Alcohol withdrawal seizures tend to occur within 48 hours after last alcohol use. Over half of patients have multiple seizures (two to six tonic-clonic seizures), but the development of status epilepticus is rare < 3%). Alcohol withdrawal seizures may be more common in patients with hypomagnesemia, respiratory alkalosis, and hypoglycemia. **Alcohol hallucinosis** is a syndrome in which vivid hallucinations (usually auditory) occur shortly after cessation of alcohol, but in the presence of an otherwise clear sensorium and with a relative paucity of autonomic symptoms. In the majority of cases, symptoms recede within a few hours to a few days, but in a small proportion of cases the symptoms become chronic. Their vividness make the hallucinations very convincing to the patient, who may act dangerously on the basis of the hallucination's content.

6. What is the medical treatment of acute alcohol withdrawal?

Benzodiazepines, a class of drugs cross-tolerant with alcohol, are the treatment of choice for moderate-to-severe alcohol withdrawal. The standard treatment for withdrawal using the longer-acting benzodiazepines, such as chlordiazepoxide (Librium) or diazepam (Valium), may be inappropriate in the ICU because patients frequently have poor hepatic metabolism and take multiple drugs; drug elmination may be slowed. In this setting the longer-acting benzodiazepines, which have multiple metabolites, may lead to prolonged obtundation, respiratory depression, and worsening or masking of a comorbid delirium. Intermediate-acting agents, such as lorazepam (Ativan) or oxazepam (Serax), may be easier to titrate because of their shorter half-lives and lack of active metabolites. Lorazepam may be given in doses of 1–4 mg every 6–8 hours and oxazepam in doses of 15–60 mg every 8 hours. Lorazepam has the added advantage of primary renal excretion and good intramuscular absorption and availability.

Benzodiazepines not only treat autonomic hyperactivity but also decrease the likelihood of alcohol withdrawal delirium (DTs) and alcohol withdrawal seizures. Anticonvulsants are not traditionally used for alcohol withdrawal (except in patients with preexisting or underlying seizure disorders), but a growing literature describes the use of valproic acid and carbamazepine in mild-to-moderate alcohol and benzodiazepine withdrawal. Antipsychotics (e.g., haloperidol) may be needed to treat alcohol hallucinosis, although theoretically they can lower the seizure threshold. Vitamin deficiencies, low levels of magnesium and phosphorus, and electrolyte disturbances should be corrected. The acute administration of thiamine, 100–200 mg IM, prior to glucose infusion may prevent the development of the potentially irreversible Wernicke-Korsakoff syndrome in patients with severe malnutrition.

7. Describe the syndrome of sedative-hypnotic withdrawal.

Sedative-hypnotic agents include benzodiazepines, barbiturates, and miscellaneous other CNS depressants (e.g., chloral hydrate, ethchlorvynol, glutethimide, meprobamate, paraldehyde). Sedative-hypnotic withdrawal is symptomatically quite similar to alcohol withdrawal, and it is not uncommon for a patient to be simultaneously dependent on alcohol and another sedative-hypnotic. The time of onset and duration of the syndrome differ in accordance with the half-life of the agent abused. With alprazolam (Xanax), for example, the onset of withdrawal is 8–12 hours, whereas for the longer-acting diazepam (Valium), the onset of withdrawal may take 5–7 days. History from the patient, family, or patient's physician is important in distinguishing between alcohol and sedative-hypnotic withdrawal. For some patients, sedative-hypnotics may be therapeutic; rather than treating withdrawal in the ICU, the agent should be continued. Patients removed from sedative-hypnotic agents frequently have withdrawal symptoms long after the period of initial agitation.

8. What is the opiate withdrawal syndrome? What are the symptoms?

Opiate withdrawal occurs in the hospital (1) when addicted patients no longer have access to their supply, (2) when narcotic overdose is treated with naloxone or naltrexone, and (3) iatrogenically when pain medications are tapered too rapidly or dose eqivalents are not correctly calculated when switching from parenteral to oral agents. Patients switched to narcotics with mixed agonist-antagonist properties, such as pentazocine, may also experience withdrawal. Symptoms include intense anxiety, rhinorrhea, lacrimation, bone pain, goose flesh, mydriasis, abdominal pain, nausea, vomiting, diarrhea, fever, and leukocytosis. Although intensely uncomfortable, opiate withdrawal is less medically serious than sedative-hypnotic and alcohol withdrawal. Opiate withdrawal can be treated through a more gradual tapering of the opiate or mitigated by adjunctive use of clonidine, a centrally acting alpha$_2$-adrenergic agonist.

9. What are the symptoms of antidepressant withdrawal?

Tricyclic antidepressants (TCAs), selective serotonin reuptake inhibitors (SSRIs, especially those with a short half-life), venlafaxine (Effexor, a norepinephrine and serotonin reuptake inhibitor [NSRI]), and monoamine oxidase inhibitors are associated with a withdrawal syndrome following abrupt cessation. Symptoms may include paresthesias, anxiety, agitation, anorexia, nausea, vomiting, abdominal pain, diarrhea, myalgias, nightmares, insomnia, hyperreflexia, akathisia, and delirium. Abrupt withdrawal from anticholinergic TCAs can lead to a syndrome of cholinergic overdrive characterized by flu-like symptoms, especially sialorrhea, abdominal cramping, and diarrhea. Symptoms generally begin 1–4 days after cessation of medication and can last for up to 2 weeks. Reinstitution of the antidepressant with more gradual tapering is effective in treating the withdrawal syndrome. For TCAs, use of diphenhydramine, 50–100 mg at bedtime, can treat the cholinergic overdrive without restarting the antidepresant.

10. Describe nonpatholgoic types of anxiety associated with ICU admission. How can they be managed?

Anxiety is to be expected among patients (and their loved ones) in the ICU. Fears of death, abandonment, isolation, loss of control, physical disability, and loss of role function are common. The seriousness of the patient's medical condition, omnipresent monitors and alarms, lack of accurate medical information, and inherent difficulties in communication may heighten anxiety further.

Each patient assigns personal meaning to the experience of illness. Psychological reactions to illness also vary with time and the defensive structure of the patient. Denial of the severity of the condition may be adaptive (and lessen anxiety) in the period immediately after a myocardial infarction but interfere with lifestyle changes later. Acutely physicians' attempts to interfere with denial usually serve to increase anxiety and are counterproductive. Questions such as "What is it like for you when …" give the patient a chance to express his or her feelings while leaving defensive structures intact. Access to family members can decrease fears of abandonment and isolation, and a sense of the physician's concern and availability can mitigate anxiety for both patient and family. A willingness to support the patient's attempts to cope, to share information, to help distinguish fantasy from reality, and to restore the patient's sense of control are also likely to be helpful.

11. How may anxiety affect the patient on a respirator?

One of the most terrifying experiences for a ventilated patient is to be conscious but unable to move. Levels of sedation should be monitored carefully for paralyzed patients. The patient who is unable to breathe in rhythm with the ventilator will also become frightened, because he or she may be trying to exhale against resistance. Lastly, weaning schedules should be monitored so that trials off the ventilator are of a comfortable length. The patient who experiences fatigue and air hunger at the end of each trial period will eventually associate weaning with failure and discomfort and become terrified about time off the ventilator.

12. What psychiatric causes of anxiety and agitation may be problematic in the ICU?

In the general population, anxiety disorders are the most common psychiatric conditions. History is generally critical in distinguishing the new onset of anxiety and agitation (which, in the ICU, should be assumed to be nonpsychiatric until proved otherwise) from preexisting psychiatric symptoms. In the acute care setting, patients with panic disorder, acute stress disorder, posttraumatic stress disorder (PTSD), and hyperventilation syndrome may be most likely to present management problems. Simple phobias are problematic only if the phobia is related to the medical setting (e.g., phobia toward blood or needles). Patients with generalized anxiety disorder, obsessive-compulsive disorder, and other phobic disorders are more likely to have chronic symptoms that will be detected only after careful interviewing.

Panic attacks are usually short-lived (5–20 minutes) but intensely uncomfortable. During an attack sufferers are afraid that they are going to die, lose control, or go crazy. A panic attack initially may be linked to a psychological or physiologic stessor, such as loss, separation, trauma, severe illness, hyperventilation, or ingestion of drugs such as cocaine and marijuana. In **panic disorder**, which affects 1.6% of the population, panic attacks recur, frequently coming "out of the blue." Patients may develop **anticipatory anxiety** as they worry about future attacks and **phobic avoidance** as they attempt to avoid situations that they fear may provoke another attack. Because of the prominence of physiologic symptoms (shortness of breath, chest pain, palpitations, nausea, vertigo), many patients seek medical help from emergency departments, cardiologists, neurologists, and pulmonary specialists. Between episodes patients with panic disorder frequently appear "highstrung" and hypochondriacal. Various effective treatments are available for panic disorder, including cognitive and behavioral therapies and SSRIs (sertraline and paroxetine are FDA-approved for this indication), an NSRI (venlaflaxine), TCAs (imipramine, nortriptyline, or desipramine), and/or high-potency benzodiazepines (typically alprazolam or clonazepam) Antidepressants usef for anxious patients must be started at the lowest dose available, because many such patients have an initial "jitteriness syndrome" that may actually be associated with eventual response.

The patient admitted to the ICU who has just suffered a rape, beating, or automobile accident may be suffering acutely from an **acute stress disorder** in addition to the medical and surgical sequelae of trauma. Problematic symptoms can include irritability, fearfulness, autonomic hyperarousal, hypervigilance, exaggerated startle, intrusive re-experiencing of the event, as in recurrent recollections, daydreams, and nightmares. Patients with chronic forms of **PTSD**, such as those that result from childhood physical or sexual abuse or neglect, are at risk for being retraumatized by the current situation and thus have difficulty in tolerating the helplessness and loss of control associated with being a critically ill patient. Potentially problematic in the management of such patients are the understandable difficulties they may have in trusting caregivers and in modulating anger and fear. Frequently, if the physician is able to deal calmly with an initial onslaught of anxiety or hostility without reacting in kind, an unintentional yet significant test has been passed. An understanding of the symptoms associated with PTSD and a willingness to share this information with the patient can be helpful. In acute PTSD, early psychiatric intervention may prevent the development of a more severe or chronic disorder. Referral to a support group with others who have suffered similar experiences can have very positive results.

Anxiety can lead to **hyperventilation**, and hyperventilation can worsen anxiety. Associated symptoms include light-headedness, weakness, paresthesias, and carpopedal spasm. Many patients are unaware that they are hyperventilating. Hyperventilation leads to respiratory alkalosis, cerebral artery constriction and substantial reductions ($\geq 40\%$) in cerebral blood flow. Some patients with panic disorder chronically hyperventilate and can have full-blown panic attacks provoked by hyperventilation. The diagnosis of hyperventilation syndrome is suspected by clinical presentation and can be confirmed by ruling out organic causes (e.g., recurrent pulmonary emboli) and by reproduction of symptoms while voluntarily overbreathing. Hyperventilation syndrome can be treated with patient education and reassurance, a conscious decrease in respiratory rate, and rebreathing (e.g,, into a paper bag) when necessary.

Anxiety is a frequent concomitant of **mood disorders**, and anxiety and agitation are particularly common in severe **depression** and **mania**. Patients with these conditions are at risk for an iatrogenic withdrawal syndrome when their anxiolytic, mood-stabilizing, or antidepressant medications are unwittingly discontinued in the ICU. Patients with other forms of **psychosis**, including schizophrenic, schizophreniform, and paranoid disorders, also may appear fearful, anxious, and agitated, especially if left unmedicated. Finally, under severe stress most people fall back on less flexible coping styles, and patients with **character disorders** show symptoms of excessive anxiety, agitation, hostility, dependence, or psychosis. Patients with narcissistic styles may feel that they are not getting the treatment that they deserve, and patients with borderline personalities may be difficult to deal with because of their unpredictability and anger.

13. What is the pharmacologic treatment of anxiety in the ICU?

In general, nonpharmacologic interventions are used to manage the normal psychological reactions to ICU admission. Exceptions may include acute coronary care patients, in whom adequate treatment of anxiety may improve survival rates, or severely agitated patients, in whom agitation interferes with necessary treatment.

In using psychotropics in the ICU, one must take care not to further impair cognition or obscure the diagnosis of developing delirium. Anxiety and agitation arising from delirium are best treated by identifying and treating the underlying disorder and, when necessary, with the symptomatic use of a high-potency antipsychotic such as risperidone or haloperidol. Benzodiazepines are used in alcohol and sedative-hypnotic withdrawal and may be used adjunctively in the treatment of severe agitation. The benzidiazepines increase levels of drugs such as phenytoin and digoxin and may potentiate respiratory depression associated with narcotics. In severely ill patients, intermediate- and short-acting benzodiazepines are preferred. Antipsychotics may also be used in the pharmacologic management of the anxious patient when respiratory depression is a concern. Patients with preexisting psychiatric disorders may have been taking antipsychotics, antidepressants, or benzodiazepines on an outpatient basis. These drugs can be associated with both psychiatric and physiologic withdrawal syndromes, and although dosages may need to be adjusted, they should be continued when possible. Other antianxiety agents of use in selected patients include beta blockers, antihistamines, and narcotics. Buspirone can be effective in long-term management but does not take effect for several weeks.

BIBLIOGRAPHY

1. American Psychiatric Association: Diagnostic and Statistical Manual of Mental Disorders, 4th ed. Washington, DC, American Psychiatric Press, 1994.
2. Boland RJ, Boldstein MG, Haltzman SD: Psychiatric management of behavioral syndromes in intensive care units. In Stoudemire A, Fogel BS, Greenberg DR (eds): Psychiatric Care of the Medical Patient, 2nd ed. New York, Oxford University Press, 2000, pp 299–314.
3. Burvill PW: Anxiety disorders after stroke: Results from the Perth Community Stroke Study. Br J Psychiatry 166:328–332, 1995.
4. Goldberg RJ, Posner DA: Anxiety in the medically ill. In Stoudemire A, Fogel BS, Greenberg DB (eds): Psychiatric Care of the Medical Patient, 2nd ed. New York, Oxford University Press, 2000, pp 165–180.
5. Mayo-Smith MF: Pharmacological management of alcohol withdrawal: A meta-analysis and evidence-based practice guideline. American Society of Addiction Medicine Working Group on Pharmacological Management of Alcohol Withdrawal. JAMA 278:144–151, 1997.
6. Roy-Byrne PP, Fann JR: Psychopharmalogic treatments for patients with neuropsychiatric disorders. In Yudofsky SC, Hale RE (eds): The American Psychiatric Press Textbook of Neuropsychiatry, 3rd ed. Washington, DC, American Psychiatric Press, 1997, pp 943–940.
7. Silverstone PH: Prevalence of psychiatric disorders in medical inpatients. J Nerv Ment Dis 184:43–51, 1996.
8. Swift RM: Alcohol and drug abuse in the medical setting. In Stoudemire A, Fogel BS, Greenberg DB (eds): Psychiatric Care of the Medical Patient, 2nd ed. New York, Oxford University Press, 2000, pp 266–281.
9. Wise MG, Griffies WS: A combined treatment approach to anxiety in the medically ill. J Clin Psychiatry 56(Suppl 2):14–19, 1995.

106. NEUROLEPTIC MALIGNANT SYNDROME

Erinn Fellner, M.D., and James L. Jacobson, M.D.

1. What is neuroleptic malignant syndrome?

Neuroleptic malignant syndrome (NMS) is a rare, potentially fatal, idiosyncratic complication of antipsychotic medications. The usual presentation consists of four primary features: (1) hyperthermia, (2) extreme generalized rigidity, (3) autonomic instability, and (4) altered mental status.

2. What are the specific criteria for diagnosis of NMS?

There are no universally accepted criteria for diagnosis of NMS. There must be a **recent history of exposure** to antipsychotic medication. Usually the exposure occurs within 7–10 days of onset of the syndrome. However, NMS can occur with chronic usage. **Temperature elevation** can be mild or severe. Labile hypertension (less often hypotension) and tachycardia indicate **autonomic**

instability. Mental status is always **altered**, typically in the form of delirium, which may progress to stupor, obtundation, and coma. Extreme **muscular rigidity** has been characterized as "lead-pipe rigidity" and is present in all skeletal muscle. **Diaphoresis** and **sialorrhea** are almost always present. **Dysphagia, tremor, tachypnea, incontinence, mutism, leukocytosis,** and **laboratory evidence of muscle injury** (e.g., elevated levels of creatinine phosphokinase [CPK]) also may be seen. Alternative causes of these symptoms must be excluded by history, examination, and laboratory studies.

3. Are there specific laboratory findings for NMS?

No laboratory findings are pathognomonic for NMS, but certain studies are important both to support the diagnosis of NMS and to exclude other systemic illnesses. Common laboratory abnormalities include massive elevation of CPK (muscle fraction) and leukocytosis. Electrolyte disturbances, such as hypernatremia, hyponatremia, hyperkalemia, hypocalcemia, hypomagnesemia, and hypophosphatemia, may occur secondaril, along with hypoxia and acid–base abnormalities. Urinalysis often reveals proteinuria and myoglobinuria from rhabdomyolysis. Blood urea nitrogen (BUN) and creatinine may be elevated, indicating renal compromise due to rhabdomyolysis. Cerebrospinal fluid (CSF) studies should be normal. An electroencephalogram (EEG) may show diffuse slowing without focal abnormalities. Structural imaging studies of the central nervous system (CNS) should be normal. To evaluate a patient with suspected NMS, the following studies should be done to exclude a systemic illness: complete blood count with a differential white blood cell count; serum electrolytes; creatinine and BUN; muscle and hepatic enzymes; blood gas analysis; thyroid function tests; urinalysis; EKG; appropriate cultures for infection; and brain imaging, EEG, and CSF studies (when indicated).

4. What is the differential diagnosis of NMS?

The differential diagnosis includes several processes that can cause increased temperature due to abnormal thermoregulation.

Differential Diagnosis of NMS

PRIMARY CNS DISORDERS	SYSTEMIC DISORDERS
Infections (viral encephalitis, post-infectious encephalitis, HIV)	Infections
	Metabolic conditions
Tumors	Endocrinopathies (thyrotoxicosis, pheochromotoma)
Cerebrovascular disease	Autoimmune disease (systemic lupus erythematosus)
Head trauma	Heat stroke
Seizures	Toxins (carbon monoxide, phenols, strychnine, tetanus)
Serotonin syndrome	Drugs (salicylates, dopamine inhibitors and antagonists,
Major psychoses (lethal catatonia)	stimulants, psychedelics, monoamine oxidase inhibitors, anesthetics, anticholinergics, alcohol or sedative withdrawal)

Modified from Caroff SN, et al: Neuroleptic malignant syndrome: Diagnostic issues. Psychiatr Ann 21: 130–147, 1991, with permission.

5. What causes NMS?

The pathophysiology of NMS is poorly understood. The mechanism thought to be responsible is central dopamine receptor antagonism in the basal ganglia and hypothalamus and peripheral dopamine antagonism in postganglionic sympathetic neurons Central dopaminergic systems are involved in thermoregulation as well as regulation of muscle tone and movement. The relatively infrequent occurrence of NMS, however, suggests the concurrence of other factors. Speculations have included imbalances with other neurotransmitter systems (gamma aminobutyric acid [GABA], serotonin, and glutamate), abnormalities in second messenger systems, and the presentation of particular risk factors. Currently, all of the antipsychotic medications have been reported to cause NMS, including recent reports implicating the atypical antipsychotic medications (clozapine, olanzapine, risperidone, quetiapine). NMS also has been reported with some antiemetic medications such as prochlorperazine maleate, metoclopramide, trimethobenzamide, and droperidol, all of which share dopamine antagonism. Abrupt cessation of antiparkinsonian drugs can cause a similar syndrome. The hallucinogen phencyclidine and the anesthetic ketamine, both antagonists of the N-methyl-D-aspartate (NMDA) receptor, can cause a similar syndrome.

6. What risk factors predispose to the development of NMS?

Suggested risk factors include dehydration, a primary diagnosis of affective disorder (especially bipolar disorder and psychotic depression), catatonia, psychomotor agitation, concurrent presence of delirium or dementia, concurrent use of other neuroactive medications, higher relative doses and parenteral administration of antipsychotics, prior history of NMS, electrolyte disturbances, any medical or neurologic illness, and a recent history of substance abuse or dependence.

7. How common is NMS?

Rates as low as 0.02% and as high as 2.5% have been reported, but overall the rate appears to be about 0.2%.

8. What is the mortality rate associated with NMS?

Mortality from NMS has been declining since its original description in 1968. The earliest reports suggested mortality rates as high as 75%. In the early 1980s mortality rates declined to 20–30%. Current studies suggest that the mortality rate declined further, probably to less than 15%. Declining mortality rates are most likely due to increased familiarity with the syndrome, which leads to more judicious use of antipsychotics and early recognition and treatment. Death results from cardiac or respiratory arrest stemming from cardiac failure, infarction, or arrhythmia; aspiration pneumonia; pulmonary emboli; myoglobinuric renal failure; or disseminated intravascular coagulation.

9. Discuss the treatments for NMS.

Early recognition and supportive treatment are crucial. Increased temperature, elevated blood pressure, tachycardia, muscle stiffness not responsive to antiparkinsonian agents, clustering of risk factors, dysphagia, sialorrhea, and severe diaphoresis early in the course of treatment with antipsychotic medication should alert the physician to the possible emergence of NMS. Antipsychotics and other neurotoxic medications must be stopped. Supportive measures to lower temperature and ensure adequate hydration are essential. Electrolyte disturbances must be corrected. The patient should be closely monitored for signs of impending respiratory failure secondary to severe muscle rigidity and inability to handle oral secretions. Cardiac and renal function should be monitored closely. Although there is no evidence that osmotic diuresis hastens recovery from NMS, it may help to maintain renal function. If renal failure occurs, dialysis may be required.

The role of pharmacologic intervention is less clear because of the lack of controlled, prospective data; it is usuall reserved for severe cases. Dopamine agonists (bromocriptine and amantadine) and/or direct muscle relaxants (dantrolene) have been used; decreased mortality rates have been reported with both types of therapy. Dosages vary widely, but doses of bromocriptine have been documented between 2.5 and 35 mg/day. Bromocriptine can be started at 2.5–5 mg three times daily given orally (or via nasogastric tube in patients with dysphagia or severely compromised mental status). Dopamine agonists, particularly in higher doses, can cause psychosis and/or vomiting, which clearly can complicate the picture and compromise the patient. The only data available on direct-acting muscle relaxants are for dantrolene. Doses of up to 10 mg/kg have been used. The goal is to decrease muscular rigidity in order to decrease the hypermetabolic state in skeletal muscle, which is partially responsible for the hyperthermia in NMS. Dantrolene can cause hepatotoxicity, which can lead to overt hepatitis and death. Combinations of dantrolene and dopamine agonists have been used, although there is no evidence that they further decrease mortality when used in combination. Anticholinergic medications commonly used to treat pseudoparkinsonism have little benefit and may further compromise thermoregulation. Recent studies suggest that benzodiazepines may reduce recovery time in NMS. Benzodiazepines also can be useful in managing an agitated, hyperactive patient once NMS has begun to resolve. Electroconvulsive therapy also may play a role in treating NMS, but further research is needed.

10. Will NMS recur with subsequent use of neuroleptic medication?

The risk of recurrence decreases with time. The recurrence rate in patients rechallenged with antipsychotics before 2 weeks after resolution of NMS is high. Patients cautiously rechallenged 2 weeks or longer after resolution of NMS often tolerated antipsychotics without difficulty. A low-potency antipsychotic agent is chosen for the rechallenge. Dosing should be conservative and increased gradually. Recent interest in the concurrent use of the calcium channel blocker nifedipine has also shown promise in prevention of recurrence, although the data are still incomplete. Some individuals are prone to NMS; of course, close attention to early symptoms is crucial.

Guidelines for Managing Patients after NMS

1. History of a previous episode of NMS confirmed?
   Yes: Go to (2).
   No: Speak with patient, family, and treating physician(s). Retrieve pertinent medical records to confirm the diagnosis of NMS.
2. Based on a careful review of the psychiatric history and previous response to treatment, is neuroleptic therapy essential?
   Yes: Go to (3).
   No: Treat accordingly, without antipsychotics.
3. Two or more episodes of NMS with more than one antipsychotic?
   Yes: Go to (4).
   No.   Wait 1–2 weeks after recovery from NMS. Rechallenge with a low-potency antipsychotic. If a low-potency antipsychotic originally causes NMS, rechallenge with a low-potency antipsychotic from a different chemical class.
4. Have prophylactic agents (e.g., bromocriptine, dantrolene) been used in conjunction with antipsychotics?
   Yes: Go to (5).
   No: Consider such a trial, or go to (5)
5. Alternatives to conventional antipsychotic therapy: (a) atypical antipsychotics, (b) benzodiazepines, (c) electroconvulsive therapy, (d) anticonvulsants, and (e) lithium.

Adapted from Lazarus A, et al: Beyond NMS: Management after the acute episode. Psychiatr Ann 21:165–174, 1991.

11. Is there any way to prevent NMS?

No. Early recognition and, when clinically warranted, lower dosing, avoidance of parenteral antipsychotic agents and rapid increases in dosage, and minimization of other risk factors (e.g., good hydration) may decrease the incidence of NMS. Catatonia may be a strong risk factor for the development of NMS; thus, antipsychotics should be avoided in catatonic patients if possible.

12. Are there alternatives to antipsychotic treatment for acutely psychotic patients?

There are a number of treatment options. Benzodiazepines may help in the management of the hyperactive psychotic patient and lower the absolute dose of antipsychotic needed. When the primary diagnosis is affective disorder (as in a significant percentage of patients developing NMS), aggressive treatment of the manic or depressive illness with antidepressants and mood stablizers is indicated. It is usually necessary to administer antipsychotic medications concomitantly when psychotic symptoms are present. Electroconvulsive therapy is a viable alternative for manic psychosis, depressive psychosis, and catatonia.

In chronic psychotic disorders (e.g., schizophrenia, schizoaffective disorder, delusional disorder) there may be no alternative to the use of antipsychotic medications. Hence, cautious rechallenging with different classes of antipsychotics (with special attention to atypical antipsychotic agents and treatment of reversible risk factors) is virtually always necessary. Avoidance of polypharmacy, if possible, is also advisable.

13. Are malignant hyperthermia (MH) and NMS related?

MH and NMS have similar clinical presentations but different pathophysiologies. MH develops after exposure to inhalation anesthetics, such as halothane, and depolarizing muscle relaxants, such as succinylcholine. MH is characterized by diffuse muscle ridigity, fever, hypermetabolism, elevated serum CK (muscle fraction), hyperkalemia, tachycardia, hypoxemia, acidosis, and myoglobinuria. It is caused by a genetic defect in a sarcoplasmic reticulum calcium channel protein, which results in excessive calcium release in skeletal muscle after exposure to triggering medications. Susceptibility to MH is diagnosed by the muscle contracture test. In susceptible people, excessive contractions occur in muscle strips exposed to varying concentrations of halothane and caffeine. Family studies and muscle contracture testing indicate that patients with NMS have the genetic defect found in patients with MH. Patients with one of the disorders do not appear to be at increased risk for the other.

14. What is serotonin syndrome (SS)? How is it differentiated from NMS?

SS is a rare but potentially fatal syndrome characterized by the triad of altered mental status, autonomic dysfunction, and neuromuscular abnormalities, which is thought to result from central and peripheral hyperserotonergic activity. The similarity between SS and NMS often leads to misdiagnosis. SS can develop after the addition of a serotonergic medication (monoamine oxidase inhibitor, tricyclic antidepressant, selective serotonin reuptake inhibitor) to a regimen that already includes serotonin-enhancing drugs or after overdoses of serotonergic drugs. The presentation is heterogeneous, but common clinical features include confusion, hypomania, agitation, restlessness, myoclonus, hyperreflexia, diaphoresis, tachycardia, blood pressure fluctuation, shivering, tremor, diarrhea, incoordination, and feer. Compared with NMS, in SS tremor and myoclonus are more prominent than muscle rigidity, fever is present less often, and the laboratory abnormalities seen in NMS (elevated CPK) are usually absent. Discontinuation of the serotonergic medications and supportive treatment are most important. As with NMS, the role of pharmacologic treatment in SS is unclear because of the lack of controlled, prospective studies. Lorazepam, propranolol, and cyproheptadine may be effective in treating symptoms. Propranolol and cyproheptadine have serotonin antagonist properties.

BIBLIOGRAPHY

1. Addonizio G, Susman VL: Neuroleptic Malignant Syndrome: A Clinical Approach. St. Louis, Mosby, 1991.
2. Brown T, Frian S, Mareth T: Pathophysiology and management of the serotonin syndrome. Ann Pharmacother 30:527–535, 1996.
3. Caroff SN, Mahn SC: Neuroleptic malignant syndrome. Contemp Clin Neurol 77:185–202, 1991.
4. Castillo E, Rubin R, Holsboer-Truacster E: Clinical differentiation between lethal catatonia and neuroleptic malignant syndrome. Am J Psychiatry 145:324–328, 1989.
5. Fink M: Neuroleptic malignant syndrome and catatonia: One entity or two? Biol Psychiatry 39:1–4, 1996.
6. Francis A, Chandragiri S, Rizvi S, et al: Is lorazepam a treatment for neuroleptic malignant syndrome? CNS Spectrum 5:54–57, 2000.
7. Gurrera RJ, Chang SS: Thermoregulatory dysfunction in neuroleptic malignant syndrome. Biol Psychiatry 39:207–212, 1996.
8. Keck PE, Caroff SN, McElroy SL: Neuroleptic malignant syndrome and malignant hyperthermia. End of a controversy? J Neuropsychiatry Clin Neurosci 7:135–144, 1995.
9. Pope JG Jr, Aizley HG, Keck PE, McElroy SL: Neuroleptic malignant syndrome: Long-term follow-up of 20 cases. J Clin Psychiatry 42:208–212, 1991.
10. Pope HG Jr, Keck JR, McElroy SL: Frequency and presentation of neuroleptic malignant syndrome in a large psychiatric hospital. Am J Psychiatry 143:1227–1232, 1986.
11. Rosenberg MR, Green M: Neuroleptic malignant syndrome: A review of response to therapy. Arch Intern Med 149:1927–1931, 1989.
12. Rosebush P, Stewart T: A prospective analysis of 24 episodes of neuroleptic malignant syndrome. Am J Psychiatry 146:717–725, 1989.
13. Rosebush PI, Stewart TD, Gelenberg AJ: Twenty neuroleptic rechallenges after neuroleptic malignant syndrome in 15 patients. J Clin Psychiatry 50:295–298, 1989.
14. Shalev A, Heresh H, Munitz H: Mortality from neuroleptic malignant syndrome. Clin Psychiatry 50:18–22, 1989.
15. Susman VL, Addonizio G: Recurrence of neuroleptic malignant syndrome. J Nerv Ment Dis 176:234–241, 1988.
16. White DA, Robins A: Analysis of 17 catatonic patients diagnosed with neuroleptic malignant syndrome. CNS Spectrum 5:58–65, 2000.

XXI. Ethics

107. ETHICS

David Shimabukuro, M.D.C.M.

1. What are the principles on which judicial decisions regarding patients' acceptance or refusal of medical care are based?

This issue tends to arise when there is a conflict among the patient, family members, and/or medical team. No legal statutes pertain to this issue, except in cases of extremis (i.e., brain death and organ transplantation), but the courts' opinions have been expressed via case law. A majority of their decisions are based on two important and distinct principles: (1) autonomy of the individual and (2) informed consent. The concept of autonomy can be defined as the fundamental right to choose one's own destiny, regardless of the eventual outcome. Of course, the choice made cannot cause harm to others. As for the principle of informed consent, it is much harder to define because it also includes the concept of competency (see below). Most experts agree, however, that informed consent is a decision made by a competent person after receiving information about available treatment options along with the risks, benefits, and consequences of these options (including the option of no treatment). Autonomy and informed consent, along with several other principles, form the basis for the concept of self-determination.

2. How does one determine the competency of a patient? What action should be taken if it is suspected that the patient is not competent to make health care decisions?

Before determining a patient's competence, one needs to know the definition of competency. In simple terms, it is the capacity to be autonomous. In legal matters, competence is a property determined by a normative standard based on current moral beliefs of society. As such, it is a value judgement that varies from moment to moment and situation to situation. Thus, there is no universal definition of competence. Practically speaking, a "functioning approach" is used to establish a patient's competence. This approach involves meeting three specific criteria: (1) free action; (2) authenticity; and (3) effective deliberation. In free action, a patient must be capable of action that is intentional and completely voluntary. It cannot be the result of coercion, duress, or undue influence. For authenticity, one must be certain that the patient is acting in character, i.e., consistent with his or her values, attitudes, and life plans ("authentically"). As for effective deliberation, the patient must realize that a decision has to be made. He or she should be aware of the alternatives and their consequences and then be able to make an informed decision based on an informed evaluation. Therefore, a competent patient should be acting freely and within character while also being able to deliberate and express the issues at hand. Given this approach, it is easy to see how determining the competence of a patient can be very difficult. When competence is not clear, a physician can request a psychiatric consultation. A psychiatrist or any other physician can deem a patient incompetent, but the decision becomes legal and binding only when it is argued in front of a judge and determined in a court of law. In most cases, it is not necessary to go to the courts, because the patient's family or other concerned people do not contest the patient's competence (i.e., comatose or heavily sedated patients). When a patient is deemed incompetent, it is necessary to appoint a surrogate to make health care decisions. This is usually done informally by designating a family member or next-of-kin to speak on behalf of the patient. When no family is available, a conservator needs to be appointed by the court.

3. Is an advance directive a legal document?

An advance directive is a document created by a competent person to express future wishes regarding medical care in the event that the person becomes incompetent or otherwise unable to make his or her preferences known. Living wills are a popular form of an advance directive. Such directives indicate what type of care a person wishes to receive and also may appoint a third party (durable power of attorney) to be responsible for making decisions if the person becomes incapacitated. Despite the lack of legal statutes, courts tend to uphold an advance directive unless there is a specific reason to doubt its validity. The Patient Self-Determination Act of 1991 (enacted by Congress in 1990) now requires all hospitals to discuss advance directives and to have forms available to patients at the time of admission.

4. What is the Ethics Committee? What is its role?

The Ethics Committee is an interdisciplinary group (physicians, nurses, risk managers, and/or other healthcare professionals) that assists in resolving ethical problems related to issues that affect the care and treatment of patients currently in the hospital. The committee commonly reviews and makes recommendations on specific cases, helps to clarify to the patient and/or the patient's surrogates the options and alternatives, and provides support to the members of the health care team who are involved in a difficult ethical dilemma. The Ethics Committee does not make decisions but provides consultation and information to guide the actual decision-makers.

5. What is the health provider's recourse when he or she morally disagrees with a patient's plan of care?

First, the provider should discuss the disputed plan with other caregivers to determine whether his or her concerns are valid. The provider should then express his or her concerns to the persons proposing the plan. An open, nonconfrontational discussion between parties allows each side to see the other's rationales and points of view. If no resolution can be achieved, consultation with the Ethics Committee is an excellent means of re-examining and reapproaching the issue. When these actions fail to reconcile the caregiver to the patient's course of treatment, a request to be removed from the case should be made. The request should be honored and the provider removed as long as others are available to care for the patient.

6. Who is ultimately responsible for determining a patient's "do-not-resuscitate" status?

The decision to withhold resuscitation attempts from a patient in cardiopulmonary arrest ideally should be a collaborative one, determined by the patient, the patient's family, and the primary physician. However, the attending physician can make a unilateral decision to withhold resuscitative efforts if he or she considers the decision inappropriate, as when the expectation of a successful resuscitation is nonexistent. If the physician makes a unilateral decision, he or she should immediately meet with the patient and family to discuss all of the issues, including alternatives, and to inform them of the decision. On most occasions, the objective medical opinion of the attending physician is the determining factor in a patient's and/or family's decision not to resuscitate. A "do-not-resuscitate" order must be signed by a physician; all other signatures, if required, are legally irrelevant. A "do-not-resuscitate" order is not synonymous with an order to withhold standard medical care.

7. What constitutes "extraordinary" measures? What about when they are futile?

Extraordinary measures are any treatments that impose a greater burden than benefit to the patient. This term is highly variable and can be applied to the same treatment for the same patient at different time points. Such interventions may cause the patient undue pain and expense for questionable gains. Does this, then, imply that extraordinary measures are futile? From a legal standpoint, there is no meaningful definition of "futility." However, physicians are not ethically obligated to deliver care that, in their best judgement, would not have a reasonable chance of benefiting the patient, even if it is demanded by the patient or his or her representative.

8. Is it ethically correct to withhold or terminate life-sustaining medical interventions?

From a legal and ethical perspective, there is no difference between withholding or terminating life-sustaining medical measures, i.e., any treatment that serves to prolong life without reversing the underlying medical condition. When treatment interventions are "futile" or unable to improve a patient's condition, they often merely prolong life and delay the patient's inevitable death. Withholding or terminating life support is often a difficult decision to make; ideally, it should be made by the patient via an advance directive. More often, however, an advance directive is not available, and the family must make this difficult decision. Regardless of who exactly decides, legally and ethically the decision should be based on what the patient would have decided (substituted judgement) or on the best interests of the patient (what outcome would most likely promote the patient's well-being).

9. Can a physician legally write an order for a "slow-code"?

A "slow-code" usually implies a short resuscitation attempt with disregard for speed and time. The decision to refrain from cardiopulmonary resuscitation should be clear and communicated to all involved parties. A "slow-code" order is a contradiction in terms and conveys a confusing message. There are only three options: full resuscitation attempt, an attempt with specific limitations, or no attempt at all. It is not legal to write a "slow-code" order.

10. Is it acceptable to provide treatment to patients based on their financial status?

It is simplistic to believe that the financial situations of the patient and health care facility do not influence patient care decisions. Nonetheless, the clinician must always have the patient's welfare as the primary objective. With that in mind, it is unacceptable to deny emergent medical care to a patient in need. However, once the patient is stable and out of imminent danger, it is legal to transfer the patient to another institution that is willing to accept the financial burden of the patient's care.

11. What is the difference between euthanasia and assisted suicide? Although illegal, are they morally and ethically acceptable?

A thorough answer to these questions would require several chapters and is beyond the scope of this book. In brief, euthanasia, or "good death," can be defined as active or passive, voluntary or involuntary, by commission or omission. From a legal and ethical standpoint, the controversy surrounds active euthanasia or the "administration of a lethal agent by [a physician] to a patient for the purpose of relieving the patient's intolerable and incurable suffering."[1] Assisted suicide occurs when "a physician facilitates a patient's death by providing the necessary means and/or information to enable a patient to perform the life-ending act."[1] The American Medical Association considers both acts to be fundamentally incompatible with the physician's role as a healer. To date, no one has been convicted for assisted suicide, even though it is a felony in many states. However, because euthanasia can be subsumed under homicide, one physician has been found guilty in a court of law; Dr. Jack Kevorkian was convicted of second-degree murder in 1999. Over the past 20 years, several physicians have pleaded guilty to euthanasia and were sentenced to probation. As of December 2001, only one state, Oregon, has legalized physician-assisted suicide. This legislation was accepted by voters in 1994 and went into effect in 1997. In November 2001, Attorney General John Ashcroft ordered the Drug Enforcement Agency (DEA) to revoke the license for prescribing controlled substances of physicians who have engaged in assisted suicide because it was not consistent with appropriate medical care and proper use of a controlled substance. The State of Oregon had acquired an injunction from the U.S. Supreme Court against this act by the federal government, but the final outcome has not been determined.

Because morals are based on societal values, one can argue that, given the acceptance of active euthanasia and physician-assisted suicide in the Netherlands and even in the United States (Oregon's Death with Dignity Act), both acts are morally acceptable. On the other hand, given the fact that these concepts are not universally accepted, their morality can be questioned. Of course, the ethics of these acts have been and continue to be debated. Of interest, less than 100 years ago, suicide itself was considered an illegal act and punishable according to the penal code.

12. How does one assess the need for increased analgesia in a dying patient? How does one provide adequate analgesia while avoiding euthanasia?

In the dying patient, prolongation of life is no longer the primary goal; rather, the primary goal is relief of pain and discomfort. To deny analgesia in such a situation, regardless of the fact that it may depress respiration or blood pressure, is to deny the patient one of the few interventions that can increase comfort at a time when it is most needed (concept of secondary effect). If the patient is conscious, attempts should be made to communicate with him or her. If the patient is unresponsive, pain medication should be administered based on physiologic responses such as heart and respiratory rate, blood pressure, and facial expression.

13. What are the various routes of administering analgesics for the dying patient?

The most common method is by intermittent bolus injection. Continuous intravenous or subcutaneous infusions of analgesics may be more effective in establishing a stable comfort level because they can be titrated to maintain a particular blood level of medication. In addition, there is less of a peak-trough effect. After bolus injections, peak levels are high and side effects may be more pronounced, whereas during the trough the patient may be in a tremendous amount of pain, awaiting sufficient analgesic effect. Because of high variability in bioavailability, the oral and transdermal routes alone are not acceptable methods for delivering analgesics for the dying patient with only hours to several days of life.

BIBLIOGRAPHY

1. American Medical Association: Council on Ethical and Judicial Affairs. Code of Medical Ethics. Chicago, American Medical Association, 1997.
2. Bone RC, Rackow EC, Weg JG: Ethical and moral guidelines for the initiation, continuation, and withdrawal of intensive care. Chest 97:949–958, 1990.
3. Greco PJ, Schulman KA, Lavizzo-Mourey R: The Patient Self-determination Act and the future of advance directives. Ann Intern Med 115:639–643, 1991.
4. Jonsen AR, Siegler M, Winslade WJ: Clinical Ethics, 2nd ed. New York, Macmillan, 1986.
5. Luce JM: Withholding and withdrawal of life support from critically ill patients. West J Med 167:411–416, 1997.
6. Nathanson JA: When does a patient have the right to refuse lifesaving medical treatment? Can Med Assoc J 150:1323–1326, 1994.
7. Stone TH, Winslade WJ: Physician-assisted suicide and euthanasia in the United States. J Leg Med 16:481–507, 1995.
8. Wear AN, Brahams D: To treat or not to treat: The legal, ethical and therapeutic implications of treatment refusal. J Med Ethics 17:131–135, 1991.

108. WITHDRAWAL OF TREATMENT

J. S. Kobayashi, M.D.

1. What are the general circumstances in which termination of critical care may be considered?

Termination of life-sustaining medical treatment may be considered when the relative burden of suffering by the patient imposed by the required medical treatment regimen outweighs the benefits in quality of life, prolongation of life, or in cases where further treatment is medically inappropriate or futile. Although quality of life considerations are solely the province of the patient, family, and/or proxy decision makers, futility is a medical decision. When a responsible consensus has been reached between the patient or proxy decision maker and the medical team that further medical intervention is inappropriate or medically inadvisable, compassionate care may continue after active treatment is terminated.

2. Why is it important to understand the issues involved in the withdrawal of treatment in the ICU?

It is important because limiting or withdrawing treatment in the ICU occurs regularly. In addition, patients' families are often dissatisfied with both pain management and communication with their physicians after the decision to withdraw treatment has been made. This decision shifts the goal of treatment from cure or recovery to "palliative care," which focuses on symptom management and allows the patient to maintain dignity while dying in a comfortable and pain-free state. According to the *Recommendations for End-of-life Care in the ICU* of the Society of Critical Care Ethics Committee, there is "an emerging perspective that palliative care and intensive care are not mutually exclusive options, but rather should be coexistent."

3. How frequently does termination of care occur in the ICU?

National survey data indicate that the proportion of deaths in the ICU setting preceded by a recommendation to withhold or withdraw life-sustaining treatment increased from 51% to 90% in the 5 years between 1988 and 1993.

4. What ethical principles are involved in decisions to terminate life-sustaining treatment?

The process of medical **informed consent** is grounded in the principle of **patient autonomy**. A competent patient may decide to refuse or consent to treatment proposed by the medical team after being informed of risks, benefits, and alternative therapies. **Professional integrity**, however, does not allow even a competent patient to demand medically inappropriate treatment, and a physician is not required to offer futile care. Either the patient (by preference) or the physician (for substantial reasons such as moral or religious grounds) may request that the care of a patient be transferred to another physician, as long as the patient is not abandoned. Finally, **institutional integrity** has been frequently invoked as a justification to withhold or withdraw treatments which are neither futile nor standard-of-care, based on cost considerations in the interests of the general principle of **distributive justice**; in theory, the intensive treatment of one patient will not jeopardize or compromise the general treatment of many.

5. Who may make the decision to terminate critical care?

A patient competent to give medical informed consent may refuse even life-sustaining treatment at any time, regardless of the opinions of family or medical team. Psychiatric consultation may help to determine clinical concerns influencing the patient's appreciation of the consequences of the decision or to determine competence. A competent patient may also establish an **advance directive** that specifies decision making preferences in the event of incapacitation.

Proxy decision makers for the incapacitated patient may consent to the termination of treatment with the preferred standard of **substituted judgment**, enabling the proxy to make the choices the patient would have made under normal circumstances. The use of the **"in the best interests of the patient"** standard is acceptable in cases in which the patient had no clearly stated preferences for end-of-life care.

In the case of medical futility, there is no ethical obligation for the physician to offer, initiate, or continue medically futile treatment. However, in order to assure the standard of care and allow a review beyond the domain of the individual medical care provider, the decision should be made in the context of an institutional policy or set of guidelines. The term **futile care** often is used when the real issue is one of medically inappropriate care, which is inadvisable even if it is not physiologically futile.

6. When a patient is incapacitated or is not competent to give informed consent, who may make decisions to terminate treatment for the patient?

In medical emergencies in which the patient has not previously identified a proxy decision maker, the physician may make treatment decisions. The need for end-of-life decision making in the critical care unit should be anticipated, however, and discussions about standard measures, such as cardiopulmonary resuscitation, should occur between the patient and family as early as feasible and as frequently as changing medical status requires. Determination of patient competence may be assessed by the medical provider, although review by a psychiatrist should be considered when impaired judgment resulting from suicidality, delirium, or other psychiatric disorders is a factor. Legal competence may ultimately be determined in the court if there is any dispute about the assessment.

Acceptable substitute decision makers vary according to statute, and medical providers should be familiar with current legislation concerning advance directives and proxy decision makers in their state. All states now allow some form of advance directive, including provisions for a **living will, durable power of attorney for health care (DPAH)**, and/or **cardiopulmonary resuscitation (CPR) directive**, and also have statutes that define surrogate or proxy decision makers or limited guardianship for health care.

7. Define the following: advance directive, living will, durable power of attorney for health care, CPR directive, and limited guardian for health care decisions.

Advance directives, which include living wills, DPAH, and CPR directives, are legal instruments established by a competent patient and become operational in the event of the patient's incapacitation. It is ultimately the responsibility of the patient to let the physician know about the existence of an advance directive and whether or not it has been revised.

A **living will** is a document that usually specifies the conditions under which a patient with an irreversible medical condition may wish to limit or terminate treatment, such as setting a time limit for ventilatory support. They are limited in comparison with DPAH, because it is difficult to anticipate all of the treatment circumstances a patient may need to address in a single document.

A **durable power of attorney for health care** (DPAH) designates a specific person as the substitute decision maker for the incapacitated patient and has the advantage of not having to specify the circumstances or conditions for termination or continuation of treatment. The DPAH can address any medical treatment decision requiring informed consent.

A **CPR directive** indicates a patient's preference about CPR and is available in some states. It requires a physician order on a document officially registered within a public health department, and may not be initiated solely by the patient. A CPR directive may be useful for a patient with a terminal illness who does not wish to be resuscitated by paramedics. Paramedics should respect the individual's wishes and refrain from initiating CPR.

A **limited guardian for health care decisions** may be appointed for an incompetent patient by the court when there is no advance directive and no clear surrogate decision maker, or when an interested party challenges the decision, competence, appropriateness, or intentions of the surrogate decision maker. If there is no dispute between medical providers and surrogate decision makers (e.g., primary family members), a petition for a guardian may not be required. Some states designate a hierarchy of substitute decision makers.

8. Are advance directives followed by physicians?

Multiple studies indicate that physicians often do not follow the stated wishes of their patients. In the multi-institutional SUPPORT study (Study to Understand Prognoses and Preferences for Outcomes and Risks of Treatments), for example, 31% of patients before intervention preferred that CPR be withheld, whereas only 47% of physicians reported this preference at the time of the first interview. DNR orders were actually written for only 49% of the 960 patients who stated they did not want CPR. Not respecting an advance directive is disrespectful of the patient as well as of the ethical principle of patient autonomy. Institutional discussions should establish procedures to identify the existence of these directives, communicate their intent to the members of the treatment team, and systematically locate these documents in the medical record.

9. What steps should be taken if a conflict about the decision to terminate treatment arises?

Despite ongoing conflict, continuing efforts to develop a consensus are important, as families often simply need time to consider or accept a recommendation to terminate treatment. A family conference may be useful to answer questions or correct misunderstandings. Psychosocial factors that may enter into the decision, such as sociocultural perceptions, family expectations, concerns about analgesia, and individual fears should be discussed. Psychiatric consultation may be obtained by either the team or family. An institutional policy should address these circumstances in advance and may include the option for a second medical opinion, or the request for transfer of treatment to another provider, team, or hospital when feasible. Finally, as a last resort, the courts may provide a legal avenue of appeal.

10. Why is it necessary to identify circumstances in which treatment may be considered medically futile?
The continuing debate about futile care developed out of efforts to limit medically inappropriate interventions as society realized that technological advances do not always guarantee that more care is better care. Physicians sought to objectify reasons to terminate care which seemed of marginal benefit despite the wishes of some patients to "do anything possible," and in agreement with other patients who felt that remaining dependent on ventilatory support was not a meaningful goal of medical treatment, being for many "more burden than benefit."

Of importance, the very few cases that may achieve any formal criteria of medical futility are among a larger group of cases in which further intervention is not medically appropriate because of small benefit to the quality or quantity of life relative to the suffering or restrictions in quality of life imposed on the patient. Nevertheless, one study found that physicians invoked "futility" as a "decisive" reason to withdraw or withhold medical treatment in a large majority (74%) of cases. The study suggested the need for standardization of the term "futility" for which physicians offered survival estimates that ranged from 0–50%.

11. Are conceptual and operational definitions of futile care useful?
Although most physicians ascribe to the concept of futile care, a universal definition remains elusive. Generally, futile care is medical treatment that serves only to prolong a dying process and offers no chance of recovery or even significant actual benefit to the patient. An irreversible condition must be present that will inevitably lead to a patient's death (either as the end result of a lethal condition or in a situation of imminent demise) where treatment will have only insignificant physiologic benefit. Physiologic futility is ultimately a medical decision, whereas decisions about futility with regard to quality of life are reserved for patients and their families. For example, although a persistent vegetative state is not a medically futile condition, the family may or may not consider continuing medical intervention futile in sustaining this state as a meaningful quality of life. Nevertheless, conceptual definitions clarify the elements of the debate and have proved useful in clinical care.

Similarly, the effort to operationalize the definition of futile care by specific criteria is far from over. Quantitative thresholds for futility as less than 1% probability of succeeding generally lack scientific outcomes research on which to base decisions. Scoring systems which attempt to estimate hospital mortality, such as the APACHE (Acute Physiology and Chronic Health Evaluation) do not consider factors such as morbidity and prognosis for the individual versus populations. Efforts to identify specific conditions that have never resulted in survival beyond a minimally defined percentage, such as certain malignancies or multiple organ failures of specific magnitude cannot be generalized. In summary, the definitional approach to medical futility cannot encompass the unique and complex aspects of the individual clinical case which are insufficiently addressed by generic concepts or criteria.

12. What advantages do procedural policies to limit medically inappropriate treatments have over policies based on definitions of futile care?
Policies that emphasize procedures to determine medically inappropriate treatments address the majority of cases in which conflicts and questions about termination of treatment occur— beyond the few case cases which may be considered medically futile. These include cases that are extremely unlikely to be beneficial, are very costly, or are of uncertain or controversial benefit, as delineated by the Ethics Committee of the Society of Critical Care Medicine.

Appropriately trained physicians may determine that a given treatment is medically unsuitable and should be withheld or withdrawn; this decision would then be subject to a process of review, rather than being required to meet definitional criteria. The institutional review process should include medical consultants as well as patients' perspectives and community values . If the decision is not disputed, a reasonable standard of care in terminating treatment may be assured. If a lack of consensus remains despite continuing and caring communication with the family and/or proxy decision maker, there also should be institutional procedures available for an appeal process that may include review by the ethics committee, or the possibility of transfer of care to another treatment team or institution.

13. Is withdrawing treatment that has already been initiated ethically different from withholding treatment that has not been started?

There is no ethical difference. In fact, it may be argued that a physician should be willing to initiate treatment without worrying about not being able to withdraw it later in order to have the opportunity to assess the clinical treatment trial that could provide the basis for a more accurate decision about the value of withholding or providing treatment. While withdrawing and withholding treatment may "feel" or seem like different actions, they are not ultimately different on ethical grounds.

14. Is withdrawal of nutrition and hydration considered the same as withdrawal of other medical treatment?

Several state court cases have defined nutrition and hydration as medical treatment that can be withdrawn when a general decision has been made to terminate all medical therapies. The notion has been challenged, opponents questioning the right of the guardian to discontinue nutrition and hydration despite current legislation allowing for the termination of other medical treatment.

A competent patient may decide this matter for him or herself. Nutrition and hydration for incapacitated patients often entail involved medical procedures such as gastrostomies and parenteral nutrition which are sometimes more complicated and technical than other aspects of the treatment plan. Although withdrawal of nutrition and hydration may not ultimately be different on ethical grounds from other medical treatment, it may have a different legal status depending on statute. This should be explored by the provider in his or her own state.

15. What are some considerations in communicating with the family about the termination of treatment?

Clear communication with the patient's family and significant others is paramount to their experience and acceptance of the decision to terminate treatment. Regular meetings that include updates about prognosis prepare the family for all eventualities. While all pertinent information should be conveyed, the family's needs, level of understanding, cultural background, and emotional status must be taken into consideration when timing the amount of information shared at each point. Proxy decision makers should be urged to represent whatever decision the patient would have been likely to make under the circumstances in order to lessen the potential burden of guilt they may carry about termination of treatment decisions. Repeated assurances regarding the medical staff's intention to attend to the continuing comfort of the patient and to minimize suffering with pain control and sedation are essential. The family should be informed that no one will be able to predict the outcome of termination of treatment. Some patients may survive after discontinuation of ventilatory support, and on occasion the patient may survive for a longer interval than anticipated. Specific opportunities to say "good-bye" to a loved one should be planned before cessation of treatment; preferences about viewing the body after death should also be discussed beforehand. Referrals to community resources should be routinely available, as well as avenues to access staff after the patient's death. Consultation with clergy, social services, counseling, and other sources of support also should be readily available.

16. What technical issues are involved in the termination of critical care?

While these issues are largely beyond the scope of this chapter, medical providers should exercise care and consideration regarding a number of issues such as: whether the patient should be moved to another area before treatment is terminated; whether the endotracheal tube should be removed; how often to suction for patient comfort; whether nutrition and hydration will be withdrawn; and how to use medications for analgesia and sedation. Comfort care measures should be continued as long as the patient is alive and analgesia may be used for adequate pain control, even if the "double effect" of suppression of respiration results. A compassionate and comforting presence is critical to address the common fear of the family that the patient will be abandoned once treatment has been terminated.

BIBLIOGRAPHY

1. Brody H, Campbell ML, Faber-Langendoen K, Ogle KS: Withdrawing intensive life-sustaining treatment—Recommendations for compassionate clinical management. N Engl J Med 336:652–657, 1997.
2. Campbell ML, Frank RR: Experience with an end-of-life practice at a university hospital. Crit Care Med 25:197–202, 1997.
3. Cleeland CS, Gonin R, Hatfield AK, et al: Pain and its treatment in outpatients with metastatic cancer. N Engl J Med 330:592–596, 1994.
4. Curtis JR, Patrick DL, Shannon SE, et al: The family conference as a focus to improve communication about end-of-life care in the intensive care unit: Opportunities for improvement. Crit Care Med 29(Suppl 2):N26–N33, 2001.
5. Daly BJ, Thomas D, Dyer MA, et al: Procedures used in withdrawal of mechanical ventilation. Am J Crit Care 5:331–338, 1996.
6. Danis M, Truog R, Devita M, et al: Consensus statement of the Society of Critical Care Medicine's Ethics Committee regarding futile and other possibly inadvisable treatments. Crit Care Med 25:887–891, 1997.
7. Gilligan T, Raffin T: How to withdraw mechanical ventilation: More studies are needed. Am J Crit Care 5:323–325, 1996.
8. Gilligan T, Raffin TA: Withdrawing life support: Extubation and prolonged terminal weans are inappropriate. Crit Care Med 24:352–353, 1996.
9. Gregory DR: VA Network Futility Guidelines: A resource for decisions about withholding and withdrawing treatment. Camb Q Health Ethics 4:546–548, 1995.
10. Halevy A, Brody BA, et al: A multi-institution collaborative policy on medical futility. JAMA 276:571–574, 1996.
11. Karlawish JH, Hall JB: Managing death and dying in the intensive care unit. Am J Respir Crit Care Med 155:1–2, 1997.
12. Levinsky NG: The purpose of advance medical planning—Autonomy for patients or limitation of care? New Engl J Med 335:741–742, 1996.
13. Luce JM: Withholding and withdrawal of life support: Ethical, legal, and critical aspects. New Horiz 5:30–37, 1997.
14. Luce JM, Alpers A: Legal aspects of withholding and withdrawing life support from critically ill patients in the United States and providing palliative care to them. Am J Respir Crit Care Med 162(6):2029–2032, 2000.
15. Luce JM, Alpers A: End-of-life care: What do the American courts say? Crit Care Med 29(Suppl 2):N40–N45, 2001.
16. O'Brien LA, Grisso JA, Maislin G, et al: Nursing home residents' preferences for life-sustaining treatments. JAMA 274:1775–1779, 1995.
17. Prendergast TJ, Luce JM: Increasing incidence of withholding and withdrawal of life support from the critically ill. Am J Respir Crit Care Med 155:15–20, 1997.
18. The SUPPORT Principal Investigators: A controlled trial to improve care for seriously ill hospitalized patients: The study to understand prognoses and preferences for outcomes and risks of treatments. JAMA 274:1591–1598, 1995.
19. Tasota FJ, Hoffman LA: Terminal weaning from mechanical ventilation: Planning and process. Crit Care Nurs Q 19(3):36–51, 1996.
20. Tomlinson T, Czlonka D: Futility and hospital policy. Hastings Cent Rep 25(3):28–35, 1995.
21. Truog RD: Recommendations for end-of-life care in the intensive care unit: The Ethics Committee of the Society of Critical Care Medicine. Crit Care Med 29(12):2332–2348, 2001.
22. Wall S, Partridge J, et al: Death in the intensive care nursery: Physician practice of withdrawing and withholding life support. Pediatrics 99:64–70, 1997.
23. Zaubler T, Viederman M, Fins J, et al: Ethical, legal, and psychiatric issues in capacity, competency, and informed consent: An annotated bibliography. J Clin Ethics 5:329–340, 1994.

XXII. Administration

109. ICU ADMINISTRATION

Christopher R. Dorothy, D.O., and Carolyn E. Bekes, M.D.

1. Must universal (standard) precautions be used with patients who have a low risk for transmission of HIV?

As noted in the Federal Register, all human blood and certain human body fluids are treated as if known to be infectious for bloodborne pathogens for **all** patients. It is the responsibility of employers and their agents to ensure that staff adhere to these regulations.

2. What diseases require respiratory isolation (negative pressure)?

Tuberculosis, chickenpox (varicella), hemorrhagic fevers (e.g., Ebola, Lassa), measles (rubeola), pneumonic plague, and disseminated shingles (zoster).

3. What role should the medical director of an ICU play in management of the unit?

There is consensus that the medical director of an ICU can play a key role in establishing and maintaining the environment in which a critically ill patient can receive high quality care with optimal resource allocation. Important aspects of medical director involvement include bed triage and efforts to contain costs by increasing efficiency of care and control of resource utilization. It has been suggested that critical care training programs incorporate a management training component.

4. Does an intensivist affect patient outcome or cost of care in the ICU?

Evidence indicates that involvement of an intensivist in patient care leads to decreased mortality rates and more effective use of resources.

5. Is there a role for a clinical pharmacist on the critical care team?

The complex pharmacologic issues of patients in the ICU warrant inclusion of a clinical pharmacist on the critical care team. Drug-drug interactions and adverse drug reactions dramatically decrease when a pharmacist is part of a multidisciplinary team.

6. Why is everyone so concerned about cutting the cost of ICU care?

On average, ICUs make up only 5–10% of a hospital's beds, but > 20% of the hospital's budget is devoted to the care of patients in these beds. Nationally, this represents 2% of the GNP.

7. Should cost be a factor in decision-making in ICUs?

In light of the high cost of critical care, physicians are challenged to document that high-cost/high-tech care results in the desired outcomes. The physician should use available resources in the most cost-effective manner for the maximal benefit of the patient.

8. Does the structure of an ICU affect the quality or cost of care?

Multidisciplinary team approaches using protocol and guidelines significantly reduce cost and improve patient outcomes. Several different models for structuring an ICU have been used. Evidence does not support any one model but clearly shows that when a formal structure is implemented, mortality rates and number of ICU days are reduced.

9. What is the role of scoring systems in an ICU?

Although it is controversial whether scoring systems can predict outcomes for individual patients, there is little question that they provide an objective description of the acuity of a population of patients. This information is useful when one attempts to compare outcomes of care between units and can be used for performance improvement projects as well as clinical research. It also may benefit the physician during familiy discussion and can be used to compare an individual case with a group of similar patients for potential outcome.

10. Describe the composition of the critical care committee.

The activities of multidisciplinary critical care units should be supervised by a hospital committee composed of representatives of those departments and divisions admitting patients to the unit. In addition, the director of nursing and nursing education for the unit together with the unit physician director and the head of the division, section, or department of critical care medicine should be committee members. It is usually appropriate for one of the latter two members to chair the committee.

11. What are the major duties of the critical care committee?

1. Define the purpose and goals of the unit. These may be incorporated in a brief mission statement.

2. Develop comprehensive policies and procedures outlining the organizational and working systems whereby the unit will achieve its goals. These policies should address, among other issues, the authorities and process for triaging (admissions and discharges) patients and admission and discharge criteria as well as the credentialing requirements and regulations for physicians, nurses, and ancillary personnel working in the unit. Policies should be developed for important aspects of patient care peculiar to the unit environment (e.g., intra- and interhospital patient transport, avoidance and control of infection).

3. Define and ensure appropriate levels of education and training for all personnel working in the unit. Ensure adequate initial orientation and ongoing in-servicing for all personnel working in the unit.

4. Recommend to the medical staff the adoption of regulations designed to allow the committee to accomplish the above tasks in an efficient manner.

5. Develop and maintain an ongoing performance improvement program designed to monitor standards of patient care and identify opportunities to improve outcomes and the efficiency of care delivery. Develop reliable benchmarking measurements permitting the comparison of outcomes achieved in the unit against results reported for similar patients in large databases.

6. Maintain an ongoing database on patient acuity, lengths of stay, utilization of resources, complications, and markers for patient outcome. Provide a mechanism for reviewing all complications and untoward events so that corrective action can be instituted where appropriate.

7. Approve and submit an annual budget for the unit designed to permit the attainment of the declared goals. The development of the budget will be the joint responsibility of the nursing and physician directorship of the unit.

12. How should disagreements between physicians and families regarding care goals for incompetent patients be resolved?

The guiding principle for determining the goals of care for any patient is the determination of the patient's wishes. In those cases in which the patient is incompetent, this may be difficult. When the patient has an advance directive it is helpful to review this and attempt to extrapolate the patient's instructions to the situation under review. Often, however, the instructions may be insufficiently detailed to permit a confident decision to be reached. If a health care surrogate has been named, discussions with this individual may often provide the necessary insight into the patient's philosophy and wishes to allow the surrogate to reach a decision based upon the information regarding prognosis and therapeutic options provided by the care team. In the great majority of cases the care team will be in agreement with these decisions. Even when no surrogate has been named, discussions with family members and friends often allow a consensus to be reached regarding what the patient would have wanted in this situation.

In a minority of cases, however, there may be disagreement between the family of an incompetent patient and the team providing care on the direction which care should take. In the past this was not uncommon because of the physician's desire to continue life-prolonging therapies and the family's view that the discomfort inflicted upon the patient was not justified. Recently there has been an increase in situations in which families press for the attainment of outcomes which the medical team believe to be unattainable, or in which family members may ask for the continuation of a situation in which there is no apparent benefit to the patient.

In these situations every effort should be made to achieve agreement by prolonged, repeated, and understanding discussions. This process is both time consuming and exhausting, but in all but the most difficult cases it will usually be successful. The offer to bring in other independent opinions may be helpful, together with the demonstration of a unanimity of opinions by all the involved consultants and caregivers. Counseling and advice offered by members of the pastoral care community should also be sought if the family is agreeable to this input. If these measures fail, consideration should be given to placing a consultation request with the hospital's bioethics committee. The family should be informed of the committee's existence and advised that they may find input from such individuals helpful. Often this intervention leads to fresh discussions, which may lead to resolution.

This phase of repeated discussions should be terminated only if and when it becomes apparent that consensus cannot be achieved. At this point, the question of how to continue becomes not only a personal issue for the team members involved, but also an institutional issue and perhaps a societal issue as well. From the individual's perspective any caregiver has the right to step down from the case if he or she finds the care plan to be immoral, but only if he or she can find a substitute caregiver (often an impossible task). The institution's risk management personnel should be notified of the situation and no change in care plan should be made without full discussion and agreement with them. Lastly, the matter can be referred to the courts.

13. What are the commonly accepted definitions of (1) an open unit, (2) a semiclosed unit, and (3) a closed unit?

In an **open unit**, patients may be admitted and cared for by all qualified physicians as defined in the hospital's credentialing policies. The patients may remain on the attendings' service and the unit director will only have clinical involvement with patients by consultative request. Triaging of patients will only take place at times of bed shortage and may be carried out by the director or on occasions by negotiation between the nursing administration and the attending physicians.

In a **semiclosed unit**, the unit director or his/her designee has the authority to approve or reject requests for admission and can request the transfer out of patients when demand exceeds resources. The director's involvement in patient care may vary, ranging from mandatory consultation or co-attending status or consultation upon request only, to consultation or involvement only in emergency situations or when there are questions regarding the standard of care.

In a **closed unit**, the director and his/her team assume responsibility for the management of all patients admitted to the unit. The patient is transferred to the service of the critical care team upon admission and transferred back to the original attending upon discharge. In most instances the patient's care is managed by the critical care team in collaboration with the admitting attending, although in some units (e.g., trauma units) the unit team may be the sole attending.

14. Does a closed vs. open unit offer benefits in terms of patient care?

Several studies have shown decreased rates of mortality and complications in closed units compared with open units. This finding may be related to the concentrated attention that the patient receives from a board-certified intensivist.

15. What are the legal requirements pertaining to the interhospital transport of patients? Where are they defined?

The legal requirements are contained in the Consolidated Omnibus Reconciliation Act (COBRA) of 1986 and the OBRA amendment of 1990. The principal requirements are as follows:

• The patient or representative must give informed consent to the transfer, which should be documented. If this is not possible, the reason should be documented.
• The sending physician must contact a physician at the receiving hospital who has the authority to admit the patient to an appropriate unit.
• The sending physician must detail the patient's condition and should receive advice regarding arrangements for stabilization and transport.
• The receiving physician must accept the patient and confirm that appropriate resources are available for the patient's management.
• Agreement must be reached on who has responsibility for management during transport if no physician accompanies the patient.
• The method of transportation shall be determined by the sending physician after consultation with the receiving physician.
• The transporting service shall be notified of the impending transfer, the patient's condition, and the support requirements.
• The receiving hospital shall secure a nurse to report on the patient's condition.
• A complete copy of the chart including all laboratory and imaging studies shall be sent with the patient.
• A minimum of two people (excluding the operator of the vehicle) shall accompany the patient and at least one shall be an R.N., M.D., or advanced E.M.T. capable of rendering ACLS and ATLS.
• If no physician accompanies the patient and if there is no means of communicating with a physician during transport, the accompanying personnel should have preauthorization to carry out lifesaving interventions.
• Equipment available during transport shall include all that is necessary to establish and maintain endotracheal ventilation, monitor BP and rhythm, defibrillate, treat arrhythmias, and provide intravenous fluid and medication support. There shall be equipment permitting communication to both the sending and receiving hospitals during transportation.
• Monitoring during transport shall be of continuous EKG, BP, respiratory rate, and whatever patient-specific parameters require observation. If the patient is being ventilated, the ventilator must have pressure and disconnect alarms, and the airway pressure must be displayed.

BIBLIOGRAPHY

1. Barie PS, Hydo LJ, Fischer E: Utility of illness severity scoring for prediction of prolonged surgical critical care. J Trauma 40:513–519.
2. Brilli RJ, Spevetz A, Branson RD, et al: Critical care delivery in the intensive care unit: Defining critical roles and the best practical model. Crit Care Med 29:2007–2019, 2001.
3. Cheng DCH, Byrick RJ, Knobel E: Structural models for intermediate care areas. Crit Care Med 27:2266–2271, 1999.
4. Civetta JM, Taylor RW, Kirby RR: Critical Care, 3rd ed. 1997, pp 127–139 and 139–146.
5. Federal Register, Vol 56, No 235, December 6, 1991, p 64175.
6. Frew SA: Patient Transfers: How to Comply with the Law. Dallas, American College of Emergency Medicine, 1995.
7. Gerber DR: Structural models for intermediate care areas: One size does not fit all. Crit Care Med 27:2321–2323, 1999.
8. Ghorra S, Reinert SE, Cioffi W, et al: Analysis of the effect of conversion from open to closed surgical intensive care unit. Ann Surg 229:163–171.
9. Kirton OC, Civetta JM, Hudson-Civetta J: Cost-effectiveness in the Intensive Care Unit. Surg Clin North Am 76:175–200, 1996.
10. Seneff M, Bojanowsky L, Zimmerman J: Improving ICU utilization by decreasing the frequency of admission and length of stay for low-risk monitor patients. Crit Care Med 27:155A, 1999.
11. Shortell SM, Zimmerman JE, Rosseau DM, et al: The performance of intensive care units: Does good management make a difference? Med Care 32:508–525, 1994.
12. Zimmerman JE, Shortell SM, Rousseau DM, et al: Improving intensive care. Observations based on organizational studies in nine intensive care units: A prospective multicenter study. Crit Care Med 21:1443–1451, 1993.

110. QUALITY ASSURANCE IN THE ICU

Christopher R. Dorothy, D.O., and Carolyn E. Bekes, M.D.

1. How is quality assessed?
The definition of quality is controversial but clearly involves meeting the expectations of the consumer. In health care, this standard usually involves the satisfaction of patients, physicians, and payers. Thus, patient satisfaction, clinical outcomes, resource utilization, and cost are key elements in the measurement of quality of care.

2. What is benchmarking?
To benchmark means to compare one's own performance-related data with similar data from another institution. The Joint Commission on Accreditation of Health Care Organizations (JCAHO) requires that hospitals benchmark with other hospitals. This process is most useful when performance-related data are compared in units with a similar patient population.

3. What is the relationship between ICU organization and quality of care?
Evidence indicates that the structure and organization of an ICU can influence outcome. A collaborative relationship among members of the health care team appears to be critical. The use of clinical protocols clearly improves patient outcomes. A multidisciplinary approach with the addition of a full-time intensivist greatly improves the quality of patient care in the ICU.

4. List the uses to which severity of illness scoring systems are commonly applied.
Stratification of the severity or acuity of illness of a number of patients with the same principal diagnosis, by such systems as the APACHE II or III, may allow comparison of outcomes related to differing therapeutic approaches and thus permit identification of the best modes of treatment. Clearly such conclusions can only be reached if the patient groups being treated are controlled for comparability.

Efficiency of care delivery can be measured only if objective measures of resource utilization together with stratification of initial acuity of illness related to likely outcome—derived from the study of results in a large variety of diverse care settings—are available. These may be provided by the APACHE and TISS systems.

Decision-making in clinical management may be aided by considering the information provided by scoring systems, as may prognostic estimates for individual patients. While such information should always be interpreted in conjunction with the clinical data pertaining to the specific patient, it may be helpful in presenting data to patients and families attempting to make informed treatment decisions.

Economics. Scoring of patients can assist in appropriate billing and reimbursement code application.

5. What are the three major components of the credentialing process identified by the Society of Critical Care Medicine in its "Guidelines for Granting Privileges for the Performance of Procedures in Critically Ill Patients"?
1. **Identification of procedures requiring credentialing** (i.e., high-risk, high-volume, risk-prone).
2. **Delineation of specific standards**, which should be defined (on a national level when possible) by practitioners who commonly perform the procedures for which the privileges are requested.
3. **Credentialing mechanism**, which should be developed individually by each institution.

6. Who should be responsible for performance improvement activities in the ICU?

Although ultimately the board of trustees is responsible for the assurance of the quality of care, the actual measurement is usually delegated to the staff of the unit. The unit director in collaboration with the nurse manager and other members of the health care team should attempt to identify areas for improvements in care delivery. A formal plan should be developed and implemented. Results should be communicated both up and down the hierarchy.

7. What database should be used for performance improvement (PI) activities?

The administrative databases available in most hospitals were designed for financial applications and do not contain the types of data usually required for performance improvement. Therefore, manual data collection is usually needed for PI. Project Impact is a national electronic database designed to assist individual institutions with improvement of clinical outcomes in an effective manner through the use of benchmarking.

8. Over the years, the terminology for delivery of quality care has changed. What is the chief conceptual difference between "quality assurance" and "performance improvement"?

The original strategy of quality assurance sought to make a series of observations (indicators) intended to ensure that the delivery of care was being carried out in compliance with the current highest standards defined at that time. The emphasis tended to be on methodology of care delivery and the avoidance of complications. The more recent term of performance improvement seeks to examine the entire care delivery system with the goal of identifying areas where improvement(s) can be instituted, even though the current system may seem adequate. This process is accomplished by familiarizing groups of personnel who will often be in a position to make valuable suggestions for improvement with an intimate knowledge of the systems under review. The impact of process change can then be examined by following predetermined markers of outcome with regard to both patient outcome and resource utilization: thus, at present, the emphasis is on outcome rather than simply on process.

9. List a number of observations on which to base assessment of outcome.

Although a variety of indicators can be used to assess outcome, the following usually provide a reasonable database and can be used for benchmarking when similar data are available from other institutions:

- **Patient satisfaction.** This should include not only the patient's subjective opinions but also some objective observations of outcome such as activities of daily living (ADL) scores. A significantly understudied aspect of this parameter is the posthospital status of the patient.
- **Length of stay (LOS).** The LOS both in the hospital and the ICU for patients who have been stratified by diagnosis, acuity, and comorbidities on admission provides valuable insight into ouctomes and an excellent database for benchmarking if followed consistently over a reasonable period.
- **Mortality indexed to severity of illness.** Although this information can provide a simple benchmarking tool, the data should be critically reviewed since death *per se* cannot always be equated with a bad outcome.
- **Incidence of unanticipated returns to the ICU during the same hospital stay.** This indicator may yield important information if examined in some detail. In addition to the actual incidence (which can be used for benchmarking), the individual cases should be reviewed. This may reveal a need to review the criteria for transferring patients from the unit or the compliance with same. Alternatively, it may stimulate consideration of the adequacy of the care capabilities of the environments receiving the patients upon discharge from the unit.
- **Incidence of complications.** Complications may be linked to procedures (e.g., line placement, endotracheal intubation) or to general management (e.g., nosocomial infection, medication errors). Of major importance are those which have a clear impact on patient welfare. The criteria for identifying these and the methodology for data collection and analysis should be defined and consistently applied.

10. How applicable to the ICU is the "clinical or critical pathway" approach to the maintenance of cost-effective care delivery?

Although the development of so-called "clinical pathways" has had considerable success in reducing costs while maintaining or improving standards of care and clinical outcomes, this methodology appears to be mainly applicable to patients with diagnoses wherein there is a fairly homogeneous group of patients who run broadly similar courses. Good examples of these diagnoses are coronary artery insufficiency and hip fractures. In the case of the patient population in a mixed adult medical-surgical ICU, however, there is no such homogeneity and it is often virtually impossible to describe an average course for a given diagnosis. Such a diversity of progression exists that relates primarily to the individual patient circumstances, that it is of little value to compare the course of an individual patient with the "clinical pathway." A much better approach in the ICU is to write treatment algorithms applicable to discrete segments of the patient's care within the continuum of the entire illness, e.g., how to manage (treat or prevent) DVT, how to wean a patient from ventilatory support principles or antibiotic selection, etc. The use of this approach maintains all the advantages of getting groups together to discuss and agree upon a unified approach toward aspects of care (thus reducing expensive diversity) without wasting time and energy on trying to create nonexistent average courses of these illnesses.

11. At what stage of the patient's stay in the ICU should the care team start thinking about the patient's discharge planning both from the ICU and from the hospital?

Although in many instances of serious illness it may seem premature, it is probably useful to give thought to the probable length of ICU stay, hospital stay, discharge status and needs, from the time of admission. In a large number of cases, unnecessary delays later in the patient's hospitalization can be averted by timely consideration of whether it is likely that the patient will ultimately be able to be discharged to home or will require a period of institutional rehabilitation and identification of rehabilitation requirements.

BIBLIOGRAPHY

1. Brilli RJ, Spevetz A, Branson RD, et al: Critical care delivery in the intensive care unit: Defining clinical roles and the best practice model. Crit Care Med 25:1007–2019, 2001.
2. Carson SS, Stocking C, Podsadecki T, et al: Effects of organizational change in the medical intensive care unit of a teaching hospital. JAMA 276:322–328, 1996.
3. Civetta JM, Taylor RW, Kirby RR: Critical Care, 3rd ed. 1997, pp 164–175.
4. Guidelines for granting privileges for the performance of procedures in critically ill patients. Guidelines Committee, Society of Critical Care Medicine. Crit Care Med 21:292, 1993.
5. Kelly WJ, O'Brien J, Baartz S, Zelcer J: Clinical information systems and quality of care in the intensive care unit. Medinfo 2:1042–1046, 1995.
6. Knaus WA, Draper EA, Wagner DP, et al: An evaluation of outcome from intensive care in major medical centers. Ann Intern Med 104:410–418, 1986.
7. Kollef MH, Shuster DP: Predicting intensive care unit outcome with scoring systems. Underlying concepts and principles. Crit Care Clin 10:1–18, 1994.
8. Parillo JE, Dellinger RP: Critical Care Medicine, 2nd ed. 2001, pp 1543–1553.
9. Rafkin HS, Hoyt JW: Objective data and quality assurance programs. Current and future trends. Crit Care Clin 10:157–177, 1994.
10. Seneff M, Knaus WA: Predicting patient outcome from intensive care: A guide to APACHE, MPM, SAPS, PRISM, and other prognostic scoring systems. J Intensive Care Med 5:33–52, 1990.
11. Shortell SM, Zimmerman JE, Rousseau DM, et al: The performance of intensive care units: Does good management make a difference? Med Care 32:508–525, 1994.
12. Teres D, Lemeshow S: Using severity measures to describe high performance units. Crit Care Clin 9:543, 1993.
13. Weissmann C: Can hospital discharge diagnoses be used for intensive care unit administrative and quality management functions? Crit Care Med 25:1320–1323, 1998.
14. Zimmerman JG, Shortell SM, Rousseau DM: Improving intensive care. Observations based on organizational studies in nine intensive care units: A prospective multicenter study. Crit Care Med 21:1443–1451, 1993.

111. SCORING SYSTEMS FOR COMPARISON OF DISEASE SEVERITY IN ICU PATIENTS

Benoit Misset, M.D.

1. What are severity scores?

Scoring systems have been developed to compare the severity of disease among patients in intesnsive care units (Icus). These scores are tabulated at admission or during the ICU stay. The scores include the assessment of several physiologic parameters that have been documented to play an independent role in predicting hospital death. The scores presented in this chapter are only those used to assess general disease severity. Other scoring systems are used to assess particular organ function (i.e., Acute Lung Injury Score for evaluation of acute respiratory distress syndrome).

2. Which scores are used for assessing the general severity of disease at ICU admission?

The three most frequently used systems are the Acute Physiology And Chronic Health Evaluation (APACHE), the Simplified Acute Physiology Score (SAPS) and the Mortality Predictive Model (MPM) . The most recent versions of each system are the APACHE II and III, the SAPS II, and the MPM II0 (at admission) and MPM II24 (at 24 hours).

3. Why were scores to assess general disease severity at ICU admission developed?

1. **To assess performance of the ICU.** The ICU patient is a medical or a surgical patient who presents either with the acute failure of one major vital function or with a high risk of developing such failure. Because the mortality rate of ICU populations is usually high and varies widely depending on patient admission policies, an objective assessment of the patients' general disease severity is necessary to ensure that the mortality rate in an ICU is consistent with the overall severity of its patient population at admission. The ratio between observed and predicted mortality, called the standardized mortality ratio (SMR), is the simplest way to assess the performance of an ICU. It allows comparisons among mortality rates of various ICUs or the mortality rates documented in one ICU over time.

2. **To assess the patient's risk of death.** The scores give an objective evaluation that helps the clinician confirm the severity of the patient's illness. However, these scores cannot be used to make decisions about individual patients (e.g., withdrawal of support).

3. **To compare or match populations in clinical studies.** In randomized, controlled studies the scores have been used to confirm that the populations obtained by randomization had a similar disease severity at admission to the ICU. In case-control studies, the scores have been used to match the control to the case patients.

4. How were scores assessing general severity at ICU admission constructed?

Scores were constructed in large, multicenter, prospective populations. The variables were selected and weighed by consensus (APACHE II) or through multiple logistic regression analyses (APACHE III, SAPS II, and MPM II) to determine whether the parameters were independent predictors of hospital death. The tested variables include age, worst values over the first 24 hours of ICU admission for certain acute physiologic abnormalities (e.g., sodium, potassium, partial arterial oxygen tension, urine output, Glasgow Coma Scale), category at admission (medical or surgical patient), and several underlying diseases (e.g., metastatic cancer, AIDS). The MPM system also includes several therapeutic items (e.g., number of venous lines) and is the only system that is collected entirely at admission to the ICU.

5. How were scores assessing general disease severity at ICU admission validated?

All of these models were validated in the initial studies in a subset of patients that were not used for construction of the scoring system. The performance of the scoring systems was considered adequate if they showed good discrimination in predicting hospital mortality and had a good calibration for the entire population under investigation. **Discrimination** in predicting hospital mortality is assessed with receiver operating characteristics (ROCs): the higher the area under the ROC curve, the more discriminative the test. The **calibration** in the entire population is measured with the goodness-of-fit test: the observed mortality must not be statistically different from the expected mortality in population deciles of equal probability intervals. The lower the H value and the higher the corresponding p value, the better the calibration.

6. Which scores have been validated adequately?

The APACHE I and II, SAPS I, and MPM I have not been constructed or validated with the current accepted methodologic standards. The SAPS II, MPM II and APACHE III scores have been shown to have good discrimination and calibration in large multicenter studies.

The **SAPS II** is well validated. The score needs to be updated with more recent ICU populations.

The **MPM II** is well validated and has the advantage of being the only score available at ICU admission rather than at 24 hours after admission. This advantage is made possible because the score includes some therapeutic items (e.g., venous lines, drainage systems). The MPM II score also needs to be updated with more recent ICU populations.

The **APACHE III** is well validated and updated regularly, but its use is limited by the fact that clinicians must pay for knowing and using its equation for calculating death probability.

7. Why were scores assessing disease severity over the ICU stay developed?

The scores measuring daily severity were developed to improve the prediction of an individual patient's death (already provided by scores at admission), to assess the activity and the performance of ICUs, and to match patients in clinical investigations. These scores are particularly useful as inclusion criteria in randomized studies in which patients are entered into the investigation several days after admission. These scores are also used as matching criteria in case control studies addressing the attributable morbidity of ICU acquired events, such as nosocomial infections.

8. Which scores have been developed for assessing severity over the ICU stay?

Various scores have been developed on ICU samples of various sizes. The scores developed on the largest ICU populations include the Organ System Failure score (OSF), the Organ Dysfunction and Infection score (ODIN), the Logistic Organ Dysfunction Score (LODS), the Sequential Organ Failure Assessment score (SOFA), and the Multiple Organ Dysfunction Score (MODS).

9. How were the scores assessing severity over the ICU stay constructed?

Sequential scores measure the number and/or the intensity of organ dysfunction. By contrast with the SAPS, MPM, and APACHE scores, they do not take age, category of admission, or underlying diseases into account, because these items do not change over the ICU stay.

The OSF, ODIN, SOFA, and MODS scores were constructed empirically. The OSF and ODIN scores assess the number of organ dysfunctions, and the SOFA and MODS scores also assess the intensity of organ dysfunction.

The MODS construction included testing of its validity, reproducibility, and sensitivity of each test item between observers.

The choice and the weight of each LODS item are derived from a multiple logistic regression model, using hospital mortality as the dependent variable. The construction was made from the data collected during the first day in the ICU.

10. How were they validated?

Discrimination for predicting mortality is better in multivariate models when the evolution of the score account and its initial values are taken into account. This principle was demonstrated with the LODS score.

11. What did these scores add to the description of ICU patients?

1. The use of the OSF score initially showed that a 100% prediction of death could be made in the most severely afflicted patients after several days. However, the same score was eventually used to demonstrate that care in the ICU had improved over years, so that published results were no longer valid 10 years later. These investigations documented that such scores are a method to assess ICU performance.

2. The mean time of occurrence of each organ failure is not the same. The peak of dysfunction for the neurologic system occurs usually before the second day; for the respiratory. cardiovascular, renal, and coagulation systems, around the third day; and for hepatic dysfunction, around the fifth day.

3. The weight of each organ failure in predicting death is not the same: hematologic and hepatic failures have less effect on mortality than respiratory, cardiovascular, renal, and neurologic failures.

4. The weight of each organ failure in predicting death is not the same over time. The same increase in respiratory dysfunction has a worse prognosis after 1 week of ICU stay. Hepatic dysfunction has an effect on mortality only after 3 weeks of ICU stay.

BIBLIOGRAPHY

1. Knaus WA, Draper EA, Wagner DP, Zimmerman JE: APACHE II: A severity of disease classification system. Crit Care Med 13: 818–829, 1985.
2. Knaus WA, Wagner DP, Draper EA, et al: The APACHE III prognostic system: Risk prediction of hospital mortality for critically ill hospitalized adults. Chest 100: 1619–1636, 1991.
3. Le Gall JR, Lemeshow S, Saulnier F: A new Simplified Acute Physiology Score (SAPS II) based on a European/North American multicenter study. JAMA 270:2957–2963, 1993.
4. Lemeshow S, Teres D, Klar J, et al: Mortality Probability Models (MPM II) based on an international cohort of intensive care unit patients. JAMA 270:2478–2486, 1993.
5. Knaus WA, Draper EA, Wagner DP., Zimmerman JE: Prognosis in acute organ-system failure. Ann Surg 202: 685, 1985.
6. Fagon J-Y, Chastre J, Novara A, et al: Characterization of intensive care unit patients using a model based on the presence or absence of organ dysfunctions and/or infection: The ODIN model. Intens Care Med 19:137–144, 1993.
7. Le Gall JR, Klar J, Lemeshow S, et al: The Logistic Organ Dysfunction system: A new way to assess organ dysfunction in the intensive care unit. JAMA 276: 802–810, 1996.
8. Vincent JL, de Mendonca A, Cantraine F, et al:. Use of the SOFA score to assess the incidence of organ dysfunction/failure in intensive care units: Results of a multicenter, prospective study. Crit Care Med 26:1793–1800, 1998.
9. Marshall JC, Cook DJ, Christou NV, et al: Multiple organ dysfunction score: A reliable descriptor of a complex clinical outcome. Crit Care Med 23:1638–1652, 1995.
10. Moreno R, Vincent JL, Matos A, et al: The use of maximum SOFA score to quantify organ failure/dysfunction in intensive care: Result of a prospective multicenter study. Intens Care Med 25:686–696, 1999.
11. Cook R, Cook D, Tilley J, et al: Multiple organ dysfunction: Baseline and serial component scores. Crit Care Med 29: 2046–2050, 2001.
12. Metnitz PG, Lang T, Valentin A, et al: Evaluation of the logistic organ dysfunction system for the assessment of organ dysfunction and mortality in critically ill patients. Intens Care Med 27: 992–998, 2001.

INDEX

Page numbers in **boldface type** indicate complete chapters.